MW01528176

LIBRARY

College of Physicians and
Surgeons
of British Columbia

INJECTION TREATMENTS IN COSMETIC SURGERY

Series in Cosmetic and Laser Therapy
Published in association with the *Journal of Cosmetic and Laser Therapy*

Already available

1. David J Goldberg
   Fillers in Cosmetic Dermatology, ISBN 9781841845098
2. Philippe Deprez
   Textbook of Chemical Peels, ISBN 9781841842954
3. C William Hanke, Gerhard Sattler, Boris Sommer
   Textbook of Liposuction, ISBN 9781841845326
4. Paul J Carniol, Neil S Sadick
   Clinical Procedures in Laser Skin Rejuvenation, ISBN 9780415414135
5. David J Goldberg
   Laser Hair Removal, Second Edition, ISBN 9780415414128

Of related interest

1. Robert Baran, Howard I Maibach
   Textbook of Cosmetic Dermatology, Third Edition, ISBN 9781841843117
2. Anthony Benedetto
   Botulinum Toxin in Clinical Dermatology, ISBN 978184214244
3. Jean Carruthers, Alastair Carruthers
   Using Botulinum Toxins Cosmetically, ISBN 9781841842172
4. David J Goldberg
   Ablative and Non-Ablative Facial Skin Rejuvenation, ISBN 9781841841755
5. David J Goldberg
   Complications in Cutaneous Laser Surgery, ISBN 9781841842455
6. Nicholas J Lowe
   Textbook of Facial Rejuvenation, ISBN 9781841840956
7. Shirley Madhere
   Aesthetic Mesotherapy and Injection Lipolysis in Clinical Practice, ISBN 9781841845531
8. Avi Shai, Howard I Maibach, Robert Baran
   Handbook of Cosmetic Skin Care, ISBN 9781841841793
9. Antonella Tosti, Maria De Padova
   Atlas of Mesotherapy in Skin Rejuvenation, ISBN 9780415419949

INJECTION TREATMENTS IN COSMETIC SURGERY

Edited by

Benjamin Ascher
Clinique Esthetic Iena
Paris, France

Co-editors

Marina Landau
Holon, Israel

Bernard Rossi
Rouen, France

informa
healthcare

2009

© 2009 Informa UK Ltd

First published in the United Kingdom in 1995

Second edition published in the United Kingdom in 2008 by Informa Healthcare, Telephone House, 69–77 Paul Street, London, EC2A 4LQ. Informa Healthcare is a trading division of Informa UK Ltd. Registered Office: 37/41 Mortimer Street, London W1T 3JH. Registered in England and Wales number 1072954

Tel: +44 (0)20 7017 5000
Fax: +44 (0)20 7017 6699
Website: www.informahealthcare.com

All rights reserved. No part of this publication may be reproduced, stored in a retrieval system, or transmitted, in any form or by any means, electronic, mechanical, photocopying, recording, or otherwise, without the prior permission of the publisher or in accordance with the provisions of the Copyright, Designs and Patents Act 1988 or under the terms of any licence permitting limited copying issued by the Copyright Licensing Agency, 90 Tottenham Court Road, London W1P 0LP.

Although every effort has been made to ensure that all owners of copyright material have been acknowledged in this publication, we would be glad to acknowledge in subsequent reprints or editions any omissions brought to our attention.

The Author has asserted his right under the Copyright, Designs and Patents Act 1988 to be identified as the Author of this Work.

A CIP record for this book is available from the British Library.

Library of Congress Cataloging-in-Publication Data
Data available on application

ISBN-13: 978–0–415–38651–7

Distributed in North and South America by
Taylor & Francis
6000 Broken Sound Parkway, NW, (Suite 300)
Boca Raton, FL 33487, USA

Within Continental USA
Tel: 1 (800) 272 7737; Fax: 1 (800) 374 3401
Outside Continental USA
Tel: (561) 994 0555; Fax: (561) 361 6018
Email: orders@crcpress.com

Book orders in the rest of the world
Paul Abrahams
Tel: +44 (0) 207 017 6917
Email: bookorders@informa.com

Composition by C&M Digitals (P) Ltd, Chennai, India
Printed and bound in India by Replika Press Pvt. Ltd

Contents

List of contributors

Claude Aharoni
Plastic Surgeon
Clinique Cornette de St Cyr
Paris
France

K Roger Aoki
Researcher
Allergan
Irvine, California
USA

Benjamin Ascher
Plastic Surgeon
Clinique Iena
Paris
France

Martine Baspeyras
Dermatologist
Bordeaux
France

Ghislaine Beilin
Family Practitioner
Paris
France

Isaac Bodokh
Dermatologist
Centre Hospitalier de Cannes
France

Anne Bouloumié
Researcher
Frankfurt am Main
Germany

Patrick Bui
Plastic Surgeon
Paris
France

Daniel Cassuto
Plastic Surgeon
University of Catania
Italy

Louis Casteilla
Researcher
CHU de Rangueil
Toulouse
France

Audrey Charrière
Researcher
INSERM
Toulouse
France

Guillaume Charrière
Researcher
INSERM
Toulouse
France

Anny Cohen-Letessier
Dermatologist
Paris
France

Béatrice Cousin
Researcher
Institut Louis Bugnard
Toulouse
France

Taciana Dal'Forno
Federal University of Rio Grande do Sul
Brazil

Mauricio De Maio
Plastic Surgeon
Sao Paulo
Brazil

Elisabeth Domergue Than Trong
Dermatologist, Hôpital Saint-Louis
Paris
France

Gérard Flageul
Plastic Surgeon
Paris
France

Timothy C Flynn
Dermatologist
Cary Skin Center and University of North Carolina
USA

Jean Louis Foyatier
Plastic Surgeon
Clinique du Val d'Ouest
Ecully
France

Nelly Gauthier
Facial Plastic Surgeon
Paris
France

David J Goldberg
Dermatologist
Skin Laser & Surgery Specialists of New York & New Jersey
USA

Ahmad Halabi
Plastic Surgeon
Clinique Iena
Paris
France

Doris Hexsel
Dermatologist
Porto Alegre
Brazil

Antoine Jaklis
Otorhinolaryngologist
Hôpital Pasteur, Nice
France

Chung Jee-Hyeok
Facial Plastic Surgeon
Gyalumhan Plastic Aesthetic Clinic
Seoul
Korea

Park Jong-Beum
Facial Plastic Surgeon
Gyalumhan Plastic Aesthetic Clinic
Seoul
Korea

Philippe Kestemont
Facial Plastic Surgeon
Nice
France

Roger Kuffer
Stomatologist
Laboratoire d'Histopathologie de la Division de Stomatologie
University of Geneva
Switzerland

Daniel Labbé
Plastic Surgeon
Caen
France

Patrick Laharrague
Researcher
Institut Louis Bugnard
Toulouse
France

Marina Landau
Dermatologist
Wolfson Medical Center
Holon
Israel

Gottfried Lemperle
Plastic Surgeon
UCSD, La Jolla
California
USA

Rosemari Mazzuco
Dermatologist
Porte Alegre
Brazil

Vladimir Mitz
Plastic Surgeon
Hôpital Boucicaud
Paris
France

Ali Mojallal
Plastic Surgeon
Centre Hospitalier St Joseph & St Luc
Lyon
France

Maryelle Moreira Lima
Dermatologist
Brazilian Center of Studies in Dermatology
Porto Alegre
Brazil

Kim Nam-Ho
Facial Plastic Surgeon
Gyalumhan Plastic Aesthetic Clinic
Seoul
Korea

Arik Nemet
Ophthalmologist
Shearei Zedek Hospital
Jerusalem
Israel

Julien Nicolas
Plastic Surgeon
Caen
France

Pierre J Nicolau
Plastic Surgeon
Paris
France

Luc Pénicaud
Researcher
Laboratoire Neurbiologie et Metabolisme
Toulouse
France

Valérie Planat
Researcher
Centre Hospitalier Universitaire
Rangueil
Toulouse
France

Françoise Plantier
Anatomopathologist, Hôpital Tarnier-Cochin
Paris
France

Annick Pons-Guiraud
Dermatologist
Hôpital St-Louis
Paris
France

Daniele Ranoux
Neurologist
CHU Dupuytren
Limoges
France

Park Rho-Hyuk
Facial Plastic Surgeon
Gyalumhan Plastic Aesthetic Clinic
Seoul
Korea

Sabrina Rodrigues Talarico
Dermatologist
Sao Paulo
Brazil

Bernard Rossi
Dermatologist
Clinique Mathilde
Rouen
France

Berthold Rzany
Dermatologist
Charité University Clinic
Berlin
Germany

Sophie Sangla
Neurologist
Clinique Bizet
Paris
France

José Santini
Facial Plastic Surgeon
Hôpital Pasteur
Nice
France

Luca Scrimali
Plastic Surgeon
University of Catania
Italy

Sergio Talarico-Filho
Dermatologist
Sao Paulo
Brazil

Daphné Thioly-Bensoussan
Dermatologist
St Louis University Hospital
Paris
France

Hananya Vaknine
Pathologist
Wolfson Medical Center
Holon
Israel

Mikaël Veber
Plastic Surgeon
Centre Hospitalier St Joseph & St Luc
Lyon
France

Catherine Wintrebert
Anesthesiologist
Clinique Turin
Paris
France

Hassan Zahouani
Researcher
Ecole Centrale de Lyon
France

Gilbert Zakine
Plastic Surgeon
Hôpital Broussais
Paris
France

Débora Zechmeister do Prado
Dermatologist
Brazilian Center of Studies in Dermatology
Porto Alegre
Brazil

Preface

Preface from Benjamin Ascher

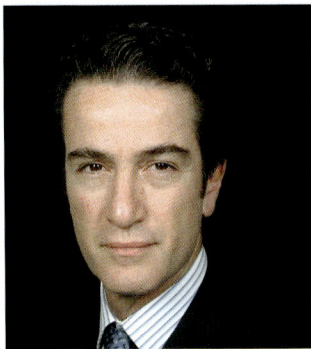

Plastic surgeons and dermatologists, as well as any other practitioner dedicated to the esthetic field, have to be concerned with every aspect of the use of injection treatments. Those training others need not only to be aware of the latest surgical developments; there is also an increasingly intense need for up to date information on the alternative medical, non-invasive treatments and accompanying procedures, which over the past 10 years have become essential aspects of our daily practice. Peelings, cutaneous lasers, bodyshaping techniques – as well as injections with botulinum toxin, fillers, volumetric implants, and fat grafts, both for face and body – are taking on an ever increasing importance which cannot be ignored if we want to optimize our clinical results.

For this reason, the first French and European University diploma dedicated to injection treatments, volumetric implants, and associated techniques in Plastic Surgery and Cosmetic Dermatology was created in 2002 by a group of doctors – Patrick Bui, Annick Pons Guiraud, and me – together with the Universities of Paris V and XII, and sponsored by Professors Jean Paul Escande (for the Dermatology field) and Laurent Lantieri (for the Plastic Surgery field). The goal of this diploma is to evaluate the use of various techniques and to offer teaching of the abovementioned practices, taking into account facial and body anatomy, semiology, and the physiology of facial and body aging. Complications and medical legal issues are broadly discussed throughout these chapters, which have largely been inspired by and developed on the basis of our courses. Further deepening the same concept, I was happy to create with Elisabeth Domergue Than Trong the first University Volumetry Unit at the Henri Mondor University Hospital Center in Paris, sponsored by Professors Martine Bagot (Dermatology) and Laurent Lantieri (Plastic Surgery). The aim of this unit is to assess different volume-enhancing products within the scope of the medical pathologies and cosmetic indications in relation to face and body lipoatrophies.

Exogenous fillers have been widely used since the development of collagen 20 years ago, and the introduction of hyaluronic acids 12 years ago. These modular injections, often reversible and efficient, must therefore be evaluated on their level of efficiency and their durability but, especially, on their safety. It seems logical to classify them according to their resorbability. The exogenous slowly and non-absorbable injection products have a significant durability and performance, notably in increase of volume, but they may produce somewhat serious complications as well as sequelae. In addition to the use of resorbable and non-resorbable products as fillers, they have been recently developed as volumetric implants and as such take an important place in our practice. In this regard chapters discussing fat as a volumetric implant, adipose tissue physiology, and survival of transplanted adipocytes are absolutely necessary additions to this book. A global approach and a technique overview of fat grafting for both face and body will be increasingly essential in the coming years.

Much attention is devoted in this book to the detection of side-effects and to their treatment and prevention. Some examples of inadequate European legislation regarding CE approval and the regulations governing production and distribution of products will be specifically described in the following chapters. In Europe CE marking is a prerequisite for any injectable products to be offered as safe; however, CE marking does not necessarily imply that the product's efficacy and side-effects have been assessed objectively during clinical studies. This marking is expected in time to fall into line with US legislation, where the marketing of any medicinal product is subject to FDA approval, based on comprehensive animal and clinical studies and on more systematic and better centralized side-effect reporting. The primary concerns involved are knowledge of the elaboration of the procedures, promotion of legal obligations, the publication of physiochemical data, and the realization of clinical studies with objective institutional results and possible medium- to long-term side-effects. All this will allow us to measure and evaluate data of actual classification, uniquely and independently obtained by industry, compared to non-clinical procedures and invalid science which are sometimes picked up in the mass media. In our specialty, which is always rapidly evolving, it is logical to combine different techniques to optimize results. This alliance of injection treatments is the best example of the evolution of our specialty today and has become the main current trend in it.

These chapters constitute a collective work independent of the esthetic industry, but have obvious economic and legal constraints inseparable from our professional activities. I would like to thank all authors, my colleagues and friends, for having agreed to contribute to this effort in spite of numerous other solicitations for their precious time. There should be particular thanks to my friends, the Co-editors Marina Landau and Bernard Rossi (two brilliant and well known dermatologists and experts in the field of cosmetic injection treatments), and to Robert Peden, Commissioning Editor for Informa Healthcare, without whom this book would have never been published.

Benjamin Ascher
Plastic Surgeon (Board Certified)
Lecturer and Clinical Assistant, Paris Academy
Member of the French Society of Plastic,
Reconstructive, and Aesthetic Surgery
Clinique Iena, 11 rue Fresnel,
75116 Paris, France
benjaminascher@wanadoo.fr

In the professional milieu new interdisciplinary interactions have been created: dermatologists and plastic surgeons meet with ENT specialists, ophthalmologists, and maxillofacial surgeons. Moreover, non-traditional specialists such as gynecologists, anesthesiologists and cardiologists have entered the field of cosmetic medicine.

All this has happened because of the introduction of a vast variety of new non-invasive technologies for skin rejuvenation and enhancement. Injectable products, such as the botulinum toxins and dermal fillers, are the main cause for this revolutionary medical as well as social trend.

Injection Treatments in Cosmetic Surgery is a team operation and creation aiming to make the work with injectable products more rewarding for both you and your patient. It gathers an enormous amount of personal knowledge and the experience of a multinational, multidisciplinary group of experts.

I would like to thank all the colleagues who enthusiastically committed themselves to this complex project. I also want to deeply thank all my patients, who over the years have continuously encouraged me to introduce into my practice the novel cosmetic and anti-aging procedures. I want to thank my family for their patience and support. And above all thanks are due to Benjamin Ascher, who artistically conducted this symphony.

Marina Landau
Dermatology, Wolfson Medical Center,
Holon President of the Israel
Society for Dermatologic Surgery
56 Joshua Ben Nun Street,
Herzlia Pituach, Israel 46763
mlandau@zahav.net.il

Preface from Marina Landau

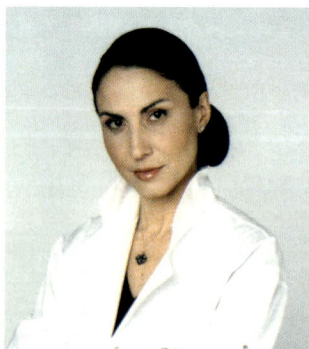

Traditionally, dermatologists were responsible for taking care of the diseased as well as for the enhancement of allegedly healthy skin, mainly by topical preparations. Plastic surgeons were involved in reconstructive and esthetic procedures using a more invasive approach.

In the last 20 years esthetic medicine and surgery have changed tremendously. From procedures being accessible for the upper socioeconomic classes exclusively, they have become achievable and possible for almost everybody; from treatments being employed in secret by middle aged wealthy women, cosmetic treatments are now consumed by almost every age group and by both genders in the open; from social 'taboo' it has became one of the most popularly discussed topics in social encounters and by the printed and digital media.

Preface from Bernard Rossi

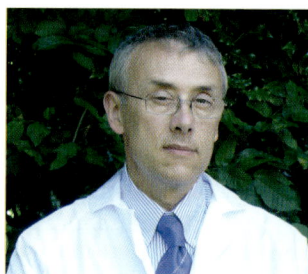

It is a pleasure to acknowledge our contributors who spent their precious time working with us on this book, contributing their insight. Their chapters will be most valuable for us in our professional life and will have a significant impact on our view of the management of aging.

I am particulary grateful to Marina Landau for her masterful insight in esthetics and the science of peels, and to Benjamin Ascher for his ability and patience in communicating his masterful insight into the use of botulinum toxins and fillers and more generally the entire esthetic area and for his leadership throughout the development process of this book.

'The deepest thing in Man, is his skin', said the famous French poet, Paul Valéry ('L'idée fixe', 1932).

Our skin reflects our age. After 20 years of research and improvement many non-invasive technologies are now able to decrease the effects or the appearance of aging, and they have become achievable for a large part of the population. However, this proliferation of methods needs to be scientifically evaluated and compared to optimize the clinical results and avoid side-effects – side-effects which may be due in large part to the lack of European legislation regarding CE approval, especially for injectable products, but are also due to the lack of training for the practitioner.

In *Injection Treatments in Cosmetic Surgery* we share our multinational and multidisciplinary experience, for our mutual benefit and also for the benefit of our patients.

Bernard Rossi
Dermatologist (Board Certified)
Member of the French Society of Dermatology
Member of the American Academy of Dermatology
Member of the American Society for Laser Medicine and Surgery Member of European Society for Laser Dermatology
Expert près la Cour d'Appel de Rouen
Expert près la Cour Administrative de Douai
Clinique Mathilde
4 rue de Lessard, 76100 Rouen, France
bernard.rossi3@wanadoo.fr

1 Practical anatomy of the face

Philippe Kestemont, Antoine Jaklis, and José Santini

Introduction

Many reference textbooks offer an exhaustive description of the head and neck anatomy. This chapter is tailored to provide the reader with a comprehensive review of the subject, highlighting the functional aspect of facial anatomy with special emphasis on practical details concerning important, simple, and more complex structures involved in facial expression. These static and dynamic subtle structures control our facial mimetic, defining the way we look to others. For that matter, it is mandatory to have a thorough knowledge of these anatomical structures before we use any method or substance that could alter their shape or modify their function, namely the botulinum toxin.

Skin and subcutaneous tissue

The face and neck can be divided into two major regions according to the texture, thickness, and quality of the skin and the underlying subcutaneous fat tissue.

The periorificial craniofacial region

This constitutes the support for the facial dynamics. The eyes, the nose, and the mouth are surrounded by the thinnest skin of the face, with an extremely poor subcutaneous fat component overlying the muscles in these areas (Figure 1.1). The tight adhesions between these superficial muscles and the overlying dermis appear as fine periorificial wrinkles known as 'expression lines'.

The eyelids are covered by thin skin almost devoid of subcutaneous fat. When present, this fat tissue should not be confused with the retro-orbital and peri-orbital (retroseptal) fat pockets (Figure 1.2).

The cervicofacial region

This is characterized by an abundant subcutaneous fat tissue and thicker skin. The underlying layer is musculoaponeurotic, comprising the superficial musculoaponeurotic system (SMAS)–platysma sheath. It is a rather static segment, usually less vulnerable to wrinkle formation.

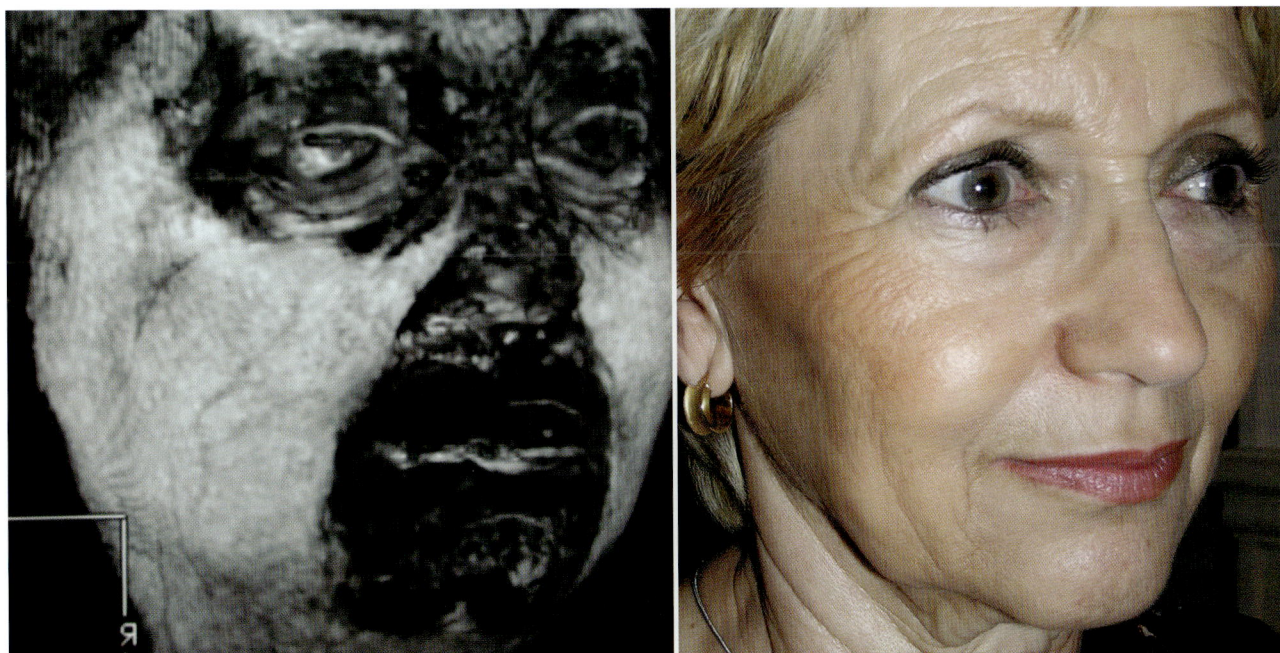

Figure 1.1 Magnetic resonance imaging (MRI): note the difference between subcutaneous fat in the periorificial craniofacial region and in the cervicofacial region.

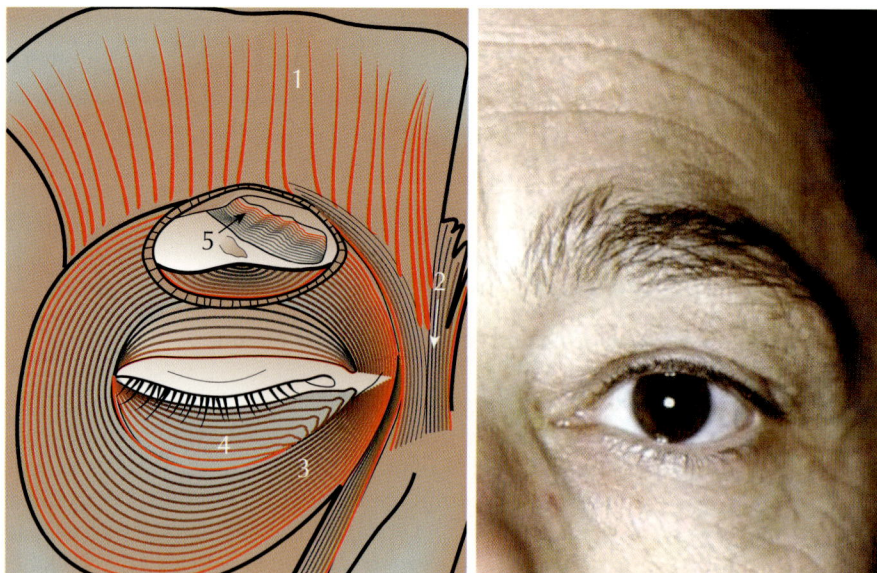

Figure 1.2 1: The frontalis muscle. 2: The procerus muscle. 3: The orbicularis oculi muscle, pars orbicularis. 4: The orbicularis oculi muscle, pars palpebralis. 5: The corrugator muscle.

The subcutaneous fat spreads all over the cheek area and the neck resulting in a homogeneous thick sheath, except in the malar area where the fat gains further volume forming the so-called 'malar fad pad' (Figure 1.1).

The subcutaneous fat plays an essential role in facial esthetics. It softens the bony landmarks, fills the facial contours, and enhances skin quality.

Platysma muscles and musculoaponeurotic structures

Periorificial and centrofacial region

This is the muscular region of the face. The perioral, perinasal, and periorbital muscles provide two essential functions:

- a primary protective function over the eye globes and the oral cavity
- a secondary dynamic function of facial mimics reflecting facial expression.

The periorbital region (Figure 1.2)

The eyebrow is a mobile structure subject to two antagonist groups of muscles: an eyebrow elevator group mainly made up by the frontalis muscle, and a depressor group made up by the orbicularis oculi muscle, the procerus muscle, and the corrugator supercilii muscle.

The musculoaponeurotic elevator group of muscles is formed by the association of the frontalis muscle, the galea aponeurotica (epicranial aponeurosis), and the occipitalis muscle.

The frontalis is a 6 × 7 cm quadrilateral-shaped muscle. Its medial fibers join at the level of the glabella where they intersect with fibers of the procerus muscle. Its central and lateral fibers overlay the corrugator

supercilii muscle and intersect with the outer fibers of the pars orbitalis component of the orbicularis oculi muscle. It is located between the galea and the skin, closely adherent to the latter. From their lower insertions on the supraorbital margin, the frontalis fibers spread over the forehead, and fuse with the galea aponeurotica to join posteriorly, in the occipital region, the occipitalis muscle. The repeated contractions of this muscle lead to the formation of horizontal forehead wrinkles.

The galea aponeurotica or epicranial aponeurosis is a broad musculoaponeurotic layer covering the calvaria. Posteriorly, it is firmly anchored to the occipital protuberance and the superior nuchal line. It is separated from the outer table of the cranium by the loose connective tissue layer. This area, also called Merkel's space, allows smooth sliding of the scalp over the cranium. Laterally, over the temporal crest, the epicranial aponeurosis is continuous with the superficial temporal fascia. We find, at that level, the superficial temporal vessels and the temporal and frontal branches of the facial nerve.

The eyebrow depressor muscles are formed by the association of three distinct muscles: the corrugator supercilii muscle, the pyramidal or procerus muscle, and the orbicularis oculi muscle.

The corrugator supercilii muscle is a deep facial muscle (Figure 1.3). It is narrow and strong, with deep medial insertions on the glabellar periosteum and another more superficial lateral transorbicular insertion on the medial portion of the eyebrow. It depresses and brings closer the inner parts of the eyebrows. Its repeated contractions result in the formation of vertical glabellar wrinkles, also called 'lion's wrinkles'.

The pyramidal or procerus muscle appears as a medial extension of the frontalis muscle. It overlaps the nasal bones in which it inserts distally along with the upper lateral cartilages. It depresses the medial

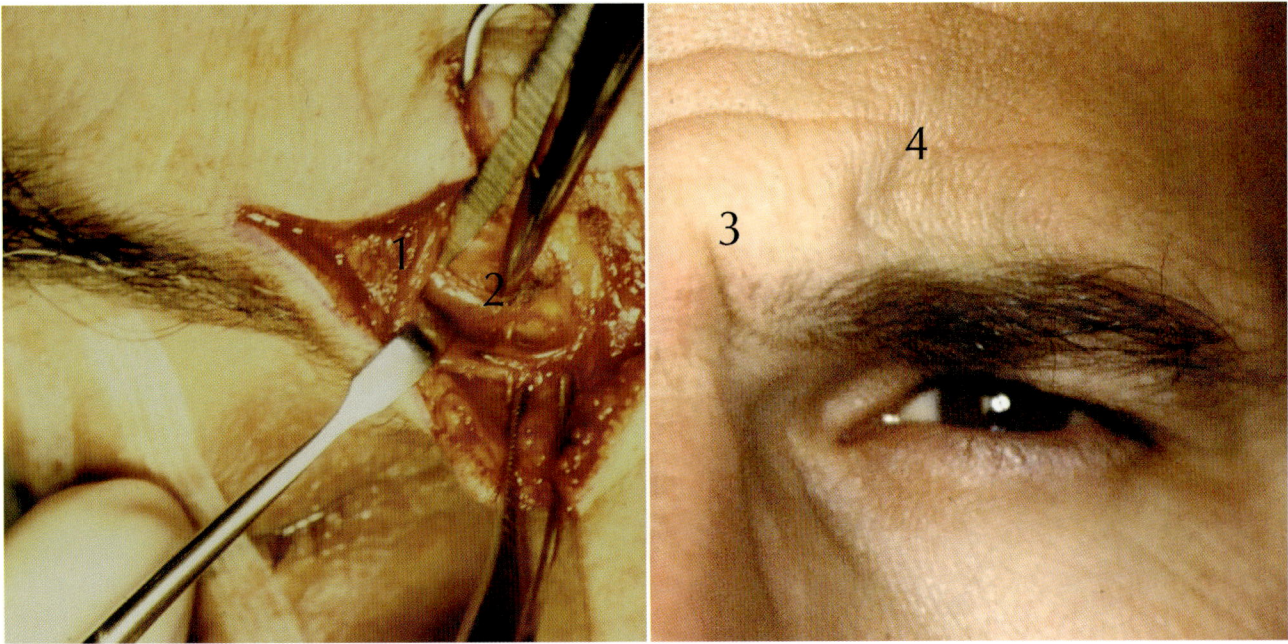

Figure 1.3 1: The procerus muscle. 2: The corrugator muscle. 3: Lion's line. 4: Corrugator's skin insertion.

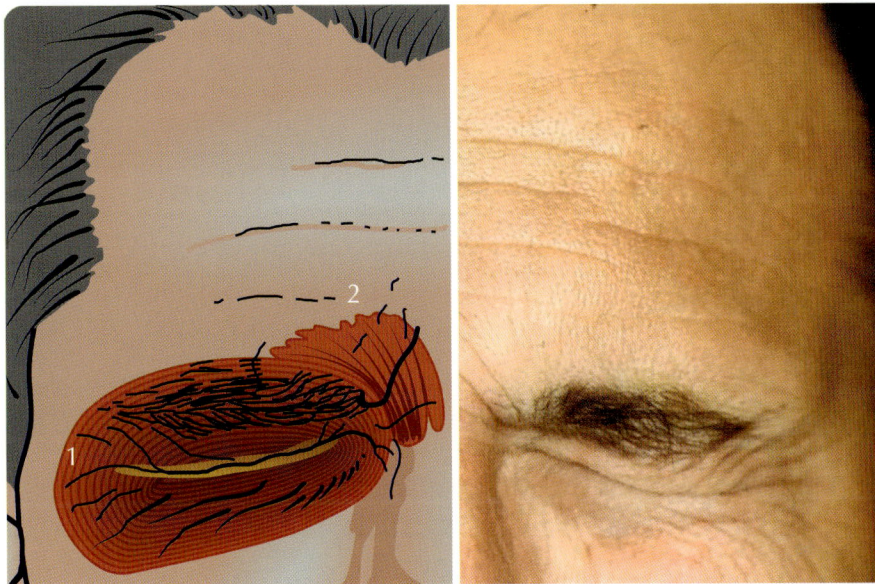

Figure 1.4 1: The orbicularis oculi muscle creates crow's feet and oblique glabellar lines. 2: The procerus muscle creates horizontal glabellar lines.

portion of the eyebrow. Its repetitive contractions lead to the formation of horizontal glabellar wrinkles.

The orbicularis oculi muscle is one of the largest muscles of facial expression. It is wide, circular, and diaphragmatic. It appears as a flat and narrow muscle sheath closely adherent to the skin. Its fibers sweep in concentric circles around the orbital margins and in the eyelids. It consists of three parts:

1. The orbital part, or pars orbicularis, is external and devoid of deep attachments. It forms a ring and inserts medially on the medial palpebral liga-ment. Its concentric fibers are often more spread

than usually represented in the classical manuals of anatomy. Its repeated contractions lead to the formation of 'crow's feet' (Figures 1.4 and 1.5) and oblique glabellar lines. These lines result from the contraction of the internal superior fibers of the pars orbicularis, also recognized by some authors as an individual muscle, the 'depressor supracilii muscle' (Figure 1.4).

2. The palpebral part, or pars palpebralis, is internal, adherent to the tarsal plates and deeply inserted in the palpebral ligament. A muscle strip known as 'Horner's muscle' detaches from the palpebral muscle and runs towards the posterior lacrimal

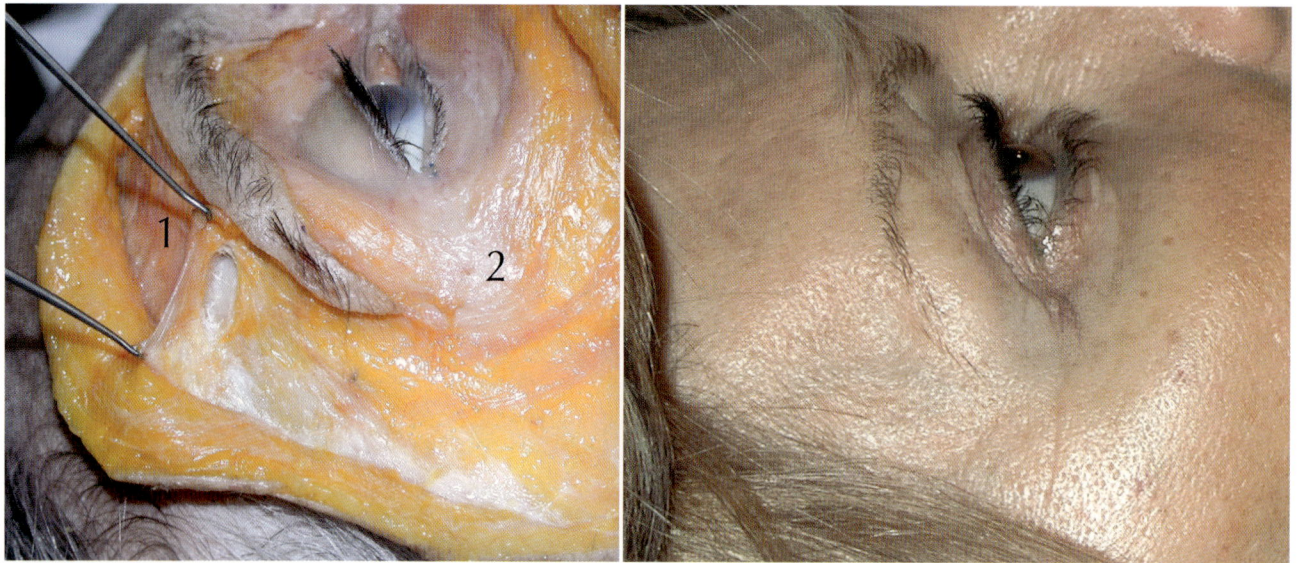

Figure 1.5   1: Frontalis muscle. 2: Orbicularis oculi muscle.

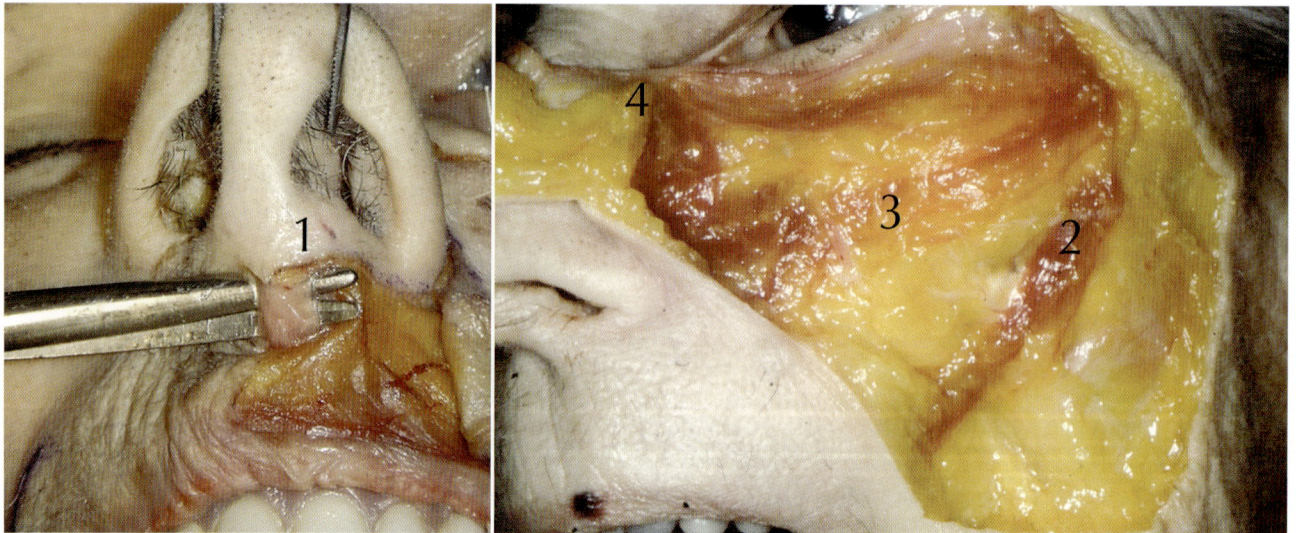

Figure 1.6   1: The depressor septi muscle. 2: The zygomatic major muscle. 3: The zygomatic minor muscle. 4: The levator labii superioris alaeque nasi muscle.

crest. This muscle encourages the emptying of the lacrimal sac and helps lymphatic drainage in the orbital region.

3. The orbitomalar crease corresponds to the inferior border of the orbicularis oculi muscle. It stands out as the limit between the orbital region and the cheek. It also delineates the superior border of the malar fad pad. Beneath the orbicularis oculi muscle there is a thin layer of fat continuous with the jugal fat called the suborbicularis oculi fat (SOOF). This layer provides a natural surgical plan of division.

The levator palpebrae superioris muscle in its retroseptal position raises the upper eyelid. It runs from its superior periosteal insertions in the orbital roof to its tight skin and tarsal insertions in the upper eyelid. Its posterior head, also called Muller's muscle, inserts in the superior border of the upper tarsal plate.

The fibroelastic layer is a continuous structure formed by the tarsus, the medial and lateral palpebral ligaments, and the orbital septum.

The nasal and perioral region (Figure 1.6)

The nasal muscles of expression are:

*   the nasalis muscle, consisting of a transverse bundle (pars transversa) that depresses the nostrils, and an alar bundle (pars alaris) that dilates the nostrils
*   the procerus muscle, a nasoglabellar muscle

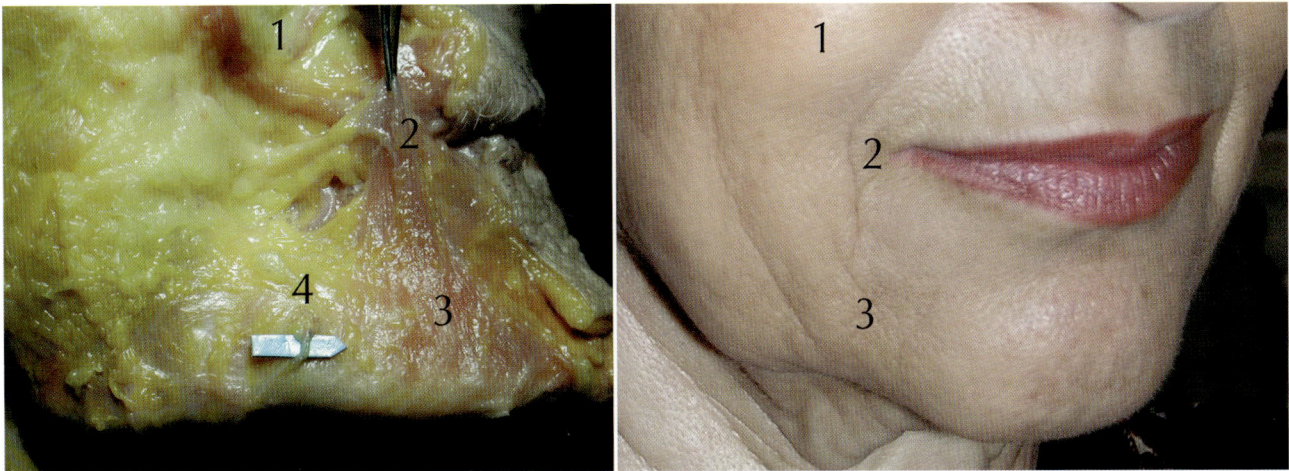

Figure 1.7 1: The zygomatic major muscle. 2: The modiolus. 3: The depressor anguli oris muscle. 4: The mandibular branch of the facial nerve.

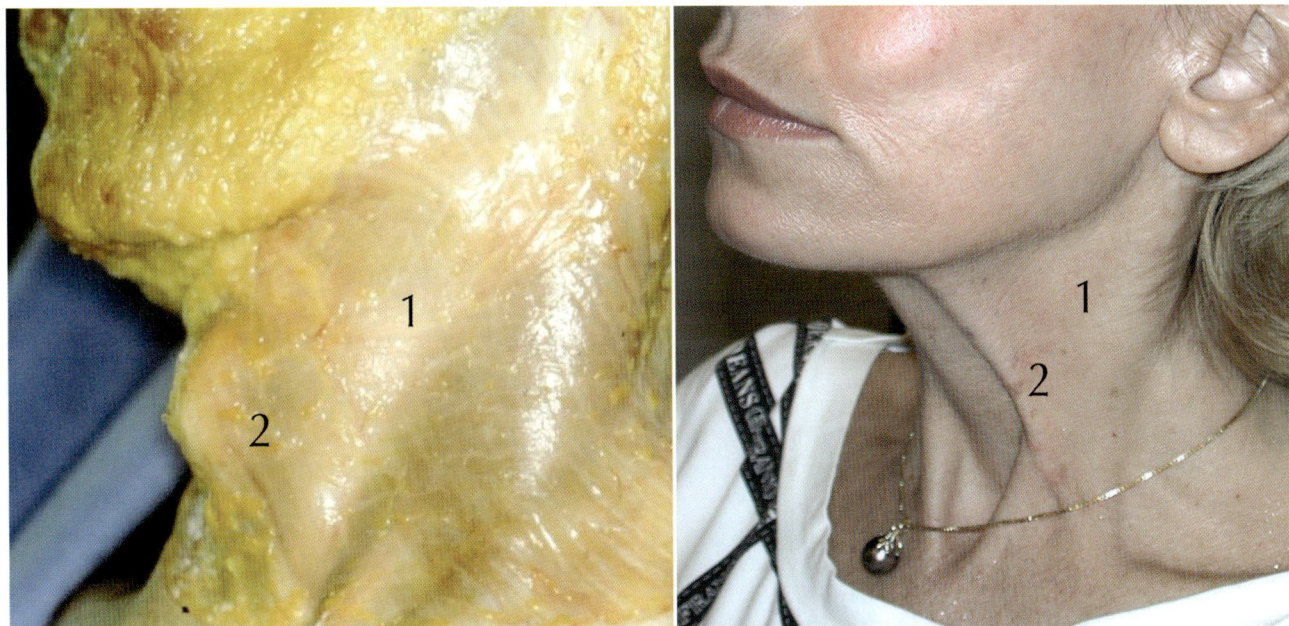

Figure 1.8 1: The platysma muscle. 2: The platysma band.

- the depressor septi or myrtiform muscle, which depresses the nasal septum
- the levator labii superioris alaeque nasi muscle, which elevates the lip and the nose.

The oromental region (Figure 1.7)

Muscles appear in layers or strata as described by Freilinger:

- a superficial layer made of the zygomaticus minor muscle, the depressor anguli oris muscle, and the orbicularis oculi muscle

- a second layer made of the zygomaticus major muscle, the risorius muscle, the platysma muscle, and the depressor anguli oris muscle
- a third layer made of the orbicularis labii muscle and the levator labii superioris muscle
- a deep layer made of the mentalis muscle, the levator anguli oris muscle, and the buccinator muscle.

The platysma (Figure 1.8) is a wide and shallow extensive sheet of vertical muscle fibers covering part of the inferior third of the face and most of the anterolateral region of the neck. It extends from the lower cheek and the perioral region down to the clavicular region. The right and left platysma muscles draw, as they diverge, an inverted V with the apex pointing towards the mandibular symphysis. The platysma is part of the SMAS–platysma sheath. The cervical component of this sheath is purely muscular (platysma muscle per se), whereas its parotid region component is mainly aponeurotic (fibrous platysma). This musculoaponeurotic sheath adheres to the underlying structures through the so-called 'facial ligaments'.

Vessels of the face

Arteries of the face

The face is mainly supplied by two distinct networks:

- a major superficial network derived from the external carotid artery
- a deep network derived from the internal carotid artery.

These two systems anastomose freely, explaining the great vitality of the facial skin.

The facial artery arises from the external carotid artery and lies superficial as it hooks around the inferior border of the mandible. In its course over the face, it runs along the nasolabial fold and follows a sinuous course between the muscle layers, running deep to the platysma and the zygomatic muscles. Near the angle of the mouth, it sends the labial and alar branches that anastomose on the midline with the contralateral arteries. Near the upper portion of the nasolabial fold it runs along the nose to the inner angle of the eye as the angular artery and anastomoses, only inconstantly, with the ophthalmic artery.

The superficial temporal artery begins in the parotid region where the external carotid artery divides into two branches, the superficial temporal artery and the internal maxillary artery. It ascends through the superficial temporal fascia, always lateral to the temporal branch of the facial nerve. Along its ascending course it gives off three collateral branches, the transverse facial artery, the zygomaticomalar artery, and the deep medial temporal artery. It ends in the scalp by dividing into two branches, an anterior frontal branch that contributes to the periorbital network of vessels and a posterior parietal branch that anastomoses with the contralateral arteries.

The internal maxillary artery contributes to the deep supply of the face. Among its 14 collateral branches we mention the buccal artery supplying the soft tissues of the cheek and the infraorbital artery emerging from the infraorbital foramen and supplying the lower eyelid and the cheek.

The ophthalmic artery branches from the internal carotid artery. It contributes to the vascular supply of the face through its terminal branching from the nasal artery, the angular artery. It has two facial branches: the supraorbital or external frontal artery, and the supratrochlear or internal frontal artery that runs upward and anastomoses with the frontal branch of the superficial temporal artery.

Veins of the face

The venous system of the face can be superposed to the arterial one. There is a superficial network made up mainly by the facial vein that arises from the union of the supratrochlear and the supraorbital veins. The facial vein runs inferiorly through the face and ends by draining into the internal jugular vein.

The superficial temporal vein drains the forehead and scalp. It unites with the maxillary vein, posterior to the neck of the mandible, to form the retromandibular vein. The retromandibular vein divides into an anterior branch that unites with the facial vein, and a posterior branch that joins the posterior auricular vein to form the external jugular vein. The external jugular vein drains into the subclavian vein.

There is a deep venous network linked to the superficial one through the angular vein that connects the cavernous sinus to the facial vein.

Nerves of the face

Motor nerves of the face: the facial nerve

Cranial nerve (CN) VII, the facial nerve, supplies the muscles of facial expression. Posteriorly, over the cheek, the extracranial portion of the facial nerve is protected by the parotid gland and then by the parotidomasseteric fascia. In fact, the facial nerve emerges from the skull through the stylomastoid foramen and runs within the parotid gland giving rise to a cervicofacial branch and a temporofacial branch. These, in turn, subdivide into five major branches. All the branches run superficially within the substance of the parotid gland before they supply the muscles of expression or mimetic muscles.

The cervical branch of the facial nerve is the most posterior and inferior of the five branches. It runs behind and below the mandibular angle and supplies the platysma muscle.

The mandibular branch of the facial nerve can be unique or divided into two branches. The inferior branch is always more significant. It runs superficially over the facial artery before giving rise to several motor branches supplying the inner surface of the mentalis muscle, the depressor labii inferioris, and the depressor anguli oris.

The buccal branch of the facial nerve divides early into two branches running over the masseter muscle just beneath the parotidomasseteric fascia:

- a superior ramus which follows an anterior and inferior oblique path, and crosses above Stensen's duct before supplying the outer surface of the buccinator muscle
- an inferior ramus supplying the inner surface of the orbicularis oris.

The zygomatic branch of the facial nerve passes transversely over the zygomatic bone before dividing into three major branches:

- the superior palpebral branch supplying the orbicularis oculi muscle and the corrugator muscle
- the inferior palpebral branch supplying again the orbicularis oculi muscle
- the infraorbital branch supplying the zygomatic muscles and muscles of the upper lip and nose.

There are many anastomoses between the buccal and zygomatic branches of the facial nerve.

The temporal branch of the facial nerve is the most vulnerable to injury during facial surgery. Its path can be outlined by drawing a line passing through a point 0.5 cm below the tragus and another 1.5 cm above the lateral border of the eyebrow. Its different branches anastomose among each other. It crosses the zygomatic arch approximately 2 cm anterior to the tragus, and reaches the superficial temporal fascia where it runs below the superficial temporal artery. It ends by supplying the inner surface of the frontal muscle.

Sensory nerves of the face: the trigeminal and the great auricular nerves

Knowledge of these is essential for the practice of local anesthesia of the face.

The trigeminal nerve provides sensory innervation of the face through its three branches:

1. The ophthalmic nerve is the superior division of the trigeminal nerve. It divides into three branches: the lacrimal, the frontal, and the nasociliary branches. The lacrimal nerve supplies the lacrimal gland, the upper eyelid, the conjunctiva, and the lateral angle of the eye. The frontal nerve further divides into two branches: supratrochlear and supraorbital. The supratrochlear nerve supplies the medial angle of the eye, the upper eyelid, the nasion, and part of the glabella. The supraorbital nerve emerges from the superior orbital margin through a foramen or a small canal before it supplies the lateral canthus, the upper eyelid, and the temporal and frontoparietal regions of the head. The nasociliary nerve in turn divides into two branches, one internal and one external supplying the nasal dorsum and the nasal tip.

2. The maxillary nerve is the intermediate division of the trigeminal nerve. In the infratemporal region, it gives off an orbital branch before it divides into a lacrimopalpebral branch supplying the lateral part of the upper eyelid and a temporomaxillary branch supplying the anterior temporal region. It emerges then below the inferior orbital margin, through the infraorbital foramen as a large terminal branch, the infraorbital nerve that supplies the the lower eyelid, the lateral aspect of the nose, the cheek, and the upper lip.

3. The mandibular nerve is the inferior division of the trigeminal nerve. It also has cutaneous sensory branches, namely, the inferior alveolar nerve. After passing through the inferior alveolar canal, the nerve emerges from the mental foramen giving the mental nerve that provides sensation to the chin and lower lip. Medial to the neck of the mandible, the mandibular nerve gives off the auriculotemporal nerve that supplies the tragus, the ear lobe, and the skin in the temporal region. These nerves arise from the posterior division of the mandibular nerve. The anterior division provides the the buccal nerve that supplies the skin over the cheek area.

The great auricular nerve belongs to the superficial cervical plexus. It is derived from the ventral rami of C2 and C3. It runs in the superficial cervical aponeurosis over the external surface of the sternocleidomastoid muscle, lateral to the external jugular vein. Below the ear, it becomes strictly subcutaneous before it supplies the ear lobe, the retroauricular region, and part of the cheek around the tragus.

Bibliography

Santini J, Krastinova-Lolov D. Chirurgie plastique de la face: rajeunissement-embellissement. Rapport de la Société Française d'ORL et de Chirurgie de la Face et du Cou. Paris: Lib Arnette, 1999.

2 Anatomy of the skin

Marina Landau and Hananya Vaknine

The skin is a complex organ with many important functions. It serves as a mechanical barrier, participates in thermoregulation, has immunological activity, protects against ultraviolet effects, and balances water loss. To fulfill all these functions, the skin has multiple cellular components and non-cellular structures.

Skin is composed of an epithelial layer of ectodermal origin, the epidermis, a layer of connective tissue of mesodermal origin, the dermis, and loose connective tissue with fat, the hypodermis. The irregular junction of the dermis and epidermis is called the dermoepidermal junction (Figure 2.1). It is created by projections of the dermis called papillae, which interdigitate with invaginations of the epidermis called epidermal ridges. Epidermal appendages include hairs, nails, and sebaceous and sweat glands.

Epidermis

Two types of cells constitute the epidermis: keratinocytes and dendritic cells.

Keratinocytes

The keratinocytes are arranged in the epidermis in four layers: the basal cell layer, the squamous cell layer, the granular cell layer, and the cornified cell layer (Figure 2.1).

Basal cells are mitotically active cells that give rise to other keratinocytes. It is assumed that once a cell is formed in the basal layer, the time required for it to travel to the surface of the granular layer is between 26 and 42 days.[1] An additional 14 days are required for passage of the cells through the normal cornified layer.[2]

The basal cells are arranged as a single row of cuboid cells (Figure 2.2). A basement membrane separates the basal layer from the dermis. It is seen by light microscopy as a PAS (periodic acid–Schiff) positive line. Basal cells are attached to the basement membrane by hemidesmosomes and to adjacent keratinocytes by desmosomes. Basal cells contain keratin filaments or tonofibrils.[3]

The squamous layer is composed of several layers of polygonal cells. This layer thickness varies accordingly to the anatomic location varies according to different

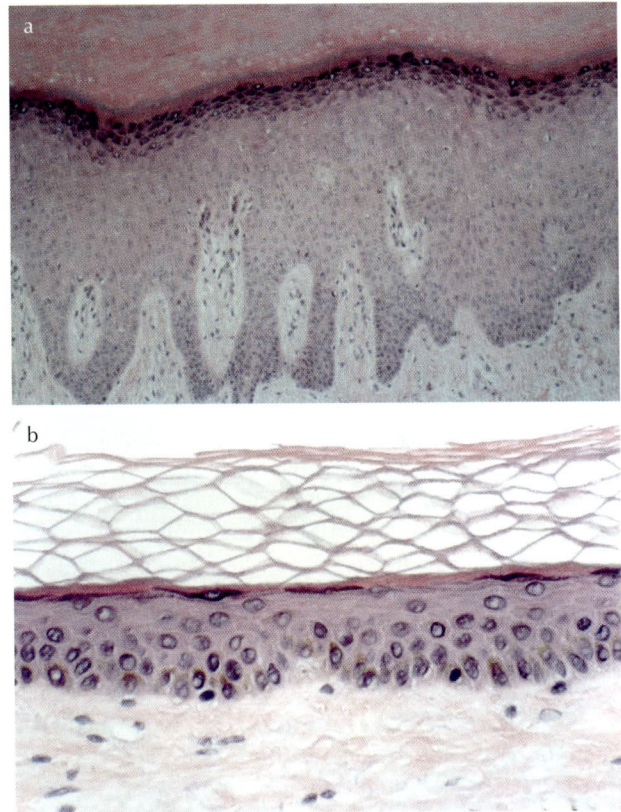

Figure 2.1 Overview of the normal epidermis. Four layers can be recognized: basal layer, squamous cell layer, granular layer, and cornified layer. (a) Thick compacted cornified layer illustrating robust interdigitating dermal papillae and epidermal ridges of acral type. (b) Thin basketweave cornified layer with only finely undulating epidermal junctional contour of thin abdominal skin.

anatomic location. Intercellular desmosomes are particularly evident between the cells in the squamous layer as short projections extending from cell to cell (Figure 2.3).

The granular layer one to three cells thick and displays flattened cells containing keratohyaline granules (Figure 2.4). These granules are precursors of fillagrin, which promotes aggregation of keratin filaments in the cornified layer. The granular cell layer represents the keratogenous zone of the epidermis, in which dissolution of the nucleus and other cell organelles begins.

The stratum corneum contains cells lacking nuclei and organelles but filed with keratin filaments embedded in a dense amorphous matrix.[4]

9

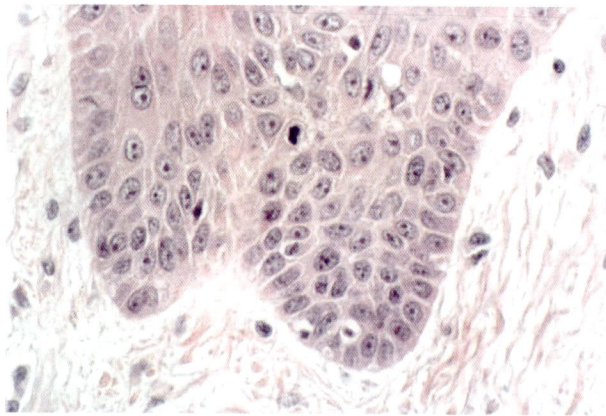

Figure 2.2   A single row of basal cells in the epidermis. Two melanocytes (cells with small dark nuclei surrounded by clear space) are present in the basal layer. Also observe a single mitotic figure in the middle of the field.

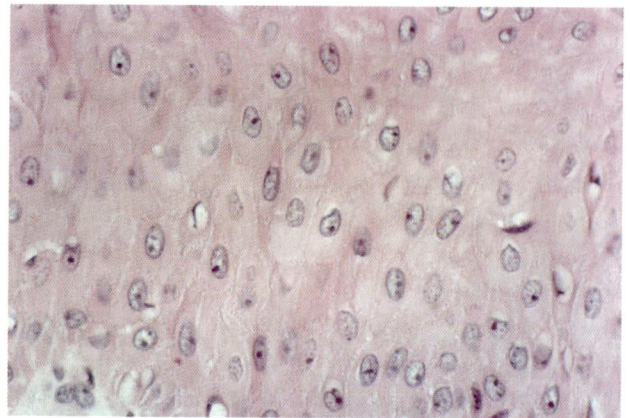

Figure 2.3   Squamous cell layer. Note the presence of intercellular bridges (desmosomes) between the cells.

Melanocytes

Melanocytes are dendritic cells derived from the neural crest. In the epidermis melanocytes are located in the basal layer, and their dendritic projections extend in all directions. In the light microscope, melanocytes appear as clear cells having a small dark-staining nucleus surrounded by a clear space, largely the result of shrinkage artifact. Melanocytes are pigment producing cells. The process of melanin production involves tyrosine as a primary substrate and includes several enzymatic and non-enzymatic steps. Once formed, melanin accumulates in granules (melanosomes) in the interior of melanocytes. These melanosomes migrate through the dendritic melanocytic projections and are transferred to the adjacent keratinocytes. The number of melanocytes in the normal skin is constant in all races: the ratio is 1 melanocyte to every 4–10 basal keratinocytes.[5] The melanocyte and the adjacent keratinocytes are called the epidermal–melanin unit.

Langerhans cells

Langerhans cells are dendritic cells derived from a precursor cell in the bone marrow. The number of Langerhans cells is similar to that of melanocytes, but they are found mainly in the stratum spinosum (squamous cell layer). Langerhans cells are the immunologic cells of the skin and function as antigen presenting cells.[6]

Merkel cells

Merkel cells are present in the undersurface of the epidermis, outer root-sheath of the hair follicle and oral mucosa. It is assumed that Merkel cells are touch receptors.

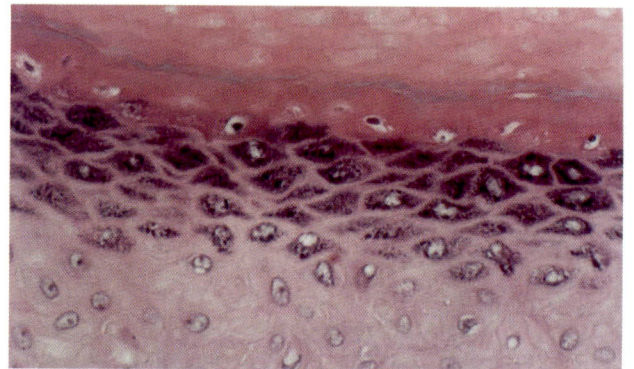

Figure 2.4   Granular cell layer with keratohyaline granules (dark dots in flat cells).

Skin adnexa

Hair

The hair follicle originates from basal keratinocytes that invaginate deep into the dermis. It is part of the pilar unit which is composed of the hair follicle, sebaceous gland, and erector pili muscle (Figure 2.5). It is divided into three segments: the infundibulum, the isthmus, and the inferior segment. The hair cycle consists of the active growth phase (anagen), involutionary stage (catagen), and resting phase (telogen).[7] The daily scalp hair growth rate averages about 0.4 mm. In the adult scalp the anagen stage lasts at least 3 years, catagen phase 3 weeks, and telogen about 3 months. At any given time approximately 84% of scalp hairs are in the anagen phase, 2% in catagen, and 14% in telogen. The histologic appearance of the hair follicle changes significantly during the hair cycle.

Three types of pigment granules are present in hair: erythromelanin granules seen in red hair, eumelanin

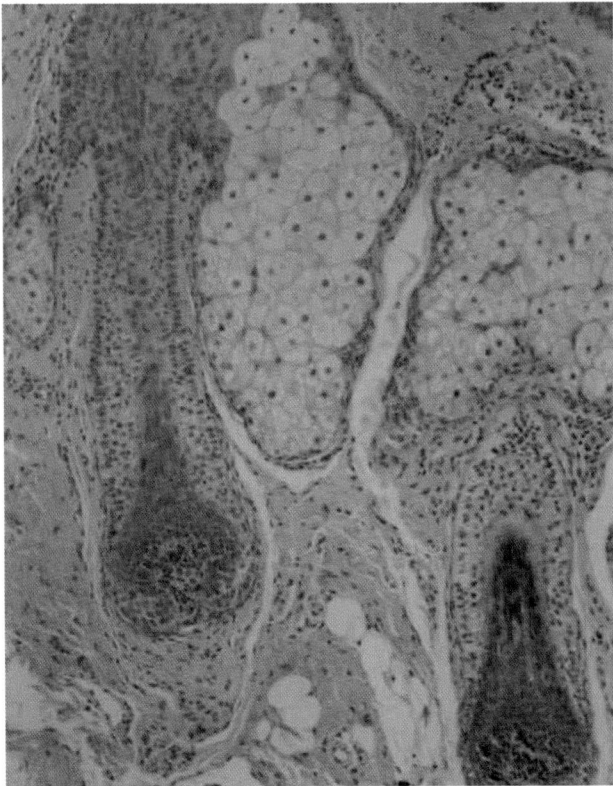

Figure 2.5 Sebaceous glands and hair follicles.

granules abundant in dark hair, and pheomelanin melanosomes that predominate in blond hair. In gray and white hair the melanocytes in the basal layer of the hair matrix are greatly reduced in number or absent.

Sebaceous glands

Sebaceous glands develop as epithelial buds emanating from the hair follicle structures, and therefore usually appear on the skin in association with the hair follicles. Sebaceous glands present everywhere on the skin except for the palms and soles. Sebaceous glands not associated with hair structures occur in the areola and nipple, labia minora, and prepuce. The meibomian glands of the eyelids are modified sebaceous glands.

A sebaceous gland consists of one to several sebaceous lobules and a single excretory duct, which leads the sebum through the hair follicle towards the skin surface. There is no relationship between the size of the sebaceous gland and the size of the associated hair. In the center of the face the sebaceous glands are large, while the associated hair is of the vellus type.

The sebaceous lobules possess a peripheral germinative layer of cuboid cells with centrally located nuclei. Sebum secretion is formed by the decomposition of sebaceous cells (holocrine secretion). Sebaceous cell disintegration is observed in portions of the lobule located closest to the duct.

Sebaceous glands respond to androgenic stimulus by discharge of the sebum to the skin surface. Sebaceous glands are well developed at birth, due to maternal hormones. They undergo atrophy during childhood and enlarge again at puberty. Sebum is composed of triglycerides, phospholipids, and waxes.

Sweat glands

Two types of sweat gland are found in the skin: eccrine and apocrine. The eccrine glands originate from the fetal epidermis and are not associated with hair follicles. They are found everywhere except for the mucocutaneous junctions. Eccrine sweat is responsible for thermoregulation. Apocrine glands are derived from the epithelium of the hair follicles, and are found mainly in the axillae, areolae, mons pubis, labia minora, prepuce, scrotum, and circumanal area. They may represent vestigial scent glands.

Dermis

The dermis is divided into two zones: papillary dermis and reticular dermis. The papillary dermis is located beneath the epidermis and around the adnexal structures. It is composed of a fine network of types I and III collagen, elastic fibers, and abundant ground substance. Reticular dermis is composed of thick bundles of collagen type I and elastic tissue.

The dermis also houses vascular plexuses, neuronal networks, ground substance and its producing dermal cells.

Dermal cells

Dermal fibroblasts produce connective tissue fibrils and dermal ground substance. Besides fibroblasts, other cells seen in normal dermis are histiocytes and mast cells. Occasionally scattered lymphocytes or neutrophils can be detected in dermis on normal skin sections.

Dermal connective tissue

Dermal connective tissue consists of collagen and elastic fibers. Collagen constitutes 70% of the dry dermis weight. A finely woven meshwork of collagen fibers is found in papillary and adventitial dermis. In reticular dermis, collagen fibers unite into thick bundles. Collagen fibers are not extensible, but their wavy arrangement in the dermis allows the skin to stretch.

The biosynthesis of collagen begins within the fibroblast by the assembly of three pro-α polypeptide chains into a triple helical procollagen molecule.[8] After excretion into the extracellular space, the procollagen molecule is

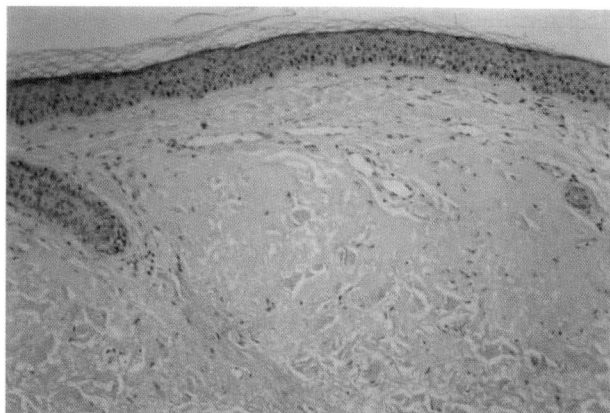

Figure 2.6 Dermal elastotic masses (bluish color) of sun-damaged skin.

converted to collagen by removal of carboxy- and amino-terminal peptides from each pro-α polypeptide chain. Collagen molecules polymerize to collagen fibrils. Collagen fibrils vary in diameter according to their age due to various degrees of polymerization. Collagenase is a rate-limiting enzyme in the collagen degradation pathway. It produces the initial cleavage of the molecule, thereby allowing it to 'unwind' and leaving it to be further digested by gelatinases.

More than 20 different types of collagen are recognized in the human body. They differ in structure and antigenicity. While collagen type I is predominant in the dermis, types III, IV, V, and VII are also found mainly in the skin.

Elastic fibers are thinner than collagen and are barely visible in routine skin sections. They are extensible like rubber, and return to their normal length after stretching. The core of elastic fibers is composed of elastin surrounded by a sheath of microfibrils, each one is composed of the glycoprotein fibrillin. The proportions of these two components change with age.

Collagen and elastic fibers in the dermis are embedded in ground substance consisting mainly of non-sulfated acid mucopolysaccharides (glycosaminoglycans), largely hyaluronic acid.

The arterioles and venules form two important plexuses in the dermis: a subpapillary plexus, supplying dermal papillae, and plexuses around hair follicles and eccrine glands.

Smooth muscle of the skin occurs as arrectores (or erectores) pilorum, attached to the hair follicle below the sebaceous glands. When contracted they pull the hair into a vertical position and produce perifollicular elevation or 'gooseflesh'.

Striated muscle is found in the skin of the neck as platysma and in the skin of the face as muscles of expression.

Subcutaneous tissue

The subcutaneous tissue is arranged into lobules of mature adipocytes. These lobules are separated by thin bands of connective tissue septae. The arteries and veins travel in the septa before reaching the deep vascular plexus.

Skin aging

Both genetic and exogenous factors contribute to the phenotypic changes of skin aging. Chronologically aged skin is dry, lax, and atrophic, with fine wrinkles and a variety of benign neoplasms. Histologically, the most consistent changes of intrinsic cutaneous aging include flattening of the dermoepidermal junction, progressive decrease in melanocyte and Langerhans cell density, loss of capillary loops and fibroblasts in the dermis, and decrease of extracellular matrix.[9]

Histological changes in photodamaged skin include thickening of the epidermis and disorganization and cytologic atypia of the keratinocytes, and uneven distribution of melanocytes in the basal layer with a significant decrease of Langerhans cells.[10] Deposition of amorphous elastic material in the papillary dermis instead of normal connective tissue is considered to be the principal element differentiating chronological aging from photoaging (Figure 2.6). Damage to the collagenous matrix is thought to underlie the coarse, rough and wrinkled appearance of photodamaged skin.

References

1. Halprin KM. Epidermal 'turnover time': a reexamination. Br J Dermatol 1972; 86: 14–19.
2. Frost P, Weinstein GD, Van Scott EJ. The ichthyosiform dermatoses: autoradiographic studies of epidermal proliferation. J Invest Dermatol 1966; 47: 561–7.
3. Lever WF. Histology of skin. In: Lever WF, Schaumberg-Lever G, eds. Histopathology of the Skin, 7th edn. Philadelphia: JB Lippincott Company, 1990.
4. Matoltsy AG. Keratinization. J Invest Dermatol 1975; 67: 20–5.
5. Cochran AJ. The incidence of melanocytes in normal skin. J Invest Dermatol 1970; 55: 65–70.
6. Wolff K, Stingl G. The Langerhans cell. J Invest Dermatol (Suppl) 1983; 80: 17–21.
7. Kligman AM. The human hair cycle. J Invest Dermatol 1959; 55: 374–8.
8. Grant ME, Prockop DJ. The biosynthesis of collagen. N Engl J Med 1972; 286: 194–9.
9. West MD. The cellular and molecular biology of skin aging. Arch Dermatol 1994; 130: 87–95.
10. Kligman LH. Photoaging. Manifestations, prevention and treatment. Clin Geriatr Med 1989; 5: 235–51.

3 Skin morphology and volume: methods of evaluation

Hassan Zahouani and Roberto Vargiolu

Introduction

The epidermis, composed of both a viable and a cornified layer (the thicknesses of which are variable), covers and slightly modifies the skin morphology. Skin relief (as well microrelief and wrinkles) is subjected to some changes due to both environmental and physiological factors. Among these factors, topical treatments by drugs and cosmetics are certainly of great importance, and their effects must be scientifically documented.

If a relatively precise definition exists for the cutaneous microrelief, this is not the case for wrinkles, where terms such as lines or furrows and the adjectives coarse, fine, small, thin, and so on are combined to qualify them. With aging, the skin microrelief changes. Some lines become more marked; they evolve progressively but very slowly to become what laypeople call wrinkles. There is no particular classification for wrinkles, even though detailed clinical study of an aged face shows wrinkles of various magnitudes. On the forehead and crow's feet areas, large wrinkles intermix with smaller ones. Others are localized on the cheeks, around the mouth, on the chin, etc. These wrinkles can be divided into small, very fine wrinkles that disappear after transverse tension, and more marked wrinkles that leave a groove after tension.

The literature dealing with the effect of retinoic acid on photoaging mentions two kinds of wrinkles (fine and coarse), without a precise definition of the categories. The only concrete proposal to qualify the wrinkle was made by Griffiths: an extension of the skin perpendicular to the axis of the wrinkle leaves a marked line, representing the bottom of the wrinkle.[1] This criterion is not used in most published papers today; hence, every scientist has his own opinion, and also the terms 'fine' and 'coarse' may have different meanings in every text.

When we look at the face of a middle-aged person, we can distinguish, in addition to the wrinkles, various types of folds, furrows, and creases, which have been described and discussed by Stegman et al.[2] These features, resulting from facial deformation, are exaggerated by the loss of subcutaneous fat, skin thinning, and gravity.

Various types of wrinkles can be seen on the face. For example, in the crow's feet region, we can distinguish 'coarse wrinkles', the structure of which has been documented by Pierard and Lapiere,[3] fine wrinkles which disappear with simple transverse distortion, and 'facial lines' depending mainly on hydration of the stratum corneum. These facial lines have been largely discussed by Packman and Gans, who also proposed a scoring system to evaluate their number and importance.[4]

One might think that there exists a continuity in the distribution of wrinkles that depends on their length or depth. This explains the difficulty in defining precisely the different types of wrinkles.

Non-invasive methods of quantification of skin topography

The last 30 years have seen a great step forward in the field of three-dimensional microscopy, especially in the analysis of the topography of surfaces. Initially the purpose was to control the quality of manufactured surfaces by measuring their roughness in a given direction, and the variables qualifying this parameter have since been standardized internationally. Unfortunately, this methodology was limited to a two-dimensional analysis that quantifies the morphology of the surface via a signal which represents the relief of a line in a given direction, not of a surface. This method was greatly improved when its principle was developed so as to make it possible to reproduce the surface relief as a three-dimensional image.[5,6]

This technological achievement allows the construction of a three-dimensional (3D) image, from the atomic scale (atomic force microscope) to macroscopic relief.

To date, most of these non-invasive methods have consisted of the use of replicas (negative) or

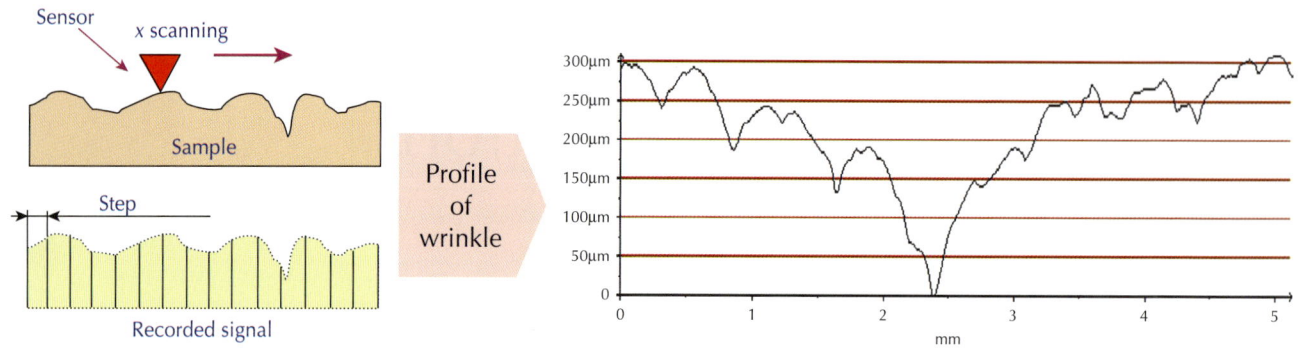

Figure 3.1   Line acquisition.

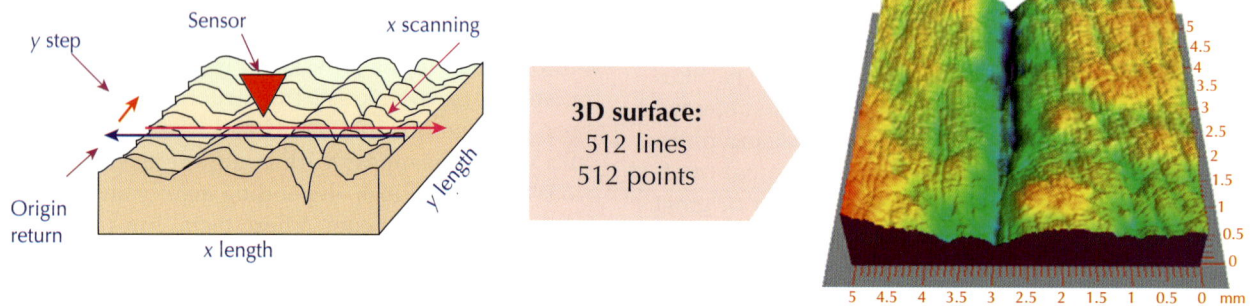

Figure 3.2   Construction of the three-dimensional relief of the face.

counter-replicas (positive) of the cutaneous surface. The relief profile is measured by either mechanical or optical microscopy techniques.

Replicas and counter-replicas

The most widely used material for skin replicas is silicone polymer. This liquid is mixed with a hardener in fixed proportions; too-slow or too-quick hardening will give a poor representation of the relief. One major pitfall is the presence of air bubbles in the replicas, especially on the surface. The presence of these bubbles depends mainly on the fluidity of the silicone polymer before hardening.[6–8]

Besides total immobility of the subject when taking the cast, body-part positioning must be perfectly controlled as it has been shown that line density, depth, and anisotropy strongly depend on skin distortion.[9] The skin surface replicas obtained are often not hard enough to allow microscope measurement using a probe; for this, one must make a hard counter-replica with cyanoacrylate resin. According to the method of evaluation used, the thickness and color of the replica may influence the quality of the measurement when an optical method is used.

Mechanical microscopy technique

This technique, based on the contact between a diamond tip and the surface, consists of scanning a line of microrelief, moving horizontally at a constant speed of around 1 mm/s. The diamond tip has a radius of curvature of 2 μm and exerts a pressure of about 10 mN on the surface. The vertical displacement of the tip is converted into an electrical signal using a transducer (capacitive or inductive), or is measured by an optical apparatus.[8]

To obtain a 3D reproduction of the cutaneous relief, the surface is scanned line by line, each line consisting of a number of points spaced out at a specified measurement step (Figure 3.1). To obtain one line, the detector moves along the x axis (perpendicular to the main axis of the cutaneous relief or wrinkle) in order to measure a certain length.

Acquisition of 3D relief

The 3D image of the surface relief is produced by placing the profiles measured at regular intervals next to each other. An example of construction of the 3D relief of the face is presented in Figure 3.2.

This early method is based on the principle schematized in Figure 3.3. It measures either a profile (2D) or

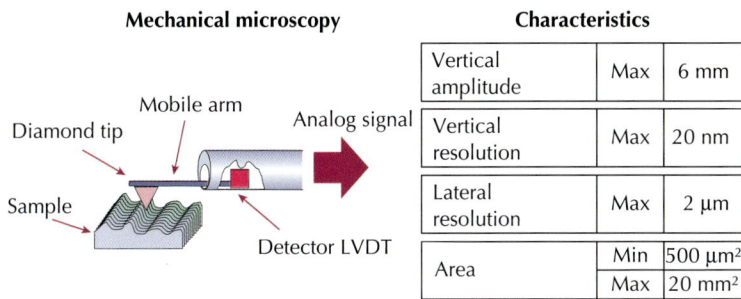

Mechanical microscopy	Characteristics		
	Vertical amplitude	Max	6 mm
	Vertical resolution	Max	20 nm
	Lateral resolution	Max	2 μm
	Area	Min	500 μm²
		Max	20 mm²

Figure 3.3   Mechanical scanning instrument.

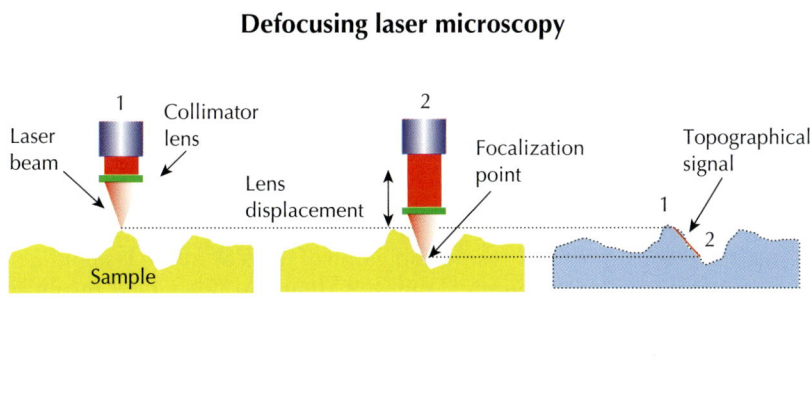

Defocusing laser microscopy	Characteristics		
	Vertical amplitude	Max	1 mm
	Vertical resolution	Max	10 nm
	Lateral resolution	Max	1 μm
	Area	Min	256 μm²
		Max	50 mm²

Figure 3.4   Defocusing laser microscope.

a surface (3D). The device consists of a tactile detector and a set of three tables (*x, y, z*). It has a mobile arm mechanically connected to an inductive detector (linear variable displacement transducer, LVDT), which transforms the variations of the relief into an analog signal.

Laser microscopy of skin relief

Defocusing laser microscopy

The negative replica of the cutaneous relief is analyzed using a defocusing laser probe with an optical measuring head, which is a servomotor operating as a transmitter–receiver. A laser diode (transmitter) sends out a beam of light to the surface, and the reflected signal is sent back to a set of four photodiodes (receiver).[10,11] The servomotor drives a lens in order to attain maximal reflected light intensity on the photodiodes. The diameter of the spot on a flat surface is 1 μm; this diameter varies when it is transmitted to a rough surface. The diameter variation of the spot in the course of measurement triggers an automatic localization control by vertical shifting of the lens. The lens is part of a vertical movement system which records the localization height that forms the topographical signal (Figure 3.4).

Laser triangulation microscopy

Triangulation microscopy uses three reference points (Figure 3.5): the fixed source, a laser diode; the point of the surface to be analyzed, whose height varies according to the local relief; and the image of this point formed by the optical system on the detector plane.[12]

When the whole measurement system is displaced relative to the surface (and parallel to the mean plane of the surface), the image formed on the detectors changes position, and the measurement of this position gives the height of the measured point relative to that of the original measured point. The advantage of this system is that it measures the relief with a wide vertical range (10 mm), with a resolution of 1 μm.

White light interferometer microscopy

The principle of vertical scanning interferometry uses two technologies to measure a wide range of surface heights. The phase-shifting interferometry (PSI) mode is used to measure smooth surfaces, while the vertical-scanning interferometry (VSI) mode can be used to measure the skin surface topography.[13] This scanning mode is a newer technique than phase-shifting interferometry. The basic interferometric principles are similar in both

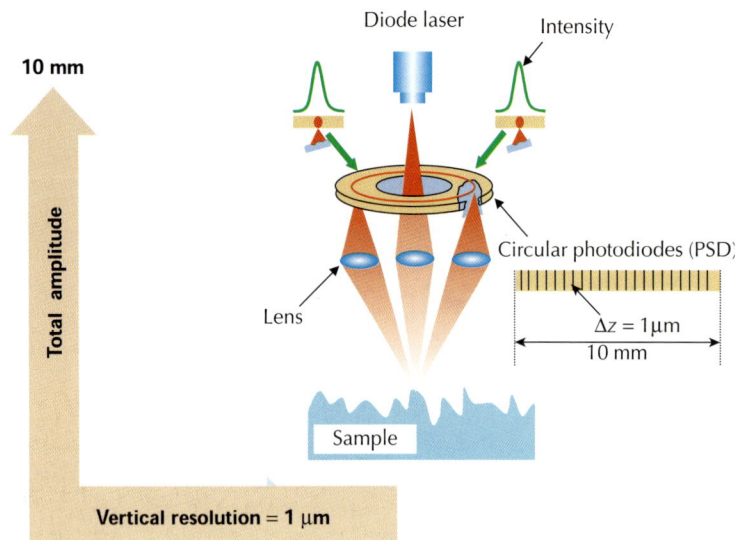

Figure 3.5   Laser triangulation microscopy. PSD, position sensing photodiode.

techniques: light reflected from the reference mirror combines with light reflected from a sample to produce interference fringes, where the best-contrast fringe occurs at best focus. In vertical-scanning interferometry, a white-light beam passes through a microscope objective to the sample surface. A beam splitter reflects half of the incident beam to a reference surface. The beams reflected from the sample and the reference surface combine at the beam splitter to form interference fringes (Figure 3.6a). During measurement, the reference arm containing the interferometric objective moves vertically to scan the surface at varying heights (Figure 3.6b). A linearized piezoelectric transducer precisely controls the motion. Because white light has a short coherence length, interference fringes are present only over a very shallow depth for each focus position. Fringe contrast at a single sample point reaches a peak as the sample is translated through focus. The VSI technique uses an algorithm that processes fringe modulation data from the intensity signal to calculate surface heights. As seen in Figure 3.6b, the fringe contrast, or modulation, increases as the sample is translated into focus, then falls as it is translated past focus. The system scans through focus (starting above focus) at evenly spaced intervals and the camera captures frames of interference data. As the system scans downward, an interference signal for each point on the surface is recorded. The system uses a series of advanced computer algorithms to demodulate the envelope of the fringe signal. Finally, the vertical position corresponding to the peak interference signal is extracted for each point on the surface.

Resolution and range of measurement

Resolution refers to the smallest distance that the interferometer surface profiler can accurately measure. It can be in terms of lateral or vertical resolution. The vertical resolution value of the VSI mode is about 3 nm with a vertical range of 1000 μm. The lateral resolution is a function of magnification objective and the chosen detector array size. The choice of magnification objective implies a fixed area zone with a high resolution, which can be scanned with the interferometer. The originality of this system is the ability to extend the area zone of analysis using a sophisticated method of stitching, while keeping the same lateral and vertical resolution. The stitching method is an automatic approach to sampling which can combine successive elementary areas in the x and y directions using a specific algorithm. The goal is to increase the range of the topographic area, with conservation of the lateral and vertical resolution. Figure 3.7 shows an example of the stitching technique used by the VSI mode.

Fringe projection microscopy

The fringe projection measuring system consists of a projection unit and a charge-coupled device (CCD) camera, which are fixed at the 'triangulation angle'. With the gray code method, gratings with a rectangular brightness distribution and differing numbers of lines are projected consecutively.[14] The number of lines is doubled with each projection run (Figure 3.8), which unambiguously defines the stripe order for each image point. When using the phase-shift technique, only one grating with sinus-shaped intensity distribution is projected, multiple times, with varying phase position (Figure 3.8).

An advantage of this combined recording technique lies in the fact that, in addition to the brightness image of the test area, the order, phase, and quality of stripe of the projected pattern can be calculated for each image point. In addition to an exact 3D

(a)

(b)

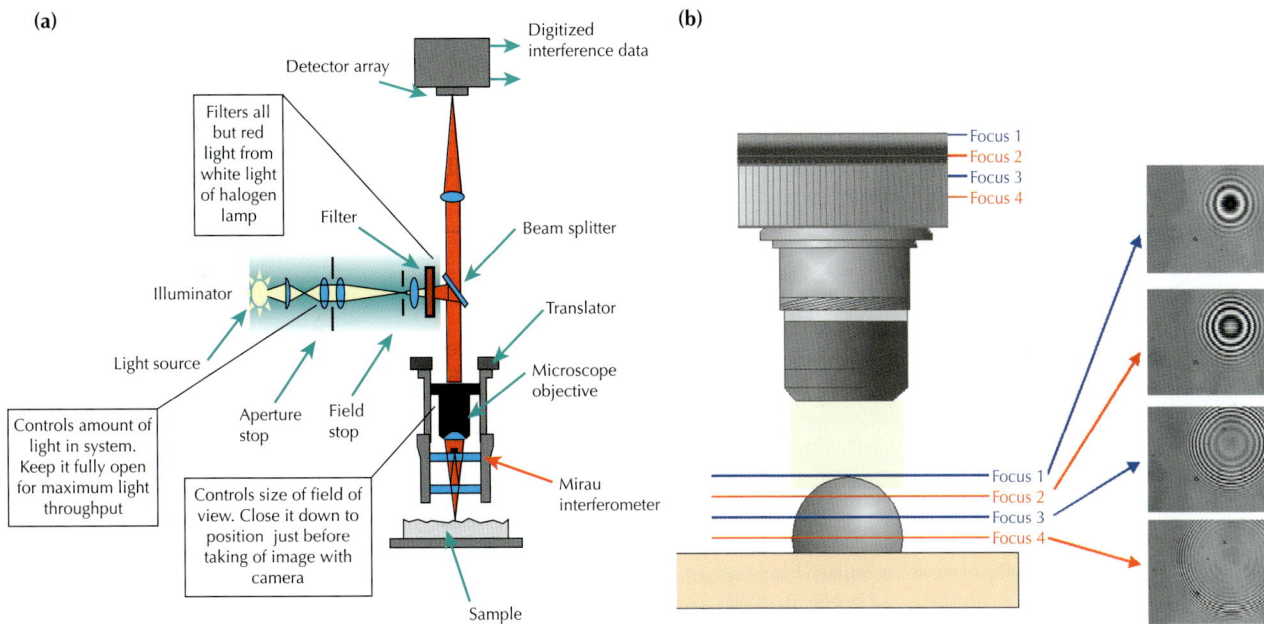

Figure 3.6   (a) White light interferometer. (b) Vertical scanning mode (VSI).

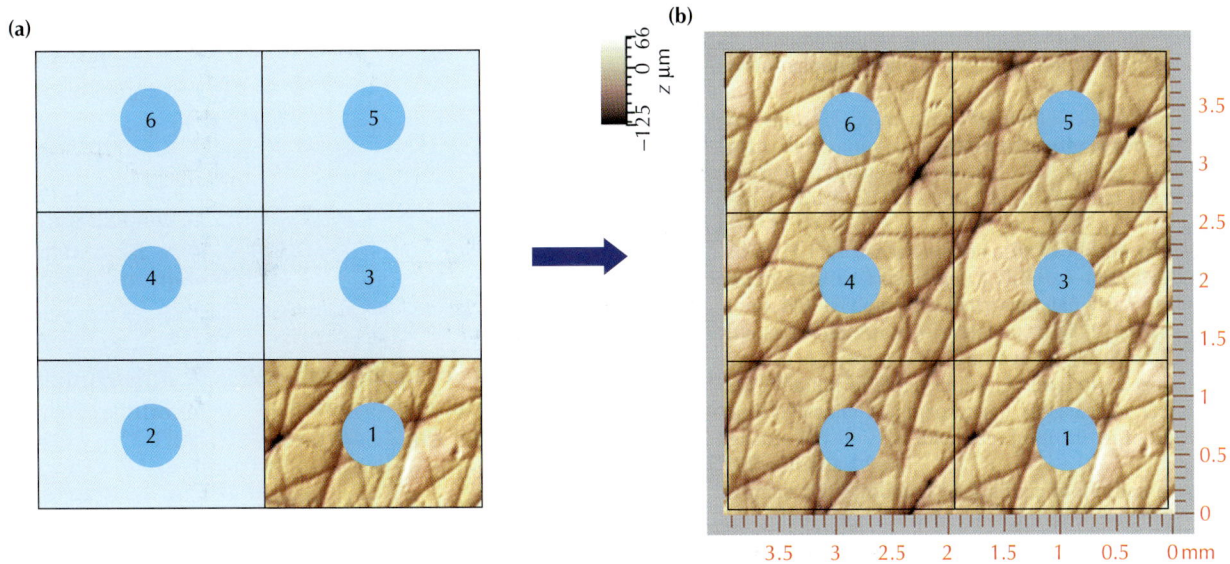

(a)

(b)

Figure 3.7   Example of stitching technique. (a) Elementary zone. (b) Large sampling by conserving high resolution.

reconstruction of the surface in which each image point is defined independently of its surrounding points, the technique enables automatic control of measuring quality. If implausible measurement points are obtained, they can be eliminated, thereby preventing incorrect interpretation.

The following aspects should be mentioned as further important experimental parameters. The fringe projection technique is able to use a depth of focus of ± 10 mm for an examination field of about 25×35 mm. Resolution in the vertical z direction within 0.2% of the measuring range leads to an actual resolution of 4 µm in the z direction. With the CCD camera type used, a horizontal resolution in the x and similarly in the y direction of 45 µm is achieved. Here, it should be stressed once again that the resolution in the z direction is not limited by the 255 gray stages of the CCD camera. On the contrary, the high resolution in the vertical direction is achieved by analysis of the intensity and phase shifts of the projected grating. The surface structure of the test area causes the intensity and phase information of the projected grating structures to deviate from the theoretically ideal structure of a flat surface. The absolute 3D coordinate of the test area

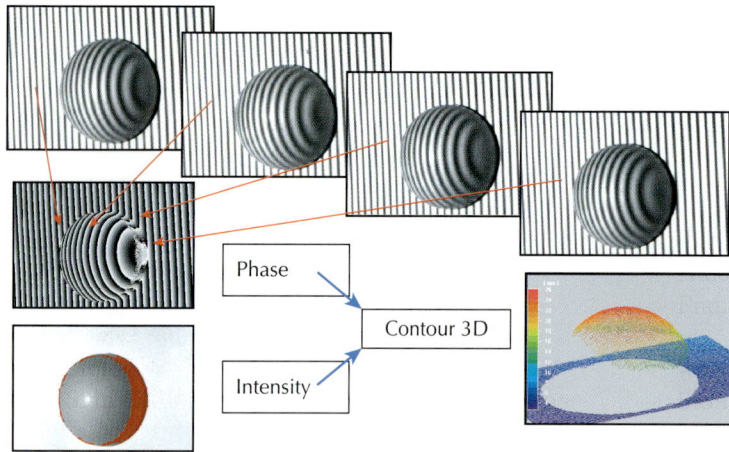

Figure 3.8 Principle of fringe projection method.

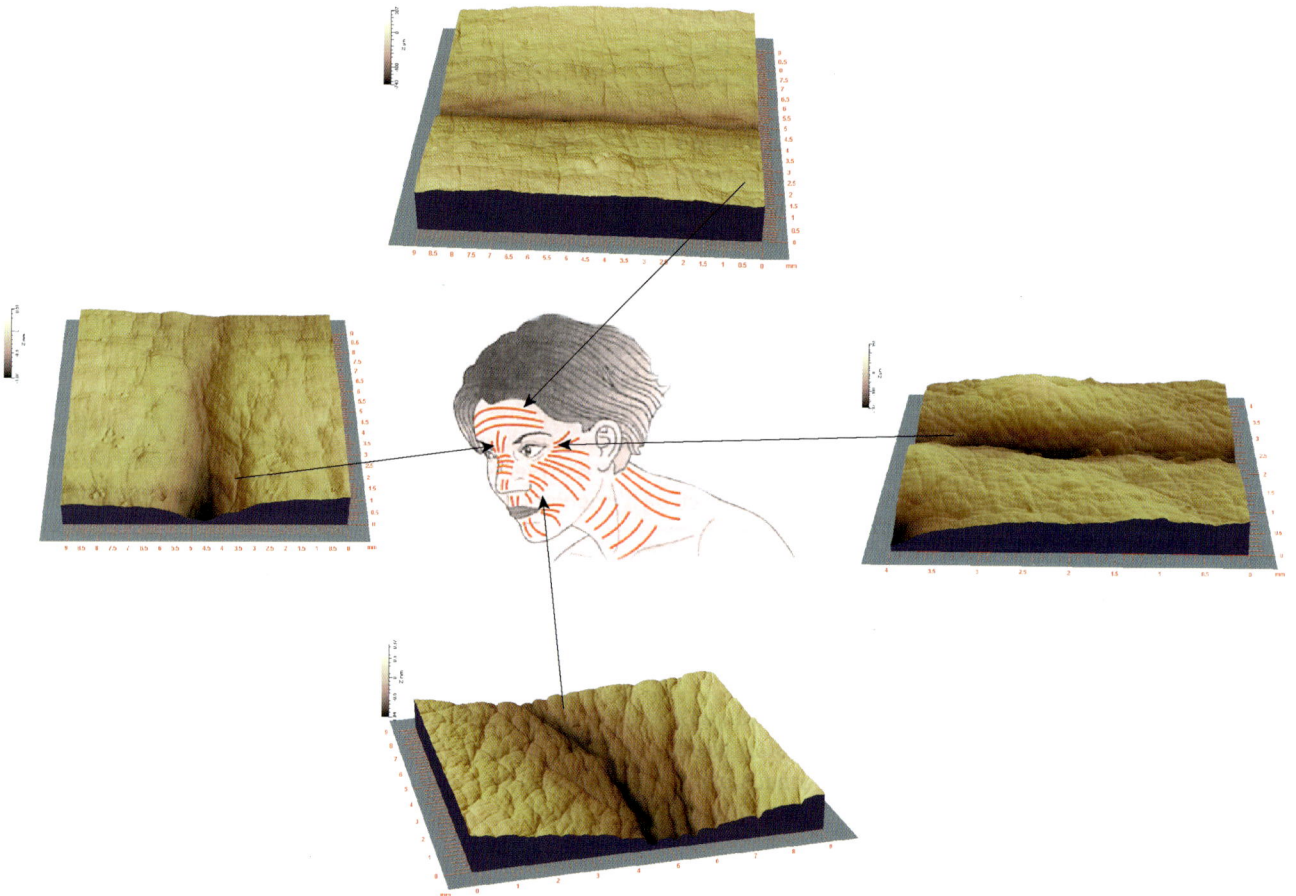

Figure 3.9 Facial wrinkles.

can then be calculated from these shifts using the corresponding mathematical algorithms.

Thanks to the computer capacity available nowadays, the image recording sequence with corresponding coordinate analysis can be carried out in less than 1 s (about 800 ms).

Facial wrinkles

As indicated in Figure 3.9, depending on the zone of the face, various types of lines can be identified according to a morphological hierarchy: deep wrinkles, fine wrinkles, and a network of microlines.

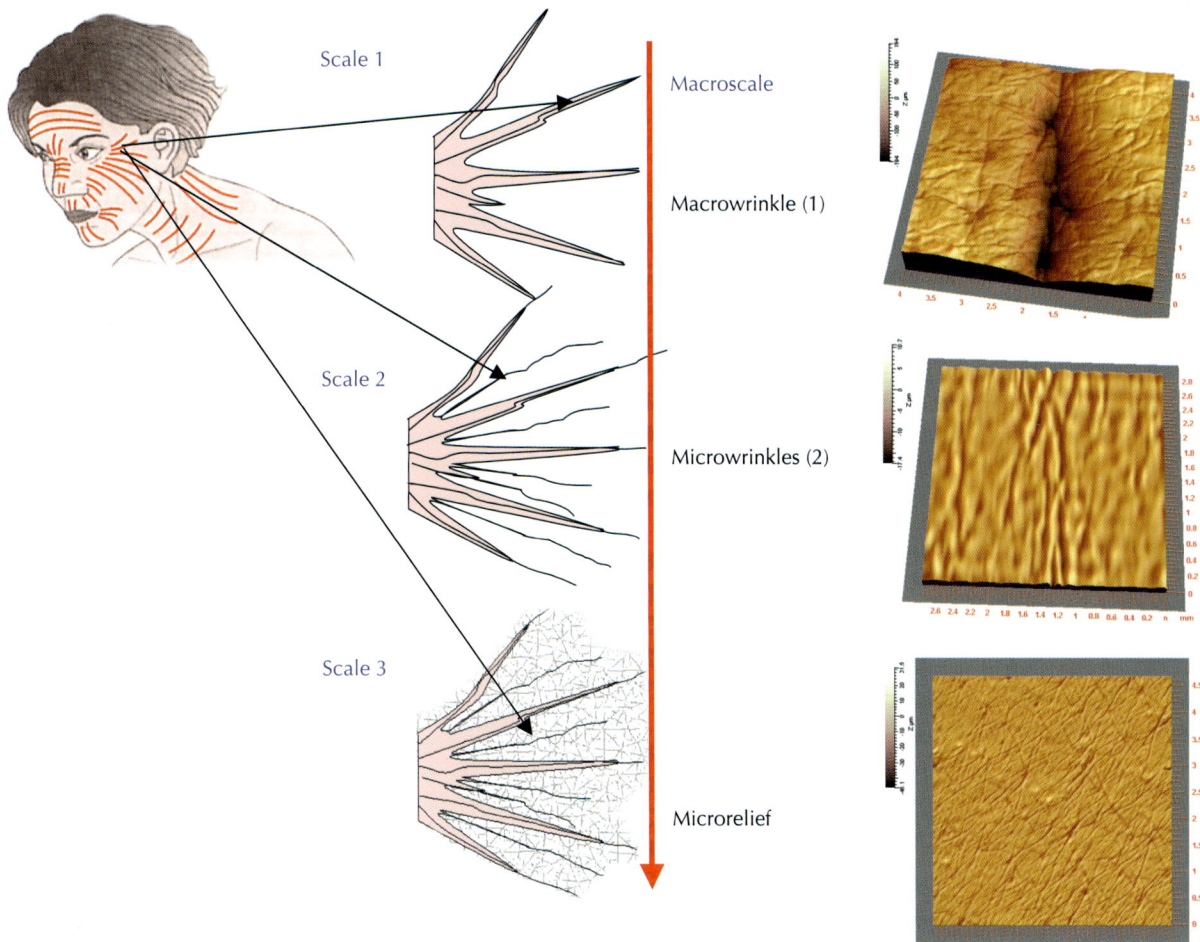

Figure 3.10 Multiscale morphology of the face.

In the absence of rigorous work on the morphology and three-dimensional scales of facial wrinkles and their evolution during aging, we studied in detail the morphology of facial wrinkles. The methodology consisted of analyzing lines using good resolution, by separating the wavelengths of the microrelief ($< 300\,\mu m$), of the fine lines, and of the principal wrinkles (Figure 3.10). The results show the existence of three or four principal axes of anisotropy: two principal axes for the micronetwork (as the volar forearm), and a vertical axis (80–110°) compared to the vertical direction of the axis of the body, in which one finds the principal direction of the wrinkle and the direction of not very deep, fine lines with a spacing which depends on the type of wrinkle and the age of the subject.

Multiscale aspect of facial lines

The study of the multiscale and anisotropic aspects of skin line morphology requires a spectral or morphological decomposition of the 3D topography. Such a decomposition will make it possible to identify the anisotropy of skin line tension, to define groups or families of lines according to their scale, and to follow their evolution during aging and their transformation after cosmetic application.

Fourier analysis is a powerful tool used to condense information represented in the spatial domain (or time domain) into the frequency domain, and to enhance the information to detail individual frequency or wavelength values. It reveals the absolute and relative contributions of different wavelength components to the mean square height of surfaces. In addition, it is more convenient to define and separate the so-called roughness and waviness components by 2D spectral analysis. In Fourier analysis the basis function is an exponential function, although Fourier series are frequently written in an alternative form using the trigonometric functions sine and cosine.

The scale and anisotropy of skin morphology components have been analyzed using 2D Fourier transformation. Determination of the spectral components of skin topography permits computation of the amplitude, direction, and wavelength of each spatial

(a)

(b)

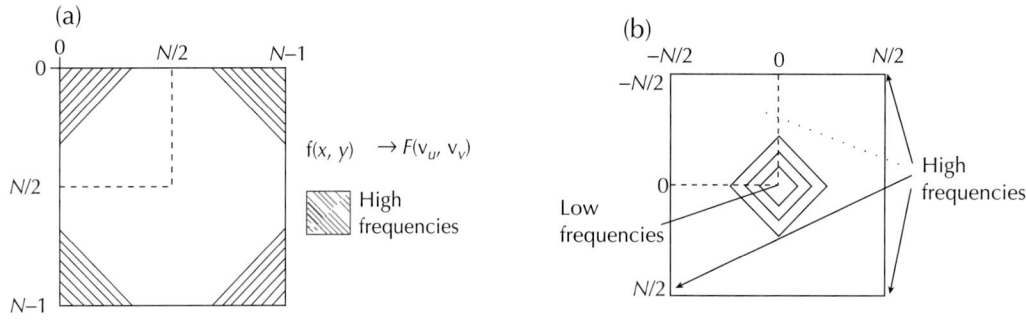

Figure 3.11 (a, b) Spatial frequency distribution.

frequency.[15–17] The complex Fourier transformation computed from scanned data is given by the relation:

$$F(v_u, v_v) = \frac{1}{N}\frac{1}{M} \sum_{j=0}^{N-1} \sum_{k=0}^{M-1} f(x_j, y_k)$$
$$\exp - 2\pi i (v_u, x_j, v_v, y_k) \tag{1}$$

which represents the spectrum of surface topography $f(x,y)$, defined in a finite bandwidth by the low and high spatial frequency limits, respectively:

$$v_{lu} = \frac{u}{N\Delta_x}, v_{lv} = \frac{v}{M\Delta_y} \text{(cycles mm}^{-1}) \quad \text{and}$$
$$v_{hu} = \frac{1}{2\Delta_x}, v_{hv} = \frac{1}{2\Delta_y} \text{(cycles mm}^{-1}) \tag{2}$$

Spatial frequency range of line network

The bandwidth of the frequency range is given by relation (3). For example, if $N = M = 512$ as the choice for the maximum sample size, if the sample intervals are fixed at $\Delta_x = \Delta_y = 10\,\mu\text{m}$, this sample size makes the sample dimensions 5.12 mm × 5.12 mm. Hence, the wavelength of the longest component of skin furrows which can be identified in the sample is approximately 5.12 mm. The frequency range of the analysis can be readily calculated from expression (3). The high frequency limit is:

$$v_{hu} = \frac{1}{2\Delta_x} = \frac{1}{2\Delta_y} = \frac{1}{2 \times 0.01} = 50 \text{ cycles mm}^{-1} \tag{3}$$

equivalent to a wavelength of $\lambda_h = 1/50 = 0.02$ mm or 20 μm. Similarly, the low frequency limit v_{lu} is given by:

$$v_{lu} = \frac{1}{N\Delta_x} = \frac{1}{M\Delta_y} = \frac{1}{512 \times 0.01}$$
$$= 0.1953 \text{ cycles mm}^{-1} \tag{4}$$

equivalent to a wavelength of $\lambda_h = 1/0.1953 = 5.12$ mm.

Fourier spectrum representation

A recorded digital image containing $N \times M$ points with an origin located at $j = k = 0$ will give rise to an $N \times M$ array or spectral coefficients under the 2D Fourier transformation. The spectral coefficients will form the pattern of the skin relief. The origin will be located at a position which corresponds to the origin of the data array. The frequency of these spectral coefficients increases along directions which correspond to the positive directions of the x and y axes of the array up to the Nyquist frequencies ($N/2$ and $M/2$). The coefficients are then repeated in inverse order. A schematic representation of this (Figure 3.11a) has no physical significance. To overcome this, the quadrants of the spectrum can be rearranged, as illustrated in Figure 3.11b. This operation moves the origin to the center of the array, and the pattern formed by the rearranged quadrants is that which would be generated by an optical Fourier transformation system, or diffraction (Fraunhoffer) type analysis.[8] In practice, the exchange of quadrants is effected by a mathematical operation rather than by physical rearrangement of the transformation coefficients. Gonzalez and Wintz[18] show that multiplying $f(x_j, y_k)$ by $(-1)^{j+k}$ is equivalent to shifting the origin to $(N/2, M/2)$ as required. So, the low frequencies of the skin relief spectrum $F(v_x, v_y)$ are located in the center of the spectrum, using the frequency translation property:[15–17]

$$TF[\exp - 2\pi i (v_{u0}x + v_{v0}y)f(x, y)]$$
$$= F(v_u - v_{u0}, v_v - v_{v0}) \tag{5}$$

for $v_{u0} = v_{v0} = \dfrac{N}{2}$ (6)

we have

$$TF[(-1)^x(-1)^y z(x, y)] = F\left(v_u - \frac{N}{2}, v_v - \frac{N}{2}\right) \tag{7}$$

Figure 3.12 shows a Fourier spectrum for volar forearm skin lines. In the above, (Δ_x, Δ_y) are the sampling steps, the subscripts u and v indicate the wavelength and orientation of a sine wave in the original data, and N and M are the numbers of data points along the x and y axes.

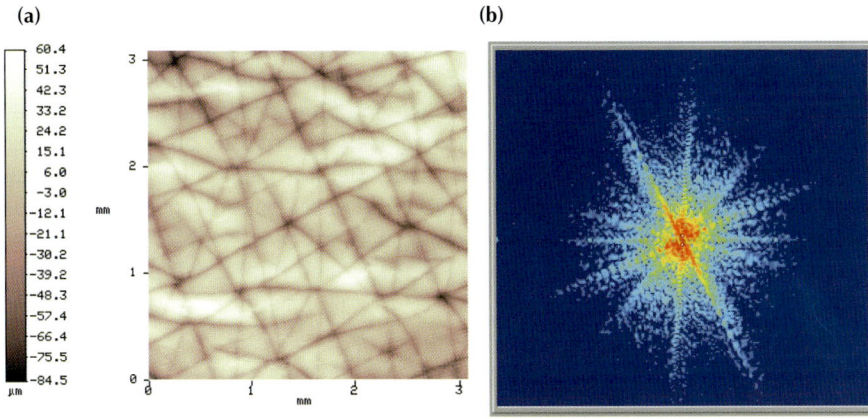

Figure 3.12 Example of Fourier spectrum for skin lines. (a) 2D view of skin line topography. (b) Spectrum.

Skin line orientation in Fourier space

The complex coefficients $F(v_u, v_v)$ of a 2D spectrum can be used to evaluate the amplitude and power spectra of the topography. The magnitude of these coefficients has the normal interpretation. The frequency domain coordinates, however, have special significance. The subscripts (u,v) indicate the wavelength and orientation of a sine wave in the original data. The axes u and v are perpendicular in Fourier space, so the frequency of a particular coefficient in the transformation is given by:

$$v = (v_u^2 + v_v^2)^{\frac{1}{2}} \tag{8}$$

whilst the orientation of the wave relative to the u axis is given by:

$$\theta = \tan^{-1}\left(\frac{u}{v}\right) \tag{9}$$

Spectral rose of skin line anisotropy

The amplitude of the skin relief spectrum is given by:

$$A(v_u, v_v) = 2\left|F(v_u, v_v)^* F(v_u, v_v)\right| \tag{10}$$

where $F(v_u, v_v)^*$ is the complex conjugate of $F(v_u, v_v)$. The amplitude spectrum can be expressed using polar coordinates $A(p, \theta)$. The various topographical components with respect to the wave direction identified in the polar spectrum can be directionally represented in the polar diagram in the form of a spectral rose:[15–17]

$$R_S(\theta), (0 \leq \theta \leq \pi) \tag{11}$$

generated with the computation of the direction of each spatial frequency, identified with respect to the x axis in the original sample.[15] The geometrical form of the spectral rose represents the global anisotropy, and permits identification of the direction of each family of lines. Figure 3.13 shows spectral roses with respect to age of the skin morphology.

Spectral decomposition of skin lines

Two fundamental sampling templates are introduced to extract the specific morphology in the frequency domain.[15] The first template is the parallel line template, which involves computation of the total power observed along a series of superimposed parallel lines across the Fourier spectrum. Consider the case of wrinkle frequencies oriented in the x or y axis of the spectrum. Extraction of the frequencies can be realized by inverse Fourier transformation of the frequencies oriented in the x or y direction as follows:

$$Z(x,y)_{wrinkles} = TF^{-1} \sum_{v=-v_X}^{+v_X} [F(v_X, v_y)]_{\theta \perp u \text{ or} // u} \tag{12}$$

Figure 3.14 shows separation of the principal wrinkle and the differently oriented furrows.

The Fourier spectrum of the image allows us to separate the various scales described in relation (11). The example of Figure 3.15 shows separation of the form and the micronetwork morphology of a face wrinkle.

The methodology can be used to evaluate the efficacy of a cosmetic product, after separation of the wrinkle and the micronetwork of lines. The example of Figure 3.16 shows the effect of a cosmetic product on the wrinkle and the micronetwork after 6 weeks of application.

Volume of wrinkle

Macroscopic volume of wrinkle

The method developed to calculate the skin or void volume of a wrinkle uses the contour height of the skin morphology; we define the skin volume as the portion enclosed in a truncation plane parallel to the mean surface and the interfacial surface. Skin volume $(V_m(h))$ is a function of the truncation depth h, and may reflect an increase in density of the skin depending on the treatment. The void volume $(V_v(h))$ is a

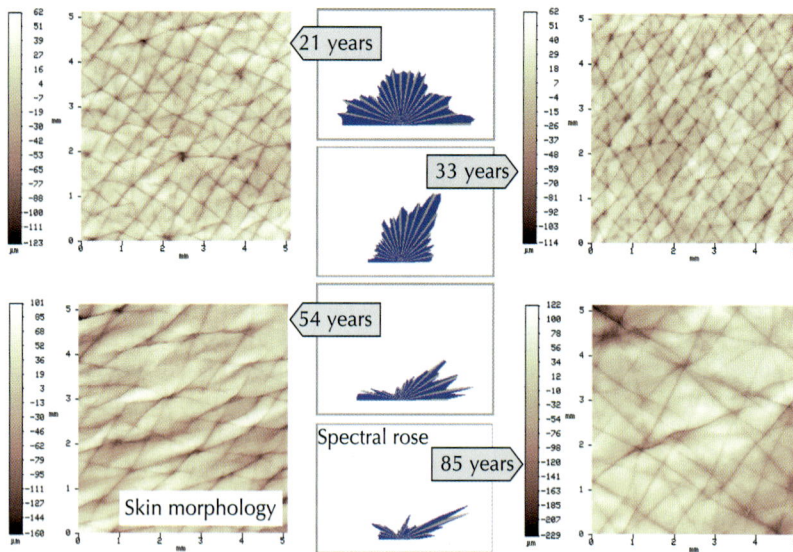

Figure 3.13 Spectral rose of skin morphology during aging.

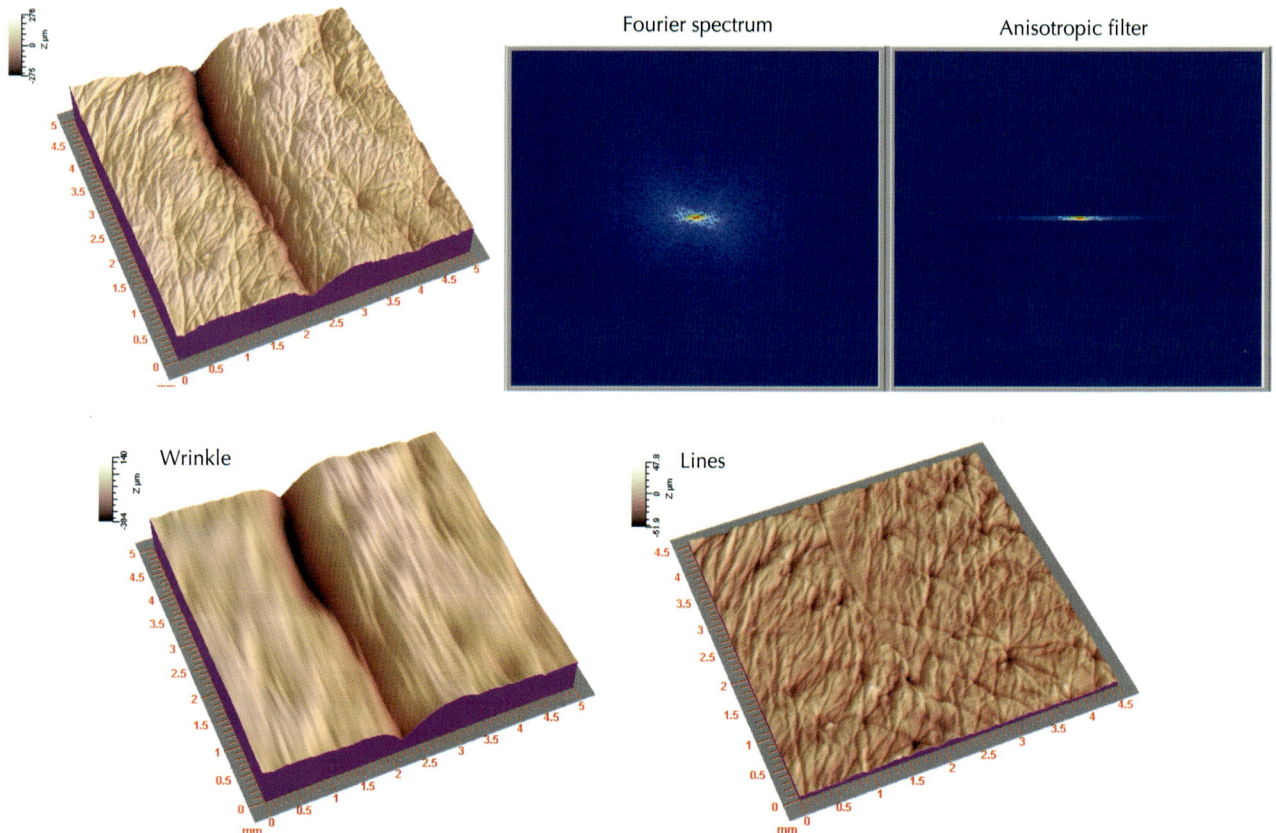

Figure 3.14 Separation of wrinkle and micronetwork of the face.

complementary function of the skin volume; it is a volume enclosed between a truncation plane at a given level parallel to the mean plane and the skin beneath the plane. The void volume reflects the geometry of the wrinkle. Figure 3.17 shows evaluation of the void volume of a wrinkle.

The geometry of the wrinkle is investigated by quantification of its volume and its projected surface. The objective of the methodology[11,15] is to find a way of locating the edge of the wrinkle automatically by assessing the sharp variation of the gradient of the relief. To locate the edge, the image is scanned line by

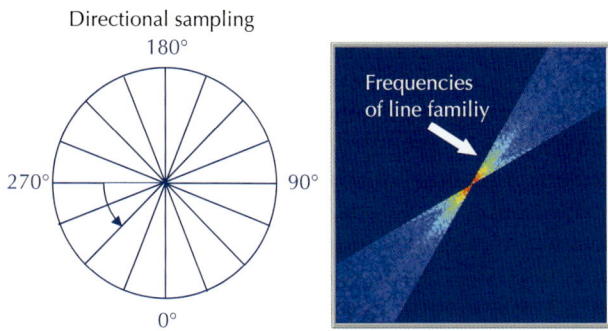

Figure 3.15   Directional spatial frequency sampling.

line and column by column in order to identify all the points which form the edge of the wrinkle. When the edge is identified, a root mean square plan is established that goes through all the points outside the wrinkle and will be the reference for calculation of the volume. Figure 3.18 shows the method used to locate the edge of the wrinkle and calculation of the surface and volume.

Assessment of cosmetic effect

The effect of the product on surface area and volume parameters is presented in Figure 3.19.

Three-dimensional morphology of skin line network

Optical skin imaging shows that the skin presents a line network: parallel furrows criss-cross, forming rectangles, squares, lozenges, trapezoids, and triangle motifs. Hashimoto proposed a simple classification into four groups of lines. Primary lines are wide and 20–100 μm deep according to site and age.[19–21] They cross to form parallelograms, rectangles, or squares. Secondary lines are narrow (depth 5–40 μm); they are branches of primary lines and form diagonals within the shapes made by the latter. Primary and secondary lines generally intersect at the points where sweat ducts and hair shafts emerge (Figure 3.20).

The main drawback of this statistical method is that it quantifies parameters of the cutaneous surface: their average value is calculated for the different morphological types of lines, which makes it impossible to

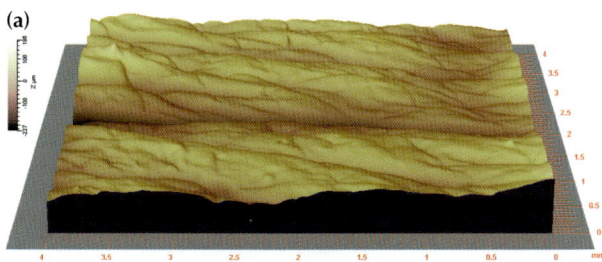

(a)

$T0$: Rz = 438 μm

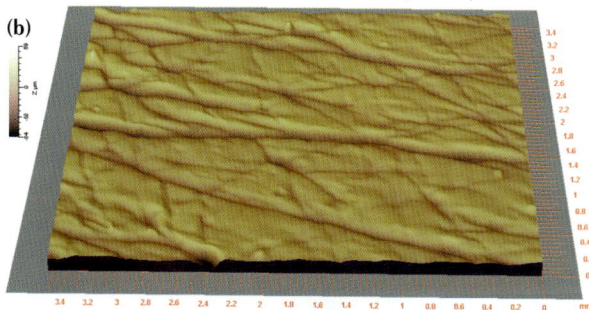

(b)

$T0$: Rz = 49.63 μm

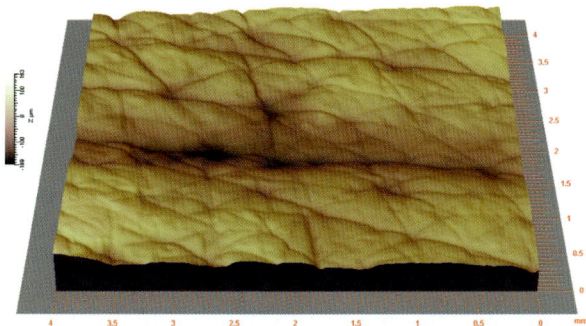

$T6$ weeks after: Rz = 276 μm

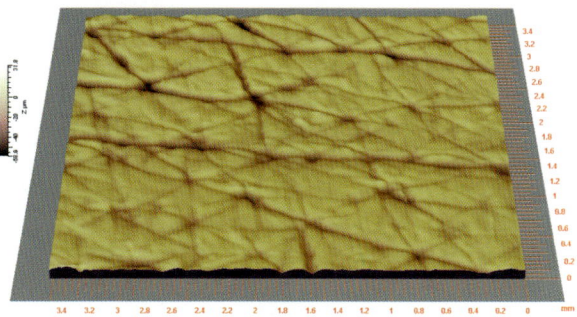

$T6$ weeks after : Rz = 37 μm

Figure 3.16   Assessment of cosmetic treatment on the morphology of (a) wrinkle and (b) micronetwork. Rz, mean value of morphology depth.

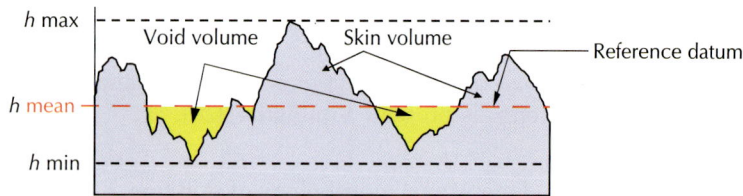

Figure 3.17   Volume evaluation of wrinkle.

distinguish the part played by each type of crease in the aging process or to identify which type of line is influenced by cosmetics.

Since 1995, a research program has been set up to develop a methodology of characterization of the cutaneous relief, the principle of which is similar to using an optical microscope, with a depth of field based on a multiresolution mathematical analysis. The main capacity of the mathematical microscope is to identify and quantify the morphological families contained in the three-dimensional image and to show the result on an absolute three-dimensional chart, demonstrating the hierarchy of the various scales of skin lines.[22,23]

Morphological assessment of the skin line network

The initial idea assumes that the texture of the cutaneous relief can be schematized by a sum of families of waves which have the following three main parameters: amplitude, wavelength, and direction:

$$
\begin{aligned}
\text{Cutaneous relief} = {} & \alpha \; secondary \; lines \; (\lambda_M, \theta_M) \\
& + \beta \; Langer's \; lines \; (\lambda_L, \theta_L) \\
& + \gamma \; wrinkles \; (\lambda_R, \theta_R)
\end{aligned}
\tag{13}
$$

The coefficients α, β, and γ are amplitude parameters that vary according to age, sex, and area of the body. The wavelengths λ_M, λ_L, and λ_R characterize the different morphological families of skin lines. The directions θ_M, θ_L, and θ_R vary according to the anisotropy of the local mechanical tension, which gives the skin a texture composed of morphological lines specific to each part of the body.

In cosmetology, it is possible to quantify the kinetics of a cosmetic product with the knowledge and follow-up of the topography of the skin, by studying the direction of the lines, their spacing, and their depth, which are associated with a mechanical effect and the aging process.

Identification of morphological features

The morphological approach developed to define and quantify skin lines is similar to methods set up in geography information systems that reproduce the topography of the earth from data provided by satellites. The method consists of the projection of an analysis grid on the relief that plays the part of the microscope lens. In line with geographical criteria

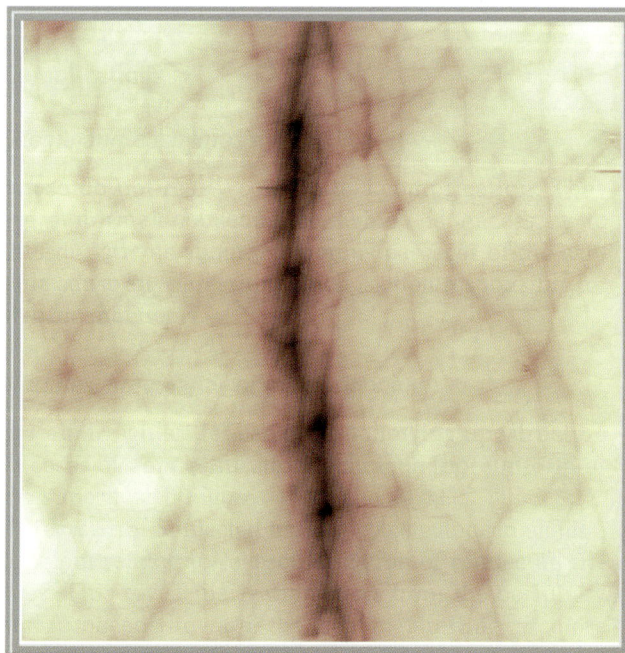

2D view

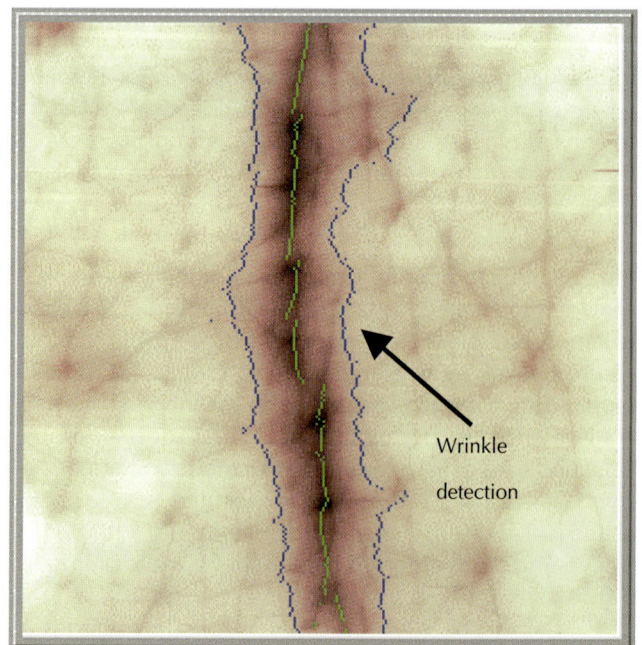

Surface: 4.635 mm^2
Volume: 0.5972 mm^3

Figure 3.18   Detection of edges of wrinkle.

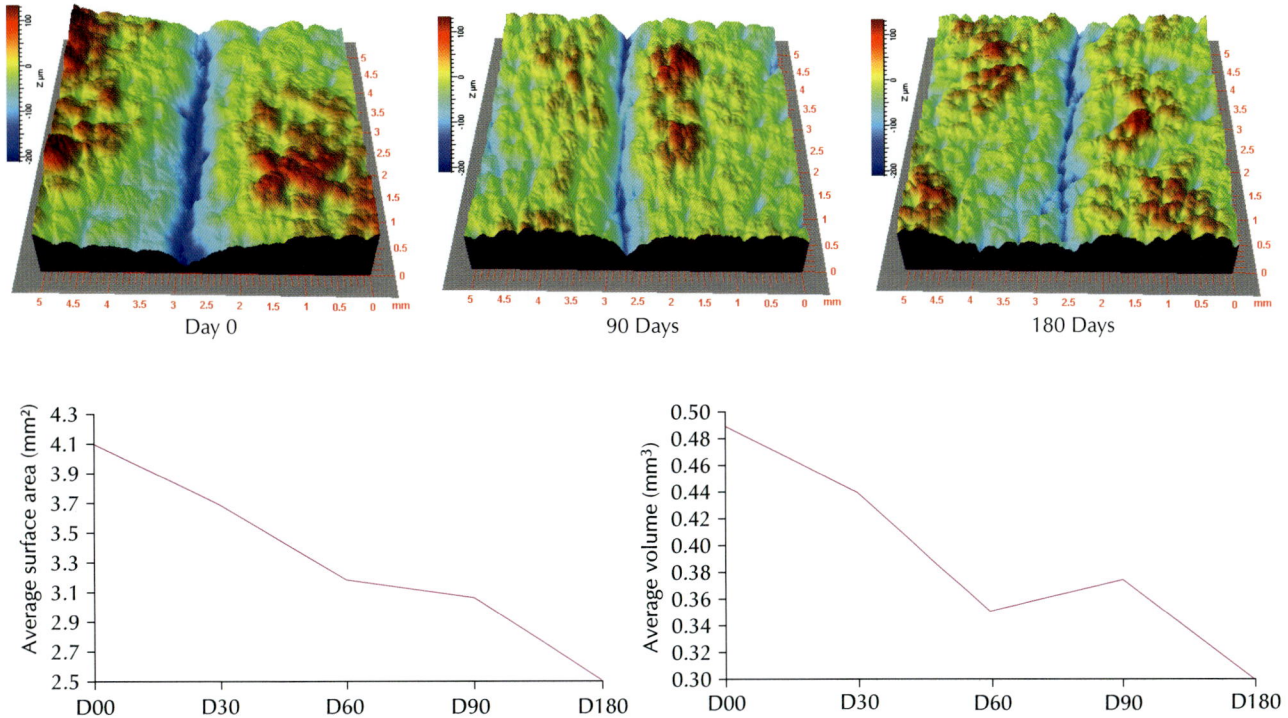

Figure 3.19   Effect of cosmetic product on surface area and volume of wrinkle.

defined by geographers, the geometrical layout of points present on the contour of the grid allow one to establish whether the point at the center of the grid is a peak, a crest, a valley, a plateau, or a hollow. Each morphological type is coded by a special positioning inside the grid and by a threshold of tolerance. The analysis grid must scan each point of the relief; each point is classified in a family according to its typology by keeping its three spatial coordinates x, y, z.

The variation of the mathematical microscope magnification is equivalent to the narrowing or dilatation of the size of the grid.[22,23]

The application of this method to the detection of volar forearm and facial skin line networks is presented in Figure 3.21.

Volumetric reconstruction of skin line network: ρ_{ij}, λ, θ

To reconstruct a skin line network in three dimensions, it is necessary to find all its local motifs. A local motif that the mathematical microscope recognizes is described by the association of two peaks separated by the hollow of a valley; the height is determined by the difference between the highest peak and the hollow of the valley. The mathematical relation that calculates the depth of the local feature is given by:

$$\rho_{ij} = \sup(Z_{peak} - Z_{hollow}) \tag{14}$$

The width of the motif is given by the distance between both peaks. The direction of the motif which coincides with the main direction of the line is defined in the orthogonal direction at the maximal variation of the local gradient. As a matter of fact, once the hollow of a valley is found, the two peaks corresponding to the maximal variation of the local relief are determined by going around the hollow in all directions.

Two constraints are used to find the direction of the motif. The direction must coincide with the local normal of the plan formed by the three features of the motif (Figures 3.22 and 3.23). If the first peak is point A, the hollow point B, and the second peak point C, the normal vector N is approximately collinear to the vectorial product:

$$\vec{N} = \vec{AB} \wedge \vec{BC} \tag{15}$$

For the direction of the motif to coincide with the direction of the valley, which is composed of a succession of motifs, it is necessary to know whether the hollow $B(i,j)$ belongs to the course of the neighboring points. To achieve this, the intersection points between half a straight line stemming from $B(i,j)$ and the nearest

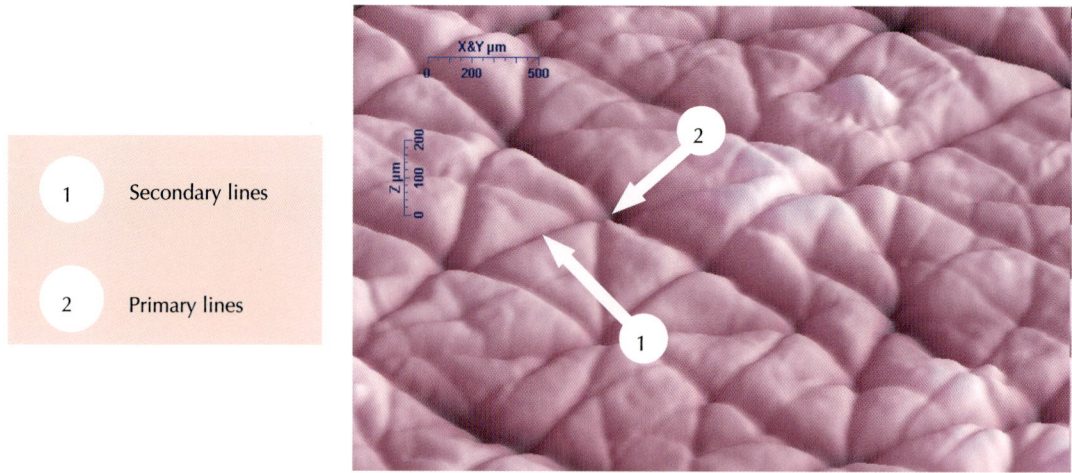

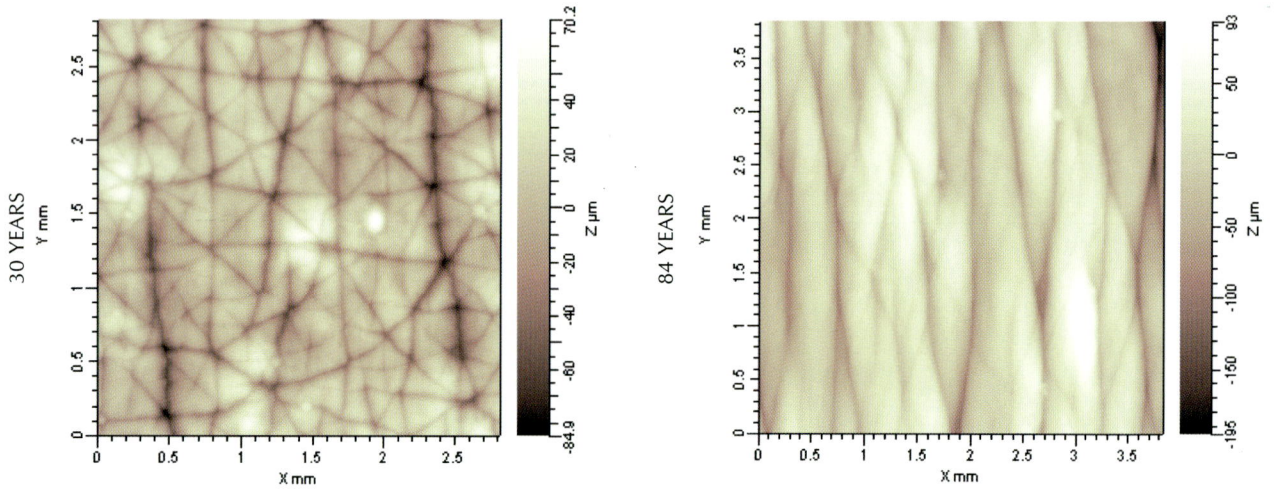

Figure 3.20   Description of skin relief morphology.

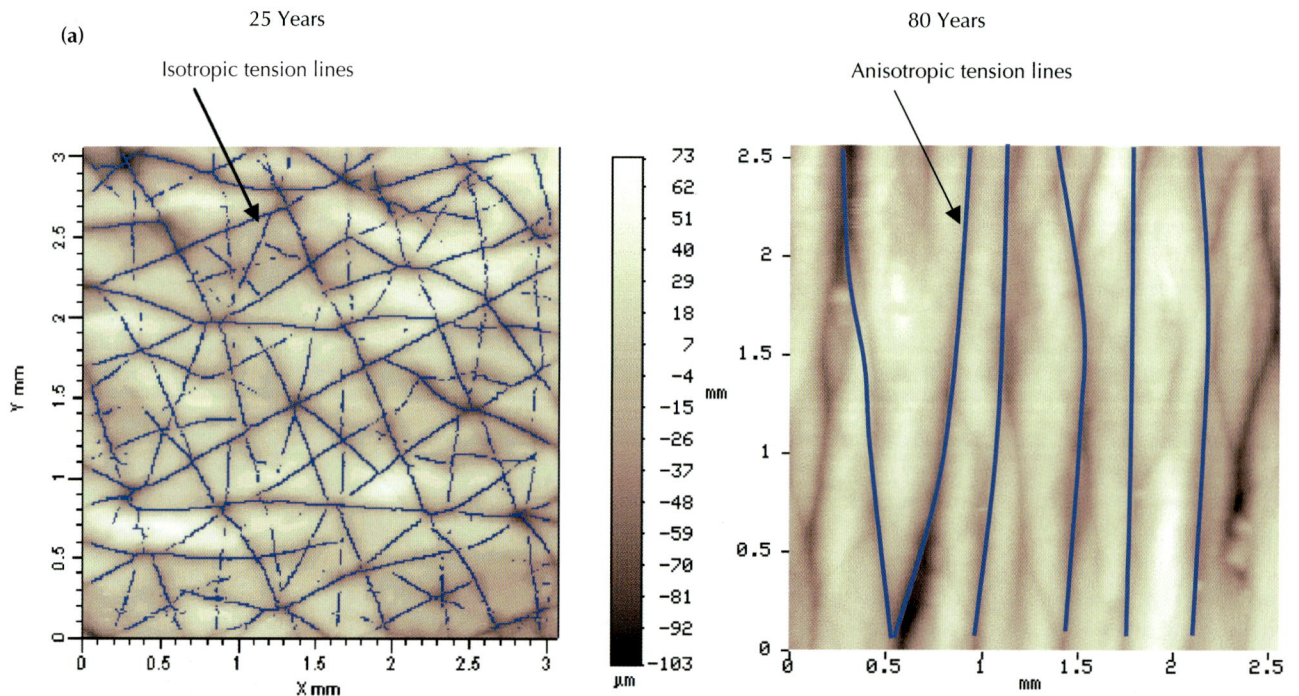

Figure 3.21   (Continued)

(b)

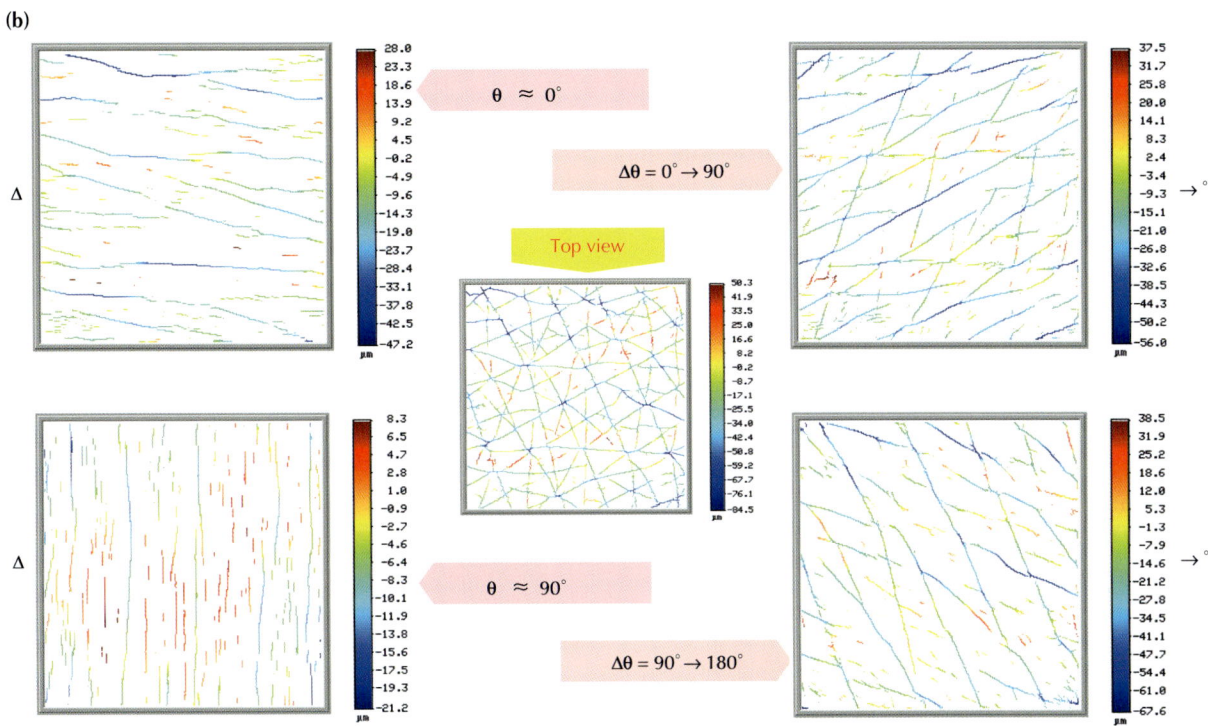

θ ≈ 0°

Δθ = 0° → 90°

Top view

→ °

θ ≈ 90°

Δθ = 90° → 180°

→ °

(c)

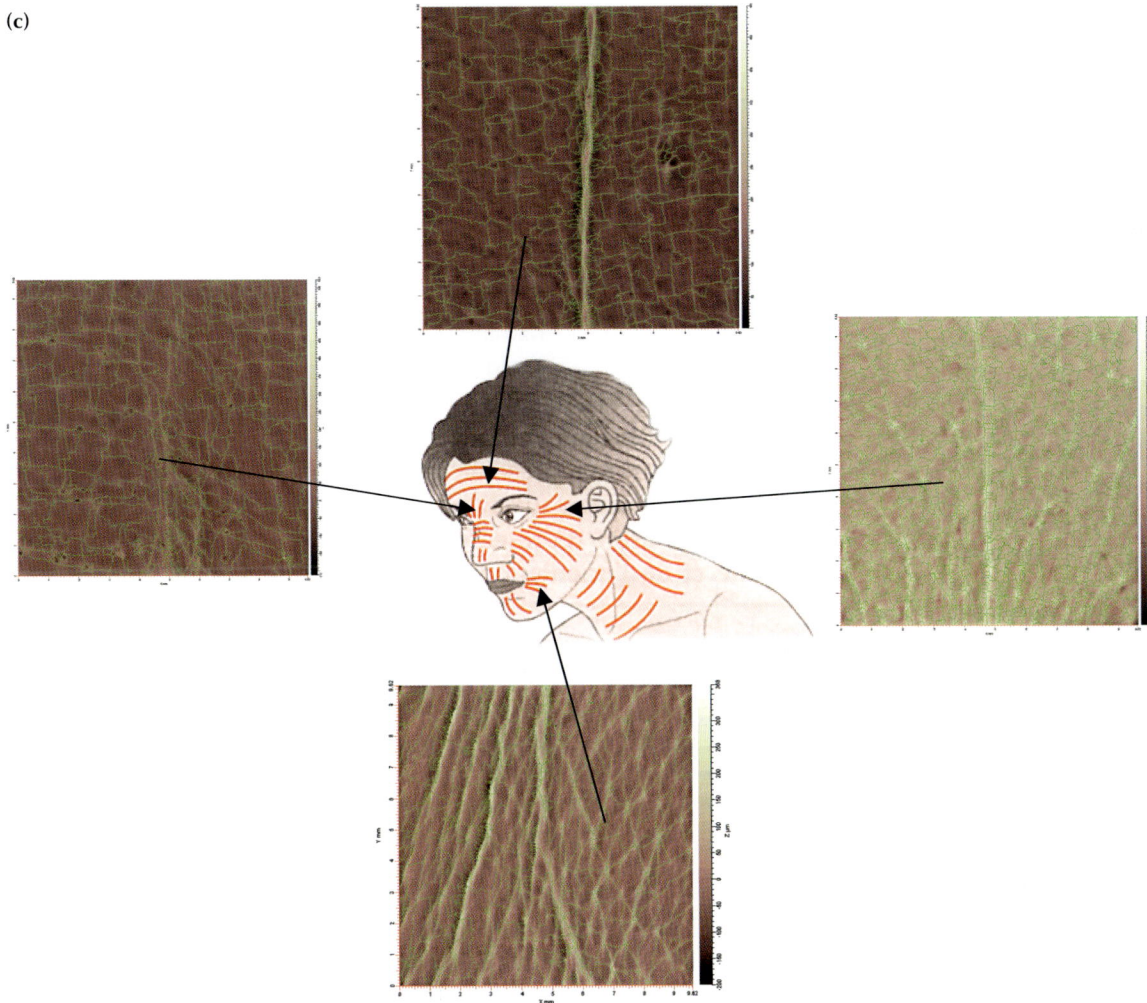

Figure 3.21 (a) Anisotropic skin line network during aging. (b) Anisotropy of volar forearm network. (c) Line network of facial morphology.

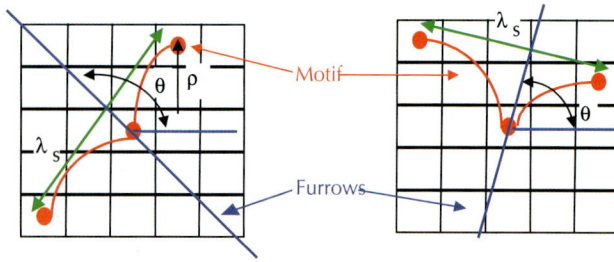

Figure 3.22   Skin line morphology.

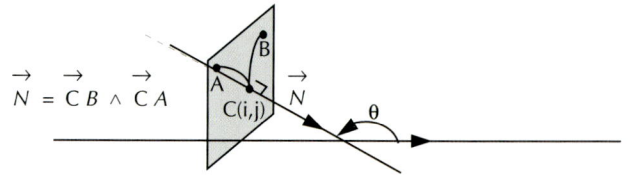

Figure 3.23   Detection of skin line direction.

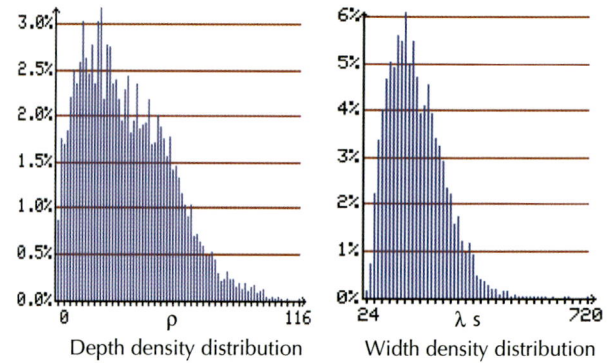

Depth density distribution   Width density distribution

Figure 3.24   Depth and width histograms.

points are noted. If there is an even number of these intersection points, then the point is outside the direction of the skin line; otherwise, the hollow is in the direction of the skin line.

The number of iterations of this procedure is equal to the number of hollow points of the detected motifs, and the three elements of the motif ρ_{ij}, λ_{ij}, and θ_{ij} are memorized in vectorial form for each motif; these three parameters will be the fundamental components of the morphological tree of the global relief.

Quantification

Distribution density of skin line depth and width

Since all the data establishing the morphologies of the skin lines are recorded, statistics regarding the depth and width of the skin lines can be presented in a form of the distribution density of each parameter (Figure 3.24).

Compass rose of skin line anisotropy

The orientation distribution of the skin lines is quantified as a compass rose; the density in a triangular part corresponds to the number of motifs of the lines which have this orientation.

To assess the evolution of skin line anisotropy during aging, it is interesting to introduce an anisotropy index from direction roses, useful to classify a particular anisotropy of skin lines. A completely anisotropic surface gives rise to a direction rose concentered into only one angular sector. Conversely, a perfectly isotropic surface leads to a circular direction rose.

So, if N is the number of angular sectors inspected between 0 and π, an anisotropy index (AI) can be defined as:[8,12]

$$AI = \frac{1}{2}\frac{\sum\limits_{i=0}^{N-1}|R_i - S/N|}{S - S/N}*100 \tag{16}$$

where R_i is the rose value corresponding to angular sector i and:

$$S = \sum_{i=0}^{N-1} R_i \tag{17}$$

S/N should be the R_i value for all i in the case of a perfectly isotropic surface, and the factor 1/2 comes from the fact that R_i values greater than S/N must be exactly compensated by lower values. The example in Figure 3.25 shows the roses of anisotropy for different morphologies of the skin.

A second presentation shows the compass rose in relation to skin line depth, which will allow one to distinguish the orientation of the line network at different scales of depth (Figure 3.26).

Tree and branches of skin line network[15,21–24]

This new concept shows the volumetric aspect of skin lines. Starting from the deepest lines up to lines marking the plateaux, each family of lines is described as a branch of a tree, in relation to its depth and direction (Figure 3.27). This new representation enables us to follow the evolution of the tree of different families of lines in relation to age, hydration, or cosmetic effect. Thanks to the originality of this representation, it is possible, for example, to assess the evolution of families of lines according to age, or under the influence of cosmetics, and above all to compare the volumetric tree of two textures on the same scale.

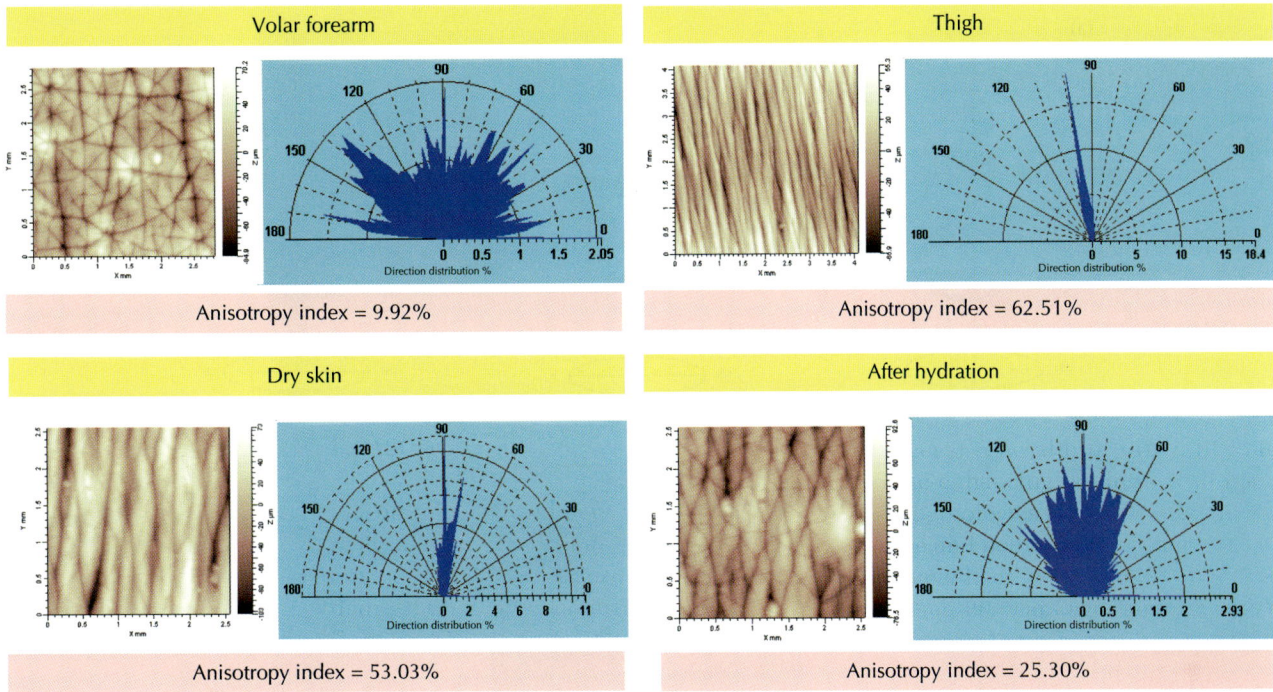

Figure 3.25   Compass roses of different morphologies.

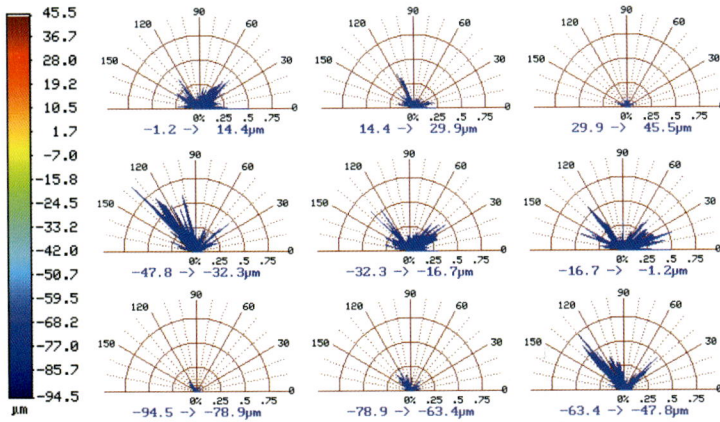

Figure 3.26   Compass rose versus depth of line.

Physiological action

With this original method, it is possible for the first time to quantify the different scales of the cutaneous lines accurately, and to follow morphological changes of the surface in relation to age. The multiresolution aspect of a morphological tree helps to quantify the effect of a cosmetic objectively and to assess the level of the tree where the cosmetic may have had an influence. The examples of Figures 3.28 and 3.29 show the use of this approach in analysis of the aging process and the effect of a hydrating product. Changes of the tree in relation to the topographical condition of the subject are worth noting.[24]

Effect of vitamin C on the upper chest[24]

In a recent study assessing the efficiency of an anti-aging product, this method demonstrated how vitamin C improved restructuring of the lines of the upper part of the chest, over a period of 6 months. The study included 20 female volunteers (50–60 years) with photoaged skin, with 6 months' daily application (low neck area) of 5% vitamin C w/o emulsion, versus placebo.

Clinical criteria comprised a global score including hydration, roughness, laxity, and small wrinkles. The relief was analyzed before application of the product and on the same area after 30 days, 60 days, and 180 days.

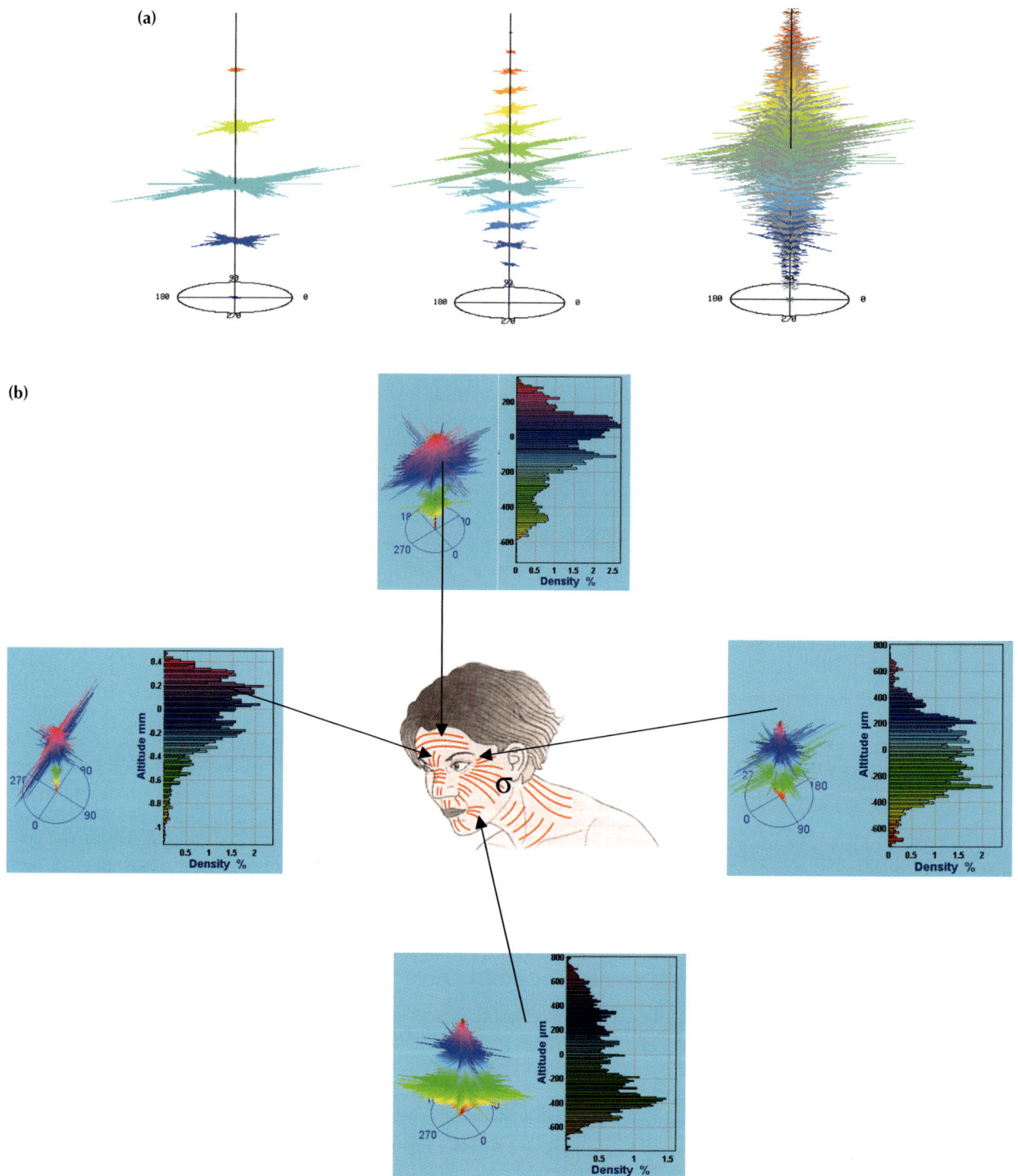

Figure 3.27   (a) Morphological tree of volar forearm network. (b) Morphological tree of facial network.

The assessment of skin lines using our morphological approach showed the following evolution of skin line density (Figure 3.30). The three families of lines (0–10 μm, 10–20 μm, 20 nm to deepest) were identified and the evolution of their density in the course of a treatment was quantified by analysis of the morphological tree branches.

In the example shown in Figure 3.19, changes to the lines after application of an antiaging product on the upper part of the chest are described. The line density (0–20 μm) increased at 3 and 6 months. A return of elasticity in the collagen fibers in several directions was confirmed by new orientations of the small lines on the plateaux. The reduction of lines of scale 10–20 μm

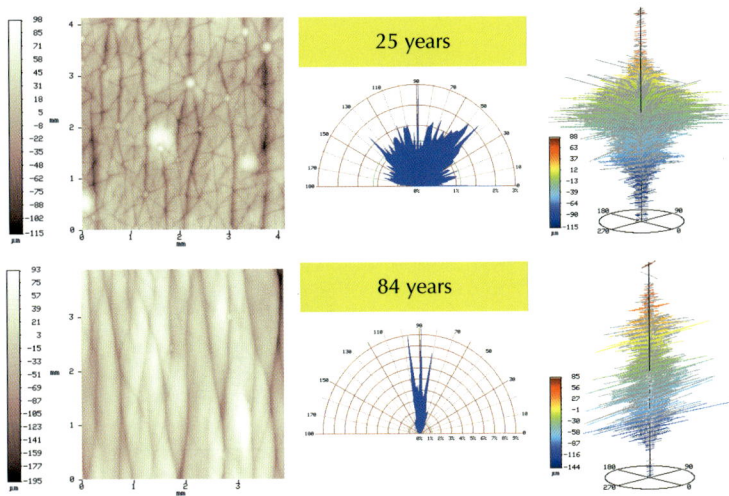

Figure 3.28 Assessment of aging morphology by 3D tree representation.

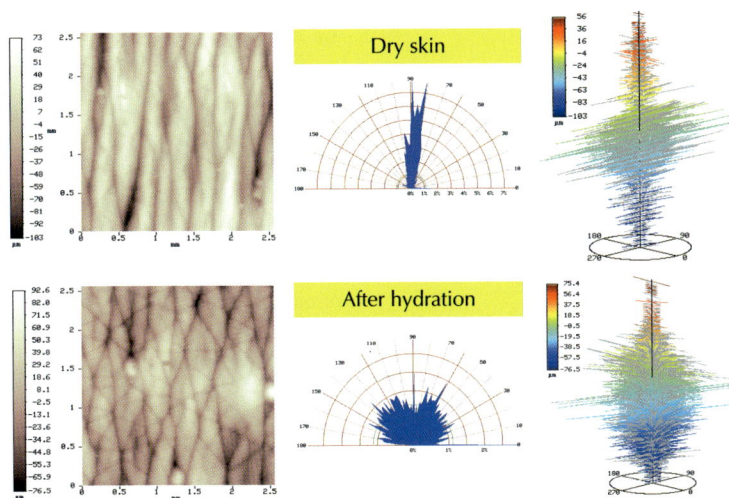

Figure 3.29 Assessment of hydration effect by 3D tree representation.

and lines over 20 μm was related to a thinning of the primary lines.

Conclusion

Since the 1980s, the study of the aging process or the effect of a cosmetic by the analysis of skin morphology has used quantification techniques developed for mechanical engineering. As mentioned above, the cutaneous morphology is not to be compared to the surface of a solid. The skin physiology seems mainly mechanical, following the dimensions of the contracted and elastic medium of the dermis.

The main lines are formed in the superficial dermis where they remain visible after separation from the epidermis, whereas the epidermis loses every trace of them. However, secondary lines marked on the plateaux of the relief can be of epidermal origin. For

this reason, an original analysis technique has been developed which is well adapted to the physiological phenomena.

The continuous development of cosmetic products and filling techniques requires metrology and characterization suited to the various scales of the cutaneous morphology according to a particular region of the body.

Two approaches are necessary to gain further expertise and investigate cosmetic efficacy. The first relates to the macroscopic geometry of the wrinkles, by computing their depth, width, surface area, and volume in a robust manner. The second approach relates to the morphology of the tension line network. This morphology represents the tension distribution of collagen fibers and matrix. A detailed morphological analysis of the skin line network and its anisotropy makes it possible to quantify degradation of the network during aging and its reorganization after cosmetic application or after plastic surgery.

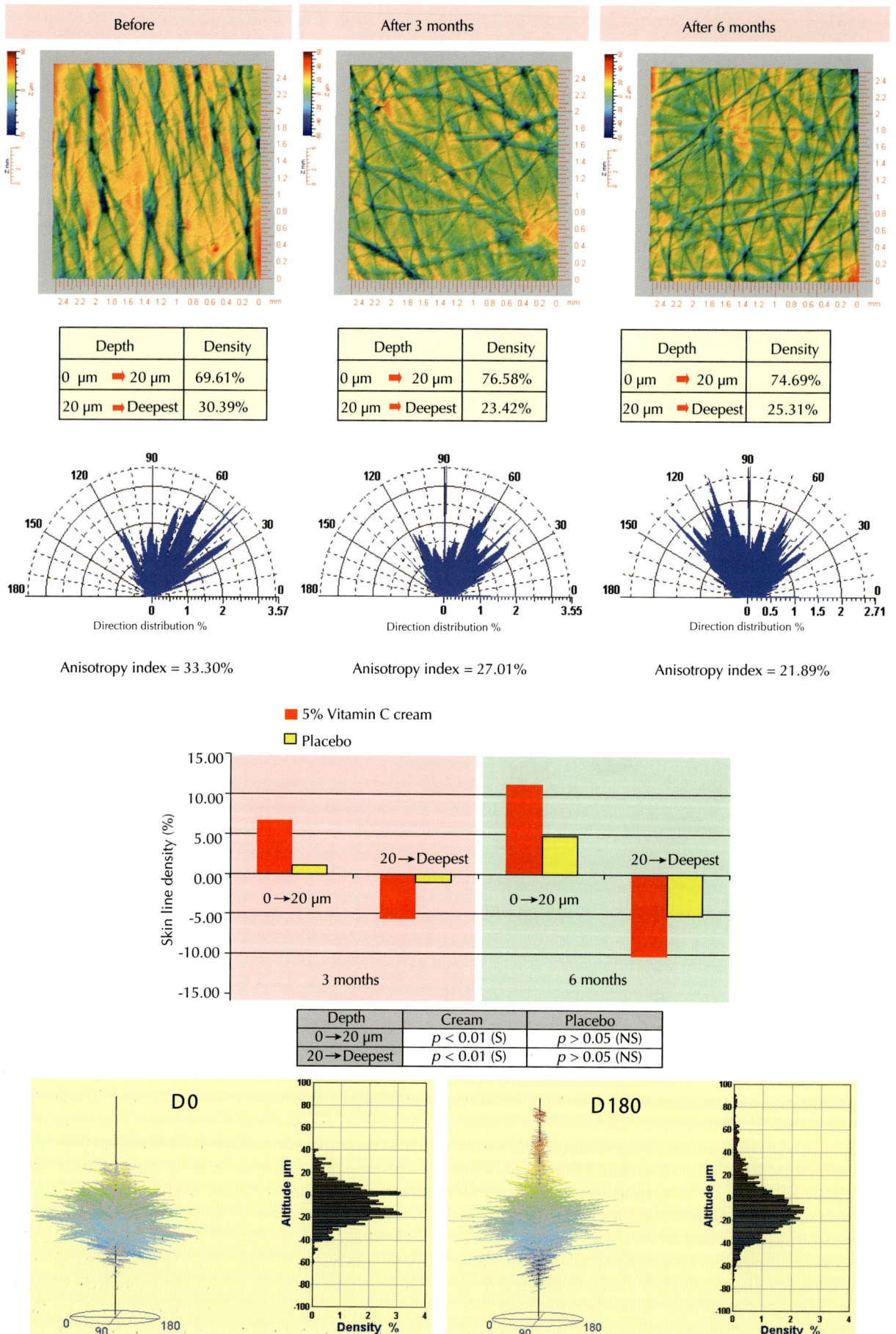

Before	After 3 months	After 6 months

Depth	Density
0 µm ➡ 20 µm	69.61%
20 µm ➡ Deepest	30.39%

Depth	Density
0 µm ➡ 20 µm	76.58%
20 µm ➡ Deepest	23.42%

Depth	Density
0 µm ➡ 20 µm	74.69%
20 µm ➡ Deepest	25.31%

Anisotropy index = 33.30%   Anisotropy index = 27.01%   Anisotropy index = 21.89%

■ 5% Vitamin C cream
□ Placebo

Depth	Cream	Placebo
0 ➡ 20 µm	$p < 0.01$ (S)	$p > 0.05$ (NS)
20 ➡ Deepest	$p < 0.01$ (S)	$p > 0.05$ (NS)

D0   D180

Figure 3.30   Effect of vitamin C on modification of skin lines.

With these new techniques, it is now possible to quantify objectively and accurately morphological changes of the skin surface during the aging process, after cosmetic injection, or after esthetic surgery. The precision of the analysis gives evidence for the influence of a cosmetic on the branches of the morphological tree by distinguishing the smoothing, restructuring, or thinning of lines and wrinkles. The current technological advances will help to disseminate the use of this technique in skin pathologies, probably usefully supplemented by video microscopy.

References

1. Griffiths CE. The clinical identification and quantification of photodamage. Br J Dermatol 1992; 127: 37–42.

2. Stegman SJ, Tromovich TA, Glocan RG. Cosmetic Dermatologic Surergy. St Louis, MO: Mosby-Year Book, 1984: 5–15.

3. Pierard GE, Lapiere CH. The microanatomical basis of facial frown lines. Arch Dermatol 1989; 125: 1090–2.

4. Packman EW, Gans EH. The panel study as a scientifically controlled investigation: moisturizers and superficial facial lines. J Soc Cosmet Chem 1978; 29: 91–8.

5. Mignot J, Zahouani H, Rondot D, Nardin P. Morphological study of human skin topography. Int J Bioeng Skin 1987; 3: 177–96.

5. Makki S, Agache P, Mignot J, Zahouani H. Statistical analysis and three dimensional representation of the human skin surface. J Soc Chem 1984; 35: 311–25.

6. Gasmueller J, Kecskes A, John P. Stylus method for skin surface contour measurement. In: Serup J, Jemec GBE, eds. Handbook of Non Invasive Methods and the Skin. Boca Raton, FL: CRC Press, 1995:

7. Makki S, Barbenel JC, Agache P. A quantitative method for the assessment of microtopography of human skin. Acta Derm Venereol 1979; 59: 285–91.

8. Cook TH. Profilometry of skin. A useful tool for the substantiation of cosmetic efficacy. J Soc Cosmet Chem 1980; 31: 339–59.

9. Corcuff P, de Lacharriere O, Leveque JL. Extension induced changes in the microrelief of the human volar forearm: varaiation with age. J Gerontol Med Sci 1991; 46: 223–7.

10. Hoppe U. Topologie der Hautoberfläche. J Soc Cosmet Chem 1979; 30: 213–39.

11. Zahouani H, Assoul M, Janod P, Mignot J. Theoretical and experimental study of wound healing: application to leg ulcers. Med Biol Eng Comput 1992; 30: 234–9.

12. Zahidi M, Assoul M, Bellaton B, Mignot J. A fast 2D/3D optical profilometer for wide range topographical measurement. Wear 1993; 65: 197–203.

13. Harashki A, Schmit J, Wyant JC. Improved vertical scanning interferometry. Appl Opt 2000; 39: 2107–15.

14. Lagarde JM, Rouvrais C, Black D. Topography and anisotropy of the skin surface with ageing. Skin Res Technol 2005; 11: 110–19.

15 Zahouani H. Spectral and 3D motifs identification of anisotropic topographical components. Analysis and filtering of anisotropic patterns by mophological rose approach. Int J Mach Tools Manuf 1998; 38: 615–23.

16. Sherrington I, Smith EH. Fourier models of the surface topography of engineering components. Surf Topogr 1988; 1: 11–25.

17. Georges G, Gordon L, Stanley L. Diffraction pattern sampling for automatic pattern recognition. Proc IEEE 1970; 58: 198–216.

18. Gonzalez, Wintz. 1997

19. Longuet-Higgins MS. Statistical properties of an isotropic random surface. Philos Trans R Soc Series A 1957; 250: 157–74.

20. Nayak PR. Some aspects of surface roughness measurement. Wear 1973; 26: 165–74.

21. Hashimoto L. New methods for surface ultrastructure. Int J Dermatol 1974; 13: 357–81.

22. Zahouani H, Vargiolu R. 3D morphological tree representation of the skin relief. A new approach of skin imaging characterisation. Presented at XX Congress of the International Federation of the Societies of Cosmetic Chemists, Cannes, France, 14–18 September, 1998: Paper 30, 69–80.

23. Zahouani H, Lee S-H, Vargiolu R. The multi-scale mathematical microscopy of surface roughness. Incidence in tribology. In: Dowson D, Priest M, Taylor A et al, eds. Lubrication at the Frontier. Amsterdam: Elsevier Science, 1999: 379–90.

24. Zahouani H, Vargiolu R. Skin tension lines morphology. In: Agache P, Humbert P, eds. Measuring the Skin. New York: Springer, 2005: 40–59.

4 Skin aging: clinical diagnosis and other factors

Anny Cohen-Letessier

According to the theory of evolution, aging is a side-effect of imperfections in the mechanisms of repair and maintenance, the process of maintenance being represented principally by preservation of telomeres and by resistance to oxidative damage (free radicals). The qualities and functions of the skin and the appendages diminish with age, and the responsibility for these alterations is attributed to the influence of numerous factors: excess exposure to solar radiation, smoking, diet, and hormonal deprivation.

Clinical characteristics of aged skin

Anatomical and physiological impairments alter the different layers of the skin from the epidermis to the hypodermis, with involvement of the subcutaneous tissue, both adipose and muscular, which plays a fundamental role and participates in the microcirculation.

The slowing down of cell turnover (28 days for a young adult, 30 days on average for an older person) gives an impression of a dull complexion and thickened skin (horny layer), owing to the accumulation and overlapping of corneal cells, revealed by an aspect and feeling of cutaneous dryness, which is often the first complaint of an aging person. Impairment of the hydrolipoprotein layer and epidermal lipids contributes to the dehydration of the skin and feeling of discomfort.

If this dryness is not corrected, wrinkles will more easily leave their imprint on the skin, with thinning of the 'living' epidermis (granular layer, stratum spinosum, and Malphighi layer) and irreversible modification of the dermoepidermal junction, which becomes flatter and loses support (impairment of collagen IV and VII and anchoring fibrils). The solidarity and communication of the dermis–epidermis is threatened.

Disordered pigmentation is expressed initially by brown spots which contribute broadly to the aged aspect of the skin, and is later translated to the appearance of white spots notably on the fronts of the legs and external surfaces of the forearms.

Vascular disturbances (cherry angiomas, microthromboses, Bateman's purpura) develop to add a colored touch to this declining picture.

Progressively, there are modifications to the macromolecules of the dermis, leading to the breakdown of collagen. Fragmentation and disorientation of elastin fibers, a fall in the rate of production of hyaluronic acid and of glycosaminoglycans, and the loss of cell cohesion in the extracellular matrix damage the fibroblasts, changing the biomechanical control of the skin and contributing to its dull aspect, and atrophy (the skin thins by 6% every 10 years). There is a loss of firmness, leading in extreme cases to a 'draped' or 'droopy' appearance.

Slackening of the skin is also influenced by the fatty and muscular layer, which thins and no longer plays a role in its support. The various volumes of the face change, and the isosceles triangle shape is reversed in comparison with a young face: the tip of the triangle becomes the base, corresponding to the rules of geometry. Mandibular folds appear, temples and cheeks become hollow, and wrinkles become more pronounced. It is necessary to consolidate, to restructure, and to avoid too much tension, otherwise we risk accentuating the bony relief and the aged aspect of the face.

It is not necessary to treat systematically expression wrinkles when they appear very early, but to treat only those that give a sad, tired aspect to the face, and to respect others, notably those associated with the smile. It is essential to understand how these wrinkles are formed. Three elements participate in this process: mechanical force, fibroblasts, and collagen fibers, referred to as '3F'.

Results of the studies of Lapierre[1] have contributed to a better understanding of the mechanism. Fibroblasts adhere to their rigid support, namely the collagen fibers, which exercise an important, stable, and regulated force of traction. The adhesion of fibroblasts to the fibrin support is caused by the intervention of integrins, inducing intracellular focal contacts.

Focal contacts and integrins are at the ends of stress fibers that are formed under tension; these stress fibers are constituted of actin and myosin (actomyosin) and represent the retractile elements of the cytoskeleton. This 'skeleton' of fibroblasts interacts permanently with the skin fibers, allowing tissue adaptation to mechanical pressures. This mechanical information is necessary to cell survival.

When tension increases, fibroblasts have an anabolic behavior (multiplication and synthesis), and when there is relaxation they have a catabolic behavior (production of proinflammatory cytokines, degradation enzymes, support lysis, cell apoptosis). From the age of 30, deformations of the surface of the skin start to appear. The iterative traction of the mimic muscles of the face on the septa of the hypodermis induces a depression of the skin by shortening and thickening the underlying muscles. The inhibition of muscular contraction allows relaxation of the hypertrophied support and diminishes the depth of wrinkles, but trying too hard to unload these muscles risks laxity, and because of the weak mechanical information, the fibroblasts assume active catabolic behavior.

To diminish wrinkles it is necessary to decrease the hypercontractility of fibroblasts and collagen fibers. Calcium plays a major role. In the case of an external stimulus there will be a massive influx of calcium into the cell, via calcium channels which act as 'locks'. This strong elevation of calcium concentration induces a response adapted to cell function, in this case muscular contraction. Certain active antagonists to the influx of calcium into the cell (e.g. manganese gluconate) and inhibitors of nerve–muscle synapses (e.g. short chain peptides) will diminish contractility.

Different factors involved in cutaneous aging

Genetic and epigenetic mechanisms are seriously involved, with large interindividual variability caused by a multiplicity of pleiotropic genes. This means that the same gene can have a beneficial effect in a young person and a negative effect in an older person, referred to as antagonistic pleiotropy.

Biological clock

The individual 'biological clock' is genetically programmed but often affected by external factors. It is expressed principally by the role of protein p53, described as the 'guardian of the genome', and by that of protein CIP1, which inhibits transition of mitotic stage G1 to stage S, and allows impairment of structural, signal, and metabolic genes, hormonal deregulation, and the shortening of telomeres.

Telomeres are nucleotide structures located at the ends of chromosomes. They shorten at every cell division; when they become too short, cells stop dividing and enter senescence. Measurement of the length of telomeres in a cell gives the age of the individual; 'cell age' can surpass 'real age', according to the degree of impairment owing to environmental factors.

A recent study of Epel et al[2] emphasizes the responsibility of chronic stress in the shortening of telomeres; the study concerned 58 women from 20 to 50 years of age, 39 of whom were mothers of seriously ill children and 19 who were mothers of healthy children. The telomeres of stressed mothers corresponded to those that were found in women 9–17 years older, and among 14 more stressed women the telomeres measured 550 base pairs (bp) less than among the others; additionally, the activity of their telomerase had been significantly reduced.

Chronic stress speeds up cutaneous aging

The publication of Valdes et al[3] shows the negative association between tobacco addiction, obesity, and cell aging; telomeres of the obese and smokers were significantly shorter than those of comparative individuals of the same age. The study concerned 1100 women in good health, from 18 to 72 years of age, 11% of whom had a body mass index of 30 or above; 47% were non-smokers, 33% were previous smokers, and 18% continued to smoke. By measuring the length of telomeres of the white blood cells of each of the women, it was found that they became shorter by 25 bp a year on average.

At the same age, slim women had longer telomeres than women with weight excess, who in turn had longer telomeres than obese women.

The women who had never smoked had longer telomeres than those who had smoked in the past, who in turn had longer telomeres than those who continued to smoke. Each pack-year smoked was equivalent to an additional 18% of telomere length loss. By smoking one packet a day for 40 years, a woman accelerated her cell aging by having telomeres equivalent in length to those of a woman 7 years older.

Tobacco use and obesity shorten the length of telomeres probably by mechanisms linked to inflammation and an increase of oxidative stress.

Mitochondria and oxidative stress

The mitochondrial theory of aging is clear. The mitochondria constitute an energy 'power station'; oxidative stress will induce mutations of mitochondrial DNA, with a reduction of the vital energy of the cell. The escape of free radicals impacts on all cell elements: cell DNA is subject to 10 000 attacks by free radicals every day.

The research of Michikawa et al[4] showed the presence of specific point mutations of mitochondrial DNA (T414G transversion) of fibroblasts in 50% of subjects of more than 65 years of age; this transversion was absent in younger subjects.

Hormones and aging

The hormonal signaling pathways play a causative and critical role in aging. The studies of Kenyon and Ruvkun and their groups[5,6] showed that in *Caenorhabditis elegans*, aging is under the influence of the DAF-2/insulin receptor-like signaling pathway. The DAF-2 receptor in *C. elegans* is equivalent to insulin-like growth factor I receptor (IGF-IR) in the human. Keratinocytes express specific insulin receptors with high affinity for insulin-like growth factors, which are anabolic peptides and mitogens partly responsible for the activity of growth hormone. Aged keratinocytes and fibroblasts lose their capacity to respond to a certain number of growth factors.

Insulin is the key hormone of metabolism; it uses nutritional energy, but will accelerate aging when it is produced in large quantities due to insulin resistance. The aim is to remain insulin-sensitive and to preserve the insulin capital.

Thyroid hormones play an essential role in aging, and a reduction of these hormones is often expressed by significant cutaneous dryness, diffuse pruritus, hair loss, and diminishing density of the body hair and eyebrows.

Sex steroids have an effect on the growth of the epidermis. In the dermis they augment the activity of fibroblasts and stimulate the production of macromolecules, collagen, elastin, and hyaluronic acid. These are reduced in the course of the hormonal deprivation of the perimenopause, resulting in acceleration of the signs of aging, including dryness, atrophy, atony, and loss of brightness.

The α-melanocyte stimulating hormone (α-MSH) is produced by epidermal keratinocytes and adheres to its receptor (MCR1) present in melanocytes, protecting against apoptosis and DNA impairment induced by UVB (ultraviolet B) radiation.

The oral intake of dehydroepiandrosterone (DHEA) has a cutaneous effect: an increase of sebaceous secretion in women aged more than 70 years and a moisturizing effect in men.

Environmental factors and aging

Sun exposure, tobacco use, pollution, and dietary factors will accelerate natural aging.

Sun exposure

'Helioderma' refers to all modifications of the skin due to sun exposure (clinical, histological, and functional manifestations in chronically exposed skin). The solar spectrum consists of UVC rays (270–290 nm) that do not reach the Earth's surface, high-energy UVB (280–320 nm) and short UVA rays (270–400 nm), low-energy long UVA rays (340–400 nm), and infrared rays. Acute effects of the sun on the skin can lead to sunburn, phototoxicity, and photoallergies. Chronic effects can lead to immunosuppression, carcinogenesis, and accelerated aging.

Pigmented and achromic actinic spots, a thickened tegument, an irregular complexion, telangiectasia, a network of wrinkles especially on the cheeks, skin extensibility, poikiloderma, and erythrosis colli are some of the many presenting signs of altered skin due to excessive sun exposure. Histologically, the epidermis is the site of development of dyskeratotic keratinocytes, with intracytoplasmic vacuoles, desmosome modifications, and tonofilaments, which can become malignant. The most substantial modifications occur in the dermis, with dermal elastoidosis, which corresponds to a deposit in the superficial dermis of thickened, degraded, abnormal elastic fibers, lysozyme deposits, and twisted, dilated vessels. Degraded collagen bundles are packed in a strip under the dermoepidermal junction as a result of elastosis. There is an increase in mastocytes and inflammatory cells that release proteases and proinflammatory cytokines, thus upsetting the balance between matrix metalloproteinases (MMPs) and their inhibitors (TIMPs).

The glycosaminoglycan (GAG) level increases. Dopa-positive melanocytes decrease (from age 30 years) with a drop in melanic pigment, whereas the melanosome density increases. Melanic pigment is poorly distributed and accumulates in clumps (senile lentigos). The keratinocyte melanogenesis–melanocyte balance is altered.

The activity and number of Langerhans cells fall sharply in sun-exposed skin, leading to immunodeficiency, with the induction of T-suppressor cells and a decrease in 'natural killers'.

Tobacco use

Smoking accentuates wrinkles, with deep lines at the angles of the lips and corners of the eyes and vertical lines on the cheeks and the jawline, and results in an atrophic and grayish skin, and a plethoric purple and red complexion. The microcirculation is disrupted, damage to macromolecules of the connective tissue (tobacco elastosis) entrains a delay of scar healing, and the age at menopause is advanced via an antiestrogenic effect. It has been found that the relative risk of wrinkling for smokers is 2.3 in men and 3.1 in women. The earlier a person starts smoking, the more dependent they become and the greater is the damage.

Nornicotine, a psychoactive metabolite of nicotine, causes the glycation of proteins via the Maillard reaction.[7] Oxidative stress is the result of the formation of numerous free radicals; tobacco smoke causes a disequilibrium between matrix metalloproteinase 1 (MMP-1), a key enzyme in the turnover of connective tissue, and its inhibitor (TIMP-1), leading to the deterioration of collagen, elastin, and glycosaminoglycans, this effect being added to that of UV radiation which stimulates the proteolytic activity of MMPs.

Tobacco use leads to premature graying of the hair and hair loss in men[8] via mechanisms of vasoconstriction of the prefollicular microcirculation, nicotine toxicity on the cell cycle of pillar cells in the papilla, and mutation of the mitochondrial DNA of the hair follicles. Oxidative stress causes perifollicular microinflammation and fibrosis. A hypoestrogenic state with the dominance of androgens augments miniaturization of the hair follicles.

Pollution

Atmospheric pollution plays a role in accelerating skin aging by diminishing its system of defense via a chronic subinflammatory state. Ozone (O_3) disrupts cutaneous lipids and vitamin E, nitrogen dioxide (NO_2) acidifies the skin (increase of lactic acid), and sulfur dioxide (SO_2) stimulates seborrhea; there is a decrease of hydration and in the desquamation enzymes of the stratum corneum.

Diet

A sedentary and stressful lifestyle, the ingestion of pollutants which change the intestinal mucous membrane, the cooking of food, which eliminates thermosoluble vitamins, the 'fast food' trend, and current ideas of fashion and beauty can all contribute to a large deficit in vitamins, β-carotene, calcium, magnesium, and iron.

The skin is an important consumer of antioxidants, but it is permanently exposed to attack (UV radiation, cigarette smoke, pollution, etc.) which can reduce the local consumption of vitamins (7 days of exposure to UV radiation, without protection, diminishes by 30% the skin take-up of vitamin A). Moreover, vitamin A promotes healthy cell turnover. The long-term consumption of a dietary supplement seems reasonable, with follow-up, in the case of insufficient intake due to poor nutrition, reduction of the bioavailability of micronutrients, and/or increase of need in physiological or pathological circumstances.

Conclusion

Healthy aging requires a good mental and physical equilibrium, a balanced diet, a hypocaloric regime (lightens the task of the mitochondria), regular and moderate exercise, and efficient protection from a noxious environment, as well as preventive and active cosmetology. Numerous factors can cause an acceleration of chronological aging, and many other mechanisms are, undoubtedly, yet to be discovered.

Beauty also feeds off the time that threatens it; it must just remain 'a polite consideration' (Colette).

References

1. Lapierre LA. The molecular structure of the tight junction. Adv Drug Deliv Rev 2000; 41: 255–64.
2. Epel ES, Blackburn EH, Lin J et al. Accelerated telomere shortening in response to stress. Proc Natl Acad Sci USA 2004; 101: 17312–15.
3. Valdes AM, Andrew T, Gardner JP et al. Obesity, smoking, and telomere length in women. Lancet 2005; 366: 662–4.
4. Michikawa Y, Mazzucchelli F, Bresolin N, Scarlato G, Attardi G. Aging-dependent large accumulation of point mutations in the human mtDNA control region for replication. Science 1999; 286: 774–9.
5. Dillin A, Crawford DK, Kenyon C. Timing requirements for insulin/IFG-I signalling in C. elegans. Science 2002; 298: 830–4.
6. Li W, Kennedy SG, Ruvkun G. Daf-28 encodes a C. elegans insulin superfamily member that is regulated by environmental cues and acts in the DAF-2 signalling pathway. Genes Dev 2003; 17: 844–58.
7. Dickerson TJ, Kanda KD. Glycation of the amyloid beta-protein by a nicotine metabolite: a fortuitous chemical dynamic between smoking and Alzheimer's disease. Proc Natl Acad Sci USA 2003; 100: 8182–7.
8. Mosley JG, Gibbs AC. Premature grey hair and hair loss among smokers: a new opportunity for health education? BMJ 1996; 313: 1616.

5A The aging face and neck

Patrick Bui and Gilbert Zakine

Aging of the face and neck

Introduction

In the course of aging, the face and neck change their morphology and appearance dramatically. Aging concerns all tissue layers composing the face and neck: the skin primarily but also the fatty masses, the musculoaponeurotic system, and the bony foundations. All levels of the face are concerned. According to the type of skin, morphotype, and exposure to certain predisposing factors, the different constituents and elements of the face will not age equally. Treatment of the esthetic consequences of aging has become an important part of medicine and plastic surgery.

Mechanisms of facial aging

Two main types of mechanism play a role: tissue modification, involving all components of the face, and a global fall of the facial tissues.[1]

Impairment of the skin is the origin of fine lines, wrinkles, and grooves and cutaneous slackening. The two main reasons for this impairment are a reduction in skin elasticity ('solar elastosis' and 'actinic damage') and repeated contraction of the fine muscles. The effects of solar elastosis, which concerns the dermis and the epidermis, become visible from the mid-20s, especially in cases of genetic predisposition (fair phenotypes). The face and neck are the zones affected first and most severely, owing to sun exposure. Wrinkles begin to appear on a woman's face around the mid-30s, at the same time that estrogen levels begin to diminish. Changes start in the epidermis and are due to the accumulation of dead keratinocytes in the stratum corneum. The amount of collagen and elastin in the dermis begins to decrease, particularly in women with excessive exposure to the sun and tobacco smoke. From the late 40s, the rate of renewal of keratinocytes begins to diminish (the life of keratinocytes will change from 100 to 48 days). The epidermis becomes thinner with a reduction of cell turnover and in the number of melanocytes (10–20% per decade) and fine, superficial wrinkles, deep wrinkles, and expression wrinkles appear. With the rapid decline of estrogen levels during the menopause, the epidermis becomes irregular; thinning of the dermis becomes more marked and the hypodermal fat layer atrophies. When the skin loses elasticity and becomes thinner, its capacity to renew itself diminishes, as does the vascularization of the dermohypodermis. The dermoepidermal junction atrophies and becomes progressively flatter. The superficial dermis atrophies, introducing a disorder of the collagen support (with modification of its tinctorial affinity), comprising degeneration with progressive reduction of elastin fibers and increased mucoid ground substance. At the same time, a further degenerative process appears that is characterized by accumulation in the dermis of colloid masses giving a yellowish color to the skin: senile elastosis. Damage caused by sun exposure can be divided into four stages.[2] Stage 1 (20–30 years), or the start of photoaging, is defined by the presence of trivial wrinkles, and the beginning of impairment of pigmentation. In stage 2 (35–50 years), expression wrinkles begin to appear, at the corners of the mouth and the eyes, and there is some keratosis. Stage 3 (from 50 years) is characterized by persistent wrinkles at rest, obvious discolorations, and marked keratosis. Finally, stage 4 is defined by deep and widespread wrinkles, a yellow shade to the skin, and increased frequency of skin malignancies. Moreover, hirsuteness is augmented by increased androgen production. The loss of elasticity is aggravated by skin dryness secondary to a reduction of sweat and sebaceous secretions.

Under the double effect of tissue impairment and gravity, prolapse becomes progressively established. It concerns the surface skin, fatty structures, and platysma muscles of the face, producing creases (skin folds) and loss of the oval. To these cutaneous impairments is added the aging of deep structures.

The basal metabolism diminishes by about 5% per decade on average from age 40, which can favor fat accumulation at the level of the abdomen, the waist, the hips, and the thighs, but also to a lesser extent the face, particularly under the chin, at the level of the cheeks, and around the eyes. Facial fat is supported by septa or fasciae, which become lax. Fat settles in the deep zones under the fasciae while it becomes thinner subcutaneously, which favors thinning and skin fragility. Slackening and atrophy of glandular tissue of the face,

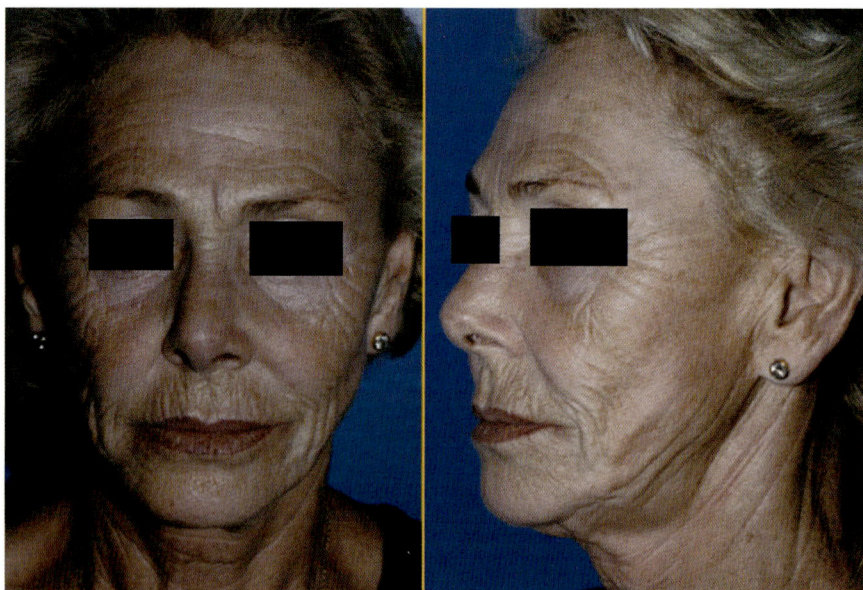

Figure 5A.1

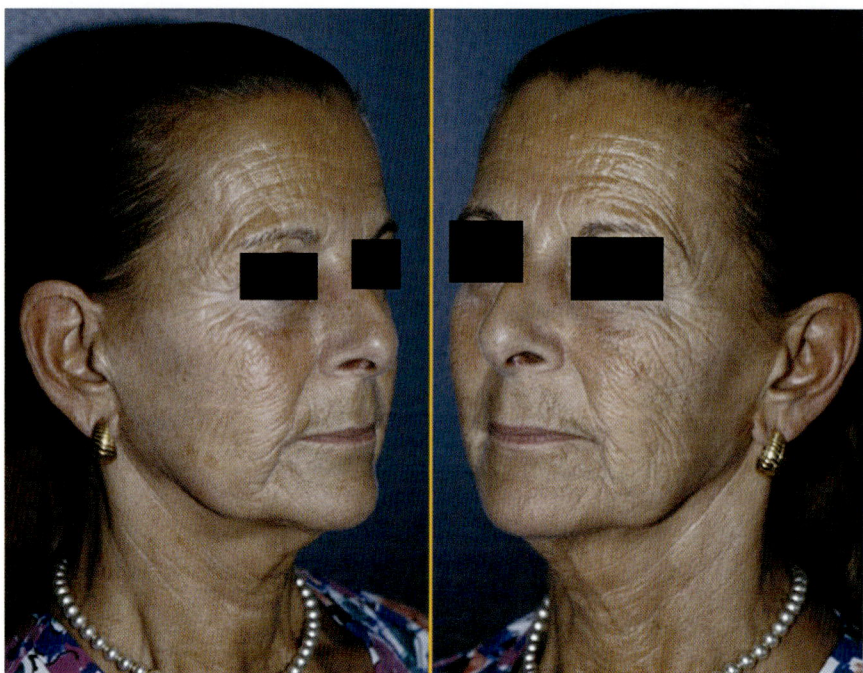

Figure 5A.2

which accelerate after the menopause, also contribute to the loss of suppleness and firmness of the skin.

Cutaneous aging: wrinkles (Figure 5A.1 and 5A.2)

The superficial skin becomes thinner, dehydrates, and progressively loses its elasticity. Subcutaneous adipose tissue becomes reduced. Muscular hypotony joins fatty hypotrophy in contributing to skin impairment.

According to the depth of wrinkles,[3] they can be differentiated into fine lines (wrinkles) and grooves (furrows). Fine wrinkles are initially isolated and discrete then converge and become multidirectional. Sometimes they are associated with repeated contraction of the muscles of the face and neck; they are then deeper and called expression wrinkles (mimic lines), such as 'crow's feet' in the orbitotemporal region. When expression wrinkles extend to the dermis, they are called grooves (skin furrows), such as 'lion's' or glabellar wrinkles (frown lines). When the skin slackens, it can be redundant in the form of excessive creases appearing on the upper eyelid. Main reasons for the appearance of wrinkles are loss of elasticity of the dermis (dermal elastosis), which depends on genetic makeup and sun exposure (actinic damage),

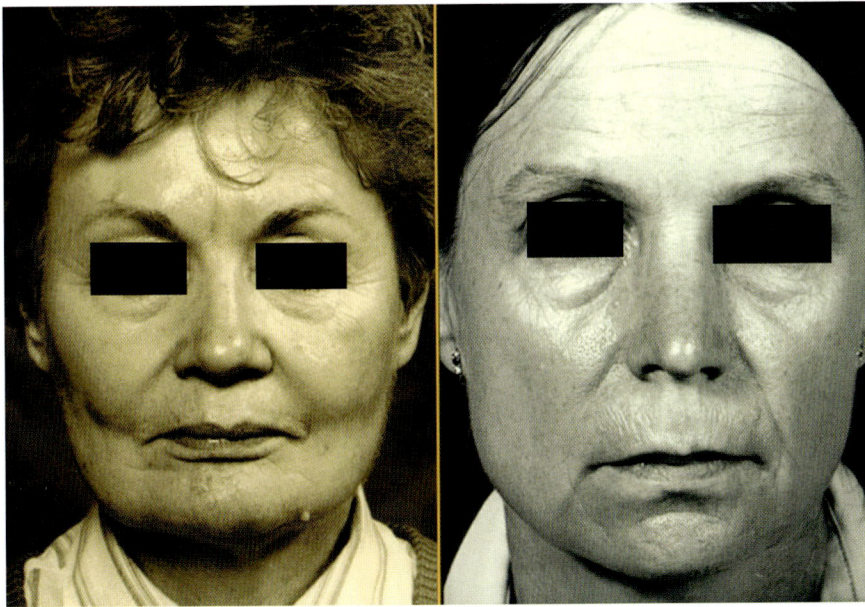

Figure 5A.3 Morphological aging depends on the osseous characteristics of the face. (a) Ptosis is predominant in a 'short' face; (b) the fat base is predominant in a 'long' face. Between the two extremes, we often find association of the two mechanisms.

and repeated contraction of the muscles of the face and neck.

Distinction must be made between, on the one hand, fine wrinkles, expression wrinkles, and grooves, and on the other hand, creases, in terms of treatment. Fine wrinkles can be treated by laser resurfacing and expression wrinkles and grooves by filler products or botulinum toxin, but creases can only be treated by cutaneous retension, cervicofacial facelift, or skin removal surgery, e.g. blepharoplasty or removal of nasolabial grooves.

Musculoaponeurotic aging

The superficial fascia, a fine muscular insertion in all mammals and limited to the deep layer of the hypodermis, has evolved in man to the point of being only a fibrous small strip, sometimes difficult to identify, at the level of the members or the trunk. Its phylogenetic-related persistence in the human face allows facial expression, and is described by Mitz and Peyronie[4] as the superficial musculoaponeurotic system (SMAS), composed of elements of muscular origin located in the same plane and forming a continuous structure. For certain authors,[5] it is a group of discontinuous structures: fine muscles of the face, parotid aponeurosis, and fine muscles of the neck or platysma are not in the same plane. Recent research[6] distinguishes two types of SMAS: type 1, a network of fibrous septa enveloping lobules of fatty tissue, found in the posterior part of the face behind the nasolabial groove, at the level of the forehead, covering the parotid, zygoma, and infraorbitary region; and type 2, a network of collagen and elastin fibers intermixed with muscular

fibers, found in front of the nasolabial groove at the levels of the upper and lower lips.

Muscular aging is characterized by a reduction in muscle mass, modification to metabolism, and excess fat. A particularly visible slackening occurs at the level of the orbicularis muscle but also around the lips. Numerous authors recommend plication, detachment with resection, or SMAS plasty. All these techniques aim to produce detachment and elevation of the SMAS, redrawing the outlines of the face and neck and diminishing tension exercised over the cutaneous sutures.[7] Retension of the orbicularis muscle at the level of the lower eyelid, with or without fixing in the periosteum of the external canthus, can be performed.

Aging of the fatty masses (Figure 5A.3)

The evolution of the fatty masses of the face can be either a decline or an increase. A reduction in fat affects the orbital, temporal, and submalar regions. In addition, the fat pad of the premalar region shows a progressive decline, with sliding of the malar region into the canine fossa, which overhangs the nasolabial groove. Some practitioners recommend repositioning of this fat pad.

A fat excess, favored by a reduction of the basal metabolism, occurs especially at the projection of the chin, in the region under the chin, and at cheek level. Direct removal or lipoaspiration can treat this mass during a cervicofacial facelift in the case of the chin projection and cheeks, or lipoaspiration can be used in the region under the chin. Numerous authors[8–15] recommend the injection of autologous fat associated with cervicofacial facelift to treat at the same time tissue prolapse and fat hypotrophy.

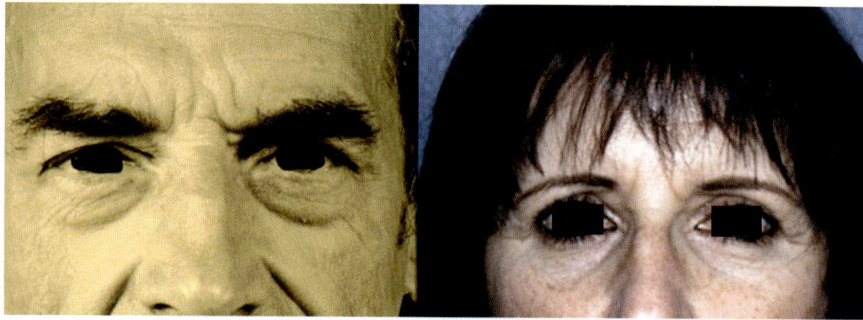

Figure 5A.4   Slackening of the upper eyelid with ptosis of the eyebrow.

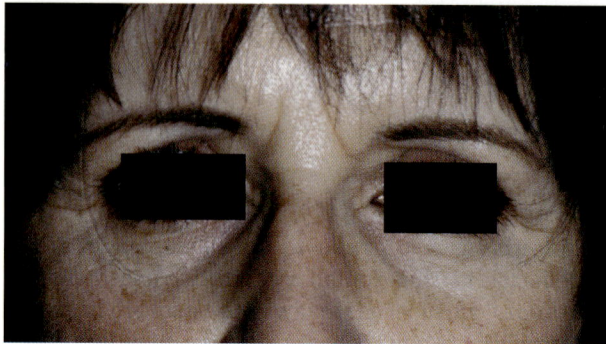

Figure 5A.5   Upper eyelid excess: in this photo the eyebrows are at a higher level to compensate the excess of eyelid.

Aging of the bony base

Expansion

Recent research has contradicted the idea that craniofacial skeletal growth is completed at the end of adolescence. To the contrary, this growth continues and is associated with an enlargement of the sinus, anticlockwise rotation of the bony structure, and clockwise rotation of the mandible. Anthropometric measurements of the skulls of aging subjects, and especially video study of aging of numerous subjects over several decades,[16] showed notable modifications. A reduction of mandibular and maxillary height, principally in relation to edentation and alveolar lysis, and a related retrusion of the jaw, appear with age.[17,18] In women, this is accompanied by an increase in depth of the upper two-thirds of the cranial arch. Every transverse dimension of the face is augmented, while the depth of the inferior third of the face is diminished. The facial skeleton is not, therefore, a static but a dynamic structure, evolving with age. The upper part of the face widens and deepens, and its projection increases by 6%, the frontal sinus from 9 to 14%, and the mandible by 7%.[19]

There is development of the prominence of the supraorbital arch, and the bony protuberances become more pronounced with prominent frontal bumps and, in men, an increase of the nasofrontal angle. Finally, the projection and form of the chin change via mandibular rotation leading to an appearance of general concavity of the facial contour. There is no reduction of the facial bony volume but, on the contrary, expansion.[20]

Demineralization

In addition, demineralization occurs. Bony structures, due to progressive demineralization (accelerated by the menopause), undergo a reduction which can, especially in very old persons, change the appearance. This reduction affects the jaw in particular. Thinning of the alveolar bone can lead to loss of teeth, and thinning of the anterior part of the upper jaw aggravates cutaneous slackening and upper lip wrinkles.

Topographic aging

The face is separated into three regions: upper, mid-, and lower. The upper face is constituted by the forehead, the glabella, the eyebrows, temporal regions, and upper eyelids. The mid-face consists of the lower eyelids, the cheeks, which are divided into anterior, mid-, and posterior zones, and the upper lip. Finally, the lower face is composed of the lower lip, the chin, and the vertical and horizontal portions of the anterior part of the neck.

Upper face (Figures 5A.4 and 5A.5)

The first signs of aging often appear in the upper third of the face. Wrinkles appear at the level of the forehead and glabella, with fine wrinkles around the temporo-orbital region (crow's feet). Slackening and thinning of the frontalis muscle leads to horizontal forehead wrinkles which, from simple expression wrinkles, can be transformed into deep grooves or even folds. Hypertrophy of the corrugator and procerus muscles is the origin of the 'lion's wrinkles' or frown lines, often wrinkles of very deep expression. The procerus is responsible for horizontal wrinkles, the corrugator for slanting wrinkles. As for the forehead, impairment can lead to simple expression wrinkles or deep grooves or folds implicating the reticular dermis. The tail of the eyebrow is subject to prolapse, due to subsidence of the orbicularis. Techniques to treat aging of the fronto-orbital region include the injection of botulinum toxin, removal of the corrugator muscle, pexy or lifting of the eyebrow by an endoscopic approach or directly, or a combination of these techniques.[21] The glabella becomes more prominent owing to a fall of frontal tissues and expansion of the sinus. The temporal pit becomes hollow, and the orbital external arch, owing to the resorption of superciliary fatty tissue and bony expansion, becomes prominent.

The upper eyelid presents excess skin which can be so marked that it interrupts the visual field. Fatty excess is often present particularly at the level of the internal pocket, particularly in a case of weakening of the orbital septum, which causes a pseudo-hernia of the fatty pocket. Sometimes, on the other hand, there is a deficiency of fat. It is not then advantageous to withdraw fat but possibly beneficial to inject, particularly to treat the lower eyelid.[8,15]

Mid-face

The lower eyelid can present in a variable manner a fatty enlargement in the form of nasal, middle, and temporal pockets, and excess skin. The convexity of these 'pockets' is due to fatty excess but also to a slackening of the septum supporting them. The orbicularis muscle loosens, favoring the appearance of fatty pockets and herniated subocularis oculi fat pads (SOOF) known as 'malar bags', while the ligament of the external canthus relaxes, sometimes leading to its fall. The slackening of fine muscles of the mid-third of the face accentuates the fall of fat under the skin, which seems to be accumulated in the lower, anterior region and diminished in the lateral, upper region. Hence, the nasolabial fold becomes a deep groove.

The malar bone becomes flattened and diminished.[18] The zygoma and malar and submalar regions lose fat, giving a skeletonized appearance of the cheekbones with submalar hollows, while 'jowls' appear from around age 30 and increase progressively. Diminishing fat is particularly notable at the level of the 'ball of Bichat', which aggravates the skeletization of the face. The cutaneous and muscular flaccidity which appears at the level of the cheeks increases the nasolabial groove and leads to the appearance of the labiomental groove. The orbicularis oris muscle atrophies and slackens, leading to thin and impaired skin of the upper lip and chronic muscular shrinkage (increased in smokers), causing the progressive appearance of the characteristic vertical wrinkles of the aging upper lip. Initially multidirectional fine lines appear, then wrinkles, which converge, then true grooves and vertical or slanting creases. The profile of the upper lip and vermilion becomes flat. Loss of teeth and osteoporosis of the anterior part of the upper maxilla increase cutaneous laxity of the upper lip. With

the descent of the labial corners, the interlabial line becomes lower than the incisal line.

The nose is also subject to the effects of aging but in an isolated manner. The quality of the skin is distrupted by solar elastosis (very exposed area) and loss of elasticity, sometimes with skin excess, and in men an increase in density of the sebaceous glands, which thickens the skin (can lead to rhinophyma). The tip loses definition and falls (under a horizontal line crossing the nasal ridge) via diminution of the alar cartilage secondary to the thinning and division of the fibrocartilage between different structures, and via weakening of the suspensory ligament, thinning of cartilage, cutaneous thickening, and decrease of the columella secondary to maxillary detachment caused by alveolar bony lysis and reduction of the nasal ridge.[22]

Lower face and neck

Aging of the cervicomental angle is particularly marked by the fall of subcutaneous fat and accumulation in the lower part of the cheeks. The oval of the face loses definition with the appearance of cutaneous and muscular prolapse, creating 'jowls' from around age 30, which are increased by fatty subsidence and can 'overflow' under the mandibular border. The apex of the chin falls and becomes lower than the mandibular line.

Hypotony and slackening of the orbicularis oris and the depressor anguli oris create vertical wrinkles at the corners of the lower lip and on the chin and increase the depth of the nasolabial groove. Atrophy of the skin favors the appearance of these wrinkles. With extension of the nasolabial groove, a labiomental wrinkle develops. Muscular hypotony is often increased by gingival retraction and resorption of the alveolar bone.

The neck presents cutaneous and muscular subsidence which can be particularly important, and which is associated with diastasis of the internal edges of the platysma muscle which also shows hypotrophy, slackening, and weakness, giving rise to the 'turkey gobbler' appearance and visible platysma bands. Weight gain that is often linked to aging causes adipose infiltration under and in front of the platysma, to varying degrees. Fat under the platysma can become visible due to separation of the platysma muscle and gives a thickened appearance to the neck. Fine, cervical wrinkles due to atrophy of the skin, solar elastosis, and a reduction of subcutaneous fat all contribute to semicircular skin creases and loss of the cervicomental angle. Finally, the cervical contour becomes convex with compaction and hyperlordosis of the cervical vertebrae leading to shortening of the neck, disappearance of the curve of the nape, lowering of the hyoid bone beneath the C5 level, and hypertrophy and protrusion of the trachea and thyroid cartilage and cricoids.

Cervicofacial facelift and other procedures are shown in Figures 5A.6–5A.11.

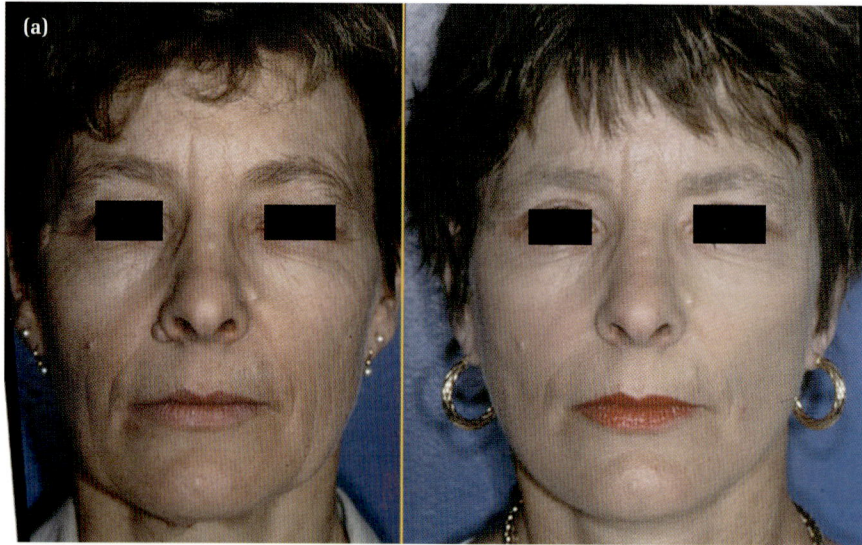

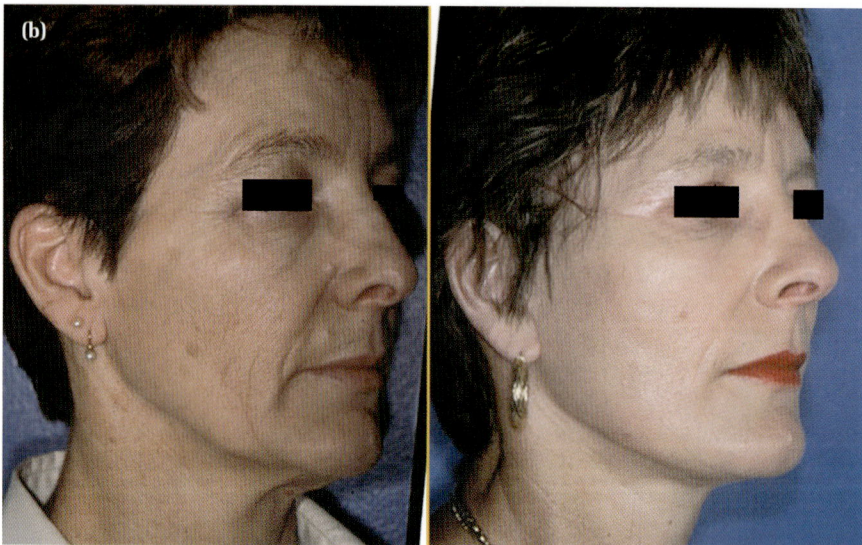

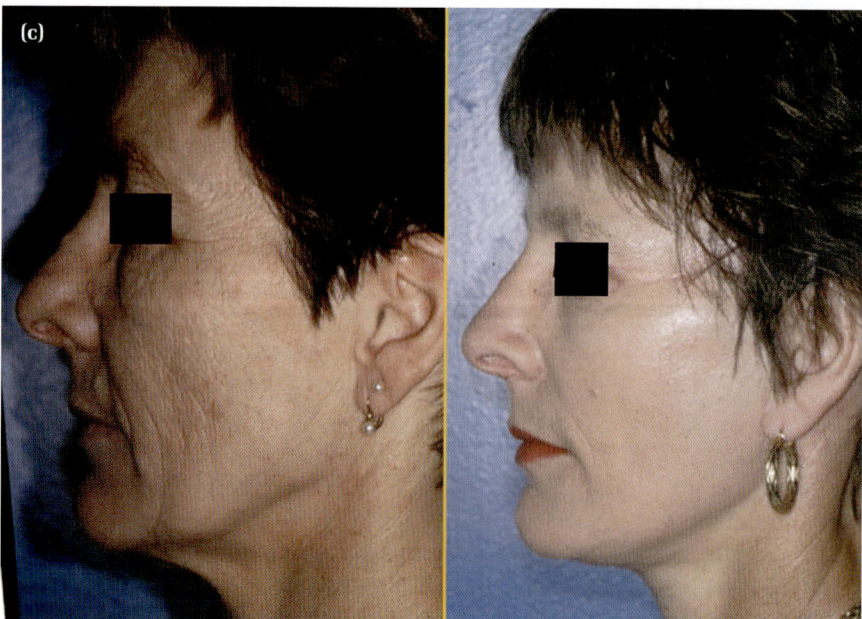

Figure 5A.6 (a–c) Associated cervicofacial facelift and dermabrasion of the full face (CO_2 ultrapulse laser).

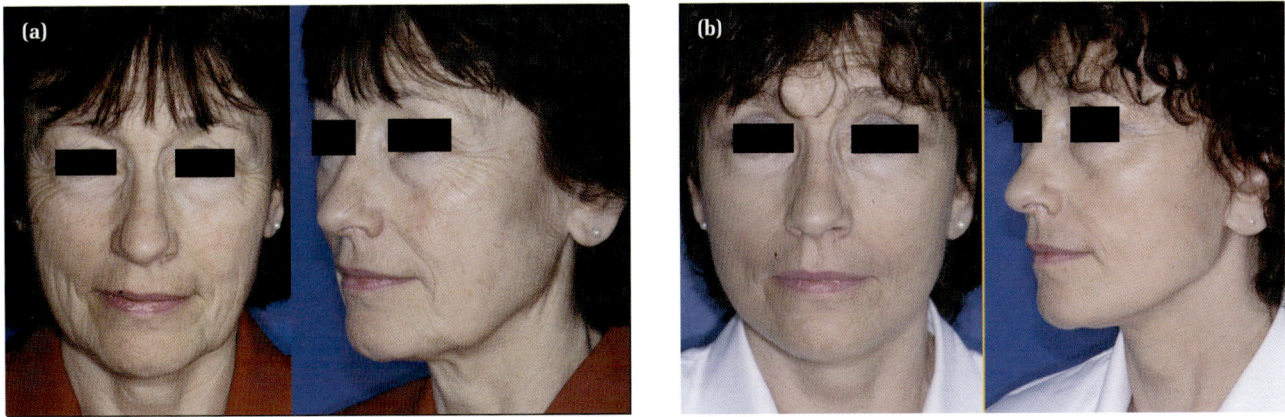

Figure 5A.7   (a, b) Associated cervicofacial facelift and peribuccal dermabrasion (CO_2 ultrapulse laser).

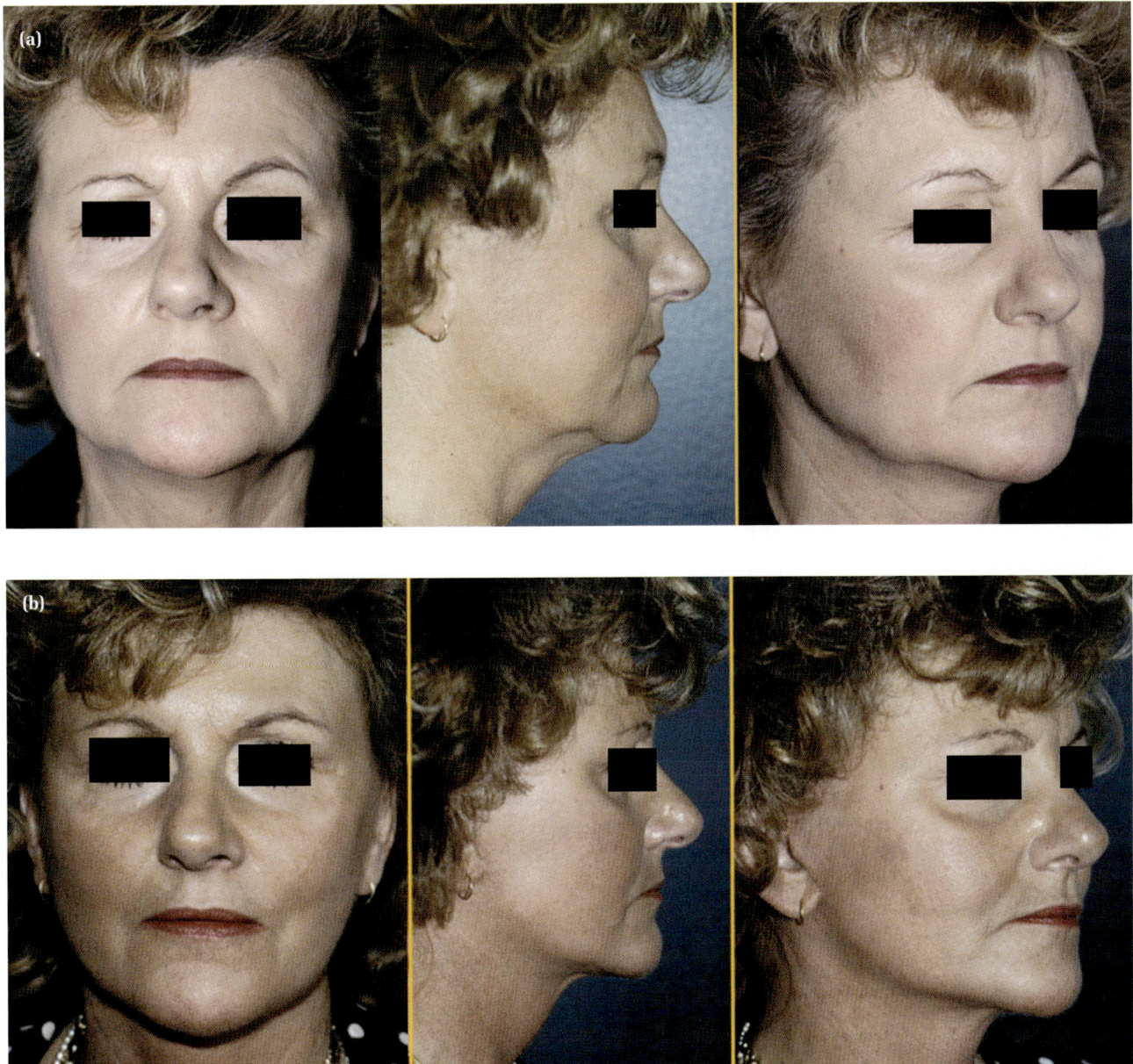

Figure 5A.8   (a, b) Short face: cervicofacial facelift and lipoaspiration under the chin.

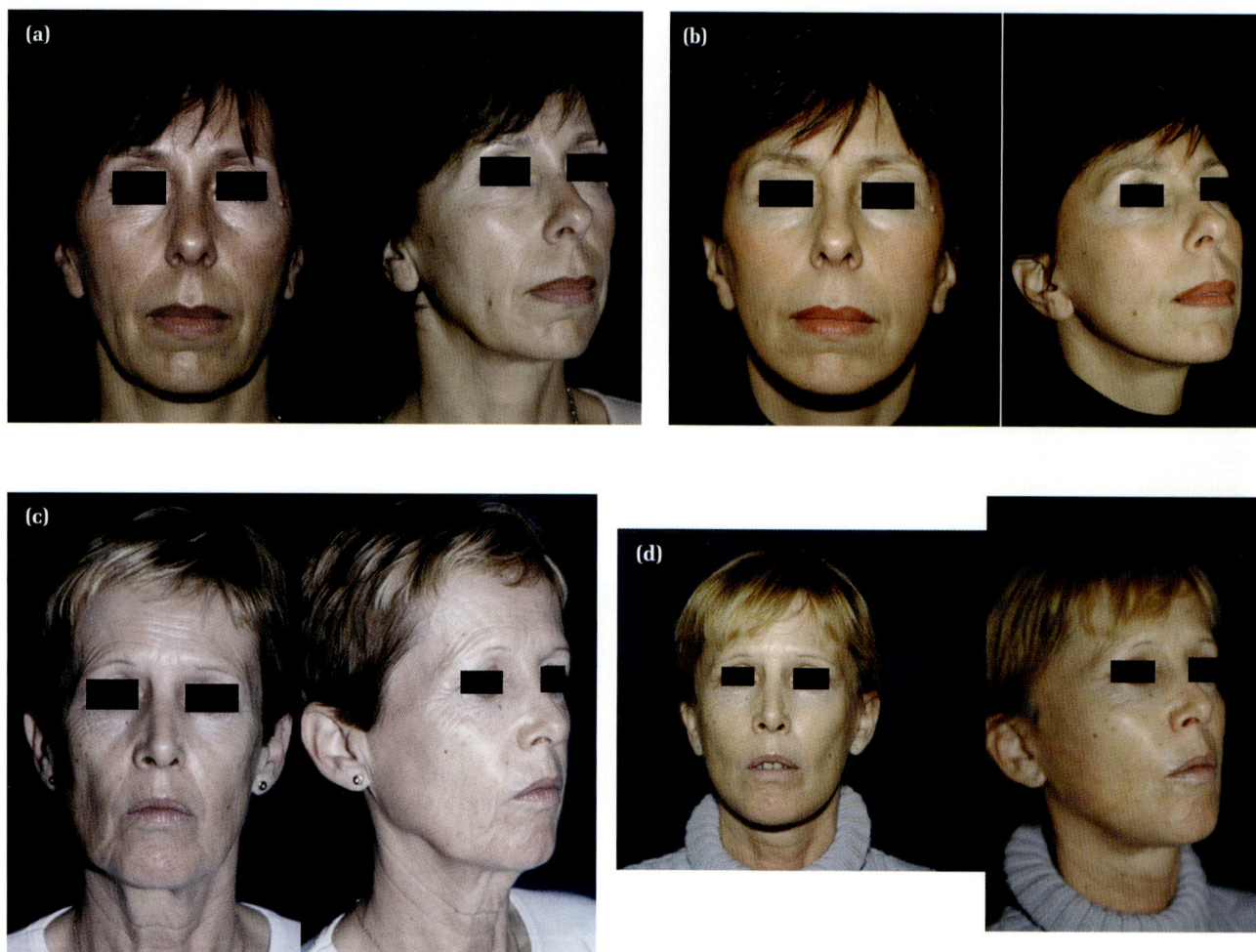

Figure 5A.9   (a–d) Long face: associated cervicofacial facelift and facial lipostructure.

Aging according to phenotype and morphotype

Ethnicity and aging

The thickness of the skin varies according to ethnicity. Dark skin has more melanin in the deep layers of the epidermis and better resistance to sun exposure. Hence, solar elastosis appears earlier and is more severe in phenotypes with pale skin, e.g. those with red or blonde hair. These phenotypes must be very vigilant regarding duration of sun exposure in relation to risk augmented by sunburn, especially for skin carcinomas: basocellular, spinocellular, and melanoma principally.

Certain ethnic groups have prominent cheekbones (especially those of Asian origin) that delay the aspect of cutaneous subsidence. When a prominent facial skeleton is associated with fine skin having a tendency to retraction more than prolapse (ethnic groups of Slavonic origin), the indication for a facelift is

rarer. In Africans, Afro-Caribbeans, and 'mestizas', with greatest thickness of the skin, an aged and wrinkled aspect of the skin is less visible and the indication for a cervicofacial facelift is reduced. In fact, the visible signs of aging are delayed on average for at least a decade in most non-Caucasian populations: Asian, Indian, Amerindian, African, Afro-American, and even Hispanic. Fine lines and expression wrinkles appear later and in a less pronounced manner. In contrast, fat prolapse and muscular slackening are equally or more important than in Caucasians.[23]

Morphotype and aging

Aging presents with important individual variations according to the predominance of skin prolapse, wrinkles, skin thickness, and exposure to environmental factors such as solar radiation or tobacco smoke.

The bony relief of the facial skeleton is particularly important, especially the malar and mandibular

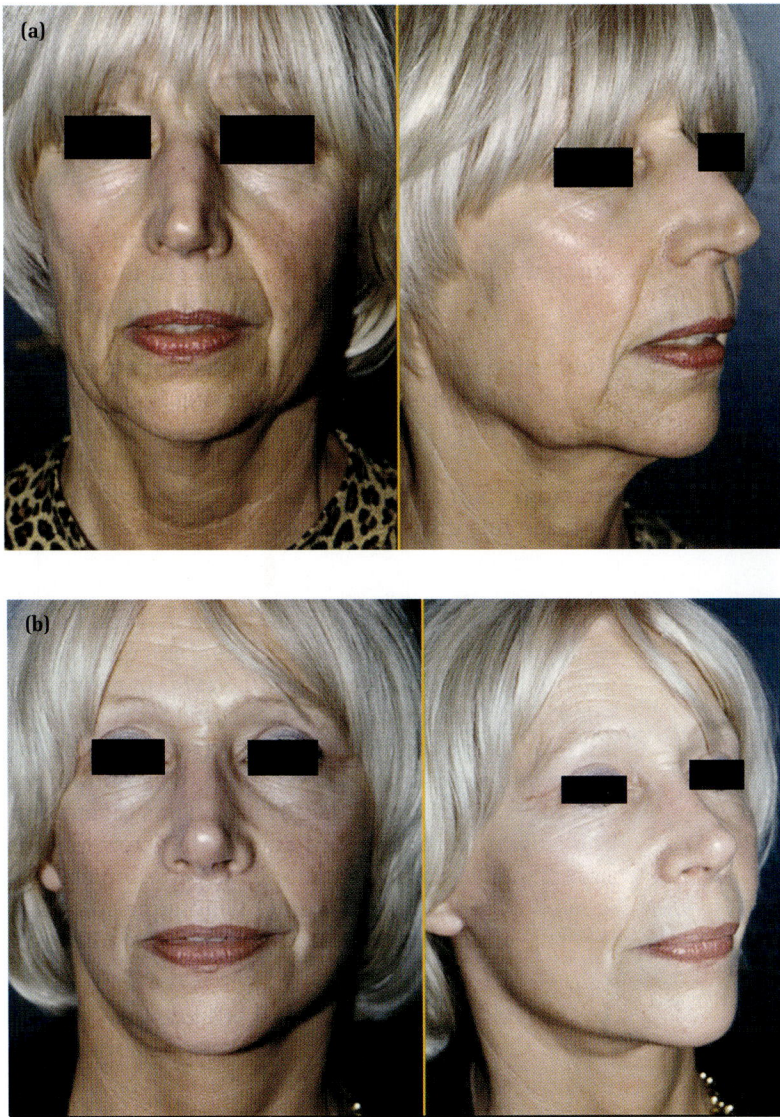

Figure 5A.10 (a, b) Ptotic face. Ptosis of tip of the nose: associated cervicofacial facelift and rhinoplasty.

regions. Prominent cheekbones will delay the effect of prolapse and a hypomandibular or 'long face' syndrome will favor the early appearance of subsidence of the inferior third of the face and neck. A rounder face associated with excess weight is an advantage, but significant weight loss will accentuate flaccidity and therefore cutaneous fall. Facial signs of aging can have a global nature or can be isolated, with the appearance and emphasis of different signs seen in a discrete manner.

Factors favoring cutaneous aging

Sun exposure, besides the obvious risks of the appearance of cutaneous cancerous lesions or transformation of precancerous lesions, favors cutaneous aging via its negative effect on elastin fibers. 'Age spots' appear, and solar elastosis develops in the skin of the face and neck, highly exposed zones which are

therefore affected most severely. These effects appear earlier for the same duration of exposure in people with a fair complexion (redheads and blondes).

Smoking is associated with well-known risks of lung cancer or chronic lung disease and cardiovascular disease, and it also contributes to cutaneous aging. Repeated contraction of the orbicularis muscle while smoking a cigarette reveals early vertical wrinkles of the upper lip. It also favors a poor buccodental state, which, as a source of infection and lysis of the alveolar bone, can change the aspect of the mouth. It also accelerates the yellowing of teeth.

Lack of sleep and psychological stress also have a harmful effect on the appearance of the skin.

A low-humidity atmosphere (frequent car or airplane travel, lengthy stay in surgical unit) can dehydrate the skin, and climatic changes can act on its physiology. Excessive blinking of the eyes (strong sunlight, use of computer screen) can favor the appearance of periorbital wrinkling.

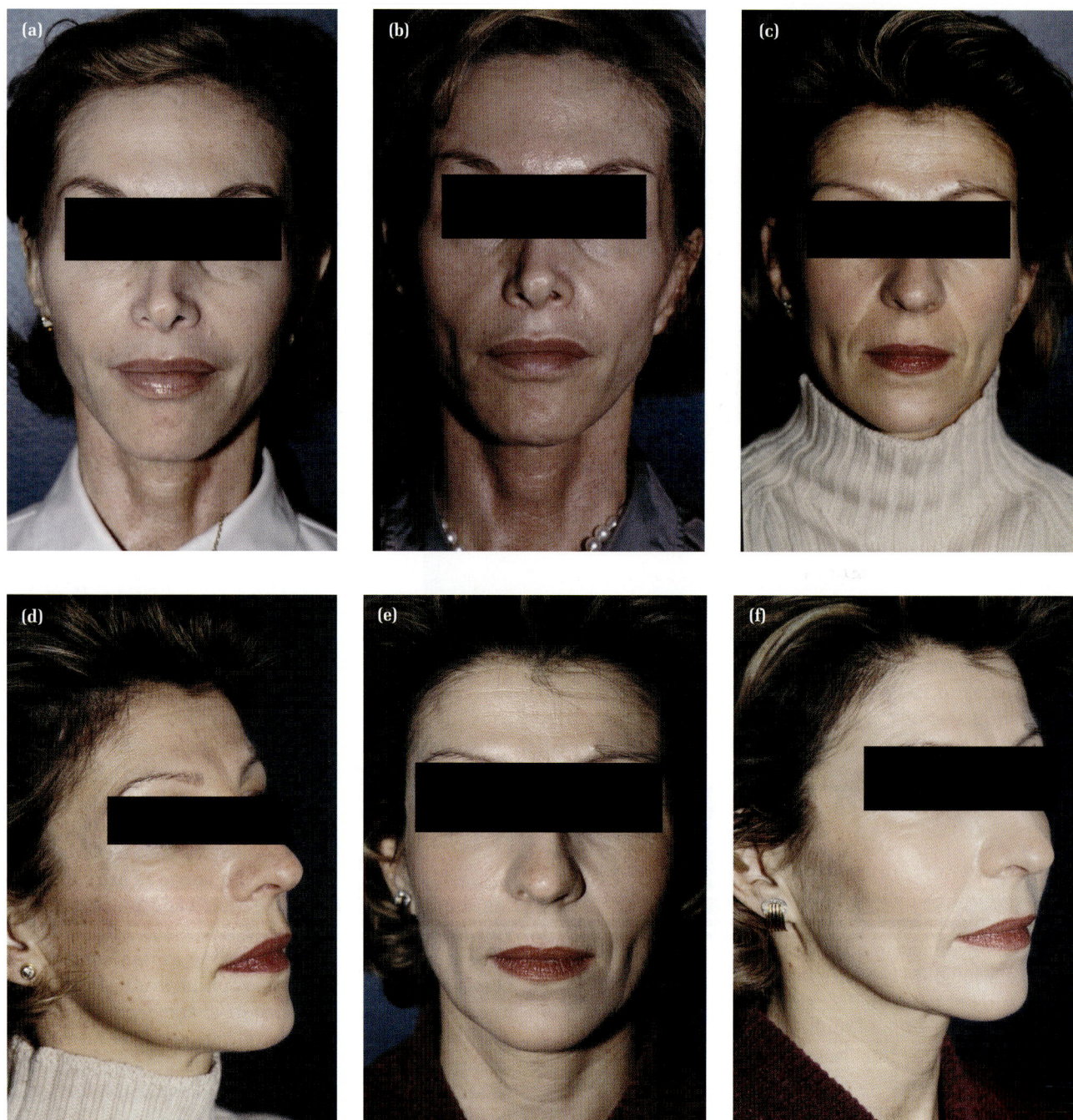

Figure 5A.11   (a–f) Lipostructure.

Large weight loss leading to slackening of the skin gives a prematurely aged appearence not only to the face but also to the rest of the body (stomach, thighs, arms, buttocks, breasts, etc.). Treatment is limited to cutaneous resection with retension.

References

1. La Trenta G. The Aging Face. Atlas of Aesthetic Face and Neck Surgery. Philadelphia: Saunders-Elsevier, 2004: 46–67.
2. Glogau RG. Physiologic and structural changes associated with aging skin. Dermatol Clin 1997; 4: 555–9.
3. Lemperle G, Holmes R, Cohen S, Lemperle S. A classification of facial wrinkles. Plast Reconstr Surg 2001; 108: 1735–50.
4. Mitz V, Peyronie M. The superficial musculo-aponeurotic system (SMAS) in the parotid and cheek area. Plast Reconstr Surg 1976; 58: 80–8.
5. Connell BF. Surgical technique of cervical lift and facial lipectomy. Aesthetic Plast Surg 1981; 5: 43–50.
6. Gassemi A, Prescher A, Riediger D, Axer H. Anatomy of the SMAS revisited. Aesthetic Plast Surg 2003; 27: 258–64.
7. Paul MD, Calvert JW, Evans GRD. The evolution of the mid-face lift in aesthetic plastic surgery. Plast Reconstr Surg 2006; 117: 1809–27.
8. Bui P. Fat as a volumetric implant. Presented at IMCAS 2006, Paris, 8 January, 2006.

9. Bui P. Complications de la lipostructure. Ann Chir Plast Esthet 2004; 49: 630–6.

10. Bui P. Facelifts: shaping the midface/malar volume enhancement. Fat aim within malar remodeling. Presented at IMCAS 2004, Paris, January, 2004.

11. Bui P. Mid and lower face: lipofilling versus polylactic acid. Presented at IMCAS 2004, Paris, January, 2004.

12. Bui P. La Lipostructure. Presented at 48th National Congress of SOFCPRE, Paris, November, 2003.

13. Bui P. Raffinements en lipofilling: lifting et lipostructure faciale antérieure. Presented at IMCAS 2002, Paris, January, 2002.

14. Guerrerosantos J. Simultaneous rhytidoplasty and lipoinjection: a comprehensive aesthetic surgical strategy. Plast Reconstr Surg 1998; 102: 191–9.

15. Trepsat F. Periorbital rejuvenation combining fat grafting and blepharoplasties. Aesthetic Plast Surg 2003; 27: 243–53.

16. Behrents RG. An Atlas of Growth in the Aging Craniofacial Skeleton. Ann Arbor, MI: Center for Human Growth and Development, 1985.

17. Pessa JE, Zadoo VP, Mutimer KL. Relative maxillary retrusion as a natural consequence of aging: combining skeletal and soft tissue changes into an integrated model of midfacial aging. Plast Reconstr Surg 1998; 102: 205–12.

18. Zadoo VP, Pessa JE. Biological arches and changes to the curvilinear form of the aging maxilla. Plast Reconstr Surg 2000; 106: 460–6.

19. Israel H. Recent knowledge concerning craniofacial aging. Angle Orthod 1973; 43: 176–84.

20. Levine RA, Garza JR, Wang PT, Hurst CL, Dev VR. Adult facial growth: application to aesthetic surgery. Aesthetic Plast Surg 2003; 27: 265–8.

21. Matarasso A, Hutchinson OHZ. Evaluating rejuvenation of the forehead and brow: an algorithm for selecting the appropriate technique. Plast Reconstr Surg 2000; 106: 687–94.

22. Rohrich RJ, Hollier LH, Janis JE, Kim J. Rhinoplasty with advancing age. Plast Reconstr Surg 2004; 7: 1936–44.

23. Matory WE. Ethnic Considerations in Facial Aesthetic Surgery. Philadelphia: Lippincott-Raven, 1998: 99–119.

24. Stuzin J, Baker T, Gordon H. The relationship of the superficial and deep facial fascias: relevance to rhytidectomy and aging. Plast Reconstr Surg 1992; 89: 441–9.

25. Knize D. An anatomically based study of the mechanism of eyebrow ptosis. Plast Reconstr Surg 1996; 97: 1321–33.

26. Yousif N, Gosain A, Matloub H et al. The nasolabial fold: an anatomic and histologic reappraisal. Plast Reconstr Surg 1994; 93: 60–9.

27. Rubin L. The anatomy of the nasolabial fold: the keystone of the smiling mechanism. Plast Reconstr Surg 1999; 103: 687–91.

28. Pessa J, Garza P, Love V et al. The anatomy of the labiomandibular fold. Plast Reconstr Surg 1998; 101: 482–6.

29. Pessa JE. An algorithm of facial aging. Plast Reconstr Surg 1998; 101: 482–6.

30. Pessa JE. An algorithm of facial aging: verification of Lambros's theory by three-dimensional stereolithography, with reference to the pathogenesis of midfacial aging, scleral show, and the lateral suborbital trough deformity. Plast Reconstr Surg 2000; 106: 479–88.

5B Hands and décolleté

Vladimir Mitz

Introduction

With their dorsal aspect which is uncovered, and their hidden palmar aspect, when they move, or when they are displayed, our hands are extremely visible in adult life. However, esthetic surgery of the hand is also functional. The hands provide a mute language via delicate moves or striking strength: to feel, to take, to caress, to break, to relax, and to express, our hands are a precious gift which deteriorates with time.

As Vilain says, the esthetics of the hand is yet a function. This is particulary true of the dorsal aspect of the hand, which gives much to see. All methods of repair must accommodate the beauty of the result with the maintenance of movement.

However, poor esthetics may have been present since childhood. In children, the most frequent pathologies are sequelae of congenital deformity, of burns, and, more rarely, of hand trauma, for instance nailbed problems, or sometimes clinodactyly. A frequent problem is represented by 'camptodactyly', which can involve the difficult terrain of lengthening the soft tissues, which are congenitally too short .

In adults, all severe mutilations of the hand produce an unesthetic appearance, but beyond trauma repair, we may consider that today there exists an esthetic need related to the aging of the population, mostly in females.

In aging, the dorsal aspect of the hand starts to get thinner, the natural fatty layer becomes atrophied, and the veins become apparent, and bulging. Dark spots cover the dorsal skin. Sometimes, there are finger deformities because of arthrosis of the proximal interphalangeal (PIP), distal interphalangeal (DIP), or metacarpophalangeal (MP) joints, or trapezometacarpal arthrosis.

It is out of the question to discuss all of these problems in this short chapter. We will only consider some anomalies, first in children then in adults.

The child

Burns

Burn sequelae to the dorsal aspect of the hand warrant esthetic repair by using the 'esthetic units' rule. Thus, only partial thickness skin grafts (and not full thickness) should be used on the dorsal side of the hand. Indeed, full thickness skin grafts first create damage at the donor site, and in addition they are too thick; they do not correspond to the future behavior and quality of partial thickness skin grafts in this area. Thus, it is convenient to restore the esthetic units of the dorsal aspect of the hand by partial thickness skin grafts taken from areas where scarring will be less conspicuous, from the inner side of the thigh, for instance. These grafts will be placed on the tendinous perimysium and above the veins, if possible preserved in order, though resembling normal skin coverage as much as possible.

The assessment of graft dimensions has to take into account the potential of rectraction in the postoperative course, and of immobilization which forces the MP joint into a 90° flexion position, with fingers extended.

It is surprising how concerned patients are about the quality of the restoration of the dorsal aspect of their hand. This must be considered when we restore the hand using flaps (inguinal, Chinese, microsurgical, etc.). These flaps have to be defatted and tailored in several stages in order to obtain the finest, most elegant dorsal skin reconstruction.

Syndactyly

We strongly advocate the avoidance of interdigital skin grafts when treating syndactyly. These grafts become dark brown and give a 'dirty' appearance. Sometimes they extend toward the palmar side of the hand, and always become dark. Raymond Vilain refers to this as a 'Lady Macbeth' sign, because she had a brown spot, ghoulish, in her palm, as a sign of her guilt.

It always seems more elegant to use simple Z-plasty, or a trident flap, or a dorsal lateral finger flap turned in the palmar area, thus leaving the raw areas for spontaneous healing without any flap. This technique has given us many satisfactory results and has been published by several authors.

Spontaneous healing in a child allows easy coverage of the lateral, and even dorsolateral side of the operated fingers, but only if care has been taken not to expose extensor and flexor tendons and the collateral vasculonervous bundle; they should remain covered by their perimysium layer.

It is indeed during the primary dissection when separating the fingers that careful attention should be paid.

This is an actual advance. In the future, no grafting should be used for repair in any case of syndactyly, be it in the hand or in the foot. We have already used this method in adults with the same good results.

Nail disorders in children are beyond the scope of this chapter. However, we have to admit that total nail reconstruction is a very difficult project, especially in children, where the anatomical structures are minute, delicate, and may even be destroyed in some cases of whitlow.

In adults

The esthetic and functional disorders caused by trauma are not dealt with here. Nowadays, three conditions are of growing interest: aging of the dorsal aspect of the hand, deformities due to arthrosis of the fingers, and skin problems.

Aging of the dorsal aspect of the hand

Currently, skin resection on the lateral cubital side of the hand, or a bracelet-like type of skin resection, is not very useful or much used. These procedures result in long scars and prolonged recovery time.

Few surgeons are now in favor of these procedures, mostly because the main problem is skin thinning with age and loss of volume of the subcutaneous compartment, reaching the point when the skin becomes almost transparent. Thus, it appears much more useful to use fat and dermofat grafts below the skin (Figure 5B.1).

It is known that only 30% of the amount of fat tissue grafted will survive after one procedure. Thus, it becomes necessary to plan at least three sets of fat grafting in order to achieve the best result.

The grafts are inserted through tiny incisions in the side of the hand; tunneling and massaging are mandatory to spread the grafts well in a monolayer below the skin, above the superficial dorsal fascia.

Centrifugation of fat does not seem useful, at least in our experience.

This operation is perfomed better under local or general anesthesia depending on patient condition and wishes (Figure 5B.2).

After 10 days, during which edema and bruising may occur, the improvement is striking. A stable result is obtained after 3–4 months, and fat grafting sessions may be scheduled to obtain the best possible result (Figure 5B.3).

This is a very satisfactory procedure, bringing a high degree of patient satisfaction with minimal risks and complications (Figure 5B.4). Complications are mostly: hematomas, infection, and inhomogeneity of the fat grafts. Appropriate treatment should be considered when complications occur, but it is always possible to repeat the operation.

Donor sites for fat harvesting are the abdominal fat (first choice) and neck and jowl fat (combining the hand improvement with a facelift procedure).

Many authors have recently published good results with this simple technique, similar to what we aim for in penoplasty and lip, cheek, or malar augmentation.

Deformities related to digital arthrosis

Operating for interdigital arthrosis is becoming more frequent, but is not yet a widespead procedure.

Two techniques are possible:

- lateral bony trimming with skin resection: this procedure gives a good esthetic result when combined with skin resection at the dorsal wedge of the DIP (operation of Romano)
- reshaping osteotomy of the DIP joint and insertion of a Swanson silicone mini-implant.

This is a good technique, but rather difficult, demanding skill. It is a 'jeweler's operation', needing careful planning of incisions, bony shaft preparation, and implant choice. The implant should be small enough not to protrude laterally, and strong enough to bring stability.

It is always necessary to tighten again the extensor apparatus, in order to avoid the 'mallet finger' deformity as a consequence of finger shortening.

These operations are carried out by devoted orthopedic and hand surgeons, but also plastic surgeons, because patients having a facelift or blepharoplasty want also to restore the hand, which can betray their true age.

There is certainly the opportunity in these conditions to improve and maybe prevent the impairment, but treating the problem is today possible.

Arthrodesis which was historically perfomed should be limited to failed procedures, in order to preserve functional movement of all joints concerned.

Hand skin problems

These are mostly treated by dermatologists rather than surgeons. Age spots are best treated by liquid nitrogen, applied once or twice a year. Laser treatment may lead to exaggerated white spots. Healing occurs within 2 weeks and brings a very discrete hypopigmentation, very acceptable in our practice. This dermatologic treatment must be repeated in order to give good results. Sun damage must be prohibited by total abstention from sun overexposure.

In conclusion, we feel that esthetic surgery of the hand is currently a major field. Previously neglected, forgotten,

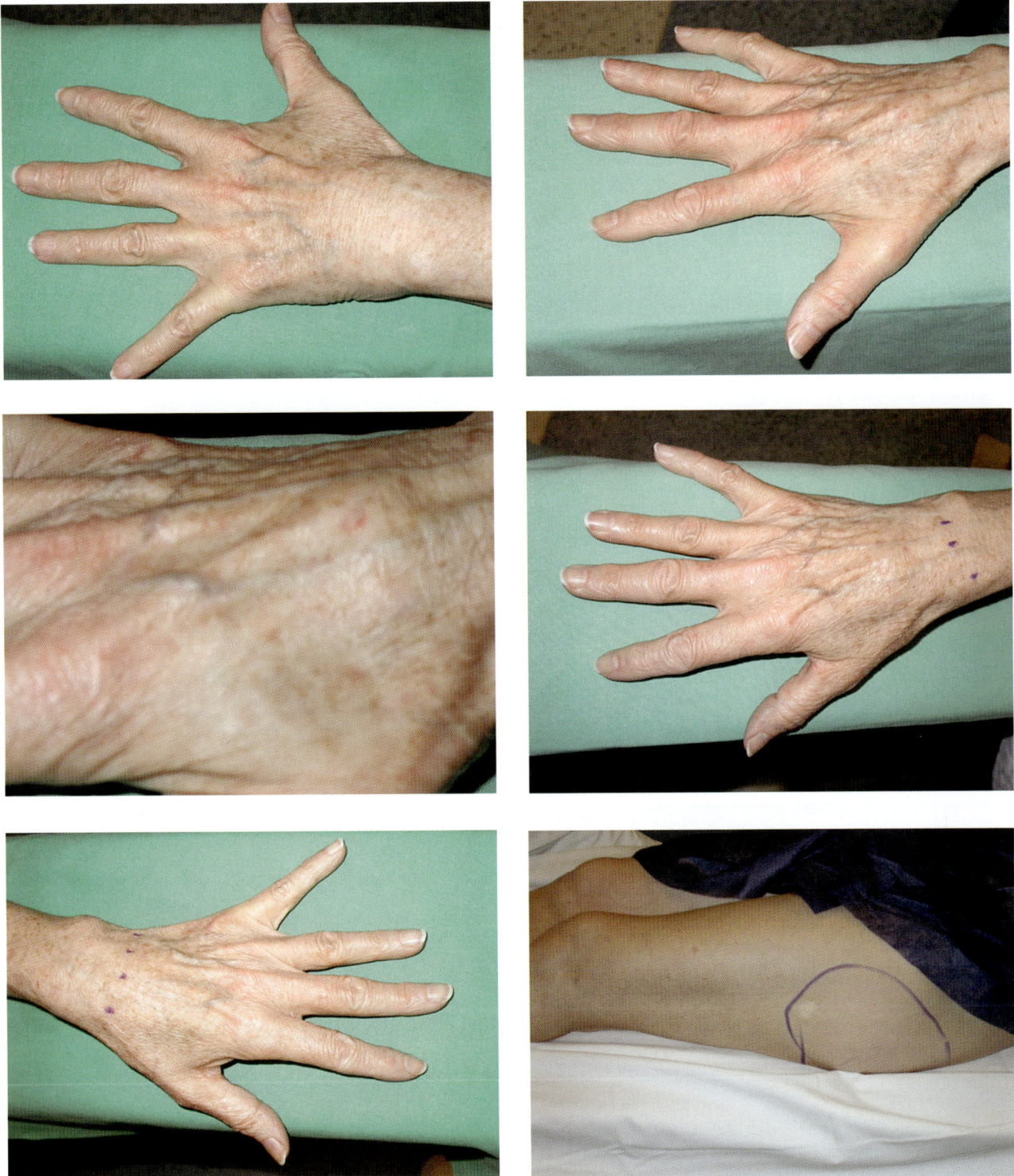

Figure 5B.1   Hands before surgery.

or badly performed, there are now new approaches offering better cosmetic appearance and function preservation. We feel that this demand is legitimate, but a stable result is difficult to obtain with only one procedure. Patient satisfaction comes about when both rheumatological pain and deformity are treated, leading to a better appearance with preservation of function.

Other pathological conditions have been excluded from this chapter: mucoid cysts, ganglia, pulp atrophy, thenar muscle atrophy, etc. We wanted here to focus on the most frequent demands of patients when complaining about poor hand esthetics, and the methods now available to treat these conditions make us more optimistic than previously and also much more daring.

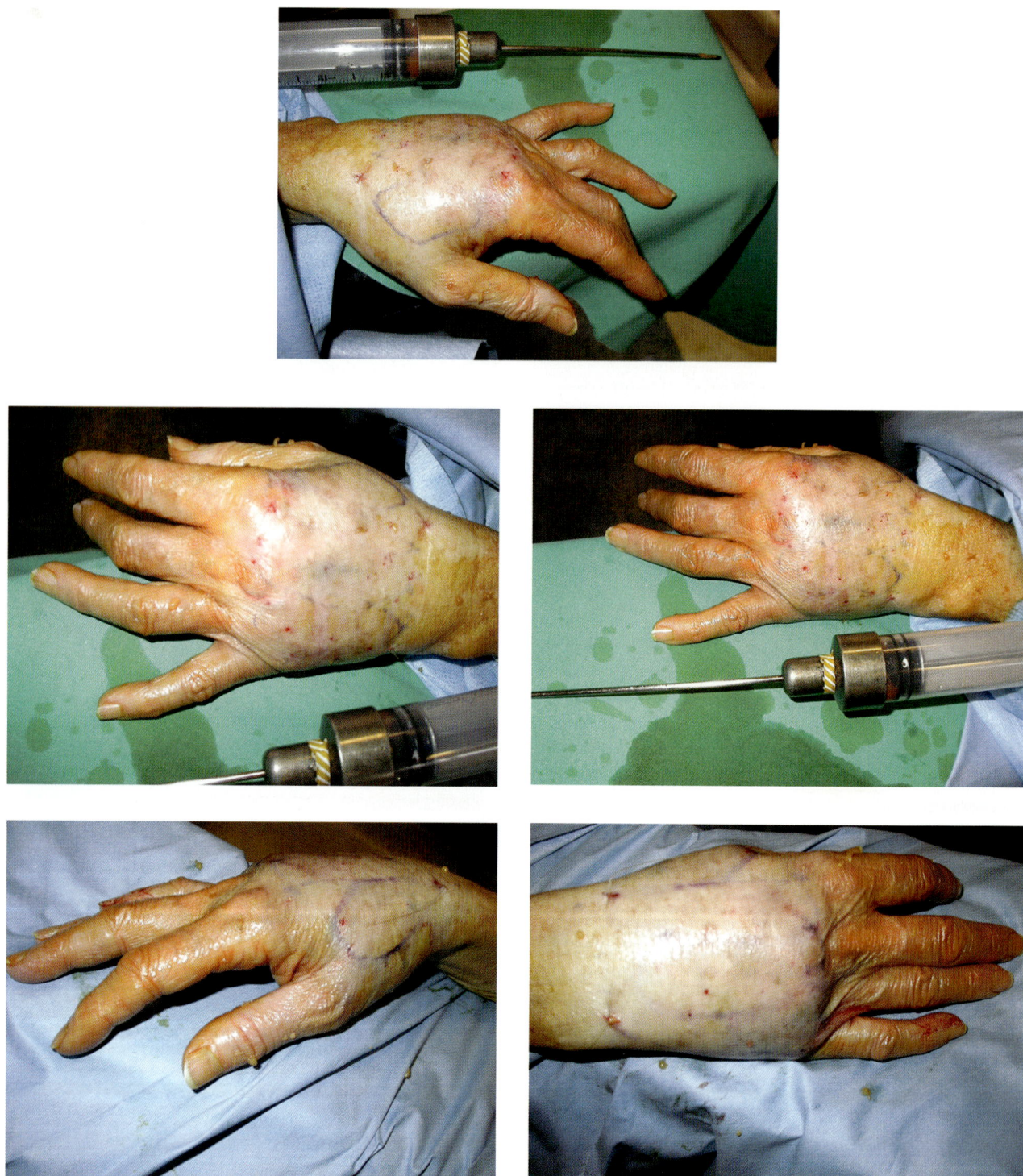

Figure 5B.2   Hands during surgery.

The décolleté

Esthetic surgery of the 'décolleté' is dominated by the demand for repair of intermammary fine wrinkles; they appear when the patient brings her shoulders together, or when she wears a tight bra.

Several anomalies may be encountered.

Dark spots

In our opinion, the best treatment is to apply carbonic snow, which seems more efficient than laser, and produces less blanching spots.

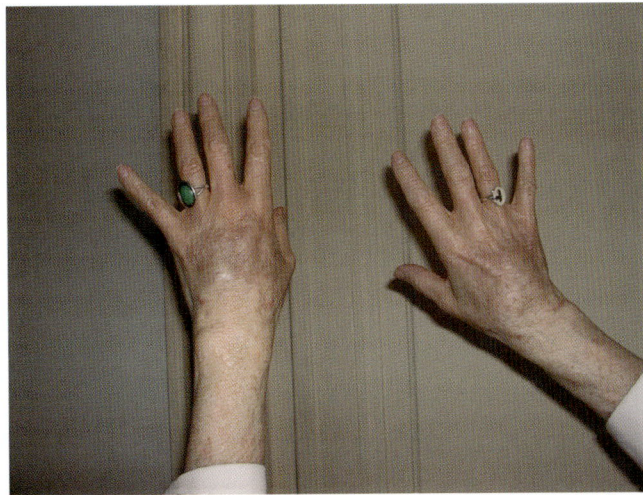

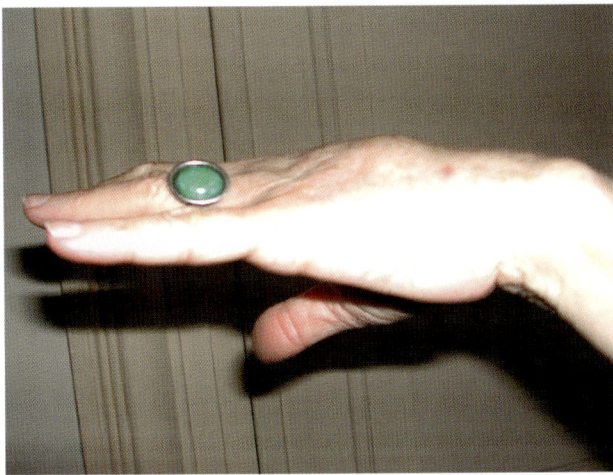

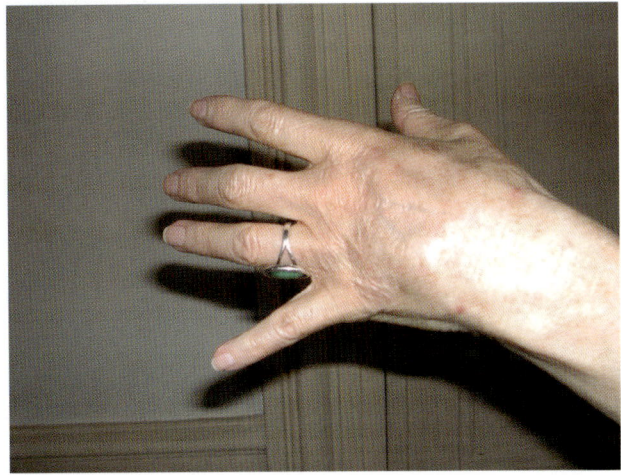

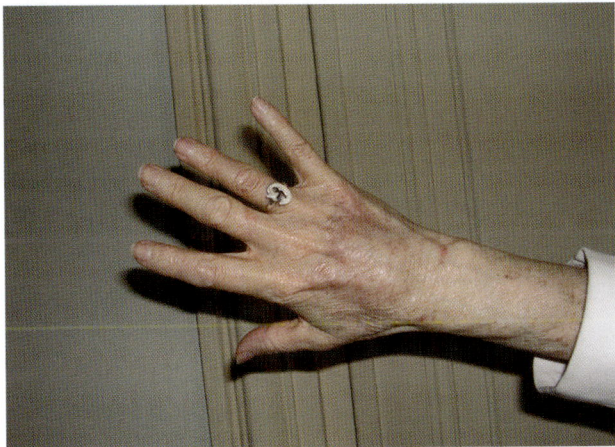

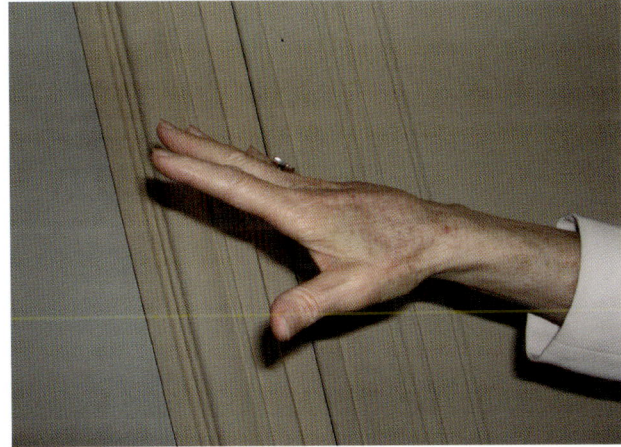

Figure 5B.3 Hands a few weeks after surgery.

Skin thinning

The skin becomes almost transparent and shows the venous necklace. Such cases are rare; fat grafting would be an effective solution.

Vertical lines in middle of sternocostal area

Two therapeutic approaches may be discussed. According to Staub, it is possible to perform a very extensive facelift, with dissection below the clavicles.

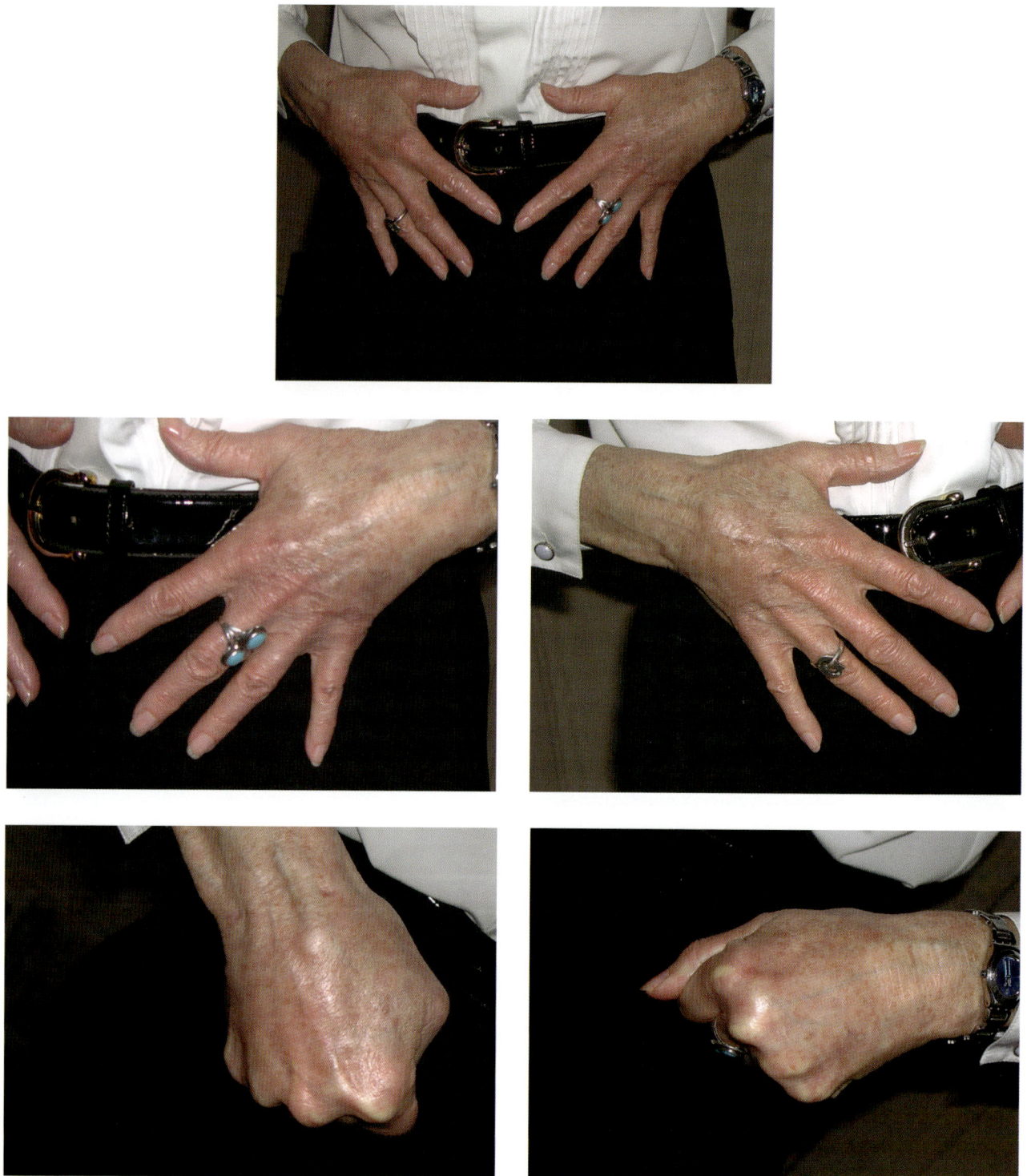

Figure 5B.4 Hands 6 months after surgery.

For this purpose, Staub infiltrates massively the sub-cutaneous area in order to produce hydrodissection, to initiate the procedure. The skin tension in the mastoid area gives a good result in diminishing décolleté lines, as he has reported at several meetings. We do not have experience with this technique.

The other technique involves the use of BOTOX® (50 u diluted in 8 ml of saline), performed in one stage by multiple punctures within the décolleté area. Such treatment has been very effective in our hands, staying stable for between 2 and 4 months. A second look after 1 month has been a good approach for achieving

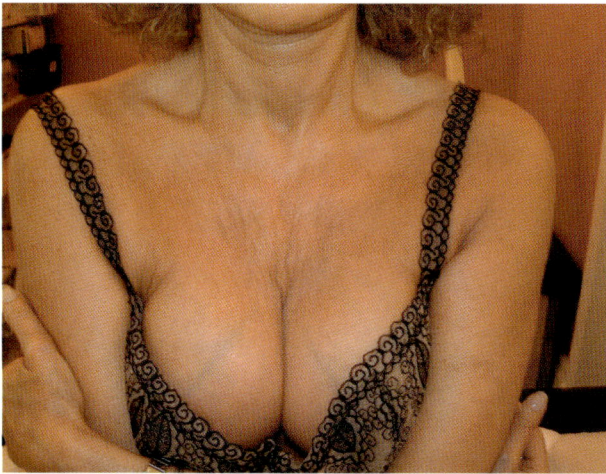

Figure 5B.5 Décolleté before surgery.

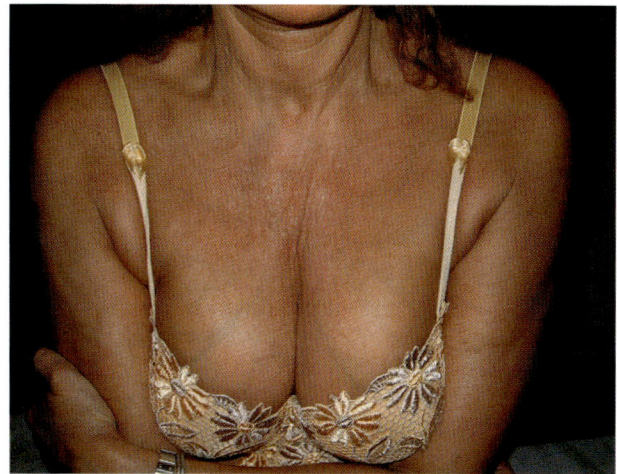

Figure 5B.6 Décolleté after surgery.

better-lasting results, by adjusting the quantity of BOTOX according to each individual case.

In conclusion, it does not seem that direct breast surgery or facelift procedures are optimum to eliminate intermammary lines. The use of BOTOX, directly injected into the area at a subcutaneous level, seems a good solution to treat this problem (Figure 5B.5 and Figure 5B.6). It probably acts on the muscle cells that are embedded in the subcutaneous fascia.

Great improvements have been found in our practice with use of this method, and we strongly recommend this treatment for the problem of intermammary wrinkles.

6 Sweat glands

Marina Landau and Hananya Vaknine

Eccrine sweat glands

The eccrine sweat glands are simple tubular glands that assist in thermoregulation of the body by compensating for heat production through evaporative water loss. They are also excretory organs that remove urea, ammonia, free amino acids, drugs, and proteolytic enzymes from the tissues.

In contrast to other mammals, in which eccrine glands are present only on the soles, in humans and anthropoid apes eccrine glands are present almost everywhere in the skin, but are most abundant on the palms, on the soles, and in the axillae.

Eccrine glands are seen first early in the fourth gestational month.[1] They begin as a group of basophilic cells in the basal layer of the epidermis. At the time of lumen formation the duct and the secretory segment are composed of two layers: the inner layer of luminal cells and the outer layer of basal cells. The ductal part keeps this structure throughout life, while in the secretory segment the luminal cells differentiate into columnar secretory cells and the basal cells differentiate into myoepithelial and secretory cells. At the time of birth, eccrine glands are completely mature in their appearance and function. It is estimated that that there are between 2 and 5 million eccrine units present at birth.[2] Their number does not increase postnatally, but complete neurologic control of sweating does not appear before the age of 2 or 3 years.

Eccrine gland anatomy

The eccrine sweat gland consists of a coiled secretory portion that is embedded deep in the reticular dermis and a duct that passes vertically through the dermis and epidermis opening to the skin surface via a sweat pore (Figure 6.1). The basal secreting coil is surrounded by fatty tissue that connects to subcutaneous fat. This portion of the gland is two cell thick, the inner (luminal) layer horbors two cell types: clear (serous) and dark (mucous) secretory cells. The luminal layer is surrounded by an outer layer composed myoepithelial cells (Figure 6.2). The dermal and epidermal portions of the duct are composed of a single cell type, organized in two layers. The intraepidermal portion is called acrosyringium (Figure 6.3). The ductal cells of acrosyringium synthesize keratohyaline, and at the sweat pore the slining becomes keratinized.

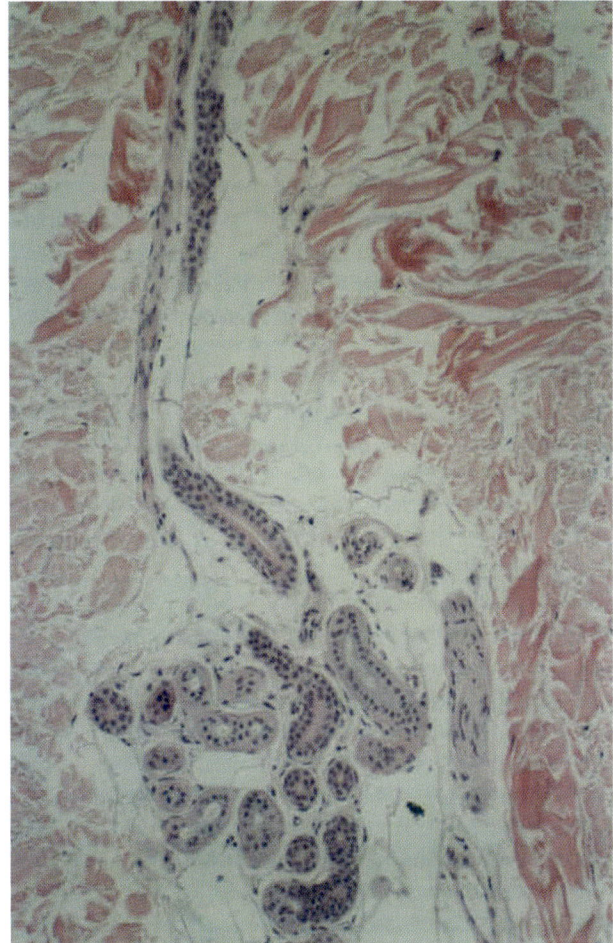

Figure 6.1 The eccrine sweat gland consists of a coiled secretory portion that is embedded deep in the reticular dermis and a duct that passes vertically through the dermis and epidermis.

Clear cells of the secreting coil have pale cytoplasm and no secretory granules. They contain glycogen, lipid, and pigment. During active sweating the glycogen in the clear cells is metabolized to lactate and hydrogen ions; lactate is secreted to the lumen together with water, Na^+, K^+, and Cl^- in a concentration that is nearly isotonic to plasma.[3] Dark cells contain large mucous granules and abundant cytoplasmatic ribosomes. Like the clear cell they also contain lipid pigment and glycogen. Myoepithelial cells are organized in a discontinuous layer at the periphery of the gland. Their function in secretion and delivery of

59

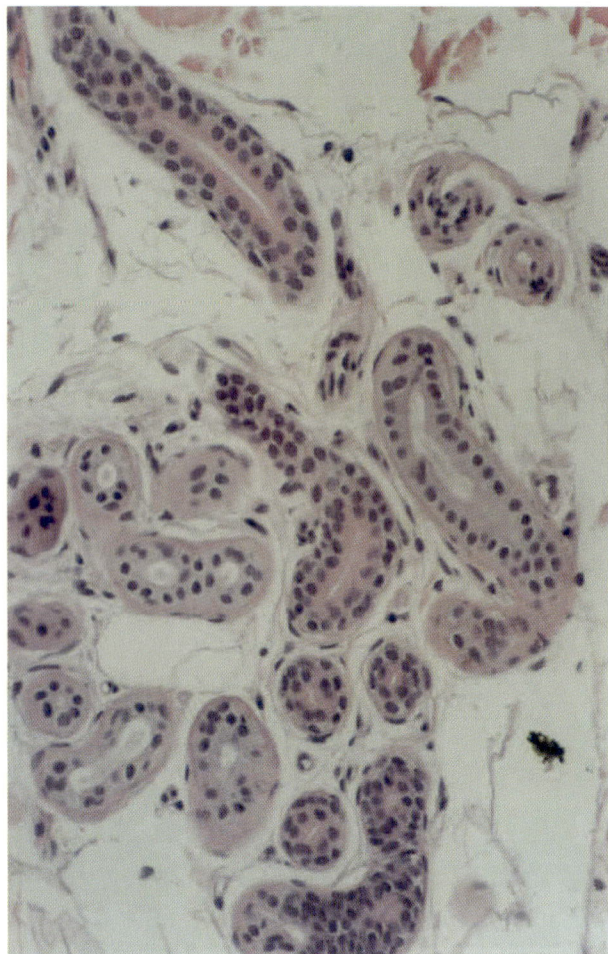

Figure 6.2 Light micrograph of sweat gland showing the secretory units (lighter profiles) and ducts with a characteristic eosinophilic appearance of the luminal aspects.

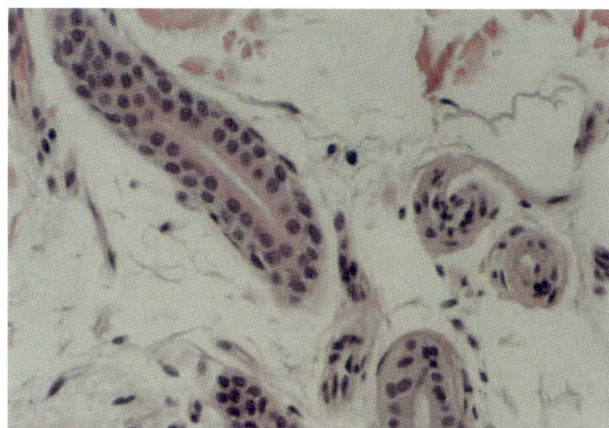

Figure 6.3 Dermal straight eccrine duct entering the epidermis as the acrosyringium.

sweat to the skin surface is not completely clear.[4] No deviation from the normal ultrastructure is found in hyperhidrotic eccrine sweat glands.[5]

Composition of eccrine sweat

The cells of the sweat duct function in the secretion and modification of sweat. Eccrine secretion, which is initially isotonic, becomes hypotonic while flowing through the eccrine duct, where NaCl and HCO_3 are actively reabsorbed.[6] The level of reabsorption depends on the sweating rhythm. When fluid flows slowly through the ductal portion of the gland, significant reabsorption of sodium and chloride occurs, which leads to a decrease of their concentration from 140 to 5 mEq/l. When sweat glands are highly stimulated and the flow is fast, the reabsorption rhythm decreases and the final concentration of the electrolytes in the sweat increases.

The concentration of lactate in sweat results from glycolysis of glucose by secretory cells. Its concentration increases with an increased sweat rate. Urea in the sweat is derived mostly from serum urea.[7] The sweat urea concentration is 2–4 times higher than in plasma at a low sweat rate and decreases at a higher sweat rate. Other sweat components are ammonia, amino acids, proteins, proteases, histamine,[8] prostaglandins,[9] amphetamine-like compounds,[10] and some orally ingested drugs.[11,12] Eccrine secretion is colorless and odorless and is composed of 99% water. All the electrolytes present in plasma are also found in sweat. Its pH is between 4.5 and 5.5 but may increase with continuous sweating.

Maximal sweat production in normal circumstances is about 700 ml per hour. However, chronic exposure to a hot environment induces acclimatization, during which sweat production can increase to up to 1.5–2 l per hour with a lower NaCl concentration. The effect of salt preservation is achieved due to a higher secretion of aldosterone.

Nervous control of eccrine sweating

Regulation of the internal body temperature is among the most important functions of the body. The preoptic hypothalamic area plays an essential role in the regulation of body temperature. The elevation of hypothalamic temperature provides the strongest stimulus for sweating response, but the glands respond also to stimuli received directly from the peripheral skin receptors.[13]

Efferent nerve fibers originating from the hypothalamic preoptic sweat center descend and synapse in the intermediolateral cell columns of the spinal cord. The myelinated axons rising from the intermediolateral horn of the spinal cord pass out in the anterior roots to reach the sympathetic chain and synapse. Unmyelinated postganglionic sympathetic class C fibers abundantly innervate the sweat glands. In contrast to other sympathetic fibers, in which noradrenaline serves as a chemical mediator, acetylcholine is a neurotransmitter of the sympathetic fibers innervating the sweat glands.

Apocrine sweat glands

Apocrine glands are linked to the upper part of the pilosebaceous unit. Like the pilosebaceous unit, they originate embryologically from the hair germ. The formation of the apocrine glands begins late in the fourth month. At the time of birth the gland structure is not complete. Apocrine glands develop their secretory portion and become functional only at puberty. They represent scent glands.

Apocrine glands are restricted to the area of the axillae, anogenital region, and as modified glands in the external ear canal (ceruminous glands), in the eyelid (Moll's glands), and in the breast (mammary glands).

Apocrine glands are composed of three segments: the secretory portion, and the intradermal and intraepidermal duct. The secretory portion of apocrine gland has a single layer of secretory cells with abundant large granules and an outer layer of myoepithelial cells. The lumen of the secretory portion of the apocrine gland is 10 times the average diameter of the eccrine gland lumen.

The ductal portion of the apocrine glands leads to the infundibular portion of the hair follicle above the sebaceous duct entrance. Occasionally, apocrine ducts may directly open to the epidermis. The apocrine duct is similar to the eccrine duct with a double layer of basophilic cells coating the lumen. The intraepidermal portion of the apocrine duct is straight and not spiral in appearance as is the intraepidermal part of the eccrine gland.

The apocrine sweat secretion was classically described as decapitation secretion. In this process, the apical part of the secretory cells is pinched off and released into the lumen. This type of secretion is continuous. After the apocrine gland is emptied there is a refractory period during which the duct is filled again with glandular secretion. More recent research indicates that the secretory process also involves a merocrine (exocytotic) process.

Apocrine secretion is more viscous and is produced in much smaller quantities compared with eccrine sweat. In marked contrast to the eccrine glands, apocrine glands are controlled by adrenergic nerves.

Apoeccrine glands

In patients with hyperhidrosis, glands sharing both eccrine and apocrine features can be found in the axilla.[14] These are called apoeccrine glands, and have a long duct that ends, as for the eccrine gland, directly on the skin surface. The secretory portion has two segments: a smaller one similar to the coiled portion of the eccrine gland and a larger one similar to the apocrine secretory segment. Its innervation is like that of the eccrine gland, but its secretion capacity is 10 times

higher. In primary hyperhidrosis the morphology of the sweat glands is normal. It appears that there is an abnormal response to nervous stimuli in hypothalamic sweat control centers.

Sweat measurements

The line between normal sweating and hyperhidrosis is poorly defined, and objective evaluations of the disease are needed. These evaluations are based on subjective assessments and objective measurements.

The iodine–starch test (Minor's test) is the oldest method used to assess sweating. It is based on the reaction between iodine, starch, and sweat that causes a purple precipitation at the site. Minor's test is performed after cleansing and drying of the test area. Alcoholic iodine solution is applied on the test site. After it is completely dry, corn or potato starch is dusted on the skin surface. When sweat is secreted, purple areas are formed (Figure 6.4). Due to its simplicity, the iodine–starch test has been the most commonly used in the entire literature. Its advantage in daily practice is related to its performance simplicity, but also to its ability to determine the size of the sweating area. Test results are sometimes striking in terms of side asymmetry and irregularity of the hyperhidrotic areas. Photography of the stained area and its change after treatment allows documentation of treatment success.[15,16] Some authors prefer to assess palmar sweat by documenting sweating points using butcher paper for a short contact time.[17]

Gravimetry is a quantitative analysis of sweat production.[18] The area to be assessed is cleansed and dried. Filter paper is weighed on a high precision laboratory scale. Then it is placed in the armpits for 60 seconds and weighed again. The rate of sweat production (in mg/min) is calculated. Normohidrosis is defined as less than 20 mg/min per area, while in hyperhidrosis cases sweat secretion is more than 50 mg/min per area. While performing this test, it should be kept in mind that evaporation, temperature, and air humidity together with stress and anxiety related to the procedure might interfere with the results.

Evaporimetry is measurement of water evaporation by an instrument that determines vapor partial pressure at different points on the skin in fixed environmental temperature and humidity. The procedure requires sophisticated equipment and is time-consuming.[19] Other objective methods for sweat assessment are the copy-paper test, Wada–Takagaki test,[20] silicone imprint test,[21] quantitative sudomotor axon reflex test,[22] dynamic operational method,[23] and capacitive humidity sensor.[24]

The subjective effect of hyperhidrosis on a patient's life can be much more significant than previously appreciated. To assess this effect, various quality of life (QOL) scales are used. The Dermatology Life

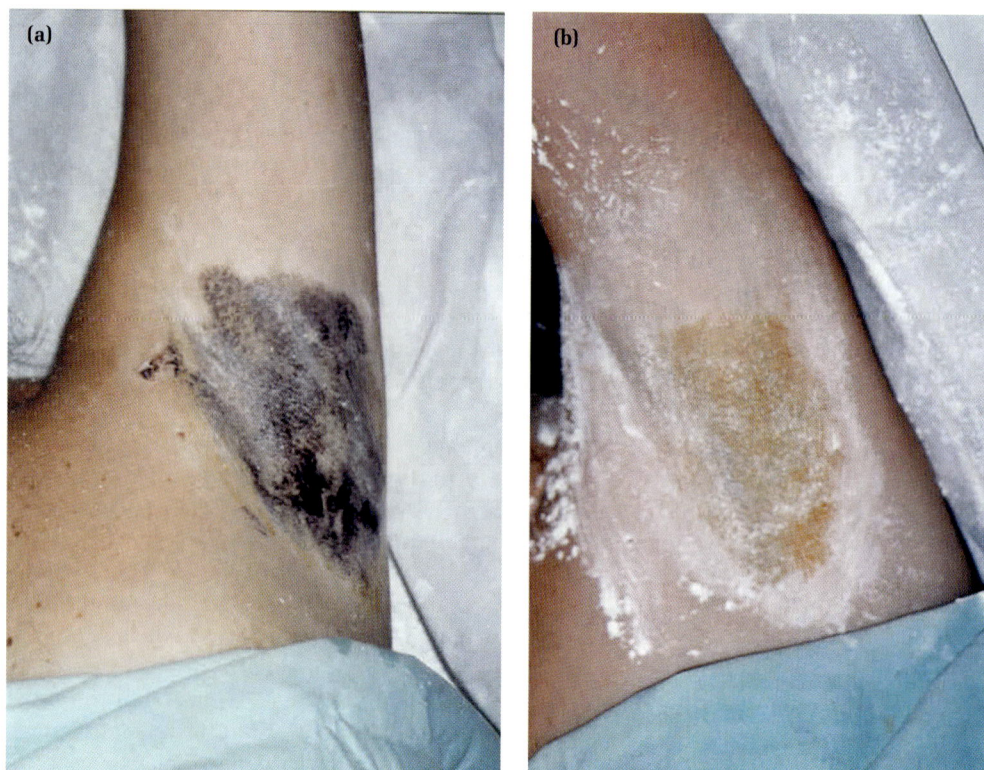

Figure 6.4 Iodine–starch test (Minor's test). (a) The reaction between iodine, starch, and sweat causes a purple precipitation at the site. (b) Two weeks after the injection of botulinum toxin A, a significant decrease in the reaction is observed.

Quality Index (DLQI) is a simple practical method of scoring of skin disease using 10 questions. It is a validated measure that allows the comparison of hyperhidrosis with other dermatological diseases.[25] The Hyperhidrosis Impact Questionnaire (HHIQ) focuses specifically on how hyperhidrosis affects patients.[26] Recently it has been demonstrated that sweat overproduction affects body odor, and can be improved by botulinum toxin A injections. The body odor is assessed by a T-shirt sniff test.[27]

References

1. Elli R. Eccrine sweat glands: electron microscopy, cytochemistry, and anatomy. In: Jadassohn J, ed. Handbuch der Haut und Geshlechtskrankheiten, Vol 1, Normale und pathologische Anatomie der Haut, 1st edn. Berlin: Springer-Verlag, 1967: 23.
2. Szabo G. The number of eccrine sweat glands in human skin. In: Montagna W, Ellis R, Silver A, eds. Advances in Biology of Skin, Vol 3. New York: Pergamon, 1962: 1.
3. Dobson RL, Sato K. The secretion of salt and water by the eccrine sweat gland. Arch Dermatol 1972; 105: 366–70.
4. Sato K, Nishiyama A, Kobayashi M. Mechanical properties and functions of the myoepithelium in the eccrine sweat gland. Am J Physiol 1979; 237: C177–84.
5. Bovell DL, Clunes MT, Elder HY, Milsom J, Jenkinson DM. Ultrastructure of the hyperhidrotic eccrine sweat gland. Br J Dermatol 2001; 145: 298–301.
6. Dobson RL, Formisano V, Lobitz WC Jr et al. Some histochemical observations on the human sweat gland. III. The effect of profuse sweating. J Invest Dermatol 1972; 31: 147–59.
7. Brusilow SW, Gordes EH. The permeability of sweat gland to nonelectrolites. Am J Dis Child 1966; 112: 328.
8. Garden JW. Plasma and sweat histamine concentrations after heat exposure and physical exercise. J Appl Physiol 1966; 21: 631–5.
9. Forstrom L, Goldyne ME, Winkelmann RK. Prostaglandin activity in human eccrine sweat. Prostaglandins 1974; 7: 459–64.
10. Vree TB, Muskens AT, van Rossum JM. Excretion of amphetamines in human sweat. Arch Int Pharmacodyn Ther 1972; 199: 311–17.
11. Shah VP, Epstein WL, Riegelman S. Role of sweat in accumulation of orally administered griseofulvin in skin. J Clin Invest 1974; 53: 1673–8.
12. Harris R, Jones HE, Artis WM. Orally administered ketoconazole: route of delivery to the human stratum corneum. Antimicrob Agents Chemother 1983; 24: 876–82.
13. Nadel ER, Bullard RW, Stolwijk JA. Importance of skin temperature in the regulation of sweating. J Appl Physiol 1971; 31: 80–7.
14. Lonsdale-Eccles A, Leonard N, Lawrence C. Axillary hyperhidrosis: eccrine or apocrine? Clin Exp Dermatol 2003; 28: 2–7.
15. Muller SA, Kierland RR. The use of a modified starch-iodine test for investigation of local sweating responses to intradermal injection of methacholine. J Invest Dermatol 1959; 32: 126–8.
16. Sato KT, Richardson A, Timm DE, Sato K. One-step iodine starch method for direct visualization of sweating. Am J Med Sci 1988; 295: 528–31.
17. Solomon BA, Hayman R. Botulinum toxin A therapy for palmar and digital hyperhidrosis. J Am Acad Dermatol 2000; 42: 1026–9.
18. Heckmann M, Breit S, Ceballos-Baumann A, Schaller M, Plewig G. Side-controlled intradermal injection of botulinum toxin A in recalcitrant axillary hyperhidrosis. J Am Acad Dermatol 1999; 41: 987–90.

19. Oberg PA, Hammarlund K, Nilsson GE et al. Measurement of water transport through the skin. Ups J Med Sci 1981; 86: 23–6.

20. Wada M, Takagaki T. A simple and accurate method for detecting the secretion of sweat. Tohoku J Exp Med 1998; 49: 284.

21. Harris DR, Polk F, Willis I. Evaluating sweat gland activity with imprint techniques. J Invest Dermatol 1972; 58: 78–84.

22. Braune G, Erbguth F, Burklein F. Dose thresholds and duration of local anhidrotic effect of botulinum toxin injections: measured by sudometry. Br J Dermatol 2001; 144: 111–17.

23. Gomez DS, Mariani U, Leirner A et al. A new method for scoring active sweat glands. Clinics 2005; 60: 505–6.

24. Ohhashi T, Sakaguchi M, Tsuda T. Human perspiration measurement. Physiol Meas 1998; 19: 449–61.

25. Finlay AY. Quality of life measurement in dermatology: a practical guide. Br J Dermatol 1997; 136: 305–14.

26. Naumann MK, Hamm H, Lowe NJ. Effect of botulinum toxin type A on quality of life measures in patients with excessive axillary sweating: a randomized controlled trial. Br J Dermatol 2002; 147: 1218–26.

27. Heckmann M, Teichmann B, Pause BM, Plewig G. Amelioration of body odor after intracutaneous axillary injection of botulinum toxin A. Arch Dermatol 2003; 139: 57–9.

7 Anesthesia in dermatology

Catherine Wintrebert

The practice of dermato-surgery is expanding with, consequently, an increasing need for anesthesia. Anesthesia in plastic surgery relies on all available techniques: local anesthesia (topical and subcutaneous), locoregional anesthesia, and general anesthesia.

Dermato-surgery can be performed as an outpatient procedure in the dermatologist's office, or in the office-based surgery setting. In this setting only local or distal locoregional anesthesia can be used, since other major plexus anesthesia and general anesthesia have to be performed by a board-certified anesthesiologist (French law 5 December 2005).

Local anesthesia

Local anesthesia is frequently used but is not devoid of risks, and implies:

- knowledge of pharmacology of the drugs used
- knowledge of locoregional anatomy
- knowledge of potential complications and their treatment
- appropriate organization of the office
- appropriate selection of and information given to the patient.

How it works

A local anesthetic is a drug which reversibly blocks the transmission of peripheral nerve impulses. Local anesthetics work by blocking membrane depolarization. Since they are injected near their sites of action, only peripheral nerves should be exposed to concentrations sufficient to produce a significant effect, but if they reach other organs via the circulation then their function will also be affected.

Local anesthetics conform to a common structural arrangement consisting of a benzene ring attached to an amine group by an intermediate chain, which incorporates either an ester or an amide linkage. The esters include chloroprocaine, cocaine, procaine, and tetracaine. (Because of its systemic toxicity and tendency to produce allergic reactions, cocacine has no place in anesthesia.) The amides include lidocaine, mepivacaine, prilocaine, etidocaine, bupivacaine, ropivacaine, and levobupivacaine.

Lidocaine is today the standard agent against which all other local anesthetics are compared (Table 7.1). It has been used safely for all types of local anesthesia. It is of moderate strength, and complications are rare and usually preceded by prodromes.

Bupivacaine is a stronger anesthetic, but complications are serious and can be cardiac and neurological, which may occur simultaneously. Ropivacaine, however, an enantiomer of bupivacaine, is a safer drug.

The pharmacokinetics is affected:

- by the dose, the concentration, and the method of administration
- by the local distribution, which depends on the site and blood supply
- by the absorption, which varies with the amount of adipose tissue and with the blood flow.

The maximal tolerable dose varies with the speed of injection and the site of absorption, and cutaneous infiltration leads to a weak plasma concentration. Absorption may be reduced by the addition of a vasoconstrictor such as epinephrine; this will allow the safe dose to be increased by 50–100%.

Several factors affect the rate of onset, potency, duration of action, and toxicity. Onset time will be decreased, and duration increased, by the use of a larger dose. The dose may be increased by increasing volume or concentration.

One of the most important decisions to be made when using a local technique is how much of a particular drug is to be injected. For lidocaine, the concentrations that are adequate to produce analgesia for skin incision are:

- infiltration: 0.5%
- minor nerve block: 1.0%
- plexus block: 1.5%
- epidural: 2.0%.

A vial of lidocaine 2% (2 mg per 100 ml) holds 400 mg in 20 ml; a vial of lidocaine 1% (1 mg per 100 ml) holds 200 mg in 20 ml; and a vial of lidocaine 0.5% (500 mg per 100 ml) holds 100 mg in 20 ml.

Topical anesthesia

Local anesthesia is delivered by superficial injection but can also be topical.

Table 7.1 Maximum tolerable doses of local anesthetics

	Lidocaine	Bupivacaine	Ropivacaine	Mepivacaine
Total maximum	200–500 mg	150 mg	200–300 mg	400 mg
Neurotoxicity	5–7 mg/kg	—	—	10 mg/kg
Cardiotoxicity	14 mg/kg	4 mg/kg	—	12 mg/kg
With epinephrine	10 mg/kg	2.5 mg/kg	—	—
Without epinephrine	7 mg/kg	2 mg/kg	4 mg/kg	—

Topical anesthesia in the form of EMLA® cream is an association of lidocaine and prilocaine in equal proportions. It is largely used as local anesthesia on normal skin before laser application to assist debridement of ulcers. It is also used on genital mucosa. In children it can be used before local infiltration of anesthetic or other painful perfusion or infiltration (except immunization).

Adverse events in relation to local anesthesia

Although adverse events are infrequent, they must be recognized so as to treat them efficiently. Most often they are the following:

1. Vagal overactivity is suspected in the case of syncope, yawning, hypersialorrhea, nausea, sweats, or pallor. The presence of bradycardia and hypotension confirms the diagnosis. Injection must be interrupted, and the physician should talk to the patient, raise the lower limbs, and, if necessary, administer atropine (10 µg/kg). This is by far the most frequent adverse event. It can be very impressive, with true syncope evidencing a low cerebral blood output.
2. Allergic adverse events are infrequent; true allergy secondary to local anesthetics of the amide family (lidocaine, bupivacaine, ropivacaine, mepivacaine) are exceptional. In most cases, allergic reaction is related to adjuvants such as parabene and, more often, sodium metabisulfite used for stabilizing adrenaline-containing solutions. They can present as a true hypersensitivity: urticaria, Quincke's edema, bronchospasm, or anaphylactic shock, or hyperreactivity, especially in asthmatic patients with Fernand–Widal syndrome; in these patients, adrenalinized lidocaine should not be used. Allergic side-effects due to local anesthetics of the ester family are more frequent, especially with para-aminobenzoic acid (chlorococaine, cocaine, procaine, tetracaine), but these are not widely used in France.
3. Systemic toxic side-effects are observed when plasma levels exceed toxic thresholds after an involuntary intravascular injection or an overdose. They are related to the concentration and the injection speed. The single most important factor in the prevention of toxicity is the avoidance of accidental intravenous injection. This can be prevented by using thin needles, by slow injection with repeated aspiration tests, after calculation of the maximum dose as a function of the patient's weight, and by keeping talking to the patient. Lidocaine toxicity can be detected by neurological symptoms which appear before cardiac symptoms, which gives a safety margin. Bupivacaine toxicity is evidenced by cardiac symptoms first, and is difficult to treat. Neurotoxicity is evidenced by logorrhea, distal limb tremor, a metallic taste, and ear ringing, and convulsions may appear quickly. Neurological events are frequent and easy to treat. In contrast, cardiac events are infrequent and severe, especially in elderly or American Society of Anesthesiologists (ASA) 3 or 4 patients. They are evidenced by ventricular rhythm or conduction abnormalities and sometimes by asystolia.

It is therefore mandatory to optimize the organization of the private practice and to established standard operating procedures for equipment maintenance and patient selection.

Basic equipment must be regularly checked:

- sphygmomanometer, saturometer, stethoscope
- oxygen bottle with debit-reducing valve and debit measurement, vacuum source (AGA, Air Liquide), and maintenance contract
- aspiration tubes, oropharyngeal cannulae
- Ambu®, facial mask
- emergency drugs: adrenaline (epinephrine;Ana-Gard®), atropine, ephedrine, Rivotril®, Solu-Medrol®, salbutamol
- a phone to call for help in case of serious problems, since initial treatment is given at the private practice.

Anamnesis allows patient selection. The physician asks about previous allergy or previous malaise, evaluates the general condition, and classifies the patient according to the ASA scale. Effort resistance must be evaluated as well as usual contraindications, taking into account that relative contraindications are known allergy, uncontrolled epilepsia, auriculoventricular conduction disorders, and porphyria.

Contraindications to adrenaline are unstable angina, recent myocardial infarction, tight aortic stenosis, obstructive cardiomyopathies, and severe hypertensive cardiomyopathy.

Patient information on the potential risks has legal implications. The Sargos case court decision (Court of Cassation 25 February 1997) indicates that the physician has to give evidence of proper information. The 9 June 1998 court decision imposes that the patient is informed of exceptional risks. Patients must be informed of the benefit to risk ratio.

One should be able to treat complications:

- oxygen therapy 100%
- convulsions: Rivotril 1 mg
- when necessary atropine, adrenaline, in order to establish satisfactory hemodynamic situation
- before all a simple procedure: lay the patient down with raised lower limbs and, if the table permits, in the Trendelenburg position.

Local anesthesia in liposuction

Local anesthesia is widely used in liposuction. Doses for liposuction are significantly larger than for other procedures because of the need to inflitrate the subcutaneous tissues with a large volume of Ringer's or saline solution containing lidocaine and epinephrine. The slow absorption of the drug in the adipose tissue is mainly due to vasoconstriction, and allows the use of doses up to 10–35 mg/kg in selected cases.

Lidocaine has been incriminated in several deaths associated with liposuction. An investigation headed by Ronald E Iverson has led to the following recommendations which reflect the collective opinion of the American Society of Plastic Surgeons.

The solution used for liposuction consists of Ringer's or saline with epinephrine, associated or not with lidocaine. There are several techniques. The wet technique involves the injection of 200–300 ml of solution. The super wet technique uses higher volumes, 1 ml of solution per ml of aspirated adipose tissue. The tumescent technique uses 3–4 ml of a solution of saline or Ringer's with 1% lidocaine and adrenaline.

Severe complications have been linked to overdoses of lidocaine, leading to a decrease in the use of this drug.

Current practice recommends the use of the wet technique, using lidocaine 30–50 ml of 1% and epinephrine 1 mg per liter of Ringer's or saline.

It is important to keep in mind that, when associated with epinephrine, lidocaine can reach its peak concentration 10–12, sometimes 24, hours after drug administration when the patient has already returned home.

Patient management needs to take into consideration risk factors linked to obesity, such as thromboembolism, but also the risks inherent to this type of surgery such as volume overload, fatty embolism, and lidocaine overdose. Multifocal procedures often requested by the patient increase the risks by increasing the duration of the surgery.

Locoregional anesthesia

Locoregional anesthesia allows a more efficient anesthesia of larger anatomic regions. Injection is done in the vicinity of a nerve or plexus or ganglion. Anesthesia of a major plexus (cervical, brachial, sacral) can only be performed in the operating room by a board-certified anesthesist (French law 5 December 1994).

More distal locoregional anesthesia such as trigeminal or at the wrist or ankle level can be done in an office setting, and is helpful for procedures on the sole of the foot and palm. Because these injections are often perivascular it is fundamental to control the extravascular nature of the injection and to use thin needles, 23G. For the sites described below, 5 ml of lidocaine is usually sufficient. Paresthesias are not needed.

Tibial nerve block allows anesthesis of the sole of the foot. Puncture is made along the posterior aspect of the inner malleolus, posterior to the tibial posterior artery, the needle in cephalad position, parallel to the Achilles tendon. Another approach is perpendicular infiltration just inferior to the tip of the malleolus in the direction of the toes, just before the contact with the bone.

Innervation of the hand is very complex. Sensitivity is given by terminal branches of the median, ulnar, radial, musculocutaneous, and median cutaneous nerves. Ulnar and median nerve block affects the palm. Ulnar block is performed through a puncture site the width of two or three fingers above the wrist along the anterior cubital tendon, the needle parallel to the direction of the tendon at a depth of 0.5–1.5 cm. Median nerve block is performed through a puncture in the space between the palmar tendons, the needle inserted distally, parallel to the axis of the long palmar tendon, 15–30° to the skin surface.

General anesthesia sedation

From the mild, awake, intravenous sedation to stronger sedations, in France all these techniques are connected with the rules of general anesthetic.

In conjunction with local anesthetic, sedation allows the performance of many procedures in plastic surgery within the framework of the day surgery, called ambulatory in France. From the viewpoint of both the surgeon and the patient it can be more reassuring than general anesthesia in that the patient is easily awakeable and the surgeon does not need to resort to ventilation techniques. It can be desired by some patients and feared by others, and will be an important point discussed during the anesthetic consultation.

The level of sedation can vary during the same intervention according to operating time, and this requires careful attention because any increase in sedation entails a risk of respiratory depression.

Although deep sedation has been a widely used technique, it is at present supplanted by the new techniques of general anesthesia, which ensure control of the airway, ventilation, and blood dynamics. Furthermore, the increasing demands of complex esthetic procedures often lead to the choice of general anesthesia.

Patients require perfect anesthetic and surgical practices and fear bad experiences during operations, whether they come from being in an uncomfortable position or from being cold besides those related to a painful event, or a surgical or anesthetic mishap: comfort and safety are required. The safety of the procedure is most important, and it is in pursuit of this that we keep modifying our practices by improving them after evaluation.

Whether mild sedation, deeper sedation, or general anesthetic, since the anesthetist participates in a surgical act, the modalities of anesthesia must follow the law of 5 December 1994. The legal aspects are as follows. For any patient whose health requires a general or locoregional anesthetic, the care centers must guarantee:

- a pre-anesthetic consultation when dealing with programmed interventions
- the necessary means for performing the anesthesia
- continuous observation after the intervention
- a system able to deal with, at any time, a complication linked to the intervention or to the performed anesthetic.

It is during the pre-anesthetic consultation that the evaluation and informing of the patient take place and the choice of a particular anesthetic in line with the surgical procedure is made.

It is of fundamental importance to correctly evaluate the patient's state, especially in those types of intervention where the patient has a dynamic profile that leads them to forget or disregard their health history. This might result in underestimating or belittling the risk of the intervention.

Adverse antecedents are sought, especially allergies, asthma, heart disease, coronary insufficiency, and other antecedents including pulmonary, hypertension-related, digestion-related, hemorrhagic, or thrombotic, or family antecedents.

Medications are considered, including those that must not be stopped, such as most antihypertension and antiangina drugs, and those that are to be paused several days before surgery, such as used for antiplatelet aggregation, as advised by a cardiovascular specialist.

The profile of the patient is determined: age, weight, height, and body mass index, keeping an eye on those patients above 30 kg/m² (overweight).

Cardiac function is evaluated with an emphasis on the ability to sustain effort. Any coronary syndrome is sought, as well as arterial hypertension. Asthma is investigated and equilibrated if found. Criteria for difficult intubations are researched: Mallampati's score, distance between the chin and the thyroid, mouth opening, snoring.

Overweight patients incur higher risks, and for these patients an in depth evaluation of all risks will have to be performed: cardiac, thromboembolic, respiratory, sleep apnea, difficult intubation. Once ascertained, these risks will have to be explained to the patient.

At the end of this consultation, the patient's state of health can be classified according to the ASA scale:

- ASA 1: normal, healthy patient
- ASA 2: patient with a moderate systemic pathology (equilibrated diabetes, controlled hypertension, anemia, chronic bronchitis, morbid obesity)
- ASA 3: patient with a severe systemic pathology, limiting activity (angina BPCO, IDM ATCD)
- ASA 4: patient whose life prognosis is permanently endangered by a severe pathology (cardiac insufficiency, renal insufficiency)
- ASA 5: patient whose life expectancy does not exceed 24 hours.

It is common practice to restrict plastic surgery to patients with a rating of ASA 1 or ASA 2. However, ASA 3 patients can be accepted under special conditions: their pathology must be stabilized by appropriate treatment, and the intervention must be as quick as possible and must not entail added constraints such as hypothermia or exaggerated positions. There must also exist an agreement between the surgeon and the anesthesiologist.

The consequences of anesthesia on the main functions are numerous:

Ventilation:

- ventilatory depression (anesthetic)
- atelectasia
- trouble swallowing
- depression of the cough reflex (morphinic)
- complications: OAP, laryngospasm, inhalation
- hypoxemia.

Circulation:

• prevention of excessive hypotension.

Hypoxemia and hypotension, if not dealt with quickly, may bring about low cerebral circulation and severe neurological problems.

Nevertheless, the safety of anesthesia has been improving since the 1980s. For patients ranked ASA 1 or ASA 2, the mean anesthetic risk is lower than one death for 100 000 anesthesias, the probability of post-surgery death being linked with the pathological state of the patient and the type of surgery.

8 History

Bernard Rossi

Over the past 25 years, our opinion of botulinum toxin has been changing. Botulinum toxin fascinates us. It is the deadliest poison known, most commonly encountered as a source of food poisoning, a poison sending shivers down our spines as a possible biological weapon, but providing hope and relief for the numerous victims of mysterious neurological conditions characterized by excessive and most often painful muscular contractions. It is able to rejuvenate our faces, but on the other hand, aerosolized or food-borne botulinum toxin could be used as a biological weapon against a civilian population.

This ambiguity, that botulinum toxin is at the same time, but not in the same place and in the same hands, a poison, a medicine, and a weapon, is a disturbing idea.

Botulinum toxin is now well known, but it has a very long history.

In AD 800, Emperor Leo VI of Byzantine forbade sausage manufacture. In 1793, a large outbreak of food poisoning occurred in Wildbad, Germany, due to the consumption of contaminated blood sausages. Hygiene standards of food production were enacted.

The Napoleonic wars brought about a decline in hygiene standards, and in 1817–1822, Justinus Kerner, a German poet and physician, identified 155 cases of food poisoning. Muller, another German physician, later described the collective symptoms as 'Kerner's disease'. In 1822 Kerner identified a fatty acid substance that he called 'sausage poison', and he published ideas for the therapeutic use of this poison to treat diseases associated with an overactive nervous system.

In 1895, during an outbreak of food poisoning due to contaminated preserved ham, Professor Emile Pierre van Ermengem, of Ellezelles, Belgium, identified the bacterium *Bacillus botulinus* (later called *Clostridium botulinum*) as the causative agent for botulism.

In 1928, Dr Herman Sommer at the University of California San Francisco isolated botulinum neurotoxin in purified form as a stable acid precipitate.

During World War II, many countries were engaged in biowarfare programs. In the USA, the National Academy of Sciences and Fred Baldwin, a bacteriologist of the University of Wisconsin, decided to set up laboratories at Camp (later Fort) Detrick, Maryland, for biowarfare research. One serviceman would soon become famous: Dr Edward Schantz.

In 1949, Burgen discovered that botulinum toxin blocked the neurotransmitter at the neuromuscular junction. In 1950, Vernon Brooks located the blockage of acetylcholine release at motor nerve endings.

In 1970, due to the 'International Biological and Toxin Weapons Convention Treaty', Fort Detrick closed its laboratories. Schantz moved to the University of Wisconsin to continue his work.

In 1960, Dr Alan B Scott appeared in the story of botulinum toxin. Alan B Scott, of the Smith-Kettlewell Eye Research Foundation, first had the idea that small doses of botulinum toxin injected directly into overactive muscles might be used to treat patients with strabismus (crossed eyes). Schantz and Scott tested botulinum toxin A in monkeys, to determine its effectiveness. Then, in 1970, Dr Scott formed a company called Oculinum to promote botulinum toxin A therapy. In 1978, the Food and Drug Administration (FDA) authorized Dr Scott to test botulinum toxin A in human volunteers.

In 1981, Dr John Elston, a British physician, treated strabismus and blepharospasm with Dysport®, a botulinum toxin A produced by CAMR (Center for Applied Micobiology and Research). A multicenter clinical trial (over 7000 patients) was carried out in 1982 to test botulinum toxin A for the treatment of strabismus.

In 1987, Dr Alastair Carruthers, a Canadian dermatologist, used botulinum toxin type A to remove wrinkles from Cathy Bickerton Swann, his receptionist.

In 1988, Allergan purchased the rights to use botulinum toxin from Oculinum, and began clinical trials for other toxin indications. In 1989, the FDA gave approval for the treatment of strabismus, blepharospasm, and hemifacial spasm associated with dystonia in patients 12 years of age and older. In 1990, in the UK approval was given for Dysport (Porton) for the indication of blepharospasm. Speywood bought Porton, and later, Ipsen bought Speywood.

In 1990, Heiner Niemann of Germany determined the DNA sequence of botulinum toxin. It was also shown to have homology with the family of zinc dependent proteases.

In 1991, Allergan bought the Oculinum company and botulinum toxin A took the name of BOTOX®.

In 1992, synaptobrevin/VAMP (vesicle-associated membrane protein) was identified as a molecular target of botulinum toxin type B. Then, in 1993, the role of synaptobrevin, syntaxin, and SNAP-25 (synapto-some-associated protein of 25 kDa) in synaptic vesicle transmission was specified; synaptobrevin was found to reside on the vesicle, while syntaxin and SNAP-25 reside on the plasma membrane. Syntaxin and SNAP-25 are molecular targets of botulinum toxin C and botulinum toxin A, respectively.

In 1997, the FDA approved a new bulk toxin source for use in the manufacture of botulinum toxin A (BTX-A). The new product, called current BOTOX, is comparable in clinical efficacy to the 'original' BOTOX, but a significant decrease of neurotoxin protein utilized leads to a reduction in the production of antibodies.

In 2000 the FDA approved BOTOX (Allergan, botulinum toxin type A) and Myobloc® (Elan Pharmaceuticals, botulinum toxin type B; named NeuroBloc in Europe) for the treatment of abnormal head position and neck pain associated with cervical dystonia.

In 2001, the UK and Canada gave approval for BOTOX (BTX-A) for axillary hyperhidrosis (excessive sweating). Canada also approved BOTOX (BTX-A) for focal muscle spasticity, and for cosmetic treatment of wrinkles at the browline.

In 2002 the FDA approved BOTOX (BTX-A) for cosmetic treatment of wrinkles at the browline. Clinical trials with BOTOX, Dysport, and Myobloc were under way for other indications such as cerebral palsy, migraine, and chronic back pain.

In 2003, French approval was given for Vistabel® for cosmetic treatment of glabellar furrows, and BOTOX for axillary hyperhidrosis.

In 2006 BOTOX or Vistabel were in use or under study as a treatment in more than 75 countries in 17 different kinds of indications, and Dysport in 70 countries.

In the future we will see more botulinum toxin A preparations on the market, and we must rank the different preparations and distinguish innovation from marketing. Also, the use of botulinum toxin A must be reserved for experienced physicians, otherwise the reputation of this powerful tool of esthetic medicine will be harmed.

9A Structure, pharmacology, and immunology of the botulinum neurotoxins

K Roger Aoki

Introduction

Botulinum toxin type A has been used for more than two decades in the treatment of strabismus and focal dystonias – movement disorders characterized by excessive, uncontrollable muscle activity.[1–3] Cosmetic use of botulinum toxin type A was reported as early as 1989 in the correction of facial asymmetry caused by facial nerve paralysis.[4] Later studies reported the beneficial effects of botulinum toxin type A for hyperfunctional facial lines.[5,6]

In the treatment of hyperfunctional facial lines, botulinum toxin type A acts by inhibiting acetylcholine release at the neuromuscular junction.[7] Its utility in facial esthetics is derived from its specific action on acetylcholine release and its localized action in the injected muscle(s). When the neurotoxin escapes from the intended muscles, unwanted weakness can occur in nearby muscles, leading to side-effects such as ptosis when treating blepharospasm. Reversibility of action is also an important therapeutic feature of botulinum neurotoxins. Even though the temporary action of botulinum neurotoxins necessitates return visits for retreatment, it allows clinicians the flexibility to refine doses and injection sites based on clinical presentation.

Botulinum neurotoxins are biological products, derived from bacteria, which are purified and processed in a series of complex steps unique to each manufacturer. These steps are critical in determining the clinical features of the botulinum neurotoxin product. In this review, the synthesis, structure, and manufacturing processes for various botulinum neurotoxins are described. The pharmacology and immunology are then considered for various botulinum neurotoxin products. A major theme of this review is that botulinum neurotoxin products are not simply interchangeable, because each is manufactured using a unique process, including synthesis by different bacteria, specific isolation and purification procedures, and the addition of distinct types and amounts of excipients.

Synthesis and structure

Botulinum neurotoxins are synthesized by anaerobic bacteria of the *Clostridium* genus, which derive their name from the Greek word *closter* or spindle, in reference to their sporulating shape.[8] The bacteria synthesize the neurotoxin protein as part of a protein complex that contains several hemagglutinin (HA) and/or non-toxin non-hemagglutinin (NTNH) proteins.[9] Different bacterial strains synthesize complexes that vary in size and protein composition, as well as neurotoxin serotype.[9]

To date, seven different botulinum neurotoxin serotypes (A, B, C1, D, E, F, and G) and three different sizes of protein complexes have been reported in the literature. The serotype and protein complex size appear to co-vary, such that each serotype is associated with a specific set of complex sizes. All of the serotypes form the smallest complex, which is approximately 300 kDa and is referred to in older literature as M or 12S toxin.[9] Serotypes A, B, C1, and hemagglutinin-positive D form the intermediate complex size of approximately 500 kDa, referred to in older literature as L or 16S toxin.[9] Type A is the only serotype that forms the largest complex of approximately 900 kDa, formerly LL or 19S toxin.[9]

Despite the variability in complex sizes, all of the bacterial strains produce single-chain neurotoxin proteins of approximately 150 kDa. This protein must be cleaved or nicked by proteases into disulfide linked di-chain molecules consisting of heavy and light chains of approximately 100 and 50 kDa, respectively, to exert its biological activity.[10,11] Some bacterial strains possess the proteolytic enzymes for this cleavage, whereas others do not.[9] Toxin produced from non-proteolytic organisms such as those that synthesize serotype E can be cleaved in vitro by trypsin.[12]

Manufacture of commercial botulinum neurotoxin products

The first botulinum neurotoxin product (now known as BOTOX®; Allergan, Inc) was developed for therapeutic

Table 9A.1 Differences in the manufacturing processes for commercially available botulinum neurotoxins. Data from references 25, 27, 29–32

	BOTOX®, BOTOX® Cosmetic/Vistabel®/ Vistabex®	Dysport®, Reloxin®	NeuroBloc®, Myobloc®	Xeomin® (NT201)
Clostridial strain	Hall (Allergan) strain	NA	Bean strain	NA
Neurotoxin complex protein size after purification	900 kDa	500 kDa, but heterogeneous	500–700 kDa	150 kDa toxin separated from complex
Excipients	900 µg sodium chloride, 500 µg serum albumin	2.5 mg lactose, 125 µg serum albumin	0.1 mol/l sodium chloride, 0.05% serum albumin, 0.01 mol/l sodium succinate	Serum albumin, sucrose (amounts NA)
Stabilization	Vacuum dried	Freeze dried	Buffered solution (pH ~5.6)	Lyophilized
Unit determination (diluent used)	Saline	Gelatin phosphate buffer	NA	NA

NA, not available.

use in the late 1970s.[1] Since then, a number of additional botulinum neurotoxin products have become commercially available. Most of these products are based on the A serotype, but one product contains the B serotype.[13,14] The effects of several other serotypes have been examined in humans, but none of these is available for commercial use. These include type F,[15,16] type E,[17,18] and type C1.[19]

Because botulinum neurotoxins are biological products, their manufacturing processes do not consist of a standardized set of chemical reactions. Indeed, each botulinum neurotoxin product is manufactured by a unique process – even those containing the same serotype. Although the manufacture of botulinum neurotoxins generally follows the series of steps outlined by Professor Schantz[20] for the original therapeutic product (BOTOX®), there are many possible methods available for each step that can ultimately affect the clinical profile of the therapeutic product.[21]

The manufacture of botulinum neurotoxins begins with synthesis of the neurotoxin complex protein by bacteria. The many different strains of *C. botulinum* determine the serotype, neurotoxin complex protein size, proteolytic activity, and other factors.[8,9] During this step, proteolytic bacterial strains activate the single-chain neurotoxin molecule.[20] The percentage activation of the neurotoxin depends on the bacterial strain.[22,23] Botulinum toxin type A is recovered from cultures approximately 95% nicked.[24] For strains with a naturally low percentage of nicked toxin, such as some strains of type B,[23] the manufacturing process may be modified to increase nicking to approximately 80%.[25,26] A high percentage of nicked or active neurotoxin is believed to be important, because inactive, single-chain neurotoxin may contribute to the overall protein content of the product without increasing its activity or effectiveness. The other factors determined by the bacterial strain – serotype and neurotoxin

complex protein size – are also likely to affect the clinical profile of botulinum neurotoxins, as discussed in the 'Pharmacology' section.

Once the neurotoxin complex protein has been synthesized by the bacteria, it must be isolated and purified. Purification of the first botulinum neurotoxin was described as a series of acid precipitation steps followed by extraction and crystallization.[20] In order to obtain approval for clinical use in the United States, Europe, Japan, and several other countries, the neurotoxin complex must be isolated and purified from the bacterial media using state of the art, pharmaceutical techniques and facilities to meet current Good Manufacturing Practices (GMP). Botulinum toxin type A manufactured by Allergan, Inc (BOTOX®, BOTOX® Cosmetic, Vistabel®, Vistabex®) contains the 900-kDa neurotoxin complex protein.[27] The botulinum toxin type A manufactured by Ipsen (Dysport® or Reloxin®) also contains the 500-kDa complex, but contains a heterogeneous mixture of complexes based on the separation procedures used during the purification phase.[28,29] The type B preparation appears to contain a 500–700-kDa complex.[25] Most of the commercially available botulinum neurotoxin preparations retain the natural protein complex structure, including the neurotoxin and its associated non-neurotoxin proteins (Table 9A.1). In one of the commercial preparations, however, the non-neurotoxin proteins are separated from the neurotoxin.[30] The worldwide availabilities of these products differ but continue to expand.

Next, excipients are added to the preparations that serve to stabilize the neurotoxin during dilution and drying.[20,33] The excipients vary among different botulinum neurotoxin products (Table 9A.1). The only ingredient common to all is serum albumin, but it is present in different amounts depending on the product (Table 9A.1). Increasing the amount of albumin has been found to alter the potency of one of the botulinum neurotoxin preparations (Dysport) in an open-label clinical study.[34] Additionally, a preclinical study found that the biological potencies of two of the type A preparations (BOTOX and Dysport) were differentially influenced by a variety of diluents.[35]

After the addition of excipients, the botulinum neurotoxin products must be stabilized. Each of the commercial preparations is stabilized using a different method: vacuum drying, freeze drying, or lyophilization (Table 9A.1). The type B preparation is stabilized in a buffered low pH (5.6) solution.[25] It is possible that the buffered low pH solution may be responsible for reports of pain on injection with type B.[13,14]

A final step in the manufacture of botulinum neurotoxins is potency testing. Because botulinum neurotoxins are biological products, their doses are given in units of biological activity instead of weight of active ingredient. In order to verify the number of units contained within a given amount of product, the biological activities of botulinum neurotoxin preparations are tested after production. For all botulinum neurotoxin preparations, one unit is defined as the median biological response after an intraperitoneal dose at 72 h in female Swiss Webster mice weighing 18–20 g. However, unlike other biological products, botulinum neurotoxins do not have an international reference standard. This has resulted in unit differences among therapeutic preparations. Unit doses vary not only among preparations containing different serotypes,[13,14,36,37] but also among those containing the same serotype.[38] In response to the differences in unit doses among products, regulatory agencies in Europe, the United States, and many other countries require statements on the product labels indicating that 'units of [specific product] are specific to the preparation and are not interchangeable with other preparations of botulinum toxin'.[31] The differences in unit potency may be due to serotype, diluent (e.g. gelatin phosphate buffer versus saline[20]), or other factors.

Overall, the biological nature of botulinum neurotoxins translates into complex manufacturing processes that vary among different products. From the different bacterial strains used to the different methods of stabilization, each process is unique and results in a botulinum neurotoxin preparation that is non-interchangeable with the others. Although this is probably most evident to clinicians in the different doses required for some of the products, it is also likely reflected in the drugs' diffusion/side-effect profiles, as will be discussed in the next section.

Pharmacology

Mechanism of action

The classic mode of action of botulinum neurotoxins is the inhibition of acetylcholine release at the neuromuscular junction. This inhibition occurs through a multistep process, generally consisting of binding, internalization, and inactivation of excitation–secretion coupling.[7] We now know that many bacterial toxins act by this general mechanism.[39]

Binding

Botulinum neurotoxins bind to specific, high-affinity acceptors/receptors located on the terminal membranes of cholinergic neurons.[40,41] The acceptor molecules for serotypes A and B are distinct,[41] and the human neuromuscular junction appears to lack acceptors for serotypes D.[42] It is possible that acceptors for the other serotypes are also distinct, but this has not been well studied. The binding step is the point at which the selectivity of action occurs, as botulinum toxin type A (and perhaps other serotypes, although they are not as well studied) inhibits vesicular exocytosis from other neuronal types if the light chain is allowed to access the intracellular compartment.[43–45]

Binding is mediated by the carboxy-terminus of the heavy chain (~100 kDa) subunit.[46] Recent studies have mapped the regions on the heavy chain of botulinum toxin type A responsible for binding to mouse brain synaptosomes.[47] These experiments identified a number of non-competing binding regions within the C-terminal domain of the heavy chain, as well some binding regions within the N-terminal domain of the heavy chain. These studies further showed that some of the binding regions within the C-terminal domain of the heavy chain, particularly within the last half of this region, completely or significantly overlapped with the antigenic regions when the molecule was considered in its three-dimensional structure.[47]

Both synaptotagmins and gangliosides are thought to be part of the botulinum neurotoxin binding structure for some of the serotypes.[48] In PC12 cells and rat diaphragm motor nerve terminals, the entry of botulinum toxin type B (but not type A or E) is mediated by synaptotagmins I and II.[49] Botulinum toxin serotypes A and B have been found to bind a single molecule of ganglioside GT1b, with critical residues located within the carboxy-terminal half of the heavy chain.[50] Although the binding of botulinum neurotoxins appears to involve both synaptotagmins and gangliosides, the entire process is not yet completely clear.[51] Some have suggested that binding may occur at microdomains on the presynaptic membrane,[52] and this hypothesis requires further study.

Internalization and translocation

Once bound to their acceptors, botulinum neurotoxins are endocytosed in vesicles and transported into the neuronal cytosol.[41,53] Internalization in an acidic compartment was hypothesized in early studies based on the finding that drugs which interfered with vesicular acidification antagonized the effects of botulinum neurotoxins.[54] Internalization does not automatically lead to translocation, as evidenced by the different fates of botulinum and tetanus toxins.[51] The low intravesicular pH is believed to be critical in translocating the neurotoxin across the vesicular membrane (summarized in reference 51). It is believed that this leads to a conformational change in the translocation domain of the heavy chain, which facilitates the translocation of the light chain to the cytoplasmic compartment.[51] The exact mechanism of this process is not known, but it has been speculated that the heavy chain can form a pore through which the light chain can pass.[55] The light chain is then exposed to the cytosol, where it can effect proteolysis.

Proteolytic cleavage of SNARE proteins

The light chains of botulinum neurotoxins are zinc-dependent endoproteases containing the conserved His-Glu-Xaa-Xaa-His zinc-binding motif.[56] Inside the cytosol, these enzymes cleave one or more of the SNARE (soluble N-ethylmaleimide-sensitive factor attachment protein receptor) proteins that form the vesicle docking and fusion apparatus.[57] Each botulinum neurotoxin serotype cleaves a specific peptide bond on one or more of the SNARE proteins. For instance, botulinum toxin type A cleaves the synaptosomal associated protein 25 kDa (SNAP-25), whereas botulinum toxin type B cleaves synaptobrevin/vesicle associated membrane protein (VAMP).[58,59] The specific site of action and the SNARE protein cleaved appear to underlie the duration of action of the various botulinum neurotoxin serotypes.[60]

The effects of botulinum neurotoxin are not permanent, and neurotransmission eventually recovers. Botulinum neurotoxin injection is followed by sprouting of nerve endings at the neuromuscular junction.[61,62] These sprouts appear to be responsible for temporary reinnervation during the early recovery phase of neurotransmission.[63] During the later phase of recovery, vesicle turnover (indicative of neuronal exocytosis) returns at the original terminal, accompanied by the retraction of neuronal sprouts.[63]

Additional sites of action

Much of the original research on botulinum neurotoxin mechanism of action was conducted on the neuromuscular junction.[7] However, it has long been known that botulinum neurotoxins also inhibit the release of acetylcholine from autonomic cholinergic terminals.[64] This has formed the basis for the therapeutic use of botulinum neurotoxins in the treatment of hyperhidrosis and other conditions that benefit from reduced autonomic activation.[65] Although it is likely that botulinum neurotoxins act by the same mechanism of action in autonomic and neuromuscular terminals, there may be slight differences that have not been investigated. This is suggested by the longer apparent duration of botulinum

toxin type A in treatment of axillary hyperhidrosis than that of focal dystonias.[36,66,67]

In addition to their effects on neurons that innervate extrafusal muscle fibers, which mediate fast synaptic neurotransmission at the neuromuscular junction, botulinum toxin type A also acts on cholinergic neurons that innervate intrafusal fibers.[68,69] Intrafusal fibers are encapsulated fibers that make up muscle spindles – the proprioceptive organs located among extrafusal, skeletal muscle fibers. Via their influence on intrafusal fibers, botulinum neurotoxins may change the sensory afferent system by reducing the Ia traffic.[68]

Finally, botulinum toxin type A has been found to inhibit the release of certain neuropeptides, including substance P and calcitonin gene-related peptide.[70,71] In addition, botulinum toxin type A has been demonstrated to inhibit experimental pain in rats and prevent the release of glutamate in response to an inflammatory stimulus.[72] Inhibition of a peripheral nociceptive response and reduction of these neuropeptides' release may at least partially mediate the observed effects of botulinum toxin type A in chronic daily headaches such as chronic migraines.[73,74]

Behavioral pharmacology

Therapeutic index

In our laboratory, we have examined the effects of botulinum neurotoxins in a preclinical model designed to determine the therapeutic indices or safety margins of various preparations.[75,76] In this model, a range of doses are injected into the mouse hindlimb muscle and the effects on muscle weakening (lower dose range to determine the median effective dose: ED_{50}) and mortality (higher dose range to determine the intramuscular lethal dose: LD_{50}) are recorded. The ratio of the ED_{50} for local muscle weakening and the LD_{50} following intramuscular injection indicate the separation between an effective dose (ED_{50}) and the dose that leaks out of the muscle to cause a distal effect in mice.

Our results indicate significant differences in the therapeutic indices (intramuscular (IM) LD_{50}/IM ED_{50}) of various botulinum neurotoxin preparations. The highest therapeutic indices have been observed for one of the type A preparations (BOTOX: 13.9 ± 1.7) and type F (16.7 ± 3.9), followed by the other type A preparation (Dysport: 7.6 ± 0.9), and type B (5.4 ± 0.3) (mean + SEM, $n = 4$–6 experiments with 10 mice per dose; significant differences observed between botulinum toxin type A preparations and type A (BOTOX) vs type B (NeuroBloc®)). These data suggest differences in the extent to which botulinum neurotoxin preparations migrate out of the treated muscles and enter the systemic circulation.

These preclinical results are consistent with clinical data showing that botulinum neurotoxin preparations exhibit different rates of adverse events.[77–80] Clinically, adverse events observed with botulinum neurotoxins tend to fall into essentially three groups: those due to expected effects of the neurotoxin (e.g. excessive muscle weakness), those due to diffusion of the neurotoxin to nearby, uninjected muscles (e.g. weakness of adjacent muscle groups), and those due to systemic distribution (e.g. distant muscle weakness). The latter two groups of adverse events are most likely attributable to migration of the neurotoxin out of the treated muscle. Therefore, it is important to have control over the amount of migration that occurs with botulinum neurotoxin injections.

The migration of botulinum neurotoxins outside the target organ depends on the structure of the molecule, the volume of injection, and diffusion. A basic principle of diffusion is that particles with greater molecular weight tend to diffuse more slowly than those of lower molecular weight through an equivalent aqueous medium, provided that charge, temperature, and general molecular structure are the same. This principle predicts that botulinum neurotoxin protein complexes of higher molecular weight will diffuse less than those of lower molecular weight.

Our preclinical results are in line with this principle. Specifically, we found that the therapeutic indices of the two botulinum toxin type A and B preparations were ordered according to their molecular weights: the highest weight preparation (BOTOX) had a higher therapeutic index (i.e. less leakage outside of the target tissue) than that of the heterogeneous preparation (Dysport), which was higher than that of the lowest weight preparation (NeuroBloc).[75,76]

Another recent publication has examined the therapeutic indices of different molecular forms of botulinum toxin type A.[81] This study reported that the lowest molecular weight complex (i.e. 300 kDa) had the highest therapeutic index, followed by the intermediate weight complex, and finally the highest molecular weight complex (900 kDa). These interesting preclinical observations will require replication and additional investigation. These results are counter to what one would expect based on the principles of diffusion, although it is possible that the presence of a hemagglutinin protein, which is contained in the two highest weight but not the lowest weight complex, may alter diffusion kinetics.[81] However, these results also run counter to clinical findings of lower adverse event rates with the 900-kDa complex preparation (BOTOX) than with the heterogeneous complex preparation (Dysport),[79,80,82–85] in addition to the recent report of a statistically significant increase in the frequency of blurred vision with Dysport over placebo in the treatment of cervical dystonia.[86]

Other recent studies have compared the largest botulinum neurotoxin type A complex (900 kDa) to the isolated 150-kDa neurotoxin.[30,87] These studies did not find significant differences in the adverse event profiles of the two preparations. Thus, these early results

also run counter to the basic principles of diffusion, suggesting that other features of the molecule or formulation may influence its migration. However, as the isolated neurotoxin product is used in clinical practice outside of the dosing and patient inclusion constraints of controlled studies, a higher rate of adverse events may be observed, particularly at higher doses. Clinical practice studies may help to clarify this issue as experience with this product accumulates.

Dose–response curves

Full dose–response curves cannot be generated with botulinum neurotoxins in humans for obvious ethical and practical reasons, and, thus, preclinical models are useful in this regard. In our murine model of muscle weakening we found that different botulinum neurotoxin preparations exhibited non-parallel dose–response curves.[75,76] These results indicate that different botulinum neurotoxin preparations behave differently in vivo, which is expected based on their complex biological nature and different manufacturing methods, including the strain of bacteria used for synthesis, serotype, complex protein size, excipients, and formulation.

These results have further implications to refute the concept that botulinum neurotoxin products can be converted using simple dose ratios. The non-parallel nature of the dose–response curves indicates that the dose ratio changes depending on the level of muscle weakening efficacy or side-effect rate specified. For instance, the preclinical ratio of ED_{50} values is not the same as the ratio of LD_{50} values for any two preparations. It is anticipated that the dose–response relationships may vary for each muscle. These results are supported by clinical studies that have found variability in the dose ratios between BOTOX and Dysport and have concluded that there is no simple ratio that can be used to convert between products.[38,84] The different side-effect profiles reported for these products also indicate that, at clinically effective doses, side-effect rates may be different.[80,85]

Immunology

Clinical immunogenicity

As bacterial proteins, botulinum neurotoxins, under specific conditions, can engender an immune response in some individuals that may reduce or abolish therapeutic effectiveness.[88] In clinical practice, neutralizing antibodies are only one possible reason for reduced clinical responsiveness, and often patients who become non-responsive may benefit from alterations in the injection procedures such as dose or location.[89] Testing for antibodies that interfere with clinical response (i.e. neutralizing antibodies) is usually done with the mouse protection assay[90,91] or, more commonly in the clinical setting, the eyebrow or frontalis test.[92]

Neutralizing antibody formation has historically been a concern for patients with conditions such as cervical dystonia that require higher doses, due to a link between dose, or amount of protein, and neutralizing antibody formation.[88] However, refinements in manufacturing procedures have led to very low rates of neutralizing antibody formation with the most-studied botulinum neurotoxin product (BOTOX), even in cervical dystonia.[89,93,94]

A few repeated treatment studies have been conducted with the other type A neurotoxin complex product (Dysport) that have examined neutralizing antibody formation. One recent study of patients treated for spasticity with three injection cycles did not find any neutralizing antibodies.[95] However, neutralizing antibodies to this type A preparation have been reported in several studies of cervical dystonia patients.[96,97] The rate of neutralizing antibody formation may be somewhat higher with the type B preparation (NeuroBloc), as the only study to follow patients treated exclusively with this product found that 44% of nine cervical dystonia patients developed neutralizing antibodies.[98] A basic finding is that higher doses (and resultant higher levels of neurotoxin complex protein) of botulinum neurotoxins are associated with a greater risk of neutralizing antibody formation.[88,90,96,99] For this reason, it would be expected that some botulinum neurotoxin preparations (e.g. Dysport, NeuroBloc) may be associated with an increased risk of neutralizing antibody formation, although comparative studies are needed to determine this unequivocally.

Epitope studies

Immunologic research has been directed at determining the portion of the 150-kDa botulinum neurotoxin molecule(s) that underlies neutralizing antibody formation. Preclinical research has localized the regions (e.g. linear epitopes) recognized by T lymphocytes and antibodies to the C-terminal domain of the botulinum toxin type A heavy chain.[100] More recently, antibody- and T-cell recognition sites have been mapped on the N-terminal portion of the heavy chain.[101] Additional studies have found that immunization with the receptor-binding region of the heavy chain C-terminal (residues 860 to 1296) prevents neurotoxin activity,[102] confirming the importance of this region in the non-response to botulinum toxin type A. Research has also shown that the switch from response to non-response in mice treated with botulinum toxin type A is associated with only slight differences in the epitope-recognition profiles (i.e. levels or affinities of the antibodies that were bound by heavy chain peptides), and these were not believed to be sufficient to mediate the response to non-response switch.[103] Research into the mechanism(s) responsible for the switch to non-response is continuing.

Conclusions

Botulinum toxin type A has been immensely useful in the treatment of selected neurologic and other disorders, and its efficacy and safety in the area of facial esthetics is well supported and accepted.[104] The efficacy and safety of botulinum neurotoxins in the management of hyperfunctional facial lines is a result of their selective inhibition of acetylcholine release in precisely targeted muscles. Distribution of the neurotoxin away from its intended site(s) can lead to unwanted side-effects, and therefore the selection of the botulinum neurotoxin product, dose, dilution, and muscles is critical for attaining optimal patient outcomes.

Botulinum neurotoxins are biological products and, as such, are manufactured in a complex series of steps that are critical in determining the final clinical profiles of the products. The different manufacturing processes used for each botulinum neurotoxin product, including the strain of bacteria used for synthesis, isolation, and purification of the neurotoxin complex, excipients added, method of stabilization, and unit determination procedures, are unique for each therapeutic preparation. These differences result in non-interchangeable products, for which clinical efficacy and safety must be independently determined.

References

1. Scott AB. Botulinum toxin injection into extraocular muscles as an alternative to strabismus surgery. Ophthalmology 1980; 87: 1044–9.
2. Scott AB, Kennedy RA, Stubbs HA. Botulinum A toxin injection as a treatment for blepharospasm. Arch Ophthalmol 1985; 103: 347–50.
3. Tsui JKC, Eisen A, Stoessl AJ, Calne S, Calne DB. Double-blind study of botulinum toxin in spasmodic torticollis. Lancet 1986; 2: 245–7.
4. Clark RP, Berris CE. Botulinum toxin: a treatment for facial asymmetry caused by facial nerve paralysis. Plast Reconstr Surg 1989; 84: 353–5.
5. Carruthers JD, Carruthers JA. Treatment of glabellar frown lines with C. botulinum-A exotoxin. J Dermatol Surg Oncol 1992; 18: 17–21.
6. Blitzer A, Brin MF, Keen MS, Aviv JE. Botulinum toxin for the treatment of hyperfunctional lines of the face. Arch Otolaryngol Head Neck Surg 1993; 119: 1018–22.
7. Simpson LL. The origin, structure, and pharmacological activity of botulinum toxin. Pharmacol Rev 1981; 33: 155–88.
8. Hatheway CL. Bacterial sources of clostridial neurotoxins. In: Simpson LL, ed. Botulinum Neurotoxin and Tetanus Toxin. San Diego: Academic Press, 1989: 3–24.
9. Sakaguchi G, Kozaki S, Ohishi I. Structure and function of botulinum toxins. In: Alouf JE, ed. Bacterial Protein Toxins. London: Academic Press, 1984: 435–43.
10. DasGupta BR. Activation of Clostridium botulinum type B toxin by an endogenous enzyme. J Bacteriol 1971; 108: 1051–7.

11. DasGupta BR, Sugiyama H. Role of a protease in natural activation of Clostridium botulinum neurotoxin. Infect Immun 1972; 6: 587–90.

12. Duff JT, Wright GG, Yarinsky A. Activation of Clostridium botulinum type E toxin by trypsin. J Bacteriol 1956; 72: 455–60.

13. Brashear A, Lew MF, Dykstra DD et al. Safety and efficacy of NeuroBloc (botulinum toxin type B) in type A-responsive cervical dystonia. Neurology 1999; 53: 1439–46.

14. Brin MF, Lew MF, Adler CH et al. Safety and efficacy of NeuroBloc (botulinum toxin type B) in type A-resistant cervical dystonia. Neurology 1999; 53: 1431–8.

15. Mezaki T, Kaji R, Kohara N et al. Comparison of therapeutic efficacies of type A and F botulinum toxins for blepharospasm: a double-blind, controlled study. Neurology 1995; 45: 506–8.

16. Greene PE, Fahn S. Use of botulinum toxin type F injections to treat torticollis in patients with immunity to botulinum toxin type A. Mov Disord 1993; 8: 479–83.

17. Washbourne P, Pellizzari R, Rossetto O et al. On the action of botulinum neurotoxins A and E at cholinergic terminals. J Physiol Paris 1998; 92: 135–9.

18. Eleopra et al. 1998.

19. Eleopra R, Tugnoli V, Rossetto O, Montecucco C, De Grandis D. Botulinum neurotoxin serotype C: a novel effective botulinum toxin therapy in human. Neurosci Lett 1997; 224: 91–4.

20. Schantz EJ, Johnson EA. Properties and use of botulinum toxin and other microbial neurotoxins in medicine. Microbiol Rev 1992; 56: 80–99.

21. Brin MF, Aoki KR, Dressler D. Pharmacology of botulinum toxin therapy. In: Brin MF, Comella C, Jankovic J, eds. Dystonia: Etiology, Clinical Features, and Treatment. Philadelphia: Lippincott, Williams & Wilkins, 2004: 93–112.

22. DasGupta BR, Sugiyama H. A common subunit structure in Clostridium botulinum type A, B and E toxins. Biochem Biophys Res Commun 1972; 48: 108–12.

23. DasGupta BR, Sugiyama H. Molecular forms of neurotoxins in proteolytic Clostridium botulinum type B cultures. Infect Immun 1976; 14: 680–6.

24. DasGupta BR, Sathyamoorthy V. Purification and amino acid composition of type A botulinum neurotoxin. Toxicon 1984; 22: 415–24.

25. Setler P. The biochemistry of botulinum toxin type B. Neurology 2000; 55 (Suppl 5): S22–8.

26. Callaway JE, Arezzo JC, Grethlein AJ. Botulinum toxin type B: an overview of its biochemistry and preclinical pharmacology. Semin Cutan Med Surg 2001; 20: 127–36.

27. Physician's Desk Reference. Botox® (Botulinum Toxin Type A). Montvale, NJ: Thomson PDR, 2003: 552–4.

28. Inoue K, Fujinaga Y, Watanabe T et al. Molecular composition of Clostridium botulinum type A progenitor toxins. Infect Immun 1996; 64: 1589–94.

29. Hambleton P et al. In: Lewis GE et al. Biomedical Aspects of Botulism. New York: Academic Press, 1981: 247–60.

30. Roggenkamper P, Jost WH, Bihari K, Comes G, Grafe S. Efficacy and safety of a new Botulinum toxin type A free of complexing proteins in the treatment of blepharospasm. J Neural Transm 2005; 113: 303–12.

31. Dysport® Product Characteristics. Available at: http://emc.medicines.org.uk/emc/assets/c/html/displaydoc.asp?documentid=870. Accessed July 31, 2005. Ipsen, Ltd, 2004.

32. Physician's Desk Reference. Myobloc® (Botulinum Toxin Type B). Montvale, NJ: Thomson PDR, 2003: 1263–5.

33. Melling J, Hambleton P, Shone CC. Clostridium botulinum toxins: nature and preparation for clinical use. Eye 1988; 2: 16–23.

34. Rollnik JD, Matzke M, Wohlfarth K, Dengler R, Bigalke H. Low-dose treatment of cervical dystonia, blepharospasm and facial hemispasm with albumin-diluted botulinum toxin type A under EMG guidance. An open label study. Eur Neurol 2000; 43: 9–12.

35. McLellan K, Das RE, Ekong TA, Sesardic D. Therapeutic botulinum type A toxin: factors affecting potency. Toxicon 1996; 34: 975–85.

36. Naumann M, Yakovleff A, Durif F; BOTOX Cervical Dystonia Prospective Study Group. A randomized, double-masked, crossover comparison of the efficacy and safety of botulinum toxin type A produced from the original bulk toxin source and current bulk toxin source for the treatment of cervical dystonia. J Neurol 2002; 249: 57–63.

37. Dressler D, Adib Saberi F, Benecke R. Botulinum toxin type B for treatment of axillar hyperhidrosis. J Neurol 2002; 249: 1729–32.

38. Marchetti A, Magar R, Findley L et al. Retrospective evaluation of the dose of Dysport and BOTOX in the management of cervical dystonia and blepharospasm: the REAL DOSE study. Mov Disord 2005; 20: 937–44.

39. Montecucco C, Papini E, Schiavo G. Bacterial protein toxins penetrate cells via a four-step mechanism. FEBS Lett 1994; 346: 92–8.

40. Black JD, Dolly JO. Interaction of 125I-labeled botulinum neurotoxins with nerve terminals. I. Ultrastructural autoradiographic localization and quantitation of distinct membrane acceptors for types A and B on motor nerves. J Cell Biol 1986; 103: 521–34.

41. Black JD, Dolly JO. Interaction of 125I-labeled botulinum neurotoxins with nerve terminals. II. Autoradiographic evidence for its uptake into motor nerves by acceptor-mediated endocytosis. J Cell Biol 1986; 103: 535–44.

42. Coffield JA, Bakry N, Zhang RD et al. In vitro characterization of botulinum toxin types A, C and D action on human tissues: combined electrophysiologic, pharmacologic and molecular biologic approaches. J Pharmacol Exp Ther 1997; 280: 1489–98.

43. O'Sullivan GA, Mohammed N, Foran PG, Lawrence GW, Dolly JO. Rescue of exocytosis in botulinum toxin A-poisoned chromaffin cells by expression of cleavage-resistant SNAP-25. Identification of the minimal essential C-terminal residues. J Biol Chem 1999; 274: 36897–904.

44. Ishikawa H, Mitsui Y, Yoshitomi T et al. Presynaptic effects of botulinum toxin type A on the neuronally evoked response of albino and pigmented rabbit iris sphincter and dilator muscles. Jpn J Ophthalmol 2000; 44: 106–9.

45. Hohne-Zell B, Galler A, Schepp W, Gratzl M, Prinz C. Functional importance of synaptobrevin and SNAP-25 during exocytosis of histamine by rat gastric enterochromaffin-like cells. Endocrinology 1997; 138: 5518–26.

46. Shone CC, Hambleton P, Melling J. Inactivation of Clostridium botulinum type A neurotoxin by trypsin and purification of two tryptic fragments. Proteolytic action near the COOH-terminus of the heavy subunit destroys toxin-binding activity. Eur J Biochem 1985; 151: 75–82.

47. Maruta T, Dolimbek BZ, Aoki KR, Steward LE, Atassi MZ. Mapping of the synaptosome-binding regions on the heavy chain of botulinum neurotoxin A by synthetic overlapping peptides encompassing the entire chain. Protein J 2004; 23: 539–52.

48. Nishiki T, Kamata Y, Nemoto Y et al. Identification of protein receptor for Clostridium botulinum type B neurotoxin in rat brain synaptosomes. J Biol Chem 1994; 269: 10498–503.

49. Dong M, Richards DA, Goodnough MC et al. Synaptotagmins I and II mediate entry of botulinum neurotoxin B into cells. J Cell Biol 2003; 162: 1293–303.

50. Rummel A, Mahrhold S, Bigalke H et al. The HCC-domain of botulinum neurotoxins A and B exhibits a singular

ganglioside binding site displaying serotype specific carbohydrate interaction. Mol Microbiol 2004; 51: 631–43.

51. Grumelli C, Verderio C, Pozzi D et al. Internalization and mechanism of action of clostridial toxins in neurons. Neurotoxicology 2005; 26: 761–7.

52. Montecucco C, Rossetto O, Schiavo G. Presynaptic receptor arrays for clostridial neurotoxins. Trends Microbiol 2004; 12: 442–6.

53. Dolly JO, Black J, Williams RS, Melling J. Acceptors for botulinum neurotoxin reside on motor nerve terminals and mediate its internalization. Nature 1984; 307: 457–60.

54. Simpson LL. The interaction between aminoquinolines and presynaptically acting neurotoxins. J Pharmacol Exp Ther 1982; 222: 43–8.

55. Pellizzari R, Rossetto O, Schiavo G et al. Tetanus and botulinum neurotoxins: mechanism of action and therapeutic uses. Philos Trans R Soc Lond B Biol Sci 1999; 354: 259–68.

56. Schiavo G, Rossetto O, Santucci A, DasGupta BR, Montecucco C. Botulinum neurotoxins are zinc proteins. J Biol Chem 1992; 267: 23479–83.

57. Montecucco C, Schiavo G. Structure and function of tetanus and botulinum neurotoxins. Q Rev Biophys 1995; 28: 423–72.

58. Schiavo G, Benfenati F, Poulain B et al. Tetanus and botulinum-B neurotoxins block neurotransmitter release by proteolytic cleavage of synaptobrevin. Nature 1992; 359: 832–5.

59. Blasi J, Chapman ER, Link E et al. Botulinum neurotoxin A selectively cleaves the synaptic protein SNAP-25. Nature 1993; 365: 160–3.

60. Foran PG, Mohammed N, Lisk GO et al. Evaluation of the therapeutic usefulness of botulinum neurotoxin B, C1, E, and F compared with the long lasting type A. Basis for distinct durations of inhibition of exocytosis in central neurons. J Biol Chem 2003; 278: 1363–71.

61. Duchen LW. Changes in the electron microscopic structure of slow and fast skeletal muscle fibres of the mouse after the local injection of botulinum toxin. J Neurol Sci 1971; 14: 61–74.

62. Angaut-Petit D, Molgo J, Comella JX, Faille L, Tabti N. Terminal sprouting in mouse neuromuscular junctions poisoned with botulinum type A toxin: morphological and electrophysiological features. Neuroscience 1990; 37: 799–808.

63. de Paiva A, Meunier FA, Molgo J et al. Functional repair of motor endplates after botulinum neurotoxin type A poisoning: biphasic switch of synaptic activity between nerve sprouts and their parent terminals. Proc Natl Acad Sci USA 1999; 96: 3200–5.

64. Ambache N. A further survey of the action of Clostridium botulinum toxin upon different types of autonomic nerve fibre. J Physiol 1951; 113: 1–17.

65. Naumann M, Jost W. Botulinum toxin treatment of secretory disorders. Mov Disord 2004; 19 (Suppl 8): S137–41.

66. Naumann MK, Hamm H, Lowe NJ; Botox Hyperhidrosis Clinical Study Group. Effect of botulinum toxin type A on quality of life measures in patients with excessive axillary sweating: a randomized controlled trial. Br J Dermatol 2002; 147: 1218–26.

67. Naumann M, Lowe NJ, Kumar CR, Hamm H; Hyperhidrosis Clinical Investigators Group. Botulinum toxin type a is a safe and effective treatment for axillary hyperhidrosis over 16 months: a prospective study. Arch Dermatol 2003; 139: 731–6.

68. Filippi GM, Errico P, Santarelli R et al. Botulinum A toxin effects on rat jaw muscle spindles. Acta Otolaryngol 1993; 113: 400–4.

69. Rosales RL, Arimura K, Takenaga S et al. Extrafusal and intrafusal muscle effects in experimental botulinum toxin-A injection. Muscle Nerve 1996; 19: 488–96.

70. Welch MJ, Purkiss JR, Foster KA. Sensitivity of embryonic rat dorsal root ganglia neurons to Clostridium botulinum neurotoxins. Toxicon 2000; 38: 245–58.

71. Durham PL, Cady R, Cady R. Regulation of calcitonin gene-related peptide secretion from trigeminal nerve cells by botulinum toxin type A: implications for migraine therapy. Headache 2004; 44: 35–42.

72. Cui M, Khanijou S, Rubino J et al. Subcutaneous administration of botulinum toxin A reduces formalin-induced pain. Pain 2004; 107: 125–33.

73. Dodick DW, Mauskop A, Elkind AH et al; BOTOX CDH Study Group. Botulinum toxin type a for the prophylaxis of chronic daily headache: subgroup analysis of patients not receiving other prophylactic medications: a randomized double-blind, placebo-controlled study. Headache 2005; 45: 315–24.

74. Mathew NT, Frishberg BM, Gawel M et al; BOTOX CDH Study Group. Botulinum toxin type A (BOTOX) for the prophylactic treatment of chronic daily headache: a randomized, double-blind, placebo-controlled trial. Headache 2005; 45: 293–307.

75. Aoki KR. A comparison of the safety margins of botulinum neurotoxin serotypes A, B, and F in mice. Toxicon 2001; 39: 1815–20.

76. Aoki KR. Botulinum neurotoxin serotypes A and B preparations have different safety margins in preclinical models of muscle weakening efficacy and systemic safety. Toxicon 2002; 40: 923–8.

77. Dressler D, Benecke R. Autonomic side effects of botulinum toxin type B treatment of cervical dystonia and hyperhidrosis. Eur Neurol 2003; 49: 34–8.

78. Dressler D. Dysport produces intrinsically more swallowing problems than Botox: unexpected results from a conversion factor study in cervical dystonia. J Neurol Neurosurg Psychiatry 2002; 73: 604.

79. Ranoux D, Gury C, Fondarai J, Mas JL, Zuber M. Respective potencies of Botox and Dysport: a double blind, randomised, crossover study in cervical dystonia. J Neurol Neurosurg Psychiatry 2002; 72: 459–62.

80. Sampaio C, Costa J, Ferreira JJ. Clinical comparability of marketed formulations of botulinum toxin. Mov Disord 2004; 19 (Suppl 8): S129–36.

81. Yoneda S, Shimazawa M, Kato M et al. Comparison of the therapeutic indexes of different molecular forms of botulinum toxin type A. Eur J Pharmacol 2005; 508: 223–9.

82. Lew H, Yun YS, Lee SY, Kim SJ. Effect of botulinum toxin A on facial wrinkle lines in Koreans. Ophthalmologica 2002; 216: 50–4.

83. Nussgens Z, Roggenkamper P. Comparison of two botulinum-toxin preparations in the treatment of essential blepharospasm. Graefes Arch Clin Exp Ophthalmol 1997; 935: 197–9.

84. Dodel RC, Kirchner A, Koehne-Volland R et al. Costs of treating dystonias and hemifacial spasm with botulinum toxin A. Pharmacoeconomics 1997; 12: 695–706.

85. Bihari K. Safety, effectiveness, and duration of effect of BOTOX after switching from Dysport for blepharospasm, cervical dystonia, and hemifacial spasm. Curr Med Res Opin 2005; 21: 433–8.

86. Truong D, Duane DD, Jankovic J et al. Efficacy and safety of botulinum type A toxin (Dysport) in cervical dystonia: results of the first US randomized, double-blind, placebo-controlled study. Mov Disord 2005; 20: 783–91.

87. Benecke R, Jost WH, Kanovsky P et al. A new botulinum toxin type A free of complexing proteins for treatment of cervical dystonia. Neurology 2005; 64: 1949–51.

88. Jankovic J, Schwartz K. Response and immunoresistance to botulinum toxin injections. Neurology 1995; 45: 1743–6.

89. Mejia NI, Vuong KD, Jankovic J. Long-term botulinum toxin efficacy, safety, and immunogenicity. Mov Disord 2005; 20: 592–7.

90. Hatheway CL, Dang C. Immunogenicity of neurotoxins of Clostridium botulinum. In: Jankovic J, Hallett M, eds. Therapy with Botulinum Toxin. New York: Marcel Dekker, 1994: 93–107.

91. Sesardic D, Jones RG, Leung T, Alsop T, Tierney R. Detection of antibodies against botulinum toxins. Mov Disord 2004; 19 (Suppl 8): S85–91.

92. Hanna PA, Jankovic J, Vincent A. Comparison of mouse bioassay and immunoprecipitation assay for botulinum toxin antibodies. J Neurol Neurosurg Psychiatry 1999; 66: 612–16.

93. Jankovic J, Vuong KD, Ahsan J. Comparison of efficacy and immunogenicity of original versus current botulinum toxin in cervical dystonia. Neurology 2003; 60: 1186–8.

94. Yablon SA, Daggett S, Brin MF. Toxin neutralizing antibody formation with botulinum toxin type A (BoNTA) treatment in neuromuscular disorders. Neurology 2005; 64 (Suppl 1): A72.

95. Bakheit AM, Fedorova NV, Skoromets AA et al. The beneficial antispasticity effect of botulinum toxin type A is maintained after repeated treatment cycles. J Neurol Neurosurg Psychiatry 2004; 75: 1558–61.

96. Goschel H, Wohlfarth K, Frevert J, Dengler R, Bigalke H. Botulinum A toxin therapy: neutralizing and nonneutralizing antibodies—therapeutic consequences. Exp Neurol 1997; 147: 96–102.

97. Kessler KR, Skutta M, Benecke R. Long-term treatment of cervical dystonia with botulinum toxin A: efficacy, safety, and antibody frequency. German Dystonia Study Group. J Neurol 1999; 246: 265–74.

98. Dressler D, Bigalke H. Botulinum toxin type B de novo therapy of cervical dystonia Frequency of antibody induced therapy failure. J Neurol 2005; 252: 904–7.

99. Herrmann J, Geth K, Mall V et al. Clinical impact of antibody formation to botulinum toxin A in children. Ann Neurol 2004; 55: 732–5.

100. Rosenberg JS, Middlebrook JL, Atassi MZ. Localization of the regions on the C-terminal domain of the heavy chain of botulinum A recognized by T lymphocytes and by antibodies after immunization of mice with pentavalent toxoid. Immunol Invest 1997; 26: 491–504.

101. Dolimbek GS, Dolimbek BZ, Aoki KR, Atassi MZ. Mapping of the antibody and T cell recognition profiles of the HN domain (residues 449–859) of the heavy chain of botulinum neurotoxin A in two high-responder mouse strains. Immunol Invest 2005; 34: 119–42.

102. Atassi MZ, Oshima M. Structure, activity, and immune (T and B cell) recognition of botulinum neurotoxins. Crit Rev Immunol 1999; 19: 219–60.

103. Atassi MZ, Dolimbek GS, Deitiker PR, Aoki KR, Dolimbek BZ. Submolecular recognition profiles in two mouse strains of non-protective and protective antibodies against botulinum neurotoxin A. Mol Immunol 2005; 42: 1509–20.

104. Kaltreider SA, Kennedy RH, Woog JJ et al. American Academy of Ophthalmology; Ophthalmic Technology Assessment Committee Oculoplastics Panel. Cosmetic oculofacial applications of botulinum toxin: a report by the American Academy of Ophthalmology. Ophthalmology 2005; 112: 1159–67.

105. Black JD, Dolly JO. Selective location of acceptors for botulinum neurotoxin A in the central and peripheral nervous systems. Neuroscience 1987; 32: 767–9.

106. Hambleton P. Clostridium botulinum toxins: a general review of involvement in disease, structure, mode of action and preparation for clinical use. J Neurol 1992; 239: 16–20.

107. Miyazaki S, Kozaki S, Sakaguchi S, Sakaguchi G. Comparison of progenitor toxins of nonproteolytic with those of proteolytic Clostridium botulinum Type B. Infect Immun 1976; 13: 987–9.

108. Rummel A, Bade S, Alves J et al. Two carbohydrate binding sites in the H(CC)-domain of tetanus neurotoxin are required for toxicity. J Mol Biol 2003; 326: 835–47.

9B The clinician's point of view

Danièle Ranoux

Clinicians should never use botulinum toxin (BTX) without knowing its mode of action, chemistry, and physiology, because they may have important consequences in terms of efficacy and safety. So, we have to be grateful to Dr Aoki for his comprehensive review of the scientific aspects of BTX (Chapter 9A). The purpose of this chapter will be to highlight the clinical implications of these fundamental data and to emphasize some issues that are of particular interest to clinicians.

Non-interchangeability

Two different serotypes and three different BTX products are now commercially available: BTX type A as BOTOX® and Dysport®, and BTX type B as Myobloc® (USA) and NeuroBloc (outside the USA). More recently introduced toxins are dealt with in Chapter 11.

As stated in all data sheets, the potency units of the different BTX formulations are not equivalent, even within the same serotype. This non-equivalence is one of the most important points to know about BTX, because an error when changing one preparation for another may account either for an overdose or for an apparent non-response, both with severe clinical consequences.[1,2]

There has been strong controversy about the conversion factor between the two formulations of BTX type A, namely BOTOX and Dysport. A dose ratio is hard to establish because it may vary according to several factors, including the type of muscle injected and the disease. In other words, a conversion factor found in one pathology may not necessarily be valid in another indication. Thus, fixed dose ratios must be interpreted with caution, and it is always preferable not to change from one formulation to another. But, when necessary, a dose ratio of 1:3 (meaning that 1 BOTOX unit equals 3 Dysport units) is an acceptable working basis.[2,3]

Diffusion/local adverse events

The diffusion of BTX to adjacent non-injected muscles is the major reason for local adverse events (for example, diplopia due to oculomotor muscle paralysis after orbicularis oculi injection), but an increased diffusion of BTX may also be desirable when injecting large muscles, in order to reach the highest possible number of neuromuscular junctions.

Thus, factors influencing BTX diffusion are important to know. In theory, as noted by Dr Aoki, botulinum neurotoxin protein complexes of greater molecular weight (i.e. BOTOX) should diffuse more slowly than those of lower molecular weight (i.e. Dysport and NeuroBloc). However, this theoretical assumption conflicts with two lines of argument. First, it is questionable whether this basic physiological rule can be simply applied to the diffusion of BTX in the human body. Indeed, after injection in a muscle, BTX does not diffuse in a homogeneous milieu. Its spread is influenced by anatomical factors such as the architecture of the injected muscles[4] and the presence of muscle fasciae, which reduces the spread of toxin by approximately 23%.[5] Second, the clinical studies available do not support the hypothesis of a difference in diffusion pattern for BOTOX and Dysport. The two studies which appropriately addressed this issue are prospective controlled studies specifically comparing the incidence of local adverse events occurring with BOTOX and Dysport in a given pathology (i.e. cervical dystonia),[2,6] with a methodology avoiding confounding factors such as volume of the injectate and dilution. Other studies did not directly compare the two products, and/or had basic methodological flaws that prevented any conclusion to be drawn. In the first study,[6] the authors failed to reveal any difference between the two products at a 1:3 ratio. In our study,[2] we found a greater efficacy of Dysport versus BOTOX at the same ratio, associated with a slight increase in dysphagia incidence in the Dysport group. Our interpretation is that the increased rate of swallowing difficulties is due to the relative overdosage of Dysport compared to BOTOX at this 1:3 ratio. Nothing allows further use of this observation as an argument for a different spreading pattern of the two products.

Apart from the above described anatomical factors, which are, by definition, non-modifiable, the spreading pattern of BTX may also vary according to factors that can be modified by the clinician: dose, volume, and technique of injection. It has been shown that the higher are the doses and the volume, the greater is the diffusion.[7,8] The number of injection points may also play a role. Several injection points distributed in the target muscle can insure that the highest possible number of neuromuscular junctions are reached, but this carries a higher risk of diffusion to adjacent muscles. In addition, the direction of the needle may have some importance when the target muscle is located in the vicinity of a functionally important muscle. For example, to inject the orbicularis oculi, it is preferable to direct the tip of the needle outwards, in order to avoid spread towards the levator palpebrae, and subsequent undesirable ptosis.

Thus, clinicians can adapt the procedure to the clinical situation. When careful selectivity is warranted (for example in cosmetic indications), it can be interesting to use a low dilution (high concentration), and/or a single injection point, and/or a lower dose. Conversely, injecting large muscles (in spasticity, for example) most often requires a higher dilution (low concentration), and/or multiple injection sites, and/or higher doses. In cosmetic uses, certain practitioners recommend using in the same session a higher volume for larger muscles such as the frontalis, and smaller volumes to treat functionally sensitive areas such as the eyelids or the mouth.[8,9]

Remote effects

Remote adverse effects are much rarer than local ones, but are potentially severe, ranging from asthenia to generalized weakness and life-threatening botulism-like syndrome. Dysphagia is considered a remote effect when the injected muscles are distant from the pharyngeal musculature, but a local side-effect when it occurs after injection of the cervical muscles. In case of doubt, distant spread of the toxin can be proved by electromyography showing increased jitter and blockings in distant muscles.[10,11]

The remote effects of BTX are not completely understood, but are supposed to be due to a hematogenous spread of the toxin. Retrograde axonal spread of toxin could be another explanation, but has never been proved in humans.

No study has examined the responsible factors, but analysis of the published cases reveals that most occurred after detrusor injections[12–14] or spasticity,[15,16] and/or after the use of high dilutions,[12] and/or in patients with underlying motor deficit. In most patients the three risk factors were present, and we can hypothesize that the conjunction of two or more risk factors may be responsible for the occurrence of such effects. Detrusor injection is probably an at-risk procedure in itself, because the bladder wall, especially between trabeculation bars, is thin, and can allow diffusion perivesically. In that particular case, but also when high doses are needed such as in spasticity, it is advisable to avoid high dilutions. Finally, distant adverse events have been reported more frequently with Dysport[12,13,15–18] than with BOTOX,[12,14] but no definite conclusion can be drawn from simple case reports. The only way to address this issue would be to perform a large, independent, prospective, controlled study to establish the mechanism and risk factors (including toxin formulation) of the distant spread of the toxin.

Immunogenicity

The use of BTX carries a risk of antibody formation, whose clinical significance is not unequivocal. Some patients with antibodies have become resistant to BTX, but others have continued to be good responders. Several risk factors have been identified, such as high doses and short intervals between two injections (including the booster technique where another dose is injected 2–3 weeks after the first injection). This supports the preventive approach, systematically using the minimum effective dose, and intervals between two injections of more than 2–3 weeks.

As far as the BTX formulations are concerned, once again there is a discrepancy between the theory and the facts. The theory, exposed by Dr Aoki, is that BTX formulations with higher levels of neurotoxin complex protein (i.e. Dysport, NeuroBloc) may be associated with an increased risk of neutralizing antibody formation. Unfortunately, no comparative study has been conducted, and the only data available are from prevalence studies performed with BOTOX, or Dysport, or NeuroBloc. To date, with a range of 3–10% for both, there is no obvious difference in antigenicity between BOTOX and Dysport.[19] By contrast, the two studies addressing BTX-B immunogenicity found antibodies in 44% and one-third of patients, respectively,[20,21] suggesting an increased antigenicity of this serotype.

Conclusion

The aim of BTX injectors is to reach the wanted therapeutic effect without side-effect. Approaching this aim warrants both good understanding of the pathology treated and mastering the multiple parameters of injection, including doses, volume, dilution, site(s) of injection, and intervals between injections.

References

1. Brin M, Blitzer A. Botulinum toxin: dangerous terminology errors. J R Soc Med 1993; 86: 493–4.
2. Ranoux D, Gury C, Fondarai J, Mas JL, Zuber M. Respective potencies of Botox and Dysport: a double blind, randomised, crossover study in cervical dystonia. J Neurol Neurosurg Psychiatry 2002; 72: 459–62.
3. Sampaio C, Costa J, Ferreira JJ. Clinical comparability of marketed formulations of botulinum toxin. Mov Disord 2004; 19 (Suppl 8): S129–36.
4. Rosales RL, Bigalke H, Dressler D. Pharmacology of botulinum toxin: differences between type A preparations. Eur J Neurol 2006; 13 (Suppl 1): 2–10.
5. Borodic GE, Ferrante R, Pearce BL, Smith K. Histologic assessment of dose-related diffusion and muscle fiber response after therapeutic botulinum-A toxin injections. Mov Disord 1994; 9: 31–9.
6. Odergren T, Hjaltason H, Kaakkola S et al. A double blind, randomised, parallel group study to investigate the dose

equivalence of Dysport and Botox in the treatment of cervical dystonia. J Neurol Neurosurg Psychiatry 1998; 64: 6–12.

7. Shaari CM, Sanders IRA. Quantifying how location and dose of botulinum toxin affect muscle paralysis. Muscle Nerve 1993; 16: 964–9.

8. Jeffrey Hsu TS, Dover JS, Arndt KA. Effect of volume and concentration on the diffusion of botulinum exotoxin A. Arch Dermatol 2004; 140: 1351–4.

9. Le Louarn C. Facial lines and wrinkles due to muscle hyperkinesia. In: Ranoux D, Gury C, eds. Practical Handbook on Botulinum Toxin. Marseille: Solal, 2007: 233–49. [in French]

10. Lange DJ, Rubin M, Greene PE et al. Distant effects of locally injected botulinum toxin: a double-blind study of single fiber EMG changes. Muscle Nerve 1991; 14: 672–5.

11. Olney RK, Aminoff MJ, Gelb DJ et al. Neuromuscular effects distant from the site of botulinum neurotoxin injection. Neurology 1988; 38: 1780–3.

12. Grosse J, Kramer G, Stöhrer M. Success of repeat detrusor injections of botulinum A toxin in patients with severe neurogenic detrusor overactivity and incontinence. Eur Urol 2005; 47: 653–9.

13. Ruffion A, Capelle O, Paparel P et al. What is the optimum dose of type A botulinum toxin for treating neurogenic bladder overactivity? BJU 2006; 97: 1030–4.

14. Wyndaele JJ, Van Dromme SA. Muscular weakness as side effect of botulinum toxin injection for neurogenic detrusor overactivity. Spinal Cord 2002; 40: 599–600.

15. Bakheit AM, Ward CD, McLellan DL. Generalised botulism-like syndrome after intramuscular toxin type A: a report of two cases. J Neurol Neurosurg Psychiatry 1997; 62: 198.

16. Bhatia KP. Generalised muscular weakness after botulinum toxin injection for dystonia: a report of two cases. J Neurol Neurosurg Psychiatry 1999; 67: 90–3.

17. Tugnoli V, Eleopra R, Quatrale R et al. Botulism-like syndrome after botulinum toxin type A injections for focal hyperhidrosis. Br J Dermatol 2002; 147: 808–9.

18. Beseler-Soto B, Sanchez-Palomares M, Santos-Serrano L et al. Iatrogenic botulism. A complication to be taken into account in the treatment of child spasticity. Rev Neurol 2003; 37: 444–6.

19. Dressler D, Hallett M. Immunological aspects of Botox, Dysport and Myobloc/Neurobloc. Eur J Neurol 2006; 13 (Suppl 1): 11–15.

20. Dressler D, Bigalke H. Botulinum toxin type B de novo therapy of cervical dystonia. Frequency of antibody induced therapy failure. J Neurol 2005; 252: 904–7.

21. Jankovic J, Hunter C, Dolimbeck BZ et al. Clinico-immunologic aspects of botulinum toxin type B treatment of cervical dystonia. Neurology 2006; 67: 2233–5.

Applications and indications

Sophie Sangla

Introduction

Botulinum toxin is the most powerful of all known neurotoxins. The first publication of its clinical use dates back to 1980, by Alan Scott,[1] an American ophthalmologist, for the treatment of strabismus in children; the Food and Drug Administration (FDA) gave its authorization for this use of the toxin in 1984. It is in neurology that the toxin has the greatest number of indications, but over 20 years its therapeutic possibilities have widened considerably. The toxin has made it possible to radically modify the quality of life of many patients having very different pathologies in many medical specialties. We will review the current principal indications for the toxin in various medical disciplines.

Indications for botulinum toxin injections

Dystonia

Dystonia is defined as involuntary muscular contractions, repeated, and causing abnormal postures or abnormal movements. Dystonias are classified according to the age at which they first begin, their distribution, and their etiology. Dystonia is called primary if it's the only symptom of the disease, it can also be one of the elements of a disorder, as in Parkinson's disease, or Wilson's disease. Botulinum toxin is the treatment of choice for focal dystonias in the adult, and it has overturned the functional prognosis for these. It can be used whatever the cause of the dystonia, with a unifocal or multifocal approach.

Blepharospasm

Blepharospasm is a focal dystonia of the orbicularis muscles of the eyes. It manifests as repeated involuntary movements closing the eyes. The age at which it usually begins ranges between 50 and 60 years, and it is more frequent in females. It often begins as an exaggerated blinking, then settles into visual impairment more marked at the time of walking, driving a car, or watching television. The closing of the eyes can be short or more constant, making the patient functionally blind.

The intensity of the blepharospasm is variable from one moment to the next, and according to the circumstances, which is an important semiological element. Blepharospasm is painless, but patients frequently report ocular 'burns', which can be related to associated dry eye syndrome.

The association of blepharospasm with an oromandibular dystonia constitutes Meige's syndrome, named after the French neurologist who described this clinical picture in 1910.[2]

There are few controlled studies, and they generally included a small number of patients and were of short duration. The majority of the studies were open, not blinded.[3–6] There is, however, a constant trend in the results which shows the superiority of toxin over placebo, and a benefit in approximately 90% of patients. A study published in 2003[6] of 178 patients followed over 20 years showed that 93% of patients were satisfied with treatment with botulinum toxin A. These results make toxin the treatment of choice in blepharospasm, in both the short and the long term. The side-effects are ptosis, diplopia, and facial asymmetry in the event of overdose or diffusion to muscles other than the targeted orbicularis. Toxin B has also been used.[7] It seems to have little effect because its duration of action is less, and the injections are painful (painless after injection with toxin A).

Spasmodic torticollis

Spasmodic torticollis (ST) is the most frequent focal dystonia in the adult; it concerns the muscles of the neck, and is responsible for an abnormal positioning of the head. Under the generic term of 'torticollis', we include several types of movement: genuine rotatory torticollis, anterocollis in flexion, retrocollis in extension, laterocollis in inclination, and procollis in looking forward with a raised chin. The beginning of ST is often insidious, with an involuntary deviation of the head which the patient can control; this positioning is intermittent, but with the passage of time it can become permanent, the patient having increasing difficulty in returning to a neutral position of the neck. To help rectify the head's position, the patient often uses a 'geste antagoniste' or sensory trick: this can take the form of stimulation of an area of skin (generally the cheek) which makes it possible to restore control.

The handicap created by ST is important because it disturbs the position of the head in walking or when writing. It is responsible for social and relational esthetic problems often compromising communal activity. The age when it begins is usually around 40; it also has a female prevalence. Botulinum toxin must be used as soon as there is any functional impairment, and in association with targeted functional rehabilitation.[8] Treatment by toxin requires a good anatomical knowledge and a precise analysis of the abnormal movement.

Several double-blind studies versus placebo have been published. Greene et al[9] showed a subjective improvement of 58% among patients treated by toxin, compared with an improvement of 4% among patients injected with placebo. There was an improvement in the ability to turn the head at rest and to walk, to a significant degree compared to the placebo group. Pain was very clearly improved (in the order of 41%) among patients receiving toxin versus 0% among patients receiving placebo. In their leading study in 1986, Tsui et al[10] demonstrated that there existed an objective improvement in the order of 63% for movement among patients injected with the toxin BOTOX® (35% for the placebo group) and about 88% for pain, compared with 15% in the placebo group. Jankovic et al,[5] in a series of 477 patients, reported improvement for 90% of the patients. A study in the United States[11] with the Dysport® toxin treated 80 patients with 500 U of toxin or placebo; there was 38% improvement in the group treated, lasting 18.5 weeks.

In the long term, over 10 years, Haussermann et al[12] found a lasting improvement in 60% of over 100 patients.

Toxin B is also used in spasmodic torticollis. Studies[13,14] carried out among patients who had already received toxin included some patients with resistance to it. The duration of improvement was 16 weeks, with an improvement of at least 20%; the amount used was 10 000 units. Side-effects were more frequent, including pain at the point of injection and dry mouth.

The most frequent side-effects are difficulties in swallowing, muscular weakness, and occasionally general tiredness. These undesirable effects commence after a delay of a few days, last 2 weeks, and are always reversible.

Writer's cramp and other functional dystonias

Writer's cramp is a task specific focal dystonia. It affects men and women equally. The age at which it begins is usually between the third and the fifth decade. There are other task specific dystonias that can appear in musicians (pianists, violinists, guitarists, harpists, saxophonists), walkers, and some sportsmen (golfers), or in certain occupations involving repetitive gestures (dressmaking, cigarette manufacturing, typing).

The dystonic posture can manifest when a pen is picked up, and continue throughout activity, sometimes with such intensity that any writing becomes impossible. The muscles to inject are located clinically by electromyographic study. Marion et al,[15] in a retrospective study in 259 patients of whom 167 benefited from botulinum toxin injections, found that 46% could return to normal writing, and 10% had only partial improvement. Side-effects include compromise of the injected muscles and/or adjacent muscles, but this is always transitory.

Oromandibular dystonia

This is a dystonia of the muscles around the mouth, and the Jaw, which hinders speech, chewing, and swallowing.

We distinguish between oromandibular dystonia of closing and that of opening, according to whether the mouth remains involuntarily impaired in closing or opening. Oromandibular dystonia manifests at the time of speech or chewing, which it impairs. The muscles used in oromandibular dystonia of closing are the temporal masseters and the internal pterygoid muscles. Impairment of closing can hinder eating.

Impairment of opening consists of abnormal movements of the jaw, which is drawn downward to a variable degree; this can sometimes result in just a tremor of the jaw. To close the mouth, patients are obliged to contract the orbicularis oris muscle, giving the face a twisted appearance. They have difficulties in eating because of this dystonia, but also because there are abnormal movements of the posterior part of the tongue. The muscles involved are the external pterygoid and the subhyoid muscles. Injection is made under electromyographic control. Difficulties in swallowing can occur after each injection and last 2–3 weeks.[16]

Meige syndrome is an oromandibular dystonia associated with blepharospasm; it is then necessary to inject the orbicularis muscles at the same session. Dystonia of the tongue is more delicate to treat because of the risks of asphyxiation, in certain cases, but it is nevertheless possible to propose toxin. Injections are carried out at the level of the genioglossus and the hypoglossus (anterior portion) under electromyographic control. Few studies have been carried out. In six patients, Charles et al reported five improvements, in eating and speaking.[17]

Spasmodic dysphonia

This focal dystonia of the larynx generally occurs in female patients aged around 40 years. Two types of dysphonia have been described.

Adduction of the vocal cords is the most frequent, whereby the voice is broken, forced, and punctuated by vocal stops. The muscles concerned are the thyroarytenoids.

Abduction of the vocal cords is much rarer. The voice is reduced to a whisper or a barely audible murmur. One often finds repeated episodes of aphony in the history. The muscles involved are the posterior cricoarytenoids.

There are also mixed forms, which require more delicate treatment and have less good clinical results.

The diagnosis of spasmodic dysphonia is often difficult because the disorder fluctuates, and otolaryngological examination is generally normal. Botulinum toxin is the treatment of choice for spasmodic dysphonia.[18] The injection is carried out percutaneously under electromyographic control. Blitzer et al, in 1989, reported their study of 901 patients,[16] with 90% improvement in the forms involving adduction and 66.7% in abduction. The side-effects were hypophonia and disorders of swallowing.

Other abnormal movements

Hemifacial spasm

Hemifacial spasm is a peripheral pathology involving the facial nerve. The average age at which it begins is around 57 years. Hemifacial spasm affects women twice as often as men, and is characterized by muscular spasms of half the face, from the frontalis muscle to the platysma of the neck. It often begins insidiously with intermittent twitches of the lower eyelid, but then the spasm extends. On the side of the face that is the origin of clonic spasms, tonic spasms can also occur, accentuating a twisted facial expression. This is primarily related to contraction of the orbicularis muscle, which produces an occlusion of varying duration; deformation of the face at the time of spasm also causes an esthetic compromise. Occurrence of the spasms is variable and uncontrolled, with the duration ranging from a few seconds to several minutes. No voluntary control is possible. The spasm persists during sleep and often obstructs drowsiness.

The results are excellent, since there is an estimated 90% improvement obtained after toxin treatment according to the various series published.[19,20]

Tremor

Botulinum toxin can be used only in rare cases, when medical care is no longer sufficiently effective and the tremor causes severe debility. Jankovic and Schwartz[21] found an improvement of 75% in the amplitude of tremors, without any functional benefit in 25 cases. On the face, isolated tremor of the chin is a good indication.[22]

Other indications

Spasticity and hypertonicity

Botulinum toxin is indicated in the treatment of spasticity of the limbs from many causes. For its application,

the spasticity must be relatively focal, because there is a limitation on the amount that can be administered, and the usual treatments must have been ineffective. The toxin can give improvement at several levels for patients presenting with spasticity: it can facilitate certain daily activities such as dressing and hygiene, decrease pain, improve range of motion, reduce abnormal postures, and allow the use of supporting equipment. It is thus necessary to lay down specific objectives for each patient that are flexible and adaptable according to the results; a multidisciplinary assumption of responsibility makes for the best therapeutic outcome. It is of course necessary to act before there are tendon retractions. Injections are generally carried out under electromyographic control with electrostimulation, which makes it possible to target the muscles since there is no voluntary contraction. The literature concerning the treatment of spasticity by botulinum toxin injection is considerable. There are many studies in the adult, some concerning the upper limbs,[23] others the lower extremities,[24] and for varied etiologies. For cerebral vascular accident, multiple sclerosis, and cranial trauma the results are satisfactory, with large amounts of toxin used and a duration of 3 months' effectiveness on average.

In the child[25] the objectives are a little different, insofar as it is necessary to act between the ages of 2 and 6 years, in order to try to correct the biomechanics of the limbs, improve mobility for the period when the child is learning motor skills, and permit growth by reducing retractions which often lead to multiple surgical operations.

Painful syndromes and headache

Botulinum toxin has been proposed as a treatment for many painful syndromes with greater or lesser involvement of muscular spasms. Lumbago,[26] tension headaches,[27] and migraines[28] have been treated by botulinum toxin with often good results. However, although the studies are numerous, their methodologies are often debatable, making it difficult to obtain a convincing level of proof. As Evers et al showed[29] in a meta-analysis carried out concerning headaches, no positive effect was demonstrable. Meta-analysis of the other indications would be desirable. Studies are necessary in order to target the patients likely to benefit from this type of treatment.

Oculomotor disorders

Strabismus Strabismus in a child was the initial indication for botulinum toxin. The treatment of convergent strabismus in a small child is surgical, but toxin could be used as a therapeutic test to indicate whether surgery is necessary, and with curative intent in the less severe forms. The toxin must be used before the age of 2. In a study[30] of 76 children (4–48 months) with strabismus treated surgically and by toxin, 90% had an improvement with non-surgical intervention (52% with only one injection).

Oculomotor paralysis Oculomotor paralyses generally regress, so recourse to surgery may sometimes be necessary, but the hyperactivity of compensatory muscles over several months makes this quite difficult. One can thus propose toxin injections to re-equilibrate the oculomotor balance, primarily with palliative intent.

Therapeutic ptosis Toxin can be proposed to avoid a traumatizing tarsorrhaphy in massive facial paralysis with complete non-occlusion, by injection into the levator palprebrae muscle which creates a ptosis which will protect the cornea.

Otolaryngological disorders

Bruxism and hypertrophy of the masseter muscles Bruxism, a pathology that happens during sleep, can be extremely invalidating, with abnormal wear on the teeth. Hypertrophy of the masseter muscles is perhaps esthetically a problem but is not so painful; temporomandibular joint pain is fairly constant. Studies showed an improvement in bruxism in 53% of patients, in pain in 64%, and in hypertrophy in 90%.[31]

Sialorrhea Sialorrhea or excessive secretion of saliva is a problem often encountered in neurology in those with cerebral palsy, amyotrophic lateral sclerosis, or Parkinson's disease, to name the most frequent.

For several years, tests of treatment of sialorrhea by botulinum toxin have been proposed using variable methods, amounts, and targets. Bhatia et al in 1999[32] treated four patients with subcutaneous injections of Dysport in the parotid muscle at the mandibular angle. This produced an improvement in three patients for 6 weeks, with side-effects of difficulties in chewing and swallowing. Porta et al[33] in 2001 conducted the first study under echographic control. In 10 treated patients, they injected the two parotid muscles (BOTOX), and also the two submaxillary muscles. In nine patients there was an improvement of 55% for a duration of 4–7 months. This more precise method increases safety.

A double-blinded versus placebo study from Mancini et al[34] in 2003 concerned 14 patients with Parkinson's disease and six patients with multisystem atrophy (MSA). The amounts used in this study were higher than those in previous studies, using Dysport in the parotid and submaxillary muscles. Toxin injection thus appears to be a good alternative for decreasing problems with drooling, but must be conducted under echographic control and by an expert.[35] Botulinum toxin B, which has a more marked antisecretory effect than does toxin A, will surely be useful, but few studies have been published.[36]

Frey's syndrome Botulinum toxin is an effective treatment for Frey's syndrome encountered after treatment of the parotid gland. This localized sweating from the gland is socially very distressing. The improvements obtained last for 6 months to 1 year.[37]

Gastrointestinal disorders

Dysphagia There has been improvement of dysphagia attributable to dysfunction of the superior esophageal sphincter (the cricopharyngeal muscle). After injection, some patients were able to resume normal oral feeding. The effectiveness of botulinum toxin was demonstrated compared to placebo among patients suffering from achalasia,[38] a rare pathology in which there is a problem in relaxing the inferior sphincter of the esophagus, which is thus injected by means of an endoscope. This type of dysphagia can also be found in patients with severe Meige's syndrome.

Anismus Anismus is an abnormal contraction of the anal striated sphincter, found in certain neurologic disorders such as Parkinson's disease. The perineal puborectalis muscle and other muscles forming the external anal sphincter cannot be relaxed any further during defecation. This results in constipation. The results of surgery are disappointing in this pathology, and it often becomes complicated by secondary anal incontinence. After electromyographic location and rectoscopy, botulinum toxin injection in the puborectalis muscle showed effectiveness.[39,40]

Chronic anal fissure This is a mucous ulceration at the lower end of the anal canal causing pain upon defecation and anal bleeding. It is associated with hypertonicity of the anal sphincter which can be alleviated by toxin injection. The rates of cicatrization vary from 44 to 96% according to the published studies. A study in 2003 compared the effectiveness of toxin with surgical sphincterotomy, with cicatrization in 6 months in 86.9% in the toxin group versus 96.4% in the operated group.[41]

Genitourinary disorders

Detrusor sphincter dyssynergia Toxin has been used to treat detrusor sphincter dyssynergia since 1988.[42] Studies were conducted among patients who had suffered medullary trauma or had multiple sclerosis. Detrusor sphincter dyssynergia occurs when there is insufficient relaxation of the sphincter when the detrusor contracts, which causes difficulty in emptying the bladder and a residue after micturation. Quantification of the results is difficult and equivocal, but several studies have shown satisfactory results with BOTOX (21 of 24 patients improved for 3–6 months[43]) and also with Dysport (10 of 17 patients improved for 2–3 months[44]).

Detrusor hyperactivity This is another indication for botulinum toxin, in patients who have had a severe attack resisting medical treatment. The technique is delicate, because one needs at least 30 sites of injection. Schurch et al in a series of 21 patients noted an improvement in 17 of them.[45]

Vaginismus When the usual methods for treating vaginismus are ineffective, toxin injections have been proposed.[46] The psychological impact of this method allows durable improvements in some cases.

Conclusion

The indications for botulinum toxin injection are very wide-ranging, in both neurology and allied specialties. The symptomatic and reversible action of botulinum toxin offers a great number of therapeutic possibilities. Although this is an extremely potent toxin, its use in expert hands presents no practical danger. Treatment should be carried out by experienced practitioners, who are familiar with the various effects of the toxin, the anatomy, and the pathologies to be treated.

References

1. Scott AB. Botulinum toxin injection into extraocular muscles as an alternative to strabismus surgery. Ophthalmology 1980; 87: 1044–9.
2. Meige H. Les convulsions de la face, une forme clinique de convulsion faciale bilatérale et médiane. Rev Neurol 1910; 21: 437–43.
3. Elston JS. The management of blepharospasm and hemifacial spasm. J Neurol 1992; 239: 5–8.
4. Grandas F, Elston J, Quinn N, Marsden CD. Blepharospasm: a review of 264 patients. J Neurol Neurosurg Psychiatry 1988; 51: 767–72.
5. Jankovic J, Schwartz K, Donovan DT. Botulinum toxin treatment of cranial cervical dystonia, spasmodic dysphonia, other focal dystonias and hemifacial spasm. J Neurol Neurosurg Psychiatry 1990; 53: 633–9.
6. Calace P, Cortese G, Piscopo R et al. Treatment of blepharospasm with botulinum neurotoxin A: long-term results. Eur J Ophthalmoel 2003; 13: 331–6.
7. Colosimo C, Chianese M, Giovannelli M, Contarino MF, Bentivoglio AR. Botulinum toxin type B in blepharospasm and hemifacial spasm. J Neurol Neurosurg Psychiatry 2003; 74: 687.
8. Bleton JP. La Rééducation de la Crampe de l'Écrivain. Marseille: Solal, 2004.
9. Greene P, Kang U, Fahn S et al. Double blind, placebo controlled trial of botulinum toxin injections for the treatment of spasmodic torticollis. Neurology 1990; 40: 1213–18.
10. Tsui JK, Eisen A, Stoessl AJ, Calne S, Calne DB. Double-blind study of botulinum toxin in spasmodic torticollis. Lancet 1986; 2: 245–7.
11. Truong D, Duane DD, Jankovic J et al. Efficacy and safety of botulinum type A toxin (Dysport) in cervical dystonia: results of the first US randomized, double-blind, placebo-controlled study. Mov Disord 2005; 20: 783–91.
12. Haussermann P, Marczoch S, Klinger C et al. Long term follow-up of cervical dystonia patients treated with botulinum toxin A. Mov Disord 2004; 19: 303–8.
13. Brashear A, Lew MF, Dykstra DD et al. Safety and efficacy of Neurobloc (botulinum toxin type B) in type A-responsive cervical dystonia. Neurology 1999; 53: 1439–46.

14. Brin MF, Lew MF, Adle CH et al. Safety and efficacy of Neurobloc (botulinum toxin type B) in type A-resistant cervical dystonia. Neurology 1999; 22: 1431–8.
15. Marion MH, Afors K, Sheehy MP. Traitement de la crampe des écrivains par la toxine botulique: efficacité et limite de cette technique basée sur 10 ans d'expérience. Rev Neurol 2003; 10: 923–7.
16. Blitzer A, Brin MF, Greene PE, Fahn S. Botulinum toxin injection for the treatment of oromandibular dystonia. Ann Otol Rhinol Laryngol 1989; 98: 93–7.
17. Charles PD, Davis TL, Shannon KM, Hook MA, Warner JS. Tongue protrusion dystonia: treatment with botulinum toxin. South Med J 1997; 90: 522–5.
18. Klap P, Cohen M, van Prooyen Keyzes S, Perrin A, Ayache D. La dystonie laryngée. Rev Neurol 2003; 159: 916–22.
19. Brin MF, Fahn S, Moskowitz C. Localized injection of botulinum toxin for the treatment of focal dystonia and hemifacial spasm. Mov Disord 1987; 2: 237–54.
20. Elston JS. Botulinum toxin treatment of hemifacial spasm. J Neurol Neurosurg Psychiatry 1986; 49: 827–9.
21. Jankovic J, Schwartz K. Botulinum toxin treatment of tremors. Neurology 1991; 41: 1185–8.
22. Babak M, Zarifoglu M, Bora I et al. Treatment of hereditary trembling chin with botulinum toxin. Mov Disord 1998; 13: 845–50.
23. Simpson DM. Botulinum toxin type A in the treatment of extremity spasticity. A randomised double blind placebo controlled trial. Neurology 1996; 46: 1306–10.
24. Burbaud P, Wiart L, Dubos JL. A randomised double blind placebo controlled trial of botulinum toxin type A in the treatment of spastic foot after stroke in hemiparetic patients. J Neurol Neurosurg Psychiatry 1996; 61: 256–9.
25. Boyd R, Graham HK. Botulinum toxin A in the management of children with cerebral palsy: identification and outcome. Eur J Neurol 1997; 4: S15–22.
26. Foster L, Clapp L, Erickson M, Jabbari B. Botulinum toxin A and chronic low back pain: a randomized, double blind study. Neurology 2002; 56: 1290–3.
27. Smuts JA, Baker MK, Smuts HM et al. Prophylactic treatment of chronic-tension type headache using botulinum toxin A. Eur J Neurol 1999; 6: 99–102.
28. Silberstein S, Mathew N, Saper J, Jenkins S. Botulinum toxin type A as a migraine preventive treatment. Headache 2000; 40: 445–50.
29. Evers S, Rahmann A, Vollmer-Haase J et al. Treatment of headache with botulinum toxin A: a review according to evidence-based medicine criteria. Cephalalgia 2002; 22: 699–710.
30. McNeer KW, Tucker MG, Spencer RF. Botulinum toxin management of essential infantile esotropia in children. Ophthalmology 1997; 115: 1411–18.
31. Moore AP, Wood GD. The medical management of masseteric hypertrophy with botulinum toxin type A. Br J Oral Maxillofac Surg 1994; 32: 26–8.
32. Bhatia KP, Munchau A, Brown P. Botulinum toxin is a useful treatment in excessive drooling in saliva. J Neurol Neurosurg Psychiatry 1999; 67: 697.
33. Porta M, Gamba M, Bertacchi G. Treatment of sialorrhoea with ultrasound guided botulinum toxin type A injection in patients with neurological disorders. J Neurol Neurosurg Psychiatry 2001; 70: 538–40.
34. Mancini F, Zangaglia R, Cristina S et al. Double-blind, placebo-controlled study to evaluate the efficacy and safety of botulinum toxin type A in the treatment of drooling in Parkinsonism. Mov Disord 2003; 18: 685–8.
35. Dogu O, Apaydin D, Sevim S, Talas DU, Aral M. Ultrasound-guided versus 'blind' intraparotid injections of botulinum toxin-A for the treatment of sialorrhea in patients with Parkinson's disease. Clin Neurol Neurosurg 2004; 106: 93–6.

36. Wan XH, Vuong KD, Jankovic J. Clinical application of botulinum toxin type B in movement disorders and autonomic symptoms. Chin Med Sci J 2005; 20: 44–7.

37. Laskawi R, Drobik C, Schonebeck C. Up to date report of botulinum toxin type A treatment in patients with gustatory sweating (Frey's syndrome). Laryngoscope 1998; 108: 381–4.

38. Pasricha PJ, Ravich WJ, Hendrix TR et al. Intrasphincteric botulinum toxin for the treatment of achalasia. N Engl J Med 1995; 332: 774–8.

39. Maria G, Brisinda G, Bentivoglio AR, Cassetta E, Albanese A. Botulinum toxin in the treatment of outlet obstruction constipation caused by puborectalis syndrome. Dis Colon Rectum 2000; 43: 376–80.

40. Ron Y, Avni Y, Lukovetski A et al. Botulinum toxin type A in therapy of patients with anismus. Dis Colon Rectum 2001; 44: 1821–6.

41. Mentes BB, Irkorucu O, Akin M et al. Comparaison of botulinum toxin injection and lateral internal sphincterectomy for treatment of chronic anal fissure. Dis Colon Rectum 2003; 46: 232–7.

42. Dysktra DD, Sidi AA, Scott AB, Pagel JM, Goldish GD. Effects of botulinum A toxin on detrusor sphincter dyssynergia in spinal cord injury patient. J Urol 1988; 139: 912–22.

43. Schurch B, Störer M, Kramer G et al. Botulinum A toxin as a treatment of detrusor-sphincter dyssynergia: a prospective study in 24 spinal cord injury patients. J Urol 1996; 155: 1023–9.

44. Petit H, Wiart L, Gaujard E et al. Botulinum A toxin treatment for detrusor-sphincter dyssynergia in spinal cord disease. Spinal Cord 1998; 36: 91–4.

45. Schurch B, Störer M, Kramer G et al. Botulinum A toxin for treating detrusor hyperreflexia in spinal cord injured patients: a new alternative to anticholinergic drugs? Preliminary results. J Urol 2000; 164: 692–7.

46. Brin MF. Treatment of vaginismus with botulinum toxin injections. Lancet 1997; 349: 252–3.

11 Variant preparations of botulinum toxin A: Purtox®, Xeomin®, and BTX-A®

David J Goldberg, Berthold Rzany, Sergio Talarico-Filho and Sabrina Rodrigues Talarico

There are now a variety of effective botulinum toxins type A available worldwide. Although the manufacturing process for each is different and the amount of associated protein content will vary from one botulinum toxin A to the next, all such toxins have in common their associated content of the type A botulinum toxin.

PurTox®

PurTox® is the botulinum toxin developed by Mentor Corporation. Studies with this toxin are ongoing in the USA and are about to enter phase III of Food and Drug Administration (FDA) trials.

In phase I of the Mentor FDA trials, PurTox was studied to determine its dose range for safety and efficacy in the treatment of glabellar rhytids. Forty subjects were examined using a dose range of the Mentor botulinum toxin from 3.125 to 25 U. Subjects were required to show a moderate forced frown to qualify for inclusion in the study. The study was a single-center, single-dose escalation study. It was an open label, randomized, double-blind, placebo-controlled study in which each subject received five injections of the toxin (or a placebo) in the glabellar area. One injection was given into the procerus muscle and two injections were given into the corrugator supercilii muscles on each side.

Subjects were assessed using a static subjective global assessment (SGA) scale of 1–100 mm; physicians used a validated photoscale of 0–3. Photodocumentation was taken throughout the study.

At the conclusion of the phase I trial, it was noted that there were no premature discontinuations from the study due to adverse events, no serious adverse events were noted, and not a single case of treatment-induced ptosis or diplopia occurred. Of note, any adverse event occurring during the study had to be reported, even if unrelated to the actual injection of PurTox. Five such adverse events (13.9%) were reported to be moderate in intensity; none were felt to be related to the study drug.

The reported summary of the phase I FDA study trial showed that the majority (86.1%) of adverse events (again, not necessarily related to drug injection) were mild in intensity. Such adverse events included injection site pain in two subjects (considered mild by the subjects), a slight headache in one subject, and a taste perversion in three subjects. As would be expected, a higher response rate was noted at higher doses. In addition, a higher response rate was sustained at higher doses of PurTox.

After completion of the phase I trial, the phase II trial was begun. Whereas the purpose of the phase I trial was to determine the dose range for safety and efficacy of PurTox in the treatment of glabellar rhytids, the purpose of the phase II study was to determine the optimal dose for efficacy of PurTox in the treatment of glabellar rhytids.

In this now expanded phase II trial, 136 subjects were assessed with a dose range of Mentor botulinum toxin at four different dose levels. Subjects were once again required to have a moderate forced frown to qualify for the phase II study. In contrast to the single-center phase I trial, the phase II trial was a multicenter (two sites), placebo-controlled, double-blind, randomized study.

Each subject received five injections of the toxin (or a placebo) in the glabellar area. Once again, one injection was given into the procerus muscle and two injections were given into the corrugator supercilii muscles on each side. Subjects used a static subjective global assessment (SGA) scale of 1–100 mm; physicians used a validated photoscale of 0–3. Photodocumentation was taken throughout the study.

The phase II trial showed a dose-dependent increase in the response rate. The highest dose tested consistently resulted in the highest response rate, which, as would be expected, was statistically significantly different from that with placebo. In addition, the duration of effect was dose-dependent, with trends of increasing duration seen with increasing toxin dose levels.

The majority of subjects noted a change in appearance within 2 days of PurTox administration, and all responders noted a change in appearance within 3–4 days of toxin administration.

The conclusions of the phase II trial were that: (1) the response rate for PurTox botulinum toxin was dose-dependent, (2) the duration of effect increased with increasing toxin dose, and (3) the highest toxin dose tested resulted in the highest degree of efficacy and longest duration of effect. The majority of subjects reported the onset of a change in appearance within 2 days of toxin administration. In general, PurTox was well tolerated, and there were no apparent dose-dependent differences in adverse events across the different toxin doses.

With the completion of the phase II trial, a multicenter phase III trial is being started. This trial will involve large numbers of subjects being treated by many investigators. The manufacturer will use the data from this study in their attempt to seek FDA approval in the USA.

Xeomin®: the German botulinum toxin A

Xeomin® (NT 201 in the scientific literature) is a new botulinum toxin A preparation from Merz Pharmaceuticals, Frankfurt/M, Germany that differs from other botulinum toxin A preparations by a decreased amount of clostridial protein. Xeomin is free of complexing proteins, which should relate clinically to less antigenicity. In contrast to other botulinum toxin preparations it can be stored at room temperature prior to dilution with saline.[1,2]

According to Medline there is one pivotal study in neurology, and one in ophthalmology.[3,4] Both studies, comprising over 700 patients, provide comparable efficacy and safety profiles of Xeomin to BOTOX®, translating into a 1:1 ratio.

Regarding esthetic indications, Xeomin is being studied in clinical trials in the treatment of glabellar frown lines. Placebo-controlled, randomized clinical trials with more than 400 patients are determining the optimal dose and investigating the efficacy and safety in this indication.

BTX-A®: the Chinese toxin from Lanzhou Institute

In 1984, a *Clostridium botulinum* type A strain was donated from the University of Wisconsin to Dr Yinchun Wang during his visit to the university. Returning to China in 1985, Dr Wang and his colleagues started research on botulinum toxin in the Lanzhou Institute of Biological Products, and 3 years later they developed a botulinum toxin in crystalline form with high toxicity, purity, and stability.

In 1989, the China National New Drug Evaluation Institute approved the beginning of clinical trials with this toxin. The trial production license was issued by the Health Ministry in 1993, and finally in 1997 the Formal Production License and the Sale Certificate

were obtained after completing clinical phase I, II, and III trials. In 2002, the product began to be exported to foreign countries, and at present it is available in South Korea, Hong Kong, India, Ukraine, Kuwait, the Philippines, Indonesia, Azerbaijan, Chile, Uzbekistan, Mexico, Paraguay, Uruguay, Colombia, and Brazil. In Brazil, the Health Ministry and Regulatory Agencies have approved the product for clinical (2003) and cosmetic use (2005).

BTX-A® is available in vials of 100 and 50 U of botulinum toxin, and each vial of 100 U has 5 mg of gelatin, 25 mg/ml of dextran, 25 mg of sucrose, and 4–5 ng of protein/100 U. The Lanzhou Institute emphasizes that the use of gelatin confers less risk of contamination compared with human serum albumin, and that the product's safety is firmly established and it is certified free of bovine spongiform encephalopathy.

We have had the opportunity to conduct a multicenter, multidisciplinary, phase III, prospective clinical trial to evaluate the efficacy and tolerability of BTX-A in the treatment of dynamic wrinkles of the upper face, enrolling 110 individuals. We included patients of both sexes, between 25 and 65 years old, with at least moderate wrinkles in the upper face, respecting the classical inclusion and exclusion criteria.

The most common adverse effects were mild, and included: headache in 6.36% (7/110), edema in 4.54% (5/110), tension of the forehead in 3.63% (4/110), and two cases of eyebrow ptosis (1.81%).

After a follow-up of 180 days, the patient levels of satisfaction (excellent or good) were 94% (day 14), 92% (day 45), 82% (day 90), 67% (day 120), 43% (day 150), and still 50% on day 180. Investigator satisfaction (excellent or good) was 97% (day 14), 88% (day 45), 67% (day 90), 32% (day 150), and 23% on day 180.

With these data we concluded that BTX-A was safe and well tolerated and could be considered one of the effective brands now available worldwide.

References

1. Jost WH, Kohl A, Brinkmann S, Comes G. Efficacy and tolerability of a botulinum toxin type A free of complexing proteins (NT 201) compared with commercially available botulinum toxin type A (BOTOX) in healthy volunteers. J Neural Transm 2005; 112: 905–13.
2. Jost W, Blümel J, Grafe S. Botulinum neurotoxin type A free of complexing proteins (XEOMIN®) in focal dystonia. Drugs 2007; 67: 669–83.
3. Benecke R, Jost WH, Kanovsky P et al. A new botulinum toxin type A free of complexing proteins for treatment of cervical dystonia. Neurology 2005; 64: 1949–51.
4. Roggenkamper P, Jost WH, Bihari K, Comes G, Grafe S; for the NT 201 Blepharospasm Study Team. Efficacy and safety of a new Botulinum Toxin Type A free of complexing proteins in the treatment of blepharospasm. J Neural Transm 2006; 113: 303–12.
5. Dressler D. [Pharmacological aspects of therapeutic botulinum toxin preparations]. Nervenarzt 2006; 77: 912–21. [in German]

12 Patient considerations

Timothy C Flynn

Introduction

Botulinum toxin treatments are currently the most popular cosmetic procedures performed in the United States. According to the American Society of Plastic Surgery (ASPS) website,[1] 4.1 million procedures were performed in 2006 alone. One reason why botulinum toxin is currently the most popular procedure is because of its remarkable effectiveness at reducing unwanted facial lines. Patient satisfaction is very high for this procedure, with many patients enthusiastically sharing their happiness with the treatment. In fact, one of the brands of botulinum toxin type A, BOTOX®, is truly a household word. Almost everyone has heard of BOTOX, and many patients have heard of it from a friend or family member who has had great results.

Patient evaluation

Patient evaluation is critical to success with botulinum toxin.[2] The physician should evaluate the aging face[3] and determine whether the wishes of the patient are appropriate for treatment with botulinum toxin. It is important to remember that there are a variety of conditions that affect the aging face. Most physicians are familiar with the effects of chronic ultraviolet light damage to the skin; however, hypertrophic muscles of facial expression cause unwanted skin folding and wrinkles. The excess activity of the memetic muscles of the face can be treated well with botulinum toxin. The progressive loss of subcutaneous fat in the face is a cause of facial aging. Patients with significant facial volume loss may need volume replacement. Facial tissue can lose elasticity leading to so-called 'gravitational effects', with the face draping more inferiorly. With age, there is a remarkable degree of remodeling of the subcutaneous bony and cartilaginous structures. This atrophying hard framework contributes significantly to the appearance of the aging face. Recent studies have documented the changes that occur in the skull.[4]

To become an expert in evaluation of the patient with an aging face can take years, and requires a significant amount of study. Paying attention to typical aging features of the face can help the physician understand facial aging progression. Good cosmetic physicians begin to understand which changes are treatable with specific products. With new products being developed in the cosmetic arena, the cosmetic surgeon must keep up to date with the current available treatments.

Many patients begin their cosmetic facial improvements by wishing to address the excessive muscular action as well as volume loss. It is important that the physician evaluates the ratio of the above factors in order to decide what the most appropriate treatment will be. For example, a patient who has an excessive amount of soft tissue draping over an atrophic hard tissue base would most likely benefit from a rhytidectomy. A woman who has noticed the appearance of moderate lines between her eyebrows, which is made worse with frowning, would benefit well from botulinum toxin treatment. A filler might be necessary to completely improve the lines.

The patient whose wrinkles occur with facial movements or are accentuated with activating the memetic muscles of the face is an excellent candidate for botulinum toxin treatment. Areas which are amenable to BOTOX are discussed in subsequent chapters, but briefly may include forehead lines, glabellar folds, periocular wrinkles ('crow's feet'), perioral rhytids, marionette lines, and dimpling of the chin. The face can be sculpted using botulinum toxin to raise eyebrows, adjust the arch of the eyebrow, improve a gummy smile, raise the corners of the mouth, correct an asymmetrical lip, and treat the platysma reducing facial descent.

The patient who has rhytids with rest (Figure 12.1) most likely will additionally need some degree of volume correction through the use of dermal filler substances. If the wrinkles are worsened with movement, a combination of BOTOX and filler substances is a commonly used approach. The patient who has excessive facial wrinkling and obvious volume loss will benefit from deep volume replacement with or without redraping of the face through a rhytidectomy. Patients who are suffering from fine wrinkles of the face and/or common aging changes of the skin will benefit from regular retinoid use, chemical peeling, and ablative or non-ablative laser resurfacing. Of course, many patients can benefit from regular skin care regimens. Treatments are tailored to individual patient problems (Table 12.1).

It is clearly the goal of the cosmetic surgeon to match the procedures with the defects that exist in

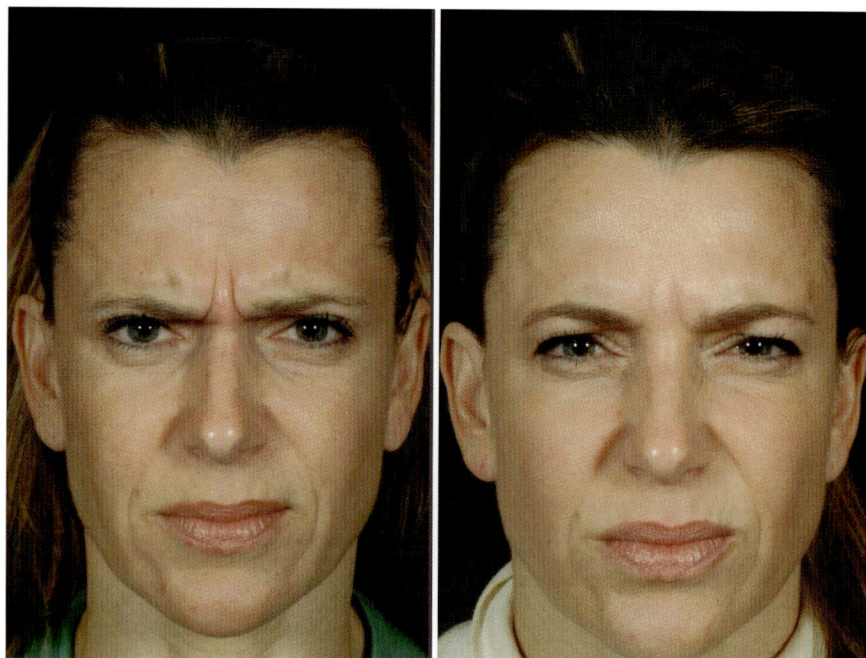

Figure 12.1 Patient with wrinkles at rest improved with botulinum toxin treatment. A filler may be needed to completely resolve the lines.

Table 12.1 Aging face treatments

Aging face symptom	Preferred treatment
Rhytids with movement	Botulinum toxin
Rhytids at rest	Filler substances ± botulinum toxin
Excessive wrinkles, volume loss	Deep volume replacements and/or redraping
Fine rhytids alone or in combination with above	Retinoids, peels, ablative or non-ablative laser surgery

each individual patient. One does not truly improve the aging face if one treats a patient with a variety of facial aging changes with only one therapy. We now know that excellent results are possible when glabellar lines are treated with botulinum toxin and a filler substance.[5] The botulinum toxin decreases the movement of the overactive glabellar complex, and the filler substance fills in the volume loss underneath the glabellar line. These agents act synergistically producing a better, long-lasting, overall effect. Similarly, patients who have photodamage consisting of fine lines, increasing dyschromia, and excessive vascularity will benefit from a cosmetic procedure such as intense pulsed-light therapy designed to address these issues.

Patient selection

Patients who are good candidates for botulinum toxin therapy are those who desire improvement of facial lines which are often the result of muscular action (wrinkles in motion) or have resting rhytids which are made worse by the underlying movement. If the patient has a wrinkle at rest which is also accentuated with muscular movement, they may need treatment with both filler substances and botulinum toxin.[6] There are many cosmetic patients who simply want an improvement in the appearance of their wrinkles at rest made worse with muscular action, or who are concerned about not having facial lines worsen with time. Many of these patients are quite satisfied with botulinum toxin; however, it is the author's experience that once patients see the improvement that is possible from the use of botulinum toxin, they are often interested in taking that next step which may be the use of a filler substance. Examples of common filler substances which are used alone or with botulinum toxin include injectable hyaluronans, collagens (human, bovine, or porcine), and semipermeable agents such as Radiesse®.

A simple tip in working with facial aging patients is to ask them directly: 'What is bothering you today?' Giving the patient time to answer and listening thoroughly will help the physician to understand exactly what the patient desires. The first-time patient may not know specifically what his or her concerns are. They may discuss a variety of concerns, necessitating the physician to pay careful attention and to make mental notes of the areas about which they have concern. After allowing the patient to completely discuss their thoughts, the doctor can usually summarize what the patient has said, showing that the physician has listened and understood the patient.

At this point, it is helpful to hand a mirror to the patient and, with the patient looking in the mirror,

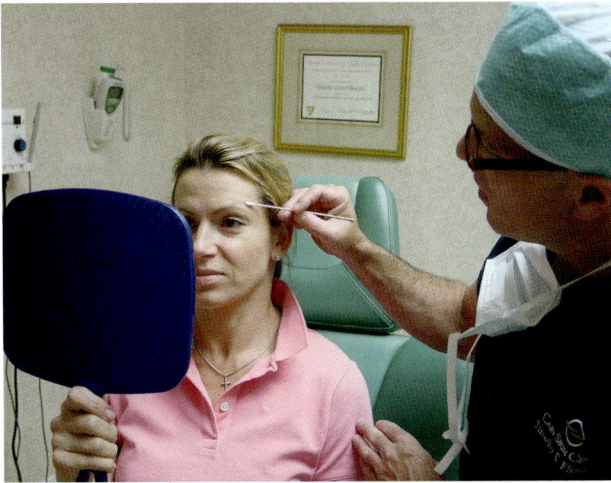

Figure 12.2 Physician and patient working with the hand mirror. In this example, the physician is demonstrating a possible brow lift which is achievable through correct use of periocular botulinum toxin.

begin the discussion of several treatment options (Figure 12.2). If it appears that the facial aging changes are amenable to botulinum toxin, the patient can accentuate their concerns by moving the muscles that produce these wrinkles. At this time, the physician can point out to the patient that these muscles will be relaxed by the protein, and the wrinkle should improve. If the patient desires some degree of sculpting with botulinum toxin, for example elevation of the lateral brow, the physician may take a cotton-tipped applicator and, with the patient looking in the mirror, show an approximate 1–2-mm elevation, and the patient can see the result. Many times patients have more than one concern, but want to start with just one treatment. The use of botulinum toxin is a good place to begin because the results are quite predictable and the patient can see an excellent result at 2 weeks. Most cosmetic surgeons routinely use botulinum toxin together with a filler substance such as hyaluronans at the same treatment session.

Another approach is to print a copy of the patient's preoperative photograph and have this available for both the patient and physician to review. All patients should have pre- and postoperative photographs taken which are valuable components of their medical record. In our clinic, all nurses take standard preoperative photographs using digital photography. They can easily print these pictures using a color laser printer in an approximately 21 × 30-cm size.

Having the patient contract the muscles which produce the wrinkles in the overlying skin helps the physician to understand the musculature. Physicians may find it helpful to palpate the contracted muscles to assess strength and the pattern of skin insertion. We then use a red 'dry erase' marker to indicate the injection sites. We have not experienced any tattooing from

the use of the markers, and any marks easily wipe off post-injection.

Contraindications

Botulinum toxin is widely used for many medical conditions in many patients. There are only a few contraindications. Patients with hypersensitivity to botulinum toxin or formulation components should not be treated. Patients with myasthenia gravis, Eaton–Lambert syndrome, or any atrophic lateral sclerosis should not be treated. Aminoglycoside antibiotics have been reported to potentiate the effects of botulinum toxin. Patients should be screened for their use. It is not advised to treat pregnant women or nursing mothers.

Patient expectations and education

Managing a patient's expectations is directly related to education about the procedure. For first-time patients, we use a cosmetic coordinator. The cosmetic coordinator is familiar with the basic science and clinical use of botulinum toxins and specifically knows how these toxins operate in the musculature. Patients are educated about how botulinum toxin works, are taught about dose and duration of the medication, and are informed about side-effects, risks, and complications. This education is supplemented by a series of pre- and postoperative photographs. We use a simple, time-tested, 'brag book' approach in which the patient is allowed to flip through a book of photographs. We have included many excellent results, and they are divided by anatomic areas that have been treated. We have also included some 'less than perfect' outcomes so that the patient is aware that they may not necessarily have a perfect result.

The issue of combination treatment is also addressed, with portions of the brag book being divided into the use of botulinum toxin alone, the use of botulinum toxin with filler substances, or the use of botulinum toxin, volume replacement, and non-ablative light sources such as IPL (intense pulsed light). This helps the patient to understand where they are headed and where they could end up with the use of multiple procedures, which are designed to address all of the changes of the aging face. Patients are often interested in knowing treatment options and seeing nice results when multiple areas are treated.

Before treatment of the patient, it is important that the physician discusses with the patient what he or she may expect and what he or she may not expect. A common statement to patients would be: 'Now remember that we are going to improve these lines, and I think that we can improve them significantly. However, we may not be able to completely erase them. I do think that you are going to look better, and I do think that you are going to like the result.'

Informed consent

It is imperative that all patients give signed informed consent before they are treated. Our informed consent is extensive, and is as much an education about the procedure as it is a legal document. Cosmetic surgeons might consider the use of such a document in their practice. The document is written in lay, common language and begins by answering questions such as: 'What is BOTOX?', 'How does botulinum toxin work?', 'How long does the treatment last?', and it ends with a thorough discussion of the risks of treatment with botulinum toxin. The risks outlined are comprehensive, and because of the American legal system and its proclivity for litigation, we must list rare risks such as scarring, diplopia, and even death. The informed consent is readdressed with every retreatment. BOTOX has a Food and Drug Administration (FDA) label for treatment of glabellar lines. If it is used in areas of the face other than the glabella it is considered an off-label use. Our consent form specifies that we may use the product off-label.

Preoperative checklist

It is helpful to have a preoperative checklist available for the staff. The botulinum toxin preoperative checklist includes a feature to document whether the patient is a new patient or a repeat patient. New patients meet with the cosmetic coordinator and are taken through the patient education system prior to meeting the physician. Repeat patients are allowed to bypass the cosmetic coordinator and meet with the regular nursing staff as well as the physician. Components of the preoperative checklist include confirmation that the patient is here for botulinum toxin treatment, preoperative photographs having been taken, discussion of pretreatment medications that the patient might be on such as aspirin or non-steroidal anti-inflammatory agents, which may increase bleeding, or aminoglycoside antibiotics, which may potentiate the effect of botulinum toxin, financial disclosure so that the patient understands exactly what the cost of the treatment will be, patient allergies, recent medical history, whether the patient requires topical anesthesia, and review of past treatment records (Table 12.2).

Treatment records

Careful recording of the treatments administered is essential for each patient. Our clinic uses a two-sided form. This form has a space available to record the patient's name, medical record number, and date of

Table 12.2   Preoperative checklist

New patient? (to see cosmetic coordinator first)
Previous treatment with botulinum toxin?
Medical records available and reviewed?
Preoperative photography taken?
Areas to be treated?
Financial forms reviewed?
Any bleeding disorders?
Use of aspirin, non-steroidal anti-inflammatory agents, Plavix®?
Use of filler substances in the area (either biodegradable or permanent)?
History of cosmetic surgery in area being treated?
Facial asymmetry?
Neuromuscular disorder such as Eaton–Lambert, myasthenia gravis, ALS?
History of motor nerve disease such as Bell's palsy?
Use of aminoglycoside antibiotics?
Known allergy to botulinum toxin or its components?
Nursing?
Pregnant?
Needs topical anesthesia?

ALS, amyotrophic lateral sclerosis.

birth for identification purposes. The botulinum product used is noted on the form as well as the lot number and expiration date. It also has a table which lists the area that was treated and a column noting the number of units used in that treatment area. It is good medical practice to record the treatment as number of units rather than volume injected, as dilution volumes may vary. The opposite side of the form contains a facial diagram, and the physician accurately marks the number of units and the exact point of injection on this 'facial map' (Figure 12.3). The form has a place for both physician and witness to sign. This way there is no question as to which areas were treated and with which type of toxin and the number of units administered. When the patient returns for repeat treatment, this form is readily available in their medical record to show exactly where the patient was treated. If the patient is pleased with their results, this operative form is available and allows the patient to be treated in exactly the same way. If there is a question as to the results that the patient achieved, it is invaluable to refer to this form and appropriate adjustments made in their treatment plan.

Postoperative care

Patients are given a written postoperative care sheet after their treatment. This written sheet is reviewed with the patient by the nurse. The postoperative checklist includes asking the patient not to manipulate the area for a period of 4 hours. It also asks the patient not to bend over or lie down for the same time period. Patients are asked to contract the musculature that was

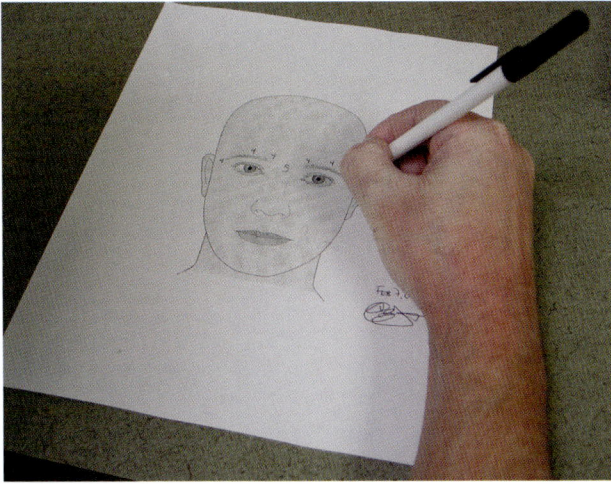

Figure 12.3   A medical record of botulinum toxin treatment showing injection points and number of units used.

injected, once every minute for a period of 2 hours, as there is some laboratory evidence in animals to suggest that active contracting of the muscle increases the uptake of the botulinum toxin. There have been no clinical studies to address any of the above issues; however, this is current common clinical practice. We also use this form to once again take the opportunity to remind the patient that they will see some effects in approximately 3–5 days, but their final effects will not be present for approximately 2 weeks. We believe that this reminder has decreased the incidence of phone calls from patients during the first week post-treatment as they are reminded that they will not have final results and they must wait 2 weeks to see them.

References

1. American Society of Plastic Surgery. Annual Statistics. Available at http://www.plasticsurgery.org/media/statistics/loader.cfm?url=/commonspot/security/getfile.cfm&PageID=2 3707.
2. Dayan SH, Bassichis BA. Evaluation of the patient for cosmetic BOTOX® Injection. Facial Plast Surg Clin N Am 2003; 11: 349–58.
3. Glogau RG. Aesthetic and anatomic analysis of the aging skin. Semin Cutan Med Surg 1996; 15: 134–8.
4. Shaw RB, Kahn DM. Aging of the midface bony elements: a three-dimensional computed comographic study. Plast Reconstr Surg 2007; 119: 675–81.
5. Carruthers J, Carruthers A. A prospective, randomized, parallel group study analyzing the effects of BTX-A (BOTOX®) and nonanimal sourced hyaluronic acid (NASHA, Restylane) in combination compared with NASHA (Restylane) alone in severe glabellar rhytids in adult female subjects: treatment of sever glabellar rhytids with a hyaluronic acid derivative compared with the derivative and BTX-A. Dermatol Surg 2003; 29: 802–9.
6. Flynn TC. Update on botulinum toxin. Semin Cutan Med Surg 2006; 25: 115–21.

Library
College of Physicians & Surgeons of B.C.
400 - 858 Beatty Street
Vancouver BC V6B 1C1

13 Legal and regulatory issues surrounding injectable dermal fillers and botulinum toxin in Europe

Martine Baspeyras

Introduction

The correction of facial skin aging with injectable products is an increasingly common medical procedure which is subject to several legal obligations: an obligation to provide due care, an obligation to inform the subject, and an obligation of continuing education for the practitioner.

There are two types of injectable products available to correct wrinkles that have different mechanisms of action: dermal fillers enhance volume, and botulinum toxin reduces muscle contraction. In 1993, dermal fillers, which had until then been considered as drugs, were included in the category of medical devices, and hence no longer required a marketing authorization. Botulinum toxin, on the other hand, is considered as an injectable drug, and as such is subject to much stricter rules and regulations, and is required to have a marketing authorization. Nevertheless, there are legal obligations that apply to both types of products: the practitioners using them must be familiar with their characteristics (doses, side-effects), must be adequately trained to use them, and must give information on the product to the subject prior to the procedure.

Legal obligations for dermal fillers

In France, since June 1998, injectable products have been required to bear a CE (Conformité Européene) marking, but this procedure does not offer any guarantee as to their efficacy or total safety. Filling is a cosmetic technique designed to correct expression or age-related wrinkles, but not skin ptosis. Broadly speaking, there are two categories of wrinkle fillers: biodegradable products and partially or non-biodegradable products.

These products are currently classed as Implantable Medical Devices (IMDs), thus differentiating them from drugs. In France, the definition of drugs is very precise (article L511 of the Public Health Code): a drug is any product that may be administered to humans to restore, correct, or modify organic functions. Before a drug reaches the market, an application must be made for a marketing authorization, which is granted according to well-defined rules regarding its manufacture, activity, and side-effects. Medical devices are different from drugs; they are considered as implants and require only a CE marking, as well as approval from the Microbiological Safety Commission (BSE) of the Health Ministry for animal-derived products.

There are several categories of implantable medical devices:

- Active implantable medical devices, intended to be totally or partially introduced, surgically or medically, into the human body or by medical intervention into a natural orifice, which are intended to remain after the procedure, and which rely for their functioning on a source of electrical energy or any source of power other than that directly generated by the human body or gravity; these devices fall under the European directive 90/385/EEC of 20 June 1990, published in the OJEC L189 of 20 July 1990.
- Medical devices other than active implantable medical devices include any instrument, apparatus, appliance, material, or other article, whether used alone or in combination, together with any accessories or software for proper functioning, intended by the manufacturer to be used in humans for the:

  - diagnosis, prevention, monitoring, treatment, or alleviation of disease or injury
  - investigation, replacement, or modification of the anatomy or of a physiological process
  - control of conception.

These devices, as well as the accessories required for operation of the device, as intended by the manufacturer, fall under the European directive 93/42/EEC of 14 June 1993 published in the OJEC L183 of 12 July 1993.

Library
College of Physicians & Surgeons of B.C.
400 - 858 Beatty Street
Vancouver BC V6B 1C1

Wrinkle filling products are currently considered as medical devices other than active implantable medical devices, and therefore must comply with directive 93/42/EEC.

Nevertheless, some publications are ambiguous; they do not consider such medical devices as being inert, and suggest that they 'stimulate tissue regeneration and neo-collagenesis'. If they do indeed have such an activity, then they become very close to being drugs.

The main criterion distinguishing a medical device from a drug lies in how the main action intended by the manufacturer is achieved:

- if it is achieved by physical means, the product is considered as a medical device (e.g. intrauterine device, suture material)
- if it is achieved by pharmacological, immunological, or metabolic means, the product is considered as a drug.

The main health and safety requirements applicable to medical devices are defined by the Public Health Code for medical devices (L665-1 to L665-9; R5274 to R5287 and R665-1 to R665-64; decree n° 95-292 of 16 March 1995 and its annexes); all these requirements are listed in the European Community (EC) declaration of conformity required to obtain a CE marking.

The European directive 93/42/EEC defines medical devices in Europe. Since 14 June 1998, it is no longer possible to sell in France or in other European countries a medical device that does not bear a CE marking. This marking represents a single, harmonized legislation applicable in all European Member States, and indicates that the device complies with the new European directives. Devices bearing a CE marking are allowed to circulate freely in all the Member States of the European Union. This European directive has two levels of application:

- a political level, as it harmonizes the various marketing procedures and reinforces the different safety levels by ensuring the compliance of all medical devices
- a technical level, as the CE marking is affixed by the manufacturer, under his own responsibility, based on various procedures and levels of control:

  - compliance with the essential performance and safety requirements, demonstrated in a technical file, including clinical data in some cases
  - specifications complying with those described in the technical file, guaranteed by the quality assurance system.

Therefore, the allocation of a CE marking is based on the product's technical file, clinical data, and quality assurance. It is designed to control risks both during its design and manufacturing stages, and after it has been placed on the market, with materiovigilance data.

A CE marking is affixed onto medical devices which comply with the essential safety and performance requirements. These essential requirements apply to the 19 countries of the European Economic Space, thus unified in terms of standards, quality, and health.

These devices must be designed and manufactured in such a way as to protect the subject's clinical condition and health:

- they must not put the users at risk
- they must attain the performances determined by the manufacturer
- their characteristics and performances must not be affected by storage
- the main risks associated with their use must be eliminated or minimized (risks associated with the toxicity of the materials, their incompatibility with biological tissues and cells, risk of infection for the subject, the user, or third parties during manipulations, risks associated with environmental conditions, such as magnetic fields, pressure etc.).

The objective of the European normalization is to detail the 'technical provisions' of the European directives.

A CE marking is not:

- a brand name
- a quality certification: it controls exclusively the safety and performances claimed by the manufacturer
- a quality assurance ISO (International Organization for Standardization) 9000 certification for the company, which is not sufficient to place a device on the market
- a voluntary, national product certification, e.g. quality labels such as NF, BS, DIN
- one of the French certification procedures that used to be compulsory for a limited number of products and devices with a preventive, diagnostic, and/or therapeutic use; the products concerned, determined by a ministerial order, were those whose use was associated with risks for the subject or the user, or whose design resulted from new technologies; this procedure was replaced on 14 June 1998 by the CE marking
- the Keymark pan-European voluntary third-party certification mark, added to the CE marking
- a reimbursement criterion for health and social services.

For animal-derived products, the 93/42/EEC directive states in article 1 that it does not apply to 'organs, tissues and cells of animal origin, unless a device is manufactured utilizing animal tissue which is rendered non-viable (i.e. not a site for metabolism or multiplication during final use), or non-viable products derived from tissues of animal origin'. Likewise, this directive does not apply to products of human origin or their derivatives.

The essential requirements are based on two main principles (annex I of the 93/42/EEC directive):

- 'Any risk associated with their use must be acceptable when weighed against the benefits to the subject and are compatible with a high level of protection of health and safety'
- 'The solutions adopted by the manufacturer for the design and construction of the devices must comply with safety principles, taking into account the generally acknowledged state of the art'.

The essential requirements include safety parameters for the subjects and the users, taking into account the benefit/risk ratios: the devices must attain the performance levels attributed to them by the manufacturer, and their characteristics and performances during their intended use must not be adversely affected during transport and storage, taking into account the instructions and information provided by the manufacturer.

There are also special requirements relative to the design and construction of the device, classed by theme, e.g. 'infection and microbial contamination'.

CE marking involves the following bodies:

- the European Commission in Brussels, guardian of the treaties, is an executive organization which has a monopoly of legislative initiative and makes propositions
- the competent authority in France is the Health Ministry; it controls application of the directives, designated by the European Commission, to the notified bodies, and has a right of inspection of the technical files, prepared and made available by the manufacturer; it makes classification decisions and holds a safeguard clause; finally, it sets up and implements the post-marketing vigilance system for the devices
- the notified bodies are 'competent bodies designated for carrying out the tasks pertaining to compliance evaluation as defined by the directive, designated by a Member State among the organizations falling under its jurisdiction, meeting the competence criteria and the requirements set in the directive and notified to the Commission and to the other Member States'.

CE marking and risks

Medical devices are currently divided into four classes (based on the US model) according to their potential risks: from class I associated with the lowest risk, to classes IIa, IIb, and III, associated with the highest risk (active implantable medical devices).

The legislation considers that wrinkle fillers are included in class III, as determined by rule 8 (implantable or invasive devices and long-term surgically invasive devices designed to have a biological effect or to be wholly or mainly absorbed), and by special rule 17 (devices manufactured using animal tissues or derivatives rendered non-viable).

There is an additional standard for the risk assessment of medical devices: standard EN 1441 provides a general methodology to identify hazards and estimate risks for the subjects, users, and third parties, associated with the use of the device, and to reduce those risks to an acceptable level.

Legislation and bovine spongiform encephalopathy

Bovine spongiform encephalopathy (BSE), also known as 'mad cow disease', has raised great concern about the use of bovine-derived products and the risk of contamination with the prion. In 1990, the literature described 15 cases (14 in England, one in France) of a new form of Creutzfeldt–Jakob disease (CJD). The rapid increase in new cases over 6 years was linked to exposure of the victims to food products derived from cattle with BSE. CJD is one of a group of diseases called transmissible spongiform encephalopathies (TSEs), which affect both animals (epizooty) and man. They are responsible for neuronal degeneration, always fatal, with a pathognomonic accumulation in the central nervous system of a transmissible (but not contagious) infectious agent called a prion (proteinaceous infectious particle). Until this new form appeared, the frequency of these diseases was low. The current form affects preferentially subjects at a young age.

Collagen was also suspected as a cause for BSE transmission to man. In the USA, numerous articles were published on the origin and control of collagen. Several safeguards were set up to eliminate the risk of contamination:

- tissue: collagen is extracted from the dermis, classed in category IV, as having 'no detectable infectivity' (annex 3)
- origin: dermis is produced from the skin of young bulls, raised exclusively in the USA, in closed lots, of direct female line since 1980; the line of each animal is known, controlled, and monitored; the animals are fed exclusively with grass, and health controls are performed regularly (every 6 weeks)
- manufacture: animals are slaughtered ethically on a specific site, without opening the cranium; collagen is isolated, concentrated, and purified, with controls all along the production chain, from the animal up to the final product, bearing a batch number and an expiry date; in addition, the collagen is sterilized using validated techniques to inactivate infectious agents
- control: defined and validated by the quality standards imposed by the Food and Drug Administration (FDA) and European directives.

This microbiological risk is assessed by the Community Health Protection for each product containing animal-derived substances; marketing is subject to the Public

Health Code (decree 95-292 of 16 March 1995 on medical devices as defined by article L665-3 of the Public Health Code, and modifying this code, annex I, A, 8-2): 'animal-derived tissues must originate from animals subjected to veterinary controls and surveillance measures adapted to the tissue's intended use [...]. Transformation, storage [...] must be performed under optimum safety conditions. Particularly, safety in terms of viruses and other transmissible agents must be guaranteed by validated techniques [...]'.

The government letter DH/EM 1 n° 96-4652 of 28 August 1996 relative to medical devices and products incorporating bovine-derived products states that, in compliance with the order of 3 May 1996, medical devices defined in articles L665-3 and L665-1 of the Public Health Code whose ingredients include bovine-derived products cannot be placed on the market and used unless the group of experts on microbiological safety has previously delivered a favorable opinion. A list, updated on 5 August 1996, of the medical devices granted a favorable opinion regarding their microbiological safety, is given in an annex. US collagen is not included in this positive list, because it had a marketing authorization in France at the time.

The order of 28 May 1998 concerned the withdrawal of implantable medical devices for cosmetic use (Official Journal of 30 May 98; annex 4):

- '[...] inasmuch as percutaneous injections of liquid silicone are associated with a risk of complications, particularly locoregional
- inasmuch as the effects and complications may have serious repercussions on the health of the people in whom such products are used
- inasmuch as the compliance with essential health and safety requirements applicable to these medical devices must be certified prior to their marketing
- the manufacture, import, export, storage, marketing, whether free of charge or not, as well as implantation of the following medical devices: [...] injectable liquid silicone for cosmetic use, are suspended for a period of 1 year as of the publication date of the present order.'

In Europe

In conclusion, a product bearing a CE marking is registered automatically and can be sold in all European countries. Although an application file must be submitted for all other countries, some non-European Union (EU) countries recognize the CE marking as a proof of quality (e.g. Switzerland, following its bilateral agreements with the EU).

In Switzerland, CE-marked devices must be registered with the agency Swissmedic, accompanied by the manufacturer's ISO 13485:2003 quality certification. Class III medical devices only require a quality certification of

the manufacturer and declaration of conformity. Swissmedic will then establish a Free Sales Certificate, granting the product the right to be sold on the Swiss market.

Legal obligations of practitioners

In France

Practitioners must be familiar with the characteristics of each product used, i.e. its chemical formula, administration route, injection technique, quantity to inject and especially the maximum quantity allowed, fate of the injected product, any side-effects, and legal aspects.

The medical procedure must not have adverse effects, and the medical risk of a cosmetic procedure must be as close to nil as possible. Under no circumstances must the condition of the subject be worsened for the purpose of achieving a cosmetic result.

Any malpractice exposes the practitioner to civil, penal, and disciplinary procedures. Medical responsibility is based on a contract (Mercier order 1936) between the physician and his client, where the practitioner agrees to provide conscientious due care, complying with current scientific data. The same rules apply to cosmetic procedures, with an even greater duty to provide information to the subject. However, there are exceptions, in particular when the physician guarantees a given result. His obligation to provide due care may then shift, from his own initiative, to an obligation to achieve a given result.

Malpractice is defined as a breach of a pre-existing obligation. There are two main categories of breaches:

- breach of medical humanism
- breach of technical duty.

The duty of humanism includes the obligation to inform, evidenced by the informed consent form.

The duty to inform is essential, and particularly important in cosmetic procedures. In the case of a dispute, the burden of proof of information lies with the practitioner since the Supreme Court issued an order to that effect on 25 February 1997 (Cousin order). Before this order was issued, it was for the subject to prove that he had not been given the necessary information (negative proof difficult to provide). This order is reminiscent of the obligation to inform as defined in article 35 of the Code of Ethics, which is reinforced for procedures aimed only at correcting simple physical imperfections (cosmetic procedures). However, this change only applies to the delivery of information and not to the relevance of its content; if the subject claims that the information was inadequate, he will have to prove it (annex 4).

Zero risk does not exist in medicine, whether cosmetic or not, and total and comprehensive information is unrealistic. Information on the major known risks, even those that are rare, is recommended. In cosmetic procedures, minor risks should be described as well. Proof of such information may be given with an informed consent form signed by the subject. However, in procedures as simple as dermal filling, evidence may be given by a third person present when oral information was given to the subject.

In the USA, datasheets are generally given to the subject for any cosmetic procedure. In France, it is compulsory to provide a detailed financial quote for procedures costing above €300, 15 days before the scheduled date (order of 17 October 1996 – Official Journal of 29 October 1996), but as it is not a surgical act, the delay can be reduced to 48 hours. This document does not list the associated risks. Some practitioners send by post a datasheet explaining the procedure and main risks, along with the scheduled date for the procedure. The fact that the subject actually comes at the appointed time is a presumption of proof that information had indeed been given. However, this raises the question of the subject's understanding of the given information and of its relevance.

The subject's consent is easy to obtain for wrinkle filling, as she has generally requested the procedure. Technical errors associated with these devices include manipulation errors (e.g. injection too deep or too superficial, infection, granuloma, necrosis), or errors in appreciation of the subject's real demand, which has not been satisfied, or an overestimation of the possibilities of correction. It is important to always err on the side of caution when it comes to promising results with cosmetic procedures. If damage has been done, the causal relationship must be demonstrated, which is often easy to do with dermal fillers. It is important to remember that although the use of silicone is currently banned, its relationship with autoimmune diseases has not been formally established, and the decision rests mostly on presumptions.

The current trend in cosmetic procedures is towards an obligation regarding the safety of the procedure. The contract between the subject and the physician means that the latter implicitly agrees not to cause any damage to the subject. This means that the physician must not worsen the subject's condition. It is very important that the subject is well informed on the risks of the procedure, so that if damage occurs, the physician is able to explain what happened. On 17 January 1991, the Supreme Court in Versailles, France, detailed some of the peculiarities of subject information in cosmetic surgery: 'In matters of cosmetic surgery, the risk must not be disproportionate compared to the expected benefits, and a balance must be struck between the injury caused by the procedure and the expected benefit. The practitioner must inform the subject of such risks. This includes intolerance to the materials used: breast implant, anti-wrinkle treatment, and lip enhancement'.

Wrinkle filling techniques correct folds considered as unsightly and aging. The result of this procedure is difficult to appreciate as is it subjective. The most important stage is the initial consultation, when the subject's actual demand must be defined. Indications must be measured

and wrinkles analyzed, explaining the limits of the correction, both physical and over time. It is also important to determine the subject's psychological profile carefully and understand her demand: even a perfect filling of wrinkles will never bring back a womanizing husband, and in this case the subject will never be satisfied.

Finally, in addition to the obligation not to cause adverse effects, provide due care, and provide extended information, the practitioner also has an obligation to keep abreast of any new development in his field. The practice of cosmetic medicine or surgery must adhere to the rules of morality, dignity, and ethics of the medical profession. Consequently, before injecting a product, the physician must also verify that it does indeed bear a CE marking. This marking is compulsory: it guarantees the product's safety and entitles it to free circulation within Europe.

A recent survey conducted among UK lawyers specialized in medical litigation provided an interesting observation: when patients were asked: 'Once the damage has occurred, what attitude would have led you not to sue?', the most common answer was 'explanations and excuses'.

Irrespective of the injectable product used, it is essential to comply strictly with the manufacturer's recommendations as specified in the instructions for use.

The skin undergoes constant deterioration and regeneration, and it may seem questionable to inject it with a permanent product which does not behave in the same way.

Subject information must include a detailed financial quote. The practitioner must allow a minimum period between this quote and the procedure. During this period, no compensation may be demanded or obtained from the person concerned, nor any commitment with the exception of fees due for the preliminary consultation. This 'grace' period is a legal requirement: its duration is determined by decree, and starts as of the date that the quote is given to the subject. A financial quote is compulsory for all cosmetic procedures in excess of €300, or which require general anesthesia. This detailed compulsory quote must be signed by the practitioner, and by the subject, who will note in his own handwriting: 'Quote received prior to procedure'.

Any failure to give a detailed quote, to forego the grace period, or to demand or obtain compensation of any nature during this period is an offense punishable by a €30 000 fine.

Fraudulent persons may be declared legally responsible under the conditions defined in article 121-2 of the Criminal Code.

Materiovigilance

Materiovigilance is poorly understood by physicians, who are more familiar with pharmacovigilance and cosmetovigilance. Like pharmacovigilance, materiovigilance is a legal requirement designed to protect public health. The national commission of materiovigilance is

Table 13.1   Availability of botulinum toxin in Europe

Country	European approved conditions of prescription, dispensation, and distribution of Vistabel®
BE – Belgium	Distribution via pharmacies (on prescription only)
	Off-label use is the responsibility of the physician
	To be confirmed: awaiting granting of marketing anthorization (MA)
CY – Cyprus*	Distribution via pharmacies
	Direct supply to physician not possible according to regulation
DK – Denmark	Distribution via pharmacies or hospitals
	Prescription restricted to specialists in dermatology, plastic surgery, and neurology, according to supplementary protection certiticate (SPC)
EE – Estonia	Classified as prescription only drug
	Not on health insurance reimbursement list
	Distribution as usual via wholesalers
EL – Greece	Not available at the moment
	Awaiting granting of MA
ES – Spain	A Spanish government letter (n° 03/2004) set the conditions of prescription, dispensation, and utilization of Vistabel
	In most cases, Allergan distributes the product directly to pharmacies. These pharmacies can store the product for clinics which do not have an internal pharmacy, or manage the stock in clinics which do not have a pharmacist in charge. The pharmacies then directly distribute the product to the qualified physicians. No specific requirement regarding physician qualifications: 'Doctors with the appropriate qualification, with experience in the treatment and with the appropriate equipment'
FI – Finland	Distribution via pharmacies or hospitals. Wholesalers can sell directly to hospitals which have a pharmacy, mainly university teaching hospitals or district hospitals. Private hospitals cannot buy directly from wholesalers
	Should only be administered by physicians with appropriate qualifications and expertise in this treatment and having the required equipment, according to national SPC – not yet approved
	Prescription not restricted
FR – France	Can be prescribed only by specialists in:
	• plastic, reconstructive, and esthetic surgery
	• dermatology
	• face and neck surgery
	• maxillofacial surgery
	• ophthalmology
	Dispensed by pharmacist or Allergan directly to the above-mentioned specialists
GE – Germany	Every physician can prescribe Vistabel
	Distribution is only through pharmacies, hospital pharmacies, or veterinary pharmacies upon prescription
HU – Hungary	Prescription only medicine, requiring special supervision by a specialist throughout the treatment after diagnosis made by a specialist or in hospital
	Standard distribution
IS – Iceland	Distribution through pharmacies with prescription restricted to specialists (dermatologists, plastic surgeons)
	Distribution from wholesalers to pharmacies, hospitals, or directly to physicians
IT – Italy	Can be prescribed only by specialists in:
	• plastic surgery
	• dermatology
	• maxillofacial surgery
	• ophthalmology
	Supplied by pharmacist or Allergan directly to the above-mentioned specialists
LT – Lithuania	Will be available only after MA has been granted
LU – Luxembourg	Distribution via pharmacies (prescription only)
	Off-label use is the responsibility of the physician
	To be confirmed: awaiting granting of MA
LV – Latvia	Not available at the moment: awaiting granting of MA
MT – Malta**	Vivian Corporation Ltd will distribute directly to trained cosmetic specialists and their respective private clinics and hospitals. Pharmacies and wholesalers are not involved in the distribution process
NO – Norway	Distribution via pharmacies. Direct distribution to physicians not possible
	Administration by physicians with appropriate qualifications and expertise in this treatment and having the required equipment, according to SPC
	Prescription not restricted, but it is recommended that the prescribing physician has the appropriate qualifications
PT – Portugal	Direct supply to physician impossible according to regulation
	Distribution via pharmacies or wholesalers to cosmetic clinics
	Prescription only medicine

(Continued)

Table 13.1   (Continued)

Country	European approved conditions of prescription, dispensation, and distribution of Vistabel®
SE – Sweden	Note: direct supply to physicians only possible for vaccines and sera
	Distribution via pharmacies, prescription only
	Administration by physicians with appropriate qualifications and expertise in this treatment and having the required equipment, according to SPC
	Prescription not restricted, but it is recommended that the prescribing physician has the appropriate qualifications
UK	Administered by physicians, surgeons, dentists, and nurses (under medical supervision)

*

**

dependent on the Ministry of Health. After products have been placed on the market, any incident is notified, then assessed and dealt with by the commission. According to the law of 18 January 1994, physicians are required to report any incident which occurred with medical devices; failure to do so exposes the practitioner to 4 years' imprisonment and/or a fine.

Botulinum toxin

Botulinum toxin is a drug, and therefore must have a marketing authorization in France. The availability of botulinum toxin for the treatment of wrinkles varies from one European country to another. The data are summarized in Table 13.1.

Table 13.1 was designed in 2006, and the data are constantly evolving. In France, botulinum toxin may become available to all physicians. However, irrespective of the distribution conditions of the drug, the importance of specific training on its use is emphasized.

Conclusion

In Europe, injectable products to correct wrinkles are subject to two legislations, depending on their classification.

Injectable products are considered as medical devices, and as such require a CE marking. This European certification means that some degree of clinical evaluation has been done, albeit limited. A CE marking is not based on uniform, strict, and rigorous rules in all countries, but it represents an attempt at harmonization.

Botulinum toxin is considered as a drug in all European countries, and must therefore be assessed in stricter clinical studies (double-blind, randomized, multicenter). Its distribution and dispensing conditions vary widely from one country to another.

14 General monitoring: conservation, dilution, and storage

Doris Hexsel, Débora Zechmeister do Prado, and Maryelle Moreira Lima

Introduction

Of the eight existing botulinum toxin (BTX) serotypes, the one designated BTX type A (BTX-A) is the purest form and was the first to be developed for clinical use.[1] Today, three commercial brands are currently marketed in Brazil, and in other countries, approved for cosmetic use: Dysport® (Ipsen, France), BOTOX® (Allergan, USA), and Prosigne® (Lanzhou Institute of Biological Products, China). A commercial brand of the botulinum toxin B (BTX-B), Myobloc®/NeuroBloc® (Elan Pharmaceuticals Inc, USA) has been granted approval by the Food and Drug Administration (FDA) for the treatment of cervical dystonia,[2] though there are few studies on the safety and effectiveness of this toxin for cosmetic use.[3,4] Additionally, studies on new preparations derived from other toxins, from both botulinum and alternatives, are under way, and they may reach the markets of several countries in the future.

The four abovementioned brand names are the ones currently commercially available and will be discussed in this chapter. Although they present the same therapeutic action, producing similar effects on muscles and sweat glands, they each have distinctive characteristics, since their methods of formulation, preservation, dilution, and storage vary.

Knowledge of the BTX formulation and handling protocols is of critical importance in order to achieve the expected cosmetic outcome.

Product formulation and presentation

While the four commercial brands are produced from purified cultures of the bacterium *Clostridium botulinum*, they each have various distinctive features, such as the number of units, chemical properties, biological action, and molecular weight.[5] While BTX-A formulations are marketed in a lyophilized form, being sterile and producing comparable and similar results after being injected, BTX-B is marketed in a diluted form in three different concentrations.

Dysport is soon to be granted approval in the USA, where it will be marketed under the trade name Reloxin®. Dysport is produced using a column based purification method.[5] The toxin complex is recovered through a series of steps, including chromatography, precipitation, dialysis, and filtration. It is then dissolved in an aqueous solution of human serum albumin and lactose, after which it is filtered and freeze-dried. The lactose acts as a bulking agent facilitating reconstitution.[6] Dysport is marketed in South America, Asia, and Europe, in vials of 500 U of BTX-A, combined with 125 µg of human serum albumin and 2.5 mg of lactose.[7]

BOTOX is produced through a technique of multiple acid precipitations until a complex is obtained consisting of proteins with a high molecular weight of the toxin, in combination with hemagglutinin protein. This complex is then redissolved in a saline and albumin solution, subjected to sterile filtration, and freeze-dried.[5] Each 100-U vial is vacuum-sealed, and contains 0.5 mg of human albumin and 0.9 mg of preservative-free sodium chloride.[5,8–10]

Because both Dysport and BOTOX use albumin as an excipient, they should not be administered to individuals with a history of allergy or intolerance to the ingredients contained in the formulation.[11]

Prosigne is processed through a series of purification procedures and then filtered by redissolving and dialysis.[12] It is marketed in vials containing 100 U of BTX-A, combined with 5 mg of gelatin, 25 mg of dextran, and 25 mg of saccharose.[12]

Myobloc/NeuroBloc is formulated in a purified liquid preparation buffered at a pH of 5.6, which provides greatly enhanced stability. Unlike the other BTX-A formulations, which are lyophilized powder preparations, BTX-B does not require reconstitution. This is considered easy and convenient by the manufacturers.[2] Size exclusion chromatography and high-performance liquid chromatography indicate that commercial preparations of type B are uniform.[4] Each single vial of formulated Myobloc/NeuroBloc contains 5000 U of botulinum toxin type B per milliliter in

0.05% human serum albumin, 0.01 mol/l sodium succinate, and 0.1 mol/l sodium chloride.[13]

Conservation

Considered unstable solutions, BTX-A preparations should be stored under refrigeration and require specific storage care. Heat will not have any damaging effect on their stability, where the recommended storage directions are observed. It is therefore recommended that BTX-A be stored under refrigeration with a thermometer to ensure the vials are maintained at the required temperature.

With relation to the storage temperatures, Dysport should be stored, before being diluted, at temperatures of 2–8°C,[8,14] according to the manufacturer's directions for use. The written directions for use provided by the manufacturers of BOTOX require it to be stored, prior to being diluted, in a freezer at a temperature of –5°C (25°F) or in a refrigerator at temperatures of 2–8°C. There are studies which have shown that BOTOX can be kept stored in a refrigerator, even prior to dilution, at the recommended temperatures of 2–8°C without any damage to its properties.[8–10,15–18] Prosigne should be stored frozen at temperatures between –20 and –5°C and, after reconstitution, should be stored under refrigeration at 2–8°C. Myobloc/NeuroBloc should be stored under refrigeration at 2–8°C, according to the manufacturer's directions for use.

As a general rule, all BTX preparations should be stored, after reconstitution and before use, under refrigeration at temperatures of 2–8°C.

Reconstitution

The recommended diluent for BTX-A reconstitution is 0.9% sterile saline, either with or without preservatives.[9,16,19–22] According to some authors, preservative use may reduce pain.[23–25] Conversely, others suggest that the presence of preservatives in the saline solution may partially inactivate the toxin, and so reduce its potency.[9,17] Nevertheless, Alam et al have demonstrated that while the addition of preservatives does not interfere with the production and the duration of effect, it acts to minimize the injection pain.[24] Carruthers and Carruthers highlight that dilution in 0.9% saline with preservatives has two advantages: the possibility of storing reconstituted BTX-A for longer, with no risk of bacterial contamination, and with an additional anesthetic effect, though mild, on the injection site, reducing the 'stinging' feeling during BTX-A injection sessions.[14] Furthermore, other studies focus on the possibility of diluting BTX-A in a solution containing xylocaine at a concentration of 1%.[17]

Prior to injecting the diluent into the vial, antisepsis of the cap on the vial with 70% alcohol is required.

For reconstitution, a 10-ml or larger vial of 0.9% saline is suggested. The desired amount should be aspirated and any residual solution discarded. This way, contamination of the BTX-A is prevented and previously opened vials can be reused.

For reconstitution, 1-ml or 3-ml syringes and 21G needles are the most commonly used equipment for BTX-A reconstitution.[23]

When injecting the diluent into the vial of BTX-A, care should be taken to ensure it is done slowly, to avoid agitation and the formation of air bubbles, which may result in protein denaturation and, consequently, loss of potency.[16,17,21,26] Trindade De Almeida et al reported no observed loss of efficacy in a preparation of BTX-A (BOTOX) after diluting two vials with and without bubble formation, injected into three patients.[27] However, for vacuum-sealed toxins it is suggested that the plunger of the syringe be locked and slowly released in order to avoid the rapid aspiration of the 0.9% saline solution. According to the manufacturer's directions for use, a vial should be discarded if the vacuum does not pull the diluent into the vial.[28]

After reconstitution, the vial may be gently rotated a few times to ensure proper homogenization of the mixture.[26,28] Prior to use, it is recommended that all reconstituted products be inspected visually. The solution should be clear, homogeneous, colorless, and free of particles.[28]

Myobloc/NeuroBloc is available as a solution and, therefore, reconstitution is not required.[2,4,29]

Dilution

There are differences in the potency of the commercial brands of BTX-A, which mean that units of a preparation of BTX-A from one manufacturer do not correspond to the units of another preparation from another manufacturer. As all BTX-A formulations present similar actions when injected into muscles and sweat glands, doses may be compared to determine the amount of units of the different formulations that produce the same results for the same length of time, in terms of the intensity of muscular relaxation and the anhydrotic effect. Establishing the dose equivalence for the different products is important in determining the doses of each product that yield the same results, and so permit the products to be diluted in such a way that they can be applied with equal volumes using the same technique. Thus, the knowledge and understanding of these equivalences provide the expertise required to perform dilution-to-injection techniques, which is critically important for obtaining the results and efficacy desired.[9,17]

There is some disagreement among authors regarding the dose equivalence of 500 and 100 U of type A botulinum toxins, with equivalences being reported of 1 U of BOTOX to 9 U[30–34] of Dysport. However, professionals skilled in the cosmetic use of the two products agree with the equivalence of 1 U of BOTOX to 2–2.5 U of Dysport.[35,36] This is the position of the authors of this chapter, who use the equivalence index of 1:2.5 U, between BOTOX and Dysport, because it yields similar results, particularly in terms of the duration and intensity of muscular paralysis and anhydrotic effect. This has been demonstrated in a recent pilot study, in which the same equivalence resulted in similar action halos,[36] and no diffusion or dispersion of the dilutions utilized (1 ml of BOTOX to 2 ml of Dysport) was observed.[36] The injected sites produced regular rounded or slightly oval action halos. Higher equivalences are contraindicated due to the high risk of causing unwanted and unnecessary potency-related effects.[37,38] To date, there are no available studies reporting dose equivalence between Prosigne and Dysport and/or BOTOX. The relative potency of Myobloc/NeuroBloc is approximately 50–125 U per 1 U of BOTOX.

Since dilutions in different volumes are utilized for cosmetic use and may vary according to the physician's preference, the toxin concentration may vary according to the therapeutic objectives. In dilutions for cosmetic applications, smaller volumes are preferable, resulting in highly concentrated products, more localized effects, minimal solution dispersion, and minimal risk of possible side-effects and complications. Usually, 100 U of BTX-A is diluted in 1 ml of 0.9% preservative-free saline, resulting in a concentration of 1 U/0.01 ml, which facilitates calculation of the appropriate dose for each injection,[15,19,39] but higher volumes may be employed, according to the physician's preference. For 500 U of BTX-A, it is suggested that either double the 0.9% saline is used in the dilution, resulting in a dose equivalence of 1:2.5 U, or dilution in 2.5 ml to obtain 200 U/ml.[16] Other dilutions may be employed, and the equivalences are shown in Table 14.1.

During recent years, researchers have been striving to deliver innovative solutions that aim to increase the efficacy and optimize the cost/benefit ratio of BTX-A therapy.[40] The options suggested are: to modify the injection technique; to increase post-injection muscle activity; to modify toxin preparation utilizing different volumes. This last option is the most commonly employed, since it requires no special skills or additional therapy.[40] There are, however, some disadvantages, undesirable for both practitioners and patients, such as the discomfort involved in the injection of high volumes and the risk of dispersion of the saline containing BTX-A into neighboring muscles. Some studies in the therapeutic field suggest that higher dilutions lead to an increase in muscular paralysis.[41,42] In the cosmetic field, some authors also advocate the use of higher volumes. Hsu et al have studied the influence of the volume injected in equivalent doses in the treatment of periorbital wrinkles, and concluded that low concentration and high volume resulted in better 'diffusion' and a more extended action within the treated area.[30] On the other hand, Fulton has

Table 14.1 The dilution suggested in order to obtain different equivalences among the commercial preparations of 100 U and 500 U of type A botulinum toxin, using different volumes

Equivalence ratio	Vial of 100 U	Vial of 500 U
1:2 U	Diluted in 1 ml	Dilute in 2.5 ml
1:2.5 U	Diluted in 1 ml	Dilute in 2 ml
1:3 U	Diluted in 1 ml	Dilute in 1.66 ml
1:2 U	Diluted in 2 ml	Dilute in 5 ml
1:2.5 U	Diluted in 2 ml	Dilute in 4 ml
1:3 U	Diluted in 2 ml	Dilute in 3.2 ml

demonstrated that BTX-A diluted in 10 ml was as effective as that diluted in 20 ml, in patients who had never received previous treatment with BTX-A.[26] Patients previously treated by Fulton required additional doses of the 10-ml dilution, in order to increase the duration of the results, showing that the 20-ml dilution was less effective.[26] Nevertheless, the choice of dilution should be based on the desired outcome, according to the specialist's preference.[30]

Another option to help optimize results is the use of adjunctive techniques, such as fillers, chemical peels, lasers, and light sources, which are the most widely used.

Myobloc/NeuroBloc is available in three vial preparations of 2500, 5000, and 10 000 U. The concentration of the product contained in each vial is 5000 U/1 ml or 500 U/0.1 ml. Many physicians choose to dilute it to reduce the pain on injection. In order to yield a final concentration of 300 U/0.1 ml for each injection, a 5000-U vial can be further diluted with preserved saline at a ratio of 0.6 ml BTX-B/0.4 ml preserved saline in a 1-ml syringe.[3] Significantly, each vial is overfilled, and contains more BTX-B than stated on the label: the vial containing 2500 U/0.5 ml actually has 4100 U in 0.82 ml; the 5000 U/1-ml vial contains 6800 U in 1.36 ml, and the 10 000 U/2-ml vial contains 12 650 U in 2.53 ml.[2]

Storage after dilution

According to the manufacturers, following reconstitution, BTX-A should be used within the shortest possible time span,[15] as its useful life is short. According to the manufacturers, BOTOX and Prosigne have a useful life of 4 hours when refrigerated at a temperature between 2 and 8°C,[1,21,39,43,44] while Dysport has a useful life of only 8 hours following reconstitution when maintained under refrigeration.

Repeated freezing and thawing of reconstituted BTX-A is not recommended, since it may lead to possible denaturation of toxin with the molecules being broken down by the ice crystals.[43] A laboratory assay by Gartlan and Hoffman demonstrated a potency loss of 69.8% of botulinum toxin (BOTOX) when frozen immediately post-dilution, for further use after 2 weeks.[45] According to these authors, toxin deterioration was statistically significant after refrigeration and storage for 12 hours, but not for 6 hours.

However, later published clinical studies challenge these findings.[43] Sloop et al compared the BTX-A (BOTOX) efficacy injected immediately post-reconstitution and after 2 weeks stored under refrigeration (4°C) or refrozen (−20°C).[43] They concluded that the BOTOX injected immediately post-dilution or after 2 weeks' storage, under refrigeration or refreezing, produced the same therapeutic effects.[43] A more recent study demonstrated a more extended duration, with no loss of efficacy of the toxin injected within up to 6 weeks after reconstitution,[46] and no contamination of the vials within up to 14 weeks afterwards.[47] Myobloc/NeuroBloc is more stable in its solution, remaining stable for 3 years when stored in a refrigerator at 2–8°C, for at least 9 months, or at room temperature (25°C).[2]

Conclusion

Knowledge of the preservation, dilution, and storage techniques is critically important in order to ensure the desired results and efficacy of the BTX treatment as well as to avoid any unwanted side-effects.

In the future, many studies will hopefully reveal more appropriate methods than those currently used for the preservation, dilution, and storage of the botulinum toxins types A and B marketed worldwide.

References

1. Carruthers J, Carruthers A. Aesthetic botulinum A toxin in the mid and lower face and neck. Dermatol Surg 2003; 29: 468–76.
2. Sadick N, Sorhaindo L. The cosmetic use of botulinum toxin type B. Int Ophthalmol Clin 2005; 45: 153–61.
3. Sadick NS. Botulinum toxin type B for glabellar wrinkles: a prospective open-label response study. Dermatol Surg 2002; 28: 817–21.
4. Spencer JM. Cosmetic uses of botulinum toxin type B. Cosmet Dermatol 2002; 15: 11–14.
5. Huang W, Foster JA, Rogachefsky AS. Pharmacolocy of botulinum toxin. J Am Acad Dermtol 2000; 43: 249–59.
6. Markey AC. Dysport. Dermatol Clin 2004; 22: 213–19.
7. Odergren T, Hjaltason H, Kaakkola S et al. A double blind, randomized, parallel group study to investigate the dose equivalence of Dysport® and Botox® in the treatment of cervical dystonia. J Neurol Neurosurg Psychiatry 1998; 64: 6–12.
8. Carruthers A, Carruthers J. The cosmetic use of botulinum A exotoxin. In: Dzubow LM (ed). Cosmetic Dermatologic Surgery. Philadelphia: Lippincott-Eaness, 1998: 1–18.
9. Benedetto AV. The cosmetic uses of botulinum toxin type A. Int J Dermatol 1999; 38: 641–55.
10. Lowe NJ. Botulinum toxin type A for facial rejuvenation. Dermatol Surg 1998; 24: 1216–18.
11. Sabatovich O, Carneiro LVJ, Zechmeister D. Aspectos fundamentais da toxina botulínica. In: Kede MPV, Sabatovich O, eds. Dermatologia Estética. São Paulo: Atheneu, 2003: 563–6.
12. Carruthers A, Carruthers JD. Toxins: new information about the botulinum neurotoxins. Dermatol Surg 2000; 26: 174–6.
13. Product literature (Package insert) on Myobloc®. Solstice Neurosciences, Inc, South San Francisco, CA, 2004.
14. Carruthers A, Carruthers J. Cosmetic uses of botulinum A exotoxin. Adv Dermatol 1997; 12: 325–48.
15. Fagien S, Brandt FS. Primary and adjunctive use of botulinum toxin type A (Botox®) in facial aesthetic surgery: beyond the glabella. Clin Plast Surg 2001; 28: 127–48.
16. Sommer B, Sattler G. Botulinum Toxin in Aesthetic Medicine. Vienna: Blackwell Science, 2001.
17. Klein AW. Dilution and storage of botulinum toxin. Dermatol Surg 1998; 24: 1179–80.
18. Klein AW. Cosmetic therapy with botulinum toxin, anecdotal memoirs. Dermatol Surg 1996; 22: 757–9.
19. Carruthers A, Carruthers J. Botulinum toxin in the treatment of glabellar frown lines and other facial wrinkles. In: Jankovic J, Hallet M, eds. Therapy with Botulinum Toxin. New York: Marcel Dekker, 1994: 577–95.
20. Khawaja HA, Hernandez-Perez E. Botox in dermatology. Int J Dermatol 2001; 40: 311–17.
21. Markey AC. Botulinum A exotoxin in cosmetic dermatology. Clin Dermatol 2000; 25: 173–5.
22. Matarasso LS. Comparison of botulinum toxin types A and B: a bilateral and double-blind randomized evaluation in the treatment of canthal rhytides. Dermatol Surg 2003; 29: 7–13.
23. Carruthers J, Fagien S, Matarazzo S. Consensus recommendations of the use of botulinum toxin type A in facial aesthtics. Plas Reconst Surg 2004; 114 (6 Suppl): 1S–21S.
24. Alam M, Dover JS, Arndt KA. Pain associated with injections of botulinum toxin A exotoxin reconstituted using isotonic sodium chloride with and without preservative: a double-blind randomized controlled trial. Arch Dermatol 2002; 138: 510–14.
25. Kwiat DM, Bersani TA, Bersani A. Increased patient comfort utilizing botulinum toxin type a reconstituted with preserved versus no preserved saline. Ophthal Plast Reconstr Surg 2004; 20: 186–9.
26. Fulton JE. Botulinum Toxin. The Newport Beach experience. Dermatol Surg 1998; 24: 1219–24.
27. Trindade De Almeida AR, Kadunc BV, Di Chiacchio N, Neto DR. Foam during reconstitution does not affect the potency of botulinum toxin type A. Dermatol Surg 2003; 29: 530–1.
28. Anderson ER. Proper dose, preparation and storage of botulinum neurotoxin serotype A. Am J Health Syst Pharm 2004; 61 (15 Suppl 6): S24–6.
29. Barnes MP. Practical aspects of using botulinum toxin type B. Eur J Neuro 2001; 8 (Suppl 4): 19–21.
30. Hsu TS, Dover JS, Arndt KA. Effect of volume and concentration on the diffusion of botulinum exotoxin A. Arch Dermatol 2004; 140: 1351–4.
31. Matarasso SL. Comparison of botulinum toxin types A and B: a bilateral and double-blind randomized evaluation in the treatment of canthal rhytides. Dermatol Surg 2003; 29: 7–13.
32. Moore P, Naumann M. General and clinical aspects of treatment with botulinum toxin. In: Moore P, Naumann M, eds. Handbook of Botulinum Toxin Treatment, 2nd edn. Oxford: Blackwell Science, 2003: 28–75.
33. Sposito MMM. New indications for botulinum toxin type A in cosmetics: mouth and neck. Plast Reconstr Surg 2002; 110: 601–11.
34. Dressler D, Rothwell JC. Electromyographic quantification of the paralysing effect of botulinum toxin in the sternocleidomastoid muscle. Eur Neurol 2000; 43: 13–16.
35. Monheit G. Advanced botulinum toxin. Presented at 63rd Annual AAD Meeting, New Orleans, 19 February, 2005.
36. Hexsel D, Dal Forno Dini T, Prado-Zechmeister D, Hexsel C. Diffusion, dispersion, or action halos of botulinum toxin? A pilot study comparing two commercial preparations of type A botulinum toxins. Am J Dermatol 2005; 52: AB2.

37. Simonetta Moreau M, Cauhepe C, Magues JP, Senard JM. A double-blind, randomized, comparative study of Dysport vs. Botox in primary palmar hyperhidrosis. Br J Dermatol 2003; 149: 1041–5.

38. Beseler-Soto B, Sanchez-Palomares M, Santos-Serrano L et al. [Iatrogenic botulism: a complication to be taken into account in the treatment of child spasticity]. Rev Neurol 2003; 37: 444–6. [in Spanish]

39. Carruthers A, Carruthers J. Botulinum toxin type A: history and current cosmetic use in the upper face. Semin Cutan Med Surg 2001; 20: 71–84.

40. Francisco GE. Botulinum toxin: dosing and dilution. Am J Phys Med Rehabil 2004; 83 (Suppl): S30–7.

41. Francisco GE, Boake C, Vaughn A. Botulinum toxin in upper limb spasticity after acquired brain injury: a randomized trial comparing dilution techniques. Am J Phys Med Rehabil 2002; 81: 355–63.

42. Gracies JM, Weisz DJ, Yang BY et al. Botulinum toxin type A in the treatment of upper limb spasticity among patients with traumatic brain injury. J Neurol Neruosurg Psychiatry 1998; 64: 419–20.

43. Sloop RR, Bradley AC, Escutin RO. Reconstituted botulinum toxin type A does not lose potency in humans if it is refrozen or refrigerated for 2 weeks before use. Neurology 1997; 48: 249–53.

44. Klein AW. Botulinum toxin: beyond cosmesis. Arch Dermatol 2000; 136: 539–41.

45. Gartlan MG, Hoffman HT. Crystalline preparation of botulinum toxin type A (Botox): degradation in potency with storage. Otolaryngol Head Neck Surg 1993; 108: 135–40.

46. Hexsel DM, Almeida AT, Rutowitsch M et al. Multicenter, double-blind study of the efficacy of injections with botulinum toxin type A reconstituted up to six consecutive weeks before application. Dermatol Surg 2003; 29: 523–9.

47. Hexsel D, Castro AI, Zechmeister D, Amaral AA. Multicenter, double-blind study of the efficacy of injections with botulinum toxin a reconstituted up to six consecutive weeks before application [Letter]. Dermatol Surg 2004; 30: 823.

15 Optimal dosing and side-effects*

Benjamin Ascher and Bernard Rossi

Introduction

Reducing the strength of muscles responsible for expression lines, through localized and selective surgical myotomy, has been used for a long time in blepharoplasty and upper and mid-facelifts.

Botulinum toxin is a potent drug, widely used for the past 30 years to treat focal dystonia in neurology and in many other medical specialties, and for the past 16 years in cosmetic dermatology and surgery. The 'chemical nerve section' achieved by botulinum toxin provides a very effective, adjustable, and lasting treatment of expression lines, particularly those in the upper third of the face, whereas surgery and alternative medical treatments are often associated with higher risks and shorter-lived effects.

Although botulinum toxin has long been considered as the 'most potent of all poisons',[1] its use has almost never been associated with severe complications, but only with reversible side-effects. Improved knowledge of local muscle anatomy, and the use, especially in our specialties, of small quantities of botulinum toxin (small volumes and few units per injection site) have reduced the risks to the extent that some have become anecdotal.[2,3]

In search of optimal dosing

Dosing and ratio

After 15 years of cosmetic development, step by step a consensus began to arise concerning an ideal dosing with the best balance between a minimal, most effective dose and a maximal but 'natural' result. The majority of practitioners have decreased both the dose per injection site and the volume of each injection, i.e. the minimal number of points. For most practitioners, the easiest injected volume seems to be between 0.05 and 0.1 ml. Most authors stress the fact that high dilutions with high volume present two disadvantages: a shorter duration of action and a risk of spreading to the neighboring muscles because of the quantity injected.

Dysport® (500 Speywood U, Beaufour Ipsen) and BOTOX® (100 U, Allergan) are the first reliable preparations of botulinum toxin, derived from the neurotoxin type A. Conversion tables have been drawn up between the two drugs, first from clinical assessments and then from both neurological and cosmetic studies. **One unit of BOTOX is approximately equivalent to 2.5 to 3 units of Dysport**. The new formulation of BOTOX for cosmetic indications, Vistabel® (50 U), has the same characteristics as BOTOX.[4,5] Botulinum Toxin type A from Ipsen for esthetic indications will be distributed in most of the world, except US territories, under the name of Azzalure® by Galderma, and in US territories under the name Reloxin® by Medicis; in Latin America, the name will remain Dysport®, and it will be distributed by Ipsen or Galderma.

The dilutions of BOTOX to 1.7 ml and Dysport to 2.5 ml produce equivalent and effective quantities and volumes: **0.05 ml is a good minimal quantity** for Dysport, i.e. 10 units per point of injection, **and** for BOTOX, i.e. 3 units per point. The neurotoxin B, NeuroBloc® (Elan Pharma), seems less effective in terms of durability and efficacy, and more painful; this product has been dropped from the cosmetic field. Xeomin® (100 U, Merz) gained German approval in two neurological indications; the first cosmetic data are expected in 2009. The dosing seems close to the BOTOX dosing.[6–8] The BOTOX and Dysport dosing per location will be studied in the 'Side-effects at the injection site' section below. It is important to inject a product with a high degree of purification, which will tend to indicate lower immunotoxicity and antigenicity. Actually, BOTOX and Dysport have a low amount of residual proteins (close to 5 ng); also, Xeomin seems free of complexing protein and PurTox® (pending product from Mentor) seems to have a high degree of purification. All products need to be approved by the most professional regulatory authorities, for example European and US.

Minimal and natural dosing

The use of both minimal dosing and minimal volume are highly necessary to avoid risks of complications,

*Portions of this chapter were previously published as 'Toxine botulique et rides' in *Annales de chirurgie plastique et esthétique* 2004; 49: 537–52, reproduced with permission of Elsevier SAS.

mainly by diffusion into inadequate adjacent muscles and resistance. For this reason, it is recommended not to inject large doses and never more than a total of 100 units of BOTOX, i.e. 500 units of Dysport, per sequence of injection (versus 1500 units in some pathologies). It would be dangerous to perform any 'booster' or short-delay total reinjection. However, it is permitted, 3–4 weeks after the global treatment, to carry out a 'touch-up' sequence with a few minimal doses, if some minor corrections are remaining. Minimal dosing avoids palsy or fixed facial expression, the hallmark of an excess quantity injected into inappropriate locations. Health is more important than beauty, whatever the cost. Dosing needs to respect a natural appearance. A more natural, more discreet botulinum toxin treatment has become the signature of the European Natural look, more in line with internal beauty and the actual demand from patients. It is required to inject just the minimal dose to obtain this natural result, and then to check the patient 3–6 weeks later.

This step-by-step approach to the treatment produces a soft rejuvenation without transformation. Long-term beauty is better than a youthful appearance at any cost. However, minimal dosing is not to be related to some micro-unit dosing regimens,[9] where the injection of a quarter to 1 unit is injected to diminish tonus at rest without diminishing its strength in maximum contraction. This treatment could produce some variability in the quality and durability of the result, and some resistance. The botulinum toxin dose has to be adjusted depending on the type of muscle being injected and its variations, type of aging and wishes of the patient (strong vs light, fixed vs natural), and the product characteristics and clinical ratio.

Side-effects and contraindications in cosmetic indications

This section includes contraindications, complications due to the injection techniques in general, the anatomical site, and sensitivity to the toxin, and systemic reactions. However, this technique **never leaves any sequelae**.

Contraindications

Contraindications include pregnancy and breast-feeding, children under 12 years old (even though no complication has ever been reported in any of these three categories), known hypersensitivity to any of the product components (particularly the protein complex or human albumin), inflammation at the injection site, neuromuscular junction disorders (myasthenia, amyotrophic lateral sclerosis (ALS), Eaton–Lambert syndrome), coagulation disorders, concomitant medication affecting neuromuscular transmission (e.g. curare, aminoglycosides, penicillamine, and quinine), or

patients with an unsuitable psychological profile, unstable, and who have not understood the indications and limits of the method.[3]

Side-effects due to injections in general

Erythema and edema

These reactions are generally moderate and last only a few hours. They are dependent on the volume injected[2] and more importantly on the diameter of the needle, and require no specific treatment.

Prevention   Introduce carefully a thin 30G needle. Inject small volumes slowly. Do not massage the injection site, and place a cold pack over it at the end of treatment.

Pain

Pain is moderate and depends on the individual sensitivity of the patient.

Prevention   Apply the same rules as above. In very rare cases, anesthetic creams such as EMLA®, a refrigerating spray, or ice pack may be used prior to the procedure.

Headaches and nausea

Headaches and nausea are the most common side-effects. Their incidence ranges from 15%[10] to 2%,[11] their intensity is generally moderate,[10–16] and they disappear after a few treatments.[3,17] They last from a few hours to 3–4 days. Local trauma, stress, and a history of migraine have been suggested as possible causes. They may require the use of painkillers or usual antimigraine drugs. Injections of botulinum toxin type A are also used to treat headaches and migraines due to muscle contractions.[3,12,18]

Bruising

Bruising is due to punctures of blood vessels, often because the latter have not been accurately located beforehand.

Prevention   According to Matarasso,[3] it is best to avoid aspirin and non-steroidal anti-inflammatory drugs (NSAIDs) for 7 days prior to the injections and to use creams containing *Arnica montana* or vitamin K.[3,12,18] Other important measures help to reduce bruising: the patient must always be in a sitting position, local veins must be identified, especially in the periorbital area, and, in areas at risk, finger pressure must be applied at the injection site after the injection, without massage.[12]

Infections

No case of infection has been reported at the injection site or other sites. The product is diluted with normal saline, irrespective of the brand, and the vial must be kept at 4°C in a refrigerator. No bacterial contamination was identified 30 days after opening.[1] However, aseptic techniques must be applied rigorously to avoid any risk.[19]

Cholinergic effects

Cholinergic effects are rare, and include mostly dry mouth and dry eye. These effects appear to be more frequent and more pronounced with the type B toxin (NeuroBloc or Myobloc®).[20,21]

Side-effects at the injection site

These side-effects are mainly associated with toxin diffusion to adjacent muscles. Their frequency has been reduced in the upper third of the face, where the indications for botulinum toxin injections are the best (glabella, forehead, eyebrows, and crow's feet), as techniques and knowledge of the anatomy of the muscles concerned have improved. Most authors agree that there are fewer indications in the middle and lower thirds of the face, and in the neck, where results are less reproducible, and more importantly more prone to complications.[1–3,12,22] Even greater caution is required in these areas.

Glabella

Blepharoptosis

The only serious complication, from a cosmetic point of view, is eyelid ptosis,[3,23,24] but it has now become increasingly rare.[11] It is caused by diffusion of the product (injected into the procerus, depressor supercilii, or corrugator) through the orbital septum toward the levator palpebrae superioris muscle.[12,15] It develops 2–15 days after the injection, is rarely transient, and lasts generally 2–8 weeks. It is, however, fully reversible.

Its treatment is exclusively symptomatic and does not shorten its course. Apraclonidine 0.5% (Iopidine®; Alcon) and phenylephrine hydrochloride (Neosynephrine® 2.5%; Ciba or Chibret) may be administered using 1–2 drops three times a day. Although they stimulate Muller's muscle, which is an agonist of the levator, these potent mydriatic agents cause serious accommodation disorders, which limit their use considerably.[3]

Prevention   We do not believe it is necessary for the patient to remain in a vertical position for 3–4 hours.[3] However, it is important to inject small volumes with a 30G needle, to avoid massage, to contract actively the treated muscles for 2–3 hours to 'fix' the product, and, more important, to inject the procerus and corrugator in the center of the glabella, away from the pupil line, and at least 1 cm outside the orbital rim.[3,22]

Furthermore, special care is recommended in patients with a history of glabellar trauma or surgery,[25,26] or in patients, often elderly, with minimal ptosis due to a deficit in the levator muscle, often masked by a

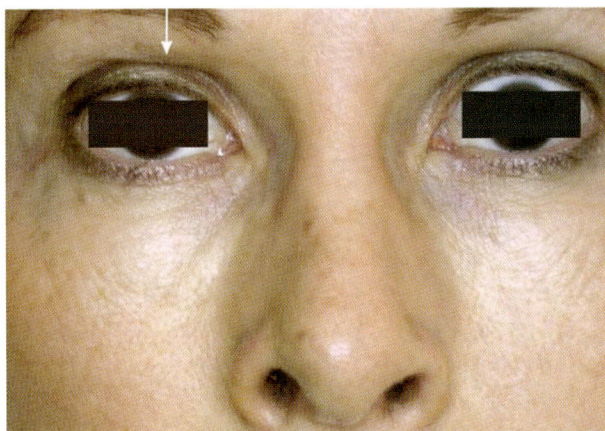

Figure 15.1   Minimal eyelid ptosis on the right, due to a deficit in the levator muscle, often masked by a resulting hypercontraction of the frontalis. It returned to normal in 1 month. Botulinum-induced ptosis is increasingly rare. In our two multicenter studies conducted between 2002 and 2004 on glabellar wrinkles, involving 102 and 100 patients, respectively, we did not report a single case of blepharoptosis.

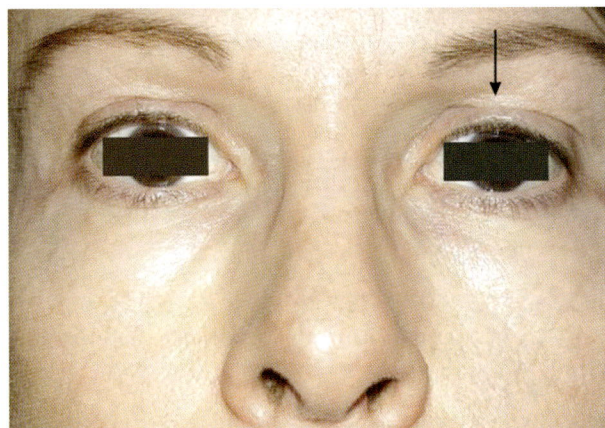

Figure 15.2   The same patient presented another minimal ptosis on the left side, following another botulinum toxin type A injection, a year later. Here again, it disappeared totally in 4 weeks. The levator palpebrae was constitutionally weak in this patient.

resulting hypercontraction of the frontalis (Figures 15.1 and 15.2). It is therefore important to take photos before the injection.[27,28]

Frequency   In 2002, A Carruthers et al observed 5.4% of blepharoptosis in 264 patients,[10] whereas JD Carruthers et al, in a similar study conducted in 2003 in 202 patients, observed only 1%. The latter reported in the literature an incidence of blepharoptosis between 0 and 20%, depending on the technique used.[29] Improved knowledge of anatomy, and improved techniques, have greatly reduced this risk. In both our studies conducted from 2002 to 2004 in 102 and 100 patients, respectively, we did not observe a single case of blepharoptosis.[11,13] We achieved the

Botulinum toxin:
Cosmetic indications
Injection points
Botox® units

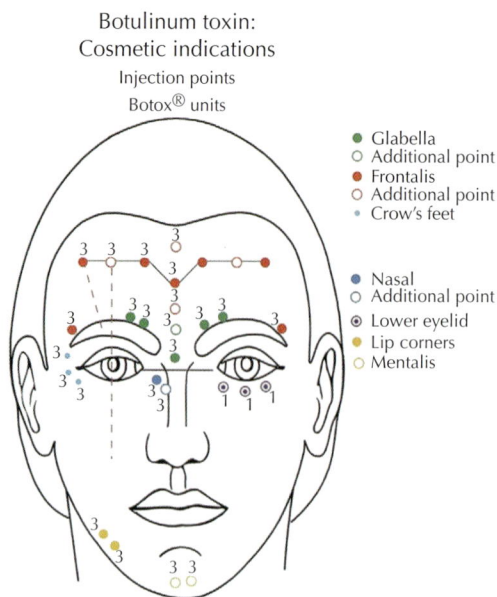

● Glabella
○ Additional point
● Frontalis
○ Additional point
● Crow's feet

● Nasal
○ Additional point
◉ Lower eyelid
● Lip corners
○ Mentalis

Figure 15.3 Facial injection points. Equivalence between the different products was established by clinical consensus only and not on a scientific basis. Generally speaking, 1 unit of BOTOX®–Vistabel® is equal to 2.5 to 3 units of Dysport® and to 50 units of NeuroBloc®. Botulinum Toxin type A from Ipsen for esthetic indications will be distributed in most of the world, except US territories, under the name of Azzalure® by Galderma, and in US territories under the name Reloxin® by Medicis; in Latin America, the name will remain Dysport®, and it will be distributed by Ipsen or Galderma.

same result in the multicenter BOTOX crow's feet study in 162 patients, co-directed with Nick Lowe,[30] and only one case in 220 subjects in our 2006 Dysport crow's feet multicenter study.[31]

Other glabellar side-effects

Immobilization of glabellar muscles may cause:

- **lymphedema** of the head of the eyebrow and adjacent eyelid. Subjects at risk must be identified: history of edema, especially in the morning, conjunctivitis, and ptosis of glabellar tissues
- **increased nasal wrinkles** due to the compensatory action of nasal muscles, especially in frowning or smiling. The problem is treated with 3 or 4 units of BOTOX (Vistabel) in one or two sites, or 10 units of Dysport (Reloxin®) per side.[12,32]

Forehead and eyebrows

Eyebrow ptosis

The frontalis muscle is thin, wide, and sensitive to small doses. If the injection line is too low, the resulting relaxation of the forehead results in a drop of the eyelids and eyebrows, which at best produces a heaviness in the forehead or discomfort in the upper eyelid, worsened by make-up, but which rarely affects vision. It lasts generally 1–4 weeks.[3]

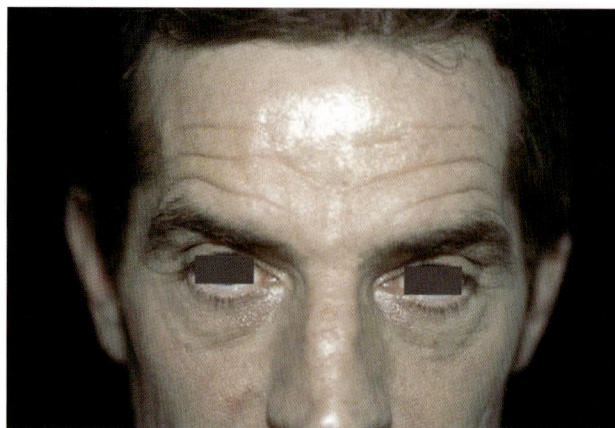

Figure 15.4 Frontoglabellar wrinkles in a 48-year-old patient, also with a ptosis of the internal section of the eyebrow, and resulting elevation of the external section due to hypercontraction of the frontalis.

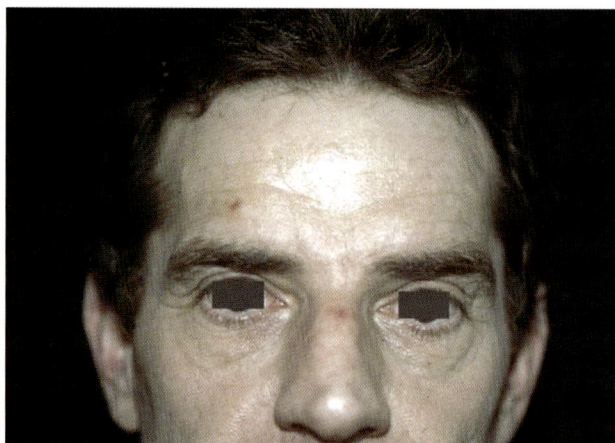

Figure 15.5 Results after four frontoglabellar botulinum toxin type A treatments, every 6 months, i.e. lasting 2 years. Not only were the wrinkles treated, but eyebrows were repositioned through balancing muscle actions.

Prevention The injection must be performed at least 1 cm above the highest forehead wrinkle. We inject along a V-shaped line, slightly obliquely upward and outward from the center, and generally 35–40 mm above the orbital wall, aligned with the pupils (Figure 15.3), thereby preserving the activity of the lower section of the frontalis.[3,28] This technique not only correctly treats forehead wrinkles, but also helps reposition the eyebrows with injections into the orbicularis oculi and glabellar muscles, depending on the muscle balance (Figures 15.4 and 15.5). Small wrinkles close to the eyebrows may persist or increase. A small dose of botulinum toxin type A (4 units of BOTOX–Vistabel), injected 3 weeks later, 1 cm above this wrinkle, treats the problem.[17]

Concomitant treatment of internal depressor muscles, procerus, depressor supercilii, and corrugator supercilii, but especially of the powerful external depressor, i.e. the external section of the orbicularis oculi, helps prevent this frontal ptosis.[32–37] This is a

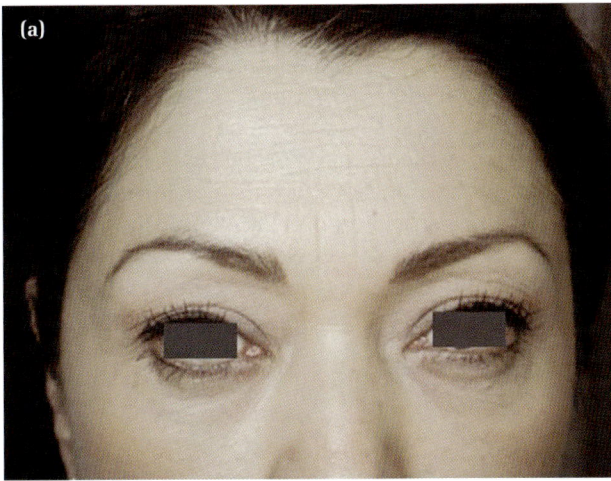

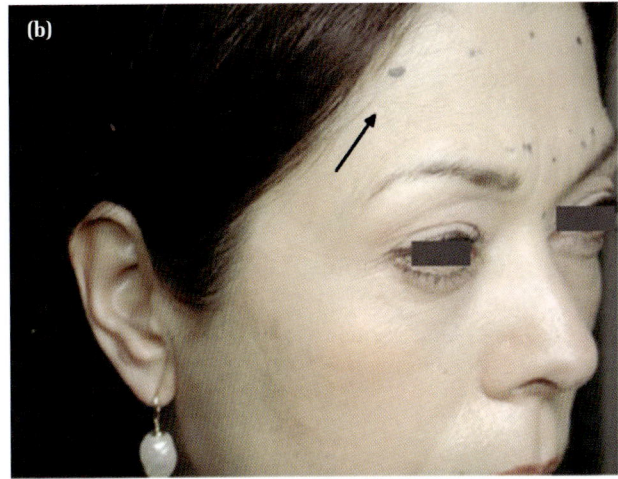

Figure 15.6 (a) A 40-year-old patient, with eyebrows seemingly in a good position, due to a compensatory hypercontraction of the frontalis. (b) In fact, the eyelid and eyebrow dropped at first, resulting in a contraction of the frontalis to lift the eyebrow higher than its normal position.

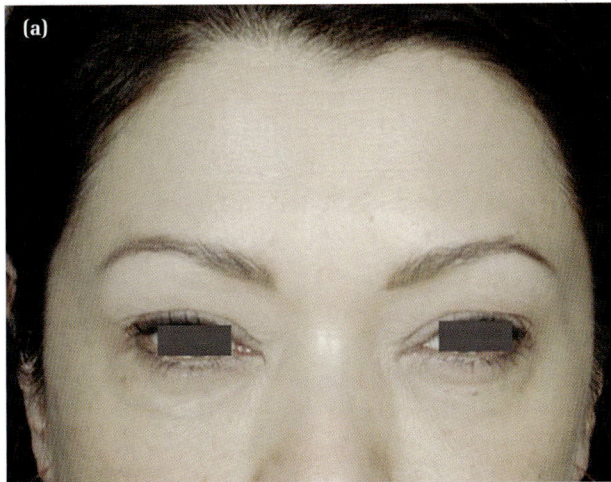

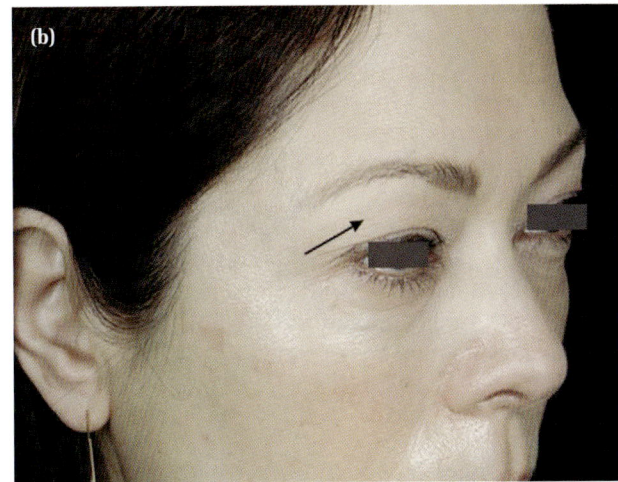

Figure 15.7 (a, b) Although the injection was performed high in the lateral section of the frontalis (Figure 15.6b), to preserve the activity of the lower section of the frontalis, it inhibited this muscle's activity, and the eyebrow dropped to its normal position (hence ptosed). This illustrates the importance of photos and explanations provided before the injections.

common complication in patients with pre-existing frontotemporal ptosis, especially in elderly people. In these cases, very small doses must be used.[38,39] Quite often, including in 30–40-year-old patients, the eyebrow seems to be correctly positioned, due to a compensatory hypercontraction of the frontalis muscle. In fact, the eyebrow drops to start with, which causes the frontalis to contract, and thus lifts the eyebrow to a position higher than normal. Such cases must be identified during the clinical examination, and here again, photos play a fundamental role (Figures 15.6 and 15.7).

Other frontal side-effects

- *Frozen look*: due to excessive treatment of the frontalis, which is sensitive to small doses. At our practice, we tend to inject only along a high line in

3–5 points, with either 4 units of Vistabel or 10 units of Dysport, and one 'locking injection' on the lateral section of the orbicularis using the same doses. Patients are reevaluated systematically at 1 month, and none of them appear 'frozen', and no further treatment is necessary in half the patients. In the other half, one or two points of 4 units of Vistabel or the equivalent dose of Dysport is enough to treat any residual hyperkinetic line and secure the effect for 5–6 months, or even more after 3–4 years of treatment (Figure 15.3).

- *'Mephisto' sign*: excessive elevation of the middle and/or external third of the eyebrow, and even in certain cases a curved center, particularly unsightly in men. This occurs when the external portion of the frontalis muscle has not been sufficiently treated. The problem is corrected with one point of 4 units of Vistabel or 10 units of Dysport, injected more externally on the same horizontal injection line.[3,15] These cases are more common in patients with strong forehead muscles and high eyebrows.[12,39]

- *Frontal tension*: very frequent after the first injections and in patients with naturally heavy eyelids. Patients just need to be warned of this minor and short-lived side-effect.

Prevention   First and foremost, measure the distances and mark injection points. Note the frequency (approximately 90%) of variations in muscle anatomy and right–left asymmetries in the forehead and eyebrow area.[3]

The eyelid region

Loose lower eyelid

The orbicularis is a superficial, thin, wide, and powerful muscle. High doses may cause excessive relaxation of the orbicularis, resulting in a herniation of infraorbital fat pads, and edema due to a lack of massage of lymph vessels by the muscles. Injections in the crow's feet must therefore be done carefully in subjects with usually puffy eyelids in the morning. Likewise, superficial lines and excessive eyelid skin may worsen after botulinum toxin injections.[32]

Prevention   Analyze signs correctly, and especially those which are not due to muscle contractions. Explain fully the limits of the method to the patient. Inject superficially and use small doses.[12,40,41]

Ptosis of lower eyelid

If the injection is too high in the pretarsal portion of the orbicularis muscle, it may cause a ptosis of the lower eyelid and hinder eye closure.[39]

Prevention   Inject at least 2 cm below the eyelashes and 1 cm from the orbital rim.

Diplopia and strabismus

Very rare, this occurs when the toxin is injected under the orbicularis and reaches the obliquus inferior oculi and when large volumes are injected close to the eye's lateral canthus, touching the rectus lateralis oculi.[3,12,42]

Prevention   Inject at least 1 cm from the orbital rim.

Ptosis of upper eyelid

This is very rare, and due to a diffusion of the toxin to the levator palpebrae superioris.

Prevention   Injections in the area of the tail of the eyebrow must be lateral, at least 1 cm from the orbital rim. Injections in the upper eyelid are contraindicated.

Lip ptosis, worsening of zygomatic wrinkles

This is rare, at 0.3% as reported by Matarasso and Matarasso.[28] It is either static, producing a droopy lip, or only dynamic, producing an asymmetrical smile. It is due to a diffusion of the toxin to the head of the zygomaticus minor and major muscles, because of injection of the crow's feet performed too low, or in the lower external portion of the eyelid. These wrinkles are very often related to underlying zygomatic wrinkles, markedly worsened, when the lower crow's feet are correctly treated. It is then tempting but risky to treat these lines.

Prevention   Never inject below the zygomatic arch, at least within the malar fat pad. Therefore, if necessary, inject these wrinkles very superficially and laterally.[12,28,32,43]

Other eyelid side-effects

Most of these are anecdotal. Temporary ectropion, with a risk of keratitis,[3] can be avoided by evaluating the laxity of the lid with the snap-back test. Dry eye can be avoided by injecting outside the lachrymal portion of the orbicularis, which lies behind the lachrymal sac.

Middle and lower thirds of the face, neck

Perioral region

The results of injections in the orbicularis oris are neither fully satisfactory nor reproducible compared to filling and resurfacing techniques. Vertical lip lines are reduced by the induced paresis of the orbicularis. These injections are often associated with the injection of an implant, such as hyaluronic acid, in the wrinkle. This combination is similar to that performed in the glabella.[44] Side-effects are common: asymmetry, difficulties in speaking and swallowing liquids due to lip dyskinesia, difficulties in smiling or playing an instrument, and sometimes drooling.[3,12,45]

Prevention   These injections must be performed with very concentrated low doses,[35] limited to 1–4 points of 1 unit of BOTOX–Vistabel or 3 or 4 units of Dysport, exclusively in the white roll of the lip, away from the Cupid's bow.

Nasolabial folds

Nasolabial folds must also be treated with care, as there is a risk of lowering mouth corners, lip ptosis, and lengthening of the upper lip[18,43,46] due to the toxin's diffusion to the zygomaticus and levator labii superioris.[39,42,47]

Lip corners and chin

Injections in the triangularis muscle help lift the lip corner, but there is a risk of transient difficulty in smiling

(a)

Botulinum toxin:
Cosmetic indications

Injections

BOTOX®, Vistabel® units

Lip corners

3 · · 3

3

2 cm

3

3   Platysma

3

(b)

Botulinum toxin:
Cosmetic indications

Injections

Dysport®

Lip corners

10 · · 10

10

2 cm

10   Platysma

10

10

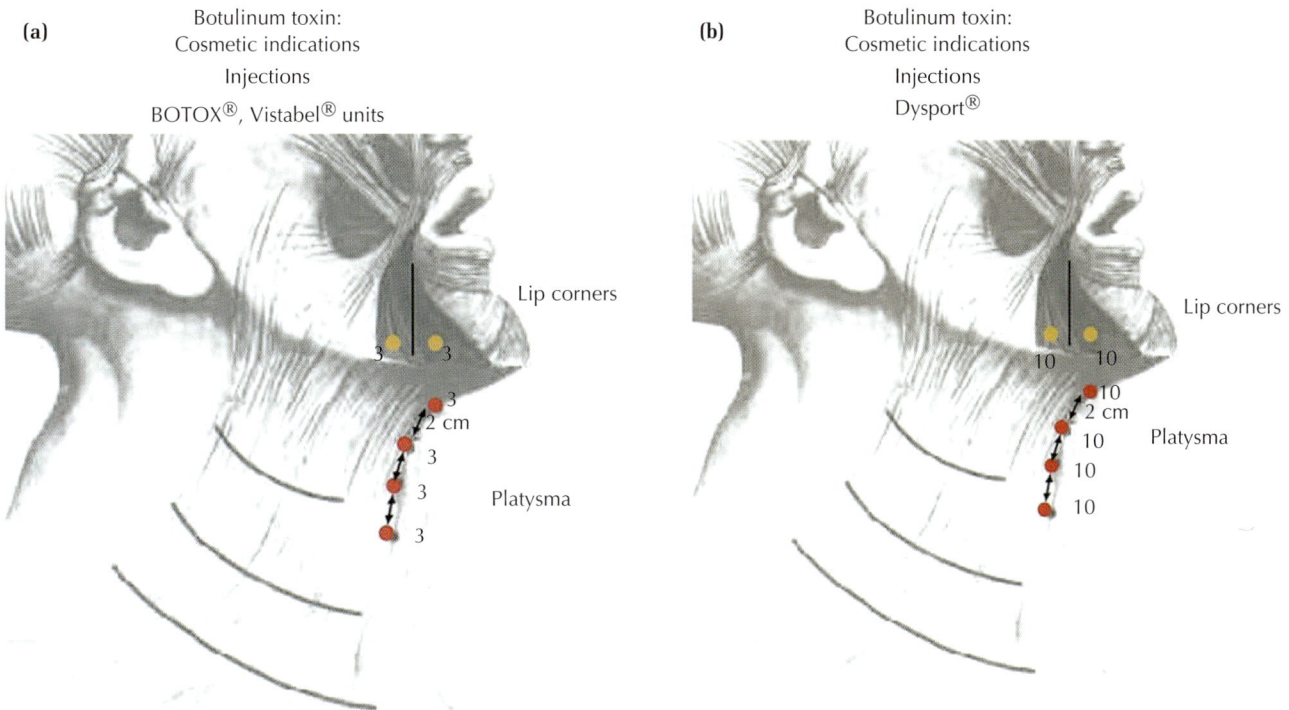

Figure 15.8 (a, b) Injections in the triangularis muscle, low at the base of the mandible, help to lift the lip corner, but may cause temporary difficulties in smiling and talking. Injections in the platysma bands are performed in 3–5 points distant by approximately 2 cm, but they are associated with risks of dysphagia, and reduced saliva secretion.

or talking due to the toxin's diffusion to the perioral muscles (Figure 15.8). Chin rhytids, horizontal or vertical wrinkles involving the mentalis muscle, are easily corrected with one or two points of 4 units of BOTOX–Vistabel or 10 units of Dysport. However, diffusion to the orbicularis muscles may cause the same difficulties when smiling, and lip dyskinesia.

Prevention   Inject low, at the base of the mandible, on a line prolonging the nasolabial fold downwards. These points also treat that area of the platysma muscle.

Neck

Horizontal neck wrinkles can be treated partially, with multiple superficial injections of Vistabel or Dysport, diluted to 4 ml. Here again, results are often only partial and not fully reproducible. Complications include dysphagia and reduced saliva secretion due to the toxin's diffusion to the subhyoid muscles following misplaced injections below the Adam's apple. Metoclopramide hydrochloride (Reglan®) may help to reduce this effect.[3] In addition, problems with flexing the neck may appear if the toxin diffuses to the sternocleidomastoid.[3,48]

The injection of the platysma bands, caused by a contraction of the anterior aspect of the platysma muscle when it is thickened and lax, is a good indication.[49] This defect occurs either at the beginning of aging before the skin has become slackened, or after a facelift which has not provided an effective solution for the front of the neck. Here again, the onset of transient

dysphagia is not rare. The recommended overall dose is 40 units of Dysport or 12–20 units of Vistabel per side, even though Matarasso et al have not reported any migration with doses up to 125 units of Vistabel–BOTOX per side[25,50,51] (Figure 15.8).

Platysma amyotrophy

This is transient and mild,[52] and clinically and histologically reversible.[53,54] It has never been described in the treatment of hyperkinetic wrinkles. In fact, the temporary reduction of the platysma thickness is compensated by dermal edema due to lymph stasis.[55] It is also clinically obvious that the strength of contraction of muscles injected several times (such as the orbicularis or frontalis) may decrease in patients who have not had any repeat injections even for several years.

Complications due to sensitivity to the toxin

No action or partial response

There may be various causes of a partial response, a short duration of action, or unchanged muscle contraction following botulinum toxin injections. First, inadequate needle positioning due to inadequate muscle identification, or dosage errors must be ruled out.[15] Electromyographic guidance may help to identify small, deep-set muscles, or those with frequent anatomical variations.[56] Drug concentrations in the vial may vary, up to about 10%, depending on the batch. In that case, contact the product manager and pharmacovigilance department of the laboratory and ask for the product's actual concentration. Second, if the correct muscles have been correctly treated, the lack of efficacy may be due to compensatory activity of adjacent muscles. For instance, when the corrugator has been adequately immobilized, the medial aspect of the orbicularis or nasal muscles may take over, giving the impression to the patient that the corrugator has been insufficiently treated, especially if hyperkinetic wrinkles persist. Last, there are variations in individual sensitivity to botulinum toxin.[3]

Prevention   Misplaced injections can be corrected easily by reinjecting the patient at least 3 weeks later. We do not consider that electromyographic guidance is essential in routine practice. It may help the diagnosis when injecting the lip triangularis muscle or platysma if the skin and hypodermis are thick. If other muscles are compensating for the induced paralysis, a mirror and pre-injection photos must be used to explain the situation to the patient. It is important to identify chronically dissatisfied patients as well as botulinum toxin 'addicts'. It is therefore very important to conduct a thorough pre-injection consultation, and obtain the patient's informed consent.[3,15]

Resistance to botulinum toxin

Resistance to botulinum toxin is rare; a few people will not respond to the toxin, even though other patients will respond well to the same product, from the same vial. These non-responders will not respond any better to repeat injections performed at least 9 weeks later. This suggests a primary resistance to botulinum toxin due to a genetic characteristic not yet identified.[32] Secondary resistance is due to rising levels of antitoxin antibodies. These antibodies have a blocking action but do not cause hypersensitivity reactions.[12,19,57] Klein reported 5% secondary resistance in patients treated for cervical dystonia with BOTOX,[12] and Kessler et al reported 2.8% with Dysport.[58] These resistances are mainly due to the use of high doses and the frequency of treatment. However, these dystonia patients were often treated with different batches of the same product, different type A toxins, or even different toxins (A, B, and F). Since 1993, we have observed only three cases out of around 15 000 patients injected for hyperkinetic wrinkles, one with BOTOX and two with Dysport. No study has ever demonstrated that doses used in cosmetic indications are associated with an antigen–antibody reaction or resistance. Of the 1600 patients treated with 50 units of Dysport in four pivotal US studies,[59] none were reported to have developed neutralizing antibodies using the mouse protection assay (MPA). None of the patients in the open-label repeat treatment study (1200 patients) developed neutralizing antibodies using the MPA. A total of 159 subjects had three BOTOX treatments and had analyzable antibody samples at day 0 of the initial double-blind trial and day 240 of the open-label study. None of these subjects were antibody-positive after three treatments.[60]

Prevention   Do not inject high doses:[57,61,62] beyond 300 units of BOTOX in total, or 40 units of BOTOX per site,[12] and avoid frequent touch-up injections. We repeat microinjections, if necessary, using 4 units of BOTOX or 10 units of Dysport at 1 month. Botulinum toxin type B, NeuroBloc from Elan Pharmaceuticals, may be preferred for touch-up injections to reduce the risk of resistance.[20] This is completely different from booster injections, which are to be avoided according to the data in the literature.[12,32] It is important to choose products with the lowest content of protein residues. This is why Allergan in 2002 developed new batches of BOTOX, with 20% less protein, 5 vs 25 ng per ml previously.[12,32] Ipsen did the same with Dysport, reducing its protein content from 12.5 to 5 ng.[63] In the past in patients with resistance, the use of botulinum toxin type F or B (NeuroBloc) was a possible solution.[20] However, systemic side-effects and effects remote from the injection site seem to be more frequent with botulinum toxin type B; this product is no longer in use in esthetic indications.[20,64]

Systemic reactions

Systemic reactions are rare. One case of psoriasis-like eruption and one case of pigmented erythema were published[65,66] and no allergic reaction was ever reported.[2] In cosmetic indications, reactions such as malaise, nausea, asthenia, flu-like syndrome, and remote electromyographic modifications have been observed,[12,34] thereby indicating that a small proportion of the product probably reaches the general circulation following the injection of massive doses, but not with the low doses used in cosmetic indications.[64] However, no crossing of the blood–brain barrier and no remote muscle paralysis have ever been observed, and no evidence has been found of pathological consequences of this diffusion[12,32,55,64,67–69] Botulinum toxin type B is associated with a greater frequency of headaches, and a greater frequency of systemic reactions, such as neck weakness, dry mouth, or dysphagia (Marion, personal communication).[70,71]

Conclusion

Dosing needs to respect a natural appearance. A more natural and more discreet botulinum toxin treatment has become the signature of the European Natural look, more in line with internal beauty and the wishes of patients. It is required to inject just the minimal dose to obtain this natural result, and then to check the patient 3–6 weeks later.

This chapter on the treatment of wrinkles does not address other treatments considered as cosmetic in Asia: hypertrophy especially of the masseters (and to a small extent the calves), particularly in Korea.[72] Park and Ahn in 2003 with 45 patients[72] and Ahn et al in 2004 with 20 patients[73] reported a significant reduction with very limited side-effects, including problems following intense mastication, and transient speech difficulties.

We insist on quality training necessary before injecting botulinum toxin, a product that is not innocuous but at the same time remarkably harmless when used correctly. In-depth knowledge of local muscle anatomy, the use of small volumes and few units per injection point, particularly in cosmetic indications, and a proper selection of indications have helped reduce the risks, which were already low, particularly in the upper third of the face. Before injecting botulinum toxin, it is essential to inform the patient about the initial and follow-up procedures, take photos, give the patient a price quote, and obtain an informed consent. It is also important to use clearly identified products, complying with marketing authorizations in each country. There are no convincing pharmacological studies nor marketing authorizations delivered in Europe and the USA for botulinum toxin type A developed as of 1990 in Lanzhou, China,[74] under the names Quick Star BTX-A® and Estetox®. The first studies on the safety and efficacy of this toxin are currently under way.

Botulinum toxin is one of the best cosmetic medical treatments currently available, particularly for upper face wrinkles. It requires no preparation, and is adjustable and reversible. Its role in the prevention of expression lines, and hence aging, appears indisputable.

References

1. Lamana C. The most poisonous poison. Science 1959; 130: 763–72.
2. Carruthers A, Kiene K, Carruthers J. Botulinum A exotoxin use in clinical dermatology. J Am Acad Dermatol 1996; 34: 788–97.
3. Matarasso SL. Complications of botulinum A exotoxin for hyperfunctional lines. Dermatol Surg 1998; 24: 1249–54.
4. Odergren T, Hjaltason H, Kaakkola S et al. A double blind, randomized, parallel group study to investigate the dose equivalence of Dysport and Botox in the treatment of cervical dystonia. J Neurol Neurosurg Psychiatry 1998; 64: 6–12.
5. Ranoux D, Gury C, Fondarai J et al. Respective potencies of Botox and Dysport: a double blind randomized crossover study in cervical dystonia. J Neurol Neurosurg Psychiatry 2002; 72: 459–62.
6. Jost WH , Kohl A, Brinkmann S et al. Efficacy and tolerability of a botulinum toxin type A free of complexing proteins (NT 201) compared with commercially available botulinum toxin type A (BOTOX) in healthy volunteers. J Neural Transm 2005; 112: 905–13.
7. Benecke R, Jost WH, Kanovsky P et al. A new botulinum toxin type A free of complexing proteins for treatment of cervical dystonia. Neurology 2005; 64: 1949–51.
8. Roggenkämper P, Jost WH, Bihari K et al. Efficacy and safety of a new botulinum toxin type A free of complexing proteins in the treatment of blepharospasm. J Neural Transm 2006; 113: 303–12.
9. Le Louarn C, Buthiau D, Buis J. Facial rejuvenation and concentric malar lift: the FACE RECURVE concept. Ann Chir Plast 2006; 51: 99–121.
10. Carruthers A, Lowe NJ, Menter MA et al. A multicenter, double-blind, randomised, placebo-controlled study of efficacy and safety of botulinum toxin type A in treatment of glabellar lines. J Am Acad Dermatol 2002; 46: 840–9.
11. Ascher B, Zakine B, Kestemont P et al. A multicenter, randomized, double blind, placebo-controlled study of botulinum toxin A in treatment of glabellar lines. J Am Acad Dermatol 2004; 512: 223–33.
12. Klein AW. Complications, adverse reactions, and insights with the use of botulinum toxin. Dermatol Surg 2003; 29: 549–56.
13. Ascher B, Zakine B, Kestemont P et al. A phase III, multicentre, randomized, double-blind, placebo-controlled study of efficacy and safety of 2 injections with 50 Speywood units of Botulinum Toxin A IPSEN in the treatment of glabellar frown lines. Cosmetic Botulinum Toxin Master Class. Paris: IMCAS, June 2004.
14. Sommer B, Sattler G. Cosmetic indications according to anatomic region. In: Botulinum Toxin in Aesthetic Medicine. Berlin: Blackwell Science, 2001, 30–55.
15. Benedetto AV. The cosmetic uses of botulinum toxin type A. Int J Dermatol 1999; 38: 641–55.
16. Sadick NS. Overview of complications of non surgical facial rejuvenation procedures. Clin Plast Surg 2001; 1: 163–76.
17. Ascher B, Klap P, Marion MH, Chanteloub B. La toxine botulique dans le traitement des rides frontoglabellaires et de la région orbitaire. Ann Chir Plast Esthet 1995; 40: 67–76.
18. Binder WJ, Blitzer A, Brin MF. Treatment of hyperfunctional lines of the face with botulinum toxin A. Dermatol Surg 1998; 24: 1198–205.
19. Klein AW. Dilution and storage of botulinum toxin. Dermatol Surg 1998; 24: 1179–80.
20. Kim EJ, Ramirez AL, Reeck JB, Maas CS. The role of botulinum toxin type B (Myobloc) in treatment of hyperkinetic lines. Plast Reconst Surg 2003; 112 (Suppl): 88S–93S.
21. Gury C. Aspects pharmacologiques du traitement par la toxine botulique. Réalités thérapeutiques en derm venero. 2004; 137: 7–12.
22. Ascher B. Toxine botulique, indications esthétiques, dermatologiques et réparatrices. In: Nieoullon A, Poulain B, Rascol O, Christen Y, eds. Les Amis du Clostridium, Tome 3, Toxine, Plasticité et Spasticité. Marseille: Solal, 2000: 11–18.
23. Markey AC. Botulinum A exotoxin in cosmetic dermatology. Clin Exp Dermatol 2000; 25: 173–5.
24. Carruthers A, Carruthers J. Treatment of glabellar frown lines with botulinum A exotoxin. J Dermatol Surg Oncol 1992; 18: 17–21.
25. Nicolau PJ, Chaouat M, Mimoun M. Skin, wrinkles and botulinum toxin. Ann Readapt Med Phys 2003; 46: 361–74.
26. Prado AC, Andrales PR. Caution in using Botox in patients with previous facial surgery. Plast Reconstr Surg 2002; 109: 1472–3.
27. Sposito MM. New indications for botulinum toxin type A in cosmetics: mouth and neck. Plast Reconstr Surg 2002; 110: 601–11; discussion 612–13.
28. Matarasso SL, Matarasso A. Treatment guidlines for botulinum toxin type A for the periocular region and a report of partial lip ptosis injections of the lateral canthus rhitids. Plast Reconstr Surg 2001; 108: 208–14; discussion 215–17.
29. Carruthers JD, Lowe NJ, Menter MA et al. Double-blind, placebo-controlled study of the efficacy and safety of botulinum toxin type A for patients with glabellar lines. Plast Reconstr Surg 2003; 112: 1089–98.
30. Lowe NJ, Ascher B, Heckmann M et al. Botulinum toxin type A (Botox) in subjects with crow's feet, multicenter study. Dermatol Surg 2005; 31: 257–62.

31. Ascher B, Rzany B; Smile Study Groupe. Botulinum toxin type A (Dysport) in subjects with crow's feet, multicenter study, a single bilateral treatment of 15, 30, 45 u. Poster presented at EADV, Rhodes, Greece, October 2006.

32. Hexsel D, Mazzuco R, Zechmeister M, Hexsel CL. Complications and adverse effects: diagnosis and treatment. In: Hexsel D, Trindade de Almeida A, eds. Cosmetic Use of Botulinum Toxin. Porto Alegre: AGE Editora, 2002, 233–39.

33. Bullstrode NW, Grobelaar AO. Long-term prospective follow-up of botulinum toxin treatment for facial rhytides. Aesthetic Plast Surg 2002; 26: 356–9.

34. Alam M, Dover JS, Klein AW. Botulinum A exotoxin for hyperfunctional facial lines. Dermatol Surg 2002; 138: 1180–5.

35. Le Louarn C. Botulinum toxin A and facial lines: the variable concentration. Aesthetic Plast Surg 2001; 25: 73–84.

36. Belhaouari L, Gassia V, Lauwers F. Frontalis muscular balance and botulinum toxin. Ann Chir Plast Esthet 2004; 49: 514–20.

37. Keen M, Blitzer A, Aviv J et al. Botulinum toxin A for hyperkinetic facial lines. Result of a double-blind, placebo-controlled study. Plast Reconstr Surg 1994; 103: 656–63.

38. Lowe NJ. Botulinum toxin A for facial rejuvenation. United States and United Kingdom perspectives. Dermatol Surg 1998; 24: 1216–18.

39. Wieder JM, Moy RL. Understanding botulinum toxin. Dermatol Surg 1998; 24: 1172–4.

40. Carruthers A, Carruthers JDA. Cosmetic uses of botulinum A exotoxin. Adv Dermatol 1997; 12: 325–48.

41. Manaloto RMP, Alster TS. Periorbital rejuvenation: a review of dermatologic treatments. Dermatol Surg 1999; 25: 1–8.

42. Garcia A, Fulton JE. Cosmetic denervation of muscles of facial expression with botulinum toxin A dose reponse study. Dermatol Surg 1996; 22: 39–43.

43. Carruthers A, Carruthers JDA. The adjunctive usage of botulinum toxin. Dermatol Surg 1998; 24: 1244–7.

44. Carruthers JDA, Carruthers A. A prospective, randomized, parallel group study analysing the effect of BTX-A (Botox) and nonanimal sourced hyaluronic acid (NASHA, Restylane®) in combination compared with NASHA (Restylane®) alone in severe glabellar rhytides in adult female subjects. Dermatol Surg 2003; 29: 802–9.

45. Edelstein C, Shorr N, Jacobs J, Balch K, Goldberg R. Oculoplastic experience with the cosmetic use of botulinum A exotoxin. Dermatol Surg 1998; 24: 1208–12.

46. Sarrabayrouse MAM. Indications and limitations for the use of botulinum toxin for the treatment of facial wrinkles. Aesthetic Plast Surg 2002; 26: 233–8.

47. Carruthers JDA, Carruthers A. Botox® use in the mid and lower face and neck. Semin Cutan Med Surg 2001; 20: 85–92.

48. Jankovic J, Brin MF. Therapeutic uses of botulinum toxin. N Engl J Med 1991; 324: 1186–93.

49. Brant FS, Bellman B. Botulinum A exotoxin for platysmal bands and rejuvenation of the ageing neck. Dermatol Surg 1998; 24: 1232–4.

50. Matarasso A, Matarassso SL, Brant FS, Bellman B. Botulinum A exotoxin for the management of the platysma bands. Plast Reconstr Surg 1999; 103: 645–52.

51. Kane MAC. Non surgical treatment of platysma bands with injection of botulinum toxin A. Plast Reconstr Surg 1999; 103: 656–63.

52. Borodic GE, Ferrante R, Pearce LB, Smith K. Histologic assessment of dose-related diffusion and muscle fiber response after therapeutic botulinum A toxin injections. Mov Disord 1994; 9: 31–9.

53. Harris CP, Alderson K, Nebeker J, Holds JB, Anderson RL. Histological features of human orbicularis oculi treated with botulinum A toxin. Arch Ophthalmol 1991; 109: 393–5.

54. Borodic GE, Gozzolino D. Pharmacology and Histology of Therapeutic Application of Botulinum Toxin. New York: Marcel Dekker, 1994.

55. Le Louarn C. The plastic surgeon and the prevention of facial aging process. Ann Chir Plast Esthet 2003; 48: 346–9.

56. Klein AW, Mantell A. Electromyographic guidance in injecting botulinum toxin. Dermatol Surg 1998; 24: 1184–6.

57. Borodic G, Johnson E, Goodnough M, Schantz E. Botulinum toxin therapy, immunologic resistance, and problems with available materials. Neurology 1996; 46: 26–9.

58. Kessler KR, Skutta M, Benecke R. Long term treatment of cervical dystonia with botulinum toxin A: efficacy, safety, and antibody frequency. J Neurol 1999; 246: 265–7.

59. Monheit G, Carruthers A, Brandt F et al. Double-blind, placebo-controlled study of efficacy and safety of botulinum toxin type A for patients with glabellar lines: determination of optimal dose. Dermatol Surg 2007; 33: 51–9.

60. FDA Medical Reviewer, 2002.

61. Carruthers A, Carruthers JDA. Cosmetic uses of botulinum A exotoxin. In: Klein AW, ed. Tissue Augmentation in Clinical Practice: Procedure and Techniques. New York: Marcel Dekker, 1998: 207–36.

62. National Institutes of Health. Clinical Use of Botulinum Toxin. NIH Consens Statement 1990; 8(8): 1–20.

63. Pickett A. Potency of type A botulinum toxin preparations in clinical use. Presented at 40th Annual Meeting of the Interagency Botulism Research Coordinating Committee (IBRCC), Atlanta, GA, 5–7 November, 2000.

64. Tugnoli Y, Eleopra R, Quartrale R et al. Botulism-like syndrome after BTX-A for local hyperhydrosis. Br J Dermatol 2002; 147: 808–9.

65. Bowden JB, Rapini RP. Psoriasiform eruption from intramuscular botulinum A toxin. Cutis 1992; 50: 415–16.

66. Cox NH, Duffey P, Royle J. Fixed drug eruption caused by lactose in an injected botulinum toxin preparation. J Am Acad Dermatol 1999; 40: 263–4.

67. Delgado MR. The use of botulinum toxin A in children with cerebral palsy: a retrospective study. Eur J Neurol 1999; 6 (Suppl 4): S11–18.

68. Boyd RN, Graham JEA, Natrass GR, Graham HK. Medium term response characterization and risk factor analysis of botulinum toxin type A in management of spasticity in children with cerebral palsy. Eur J Neurol 1999; 6 (Suppl 4): S37–45.

69. Smuts JA, Baker MK, Smuts HM et al. Prophylactic treatment of chronic tension-type headache using botulinum toxin type A. Eur J Neurol 1999; 6 (Suppl 4): S99–102.

70. Racette BA, Lopate G, Good L, Sagitto S, Perlmutter JS. Ptosis as a remote effect of therapeutic botulinum B injection. Neurology 2002; 59: 1445–7.

71. Lange DI, Brin MF, Warner C et al. Distant effects of locally injected botulinum toxin. Muscle Nerve 1987; 10: 552–5.

72. Park MY, Ahn KY. Botulinum toxin A for the treatment of hyperkinetic wrinkle lines. Plast Reconstr Surg 2003; 112 (Suppl): 148S–50S.

73. Ahn J, Horn C, Blitzer A. Botulinum toxin for masseter reduction in Asian patients. Arch Facial Plast Surg 2004; 6: 188–91.

74. Wang Y et al. Preparation of type A crystalline botulinum toxin for therapeutic and establishment of an experimental animal model. J Biol Prod 1990; 3: 121–5.

16 The periorbital area

Marina Landau and Arik Nemet

Anatomy

The orbicularis oculi is a ring-shaped muscle that lies immediately under the skin in the periorbital zone. It is composed of three parts: the preorbital (the most external), preseptal, and pretarsal (closest to the eyelashes) portions (Figure 16.1). Repeated contraction of the lateral parts of the preseptal and preorbital portions of the orbicularis muscle causes the formation of 'crow's feet' or 'smile lines', wrinkles extending radially from the region of the lateral canthus (Figure 16.2).[1]

Clinical indications for botulinum toxin A injection

Botulinum toxin is used widely in the orbital area, including in dystonic movement disorders, strabismus, nystagmus, lacrimal hypersecretion syndromes, eyelid retraction, spastic entropion, and compressive optic neuropathy. All these indications are beyond the scope of this chapter, which covers the cosmetic indications only. The main cosmetic indications in the periorbital area include: crow's feet, hypertrophic low eyelid orbicularis and narrow eye aperture, and for eyebrow elevation. In all these indications, botulinum toxin A (BTX-A) has been shown to have transient clinical effect with no permanent histological changes.[2]

Periorbital lines are a result of intrinsic skin aging, ultraviolet damage, and repetitive action of the periorbital muscles. Mimetic lines in this area represent one of the earliest facial stigmata of aging. Several different patterns of animation in this area have been observed.[3] The first report regarding the possibility to treat these wrinkles by BTX-A was published in 1990.[4] Periorbital wrinkles respond well to BTX-A injections, but they are still partially visible while a patient is smiling. Younger patients with a minimal degree of solar elastosis usually have better results than older ones (Figure 16.3).

In some individuals there is hypertrophy of the pretarsal orbicularis in the lower eyelid, causing a 'jelly roll' appearance on a full smile (Figure 16.4).[5] In addition, individuals of Asian ethnic origin have narrower palpebral apertures, which cause the eyes almost to close while smiling.[6] These conditions, as well as cases of mimetic wrinkles under the lower eyelid, are

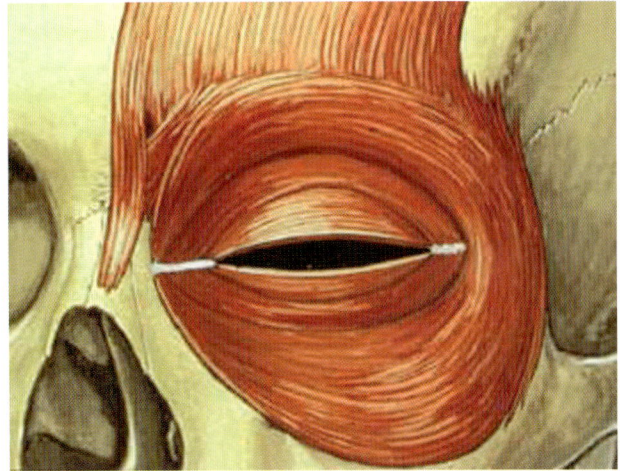

Figure 16.1 Orbicularis oculi muscle is composed of three parts: the pre-orbital (the most external), the pre-septal, and the pre-tarsal portions (the closest to eyelashes).

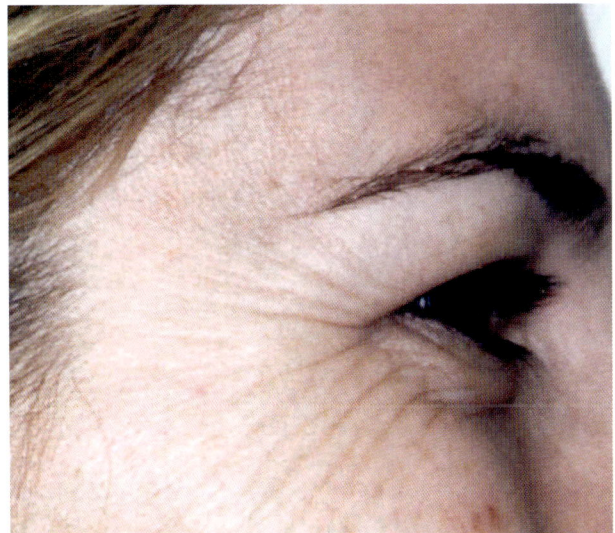

Figure 16.2 Repeated contraction of the lateral parts of the pre-septal and preorbital portions of the orbicularis muscle causes the formation of smile lines.

beneficially affected by BTX-A injections in the suborbital area. Suborbital treatment produces a more subtle effect than in the periorbital area; nonetheless, after treatment, the subject has a more 'open eye' look and rounder eye appearance.[7]

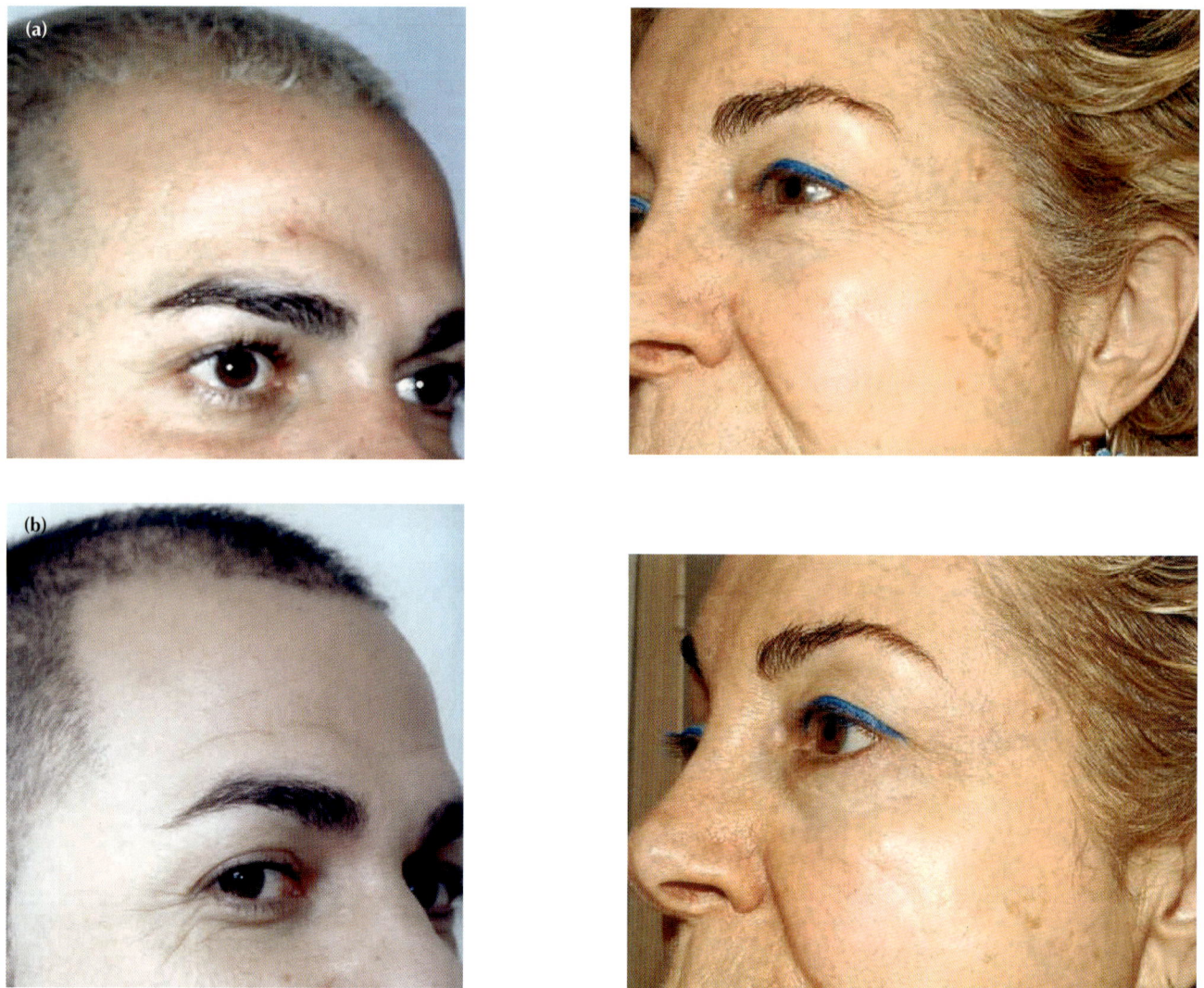

Figure 16.3   The effect of periorbital botulinum toxin A (BTX-A) injection in female and male patients: (a) patient 1; (b) patient 2: left hand images before, right hand images after treatment.

The eyebrows are constantly under the influence of downward forces such as the static force of gravity and the dynamic force of depressor muscles (e.g. corrugator supercilii, procerus, orbicularis oculi). As a result of these forces, with aging, brow ptosis develops. Clinical observations show that the lateral eyebrow becomes ptotic earlier than the medial eyebrow.[8] In addition to the ability of BTX-A treatment to efface hyperfunctional lines, it has been reported that by treatment of brow depressors, elevation of the eyebrows is achieved in the majority of patients.[9,10]

Injection technique

In the periorbital region various techniques have been described, but in most cases 2–4 injection points located 1–1.5 cm apart from each other are sufficient. We recommend marking the injection points while the patient is smiling or squinting (Figure 16.5). The injection

sites are located 1 cm lateral to the orbit with the needle tip pointing away from it. The injection is performed superficially with the patient in a relaxed state, to visualize the blood vessels and thus minimize bruising. All injection sites should be situated above the zygomatic bone to avoid lip drooping.

In a parallel group, double-blind study assessing the efficacy of four different doses of BTX-A (BOTOX®; Allergan, Inc) in the periorbital area, 12 U per side was found to be the most effective and safe.[11] The duration of the antiwrinkle effect of BTX-A, as assessed by blinded observers using standard photography and three-dimensional in vivo profilometry, was shown to last up to 6 months.[12] With repeated treatments the benefits are more sustained.[13] Botulinum toxin B is now commercially available, but information regarding its diffusion, dose equivalence, and effect duration is still lacking. When comparing the effects of BTX-A and BTX-B, using an effective ratio of 1:50, it was found that BTX-B was associated with slightly more

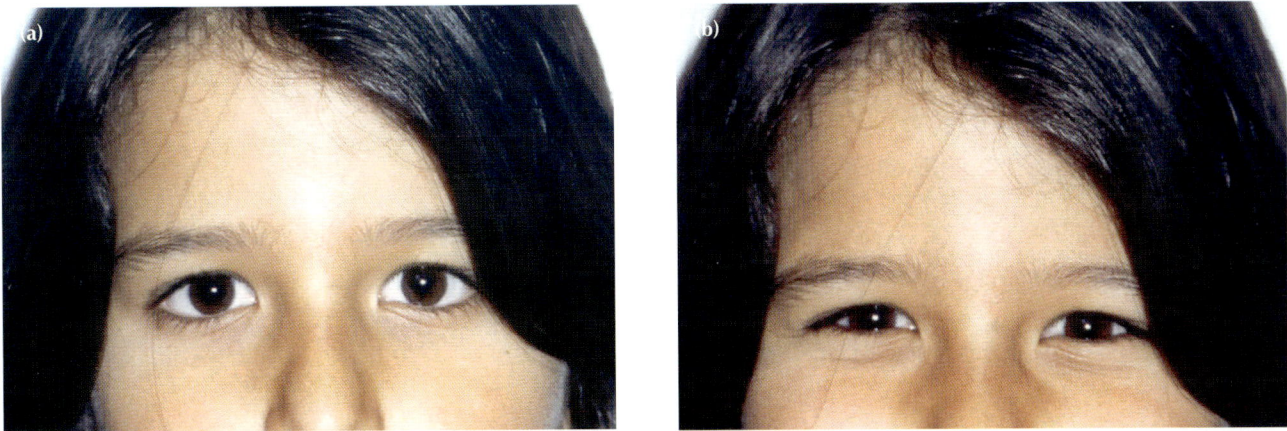

Figure 16.4 Hypertrophy of pretarsal orbicularis in the lower eyelid causes a 'jelly roll' appearance on rest (a) and full smile (b).

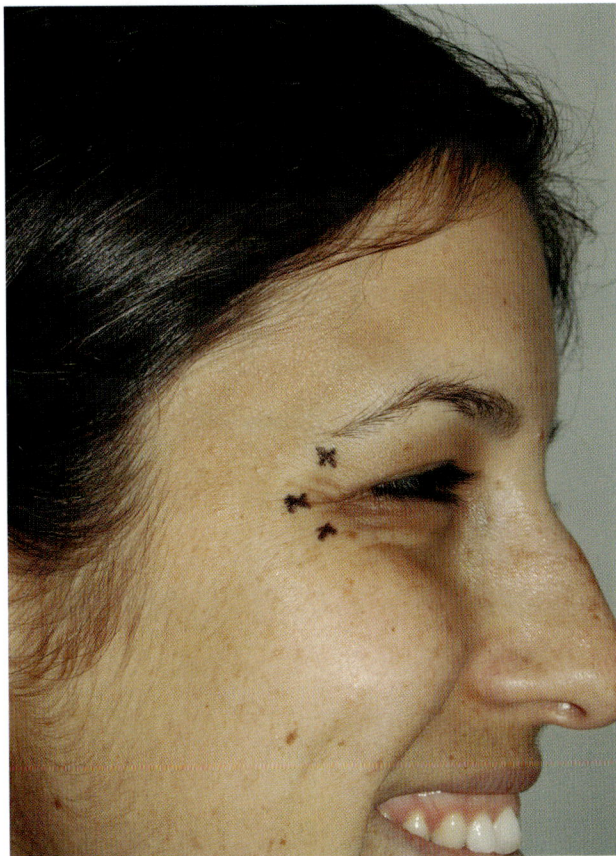

Figure 16.5 In the periorbital region, 2–4 injection points located 1–1.5 cm apart are sufficient. The injection sites are located 1 cm lateral to the orbit. All injection sites should be situated above the zygomatic bone to avoid lip drooping.

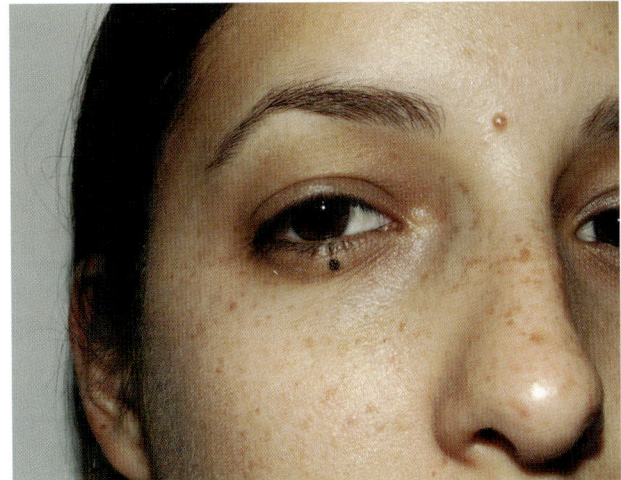

Figure 16.6 Injection of the suborbital region is performed 3 mm below the inferior ciliary margin in the mid-pupillary line, with the needle held tangential to the globe to prevent accidental perforation: 2–4 U.

discomfort upon injection, quicker onset of action, and briefer duration of muscle paralysis.[14]

Injection into the suborbital region is usually combined with lateral orbital area treatment, in a synergistic fashion.[6] This treatment should not be performed in patients with a positive snap test, because they are predisposed to develop ectropion and lagophthalmos. The injection is performed 3 mm below the inferior ciliary margin in the mid-pupillary line, with a needle held tangential to the globe to prevent accidental perforation. Between 2 and 4 U of BTX-A are injected (Figure 16.6). If a higher dosage is used, the incidence of lower eyelid edema and incomplete sphincter function is extremely high.[15]

To create eyebrow elevation by injecting the periorbital area, in addition to two regular periorbital sites, 2.5 U of BTX-A are injected into two points of the superolateral portion of the orbicularis oculi below the lateral third of the brow. As a result the brow is elevated with the central and lateral part showing maximal elevation (Figure 16.7).[10]

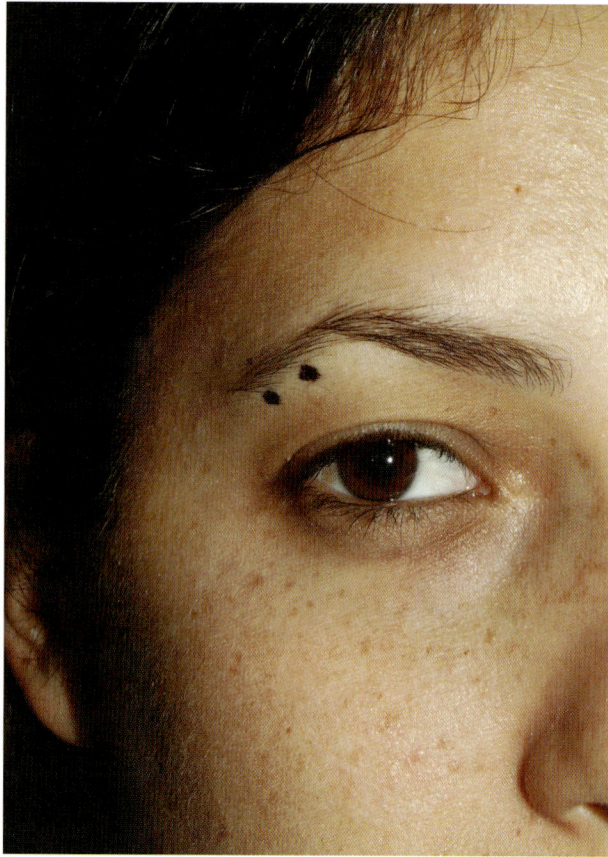

Figure 16.7   For eyebrow elevation, 2.5 U of BTX-A are injected into two points of the superolateral portion of the orbicularis oculi below the lateral third of the brow.

Combination treatment

A combination of minimally invasive procedures for facial rejuvenation meets our improved understanding of the mechanisms involved in skin aging. For this reason, combined use of BTX-A with other ablative and non-ablative techniques for periorbital rejuvenation have become popular in recent years (Figure 16.8). When facial muscles are weakened by BTX-A, the immobilized skin can regenerate more efficiently after light treatments and chemical peels. Therefore, when these techniques are combined, the results are superior to the use of individual therapies alone.[16,17]

Adverse effects

Local untoward reactions caused by percutaneous injection of BTX-A include pain, edema, erythema, ecchymosis, headache, and hypesthesia. These are generally mild and transient. When not contraindicated, patients should avoid platelet inhibitors, including aspirin and non-steroidal anti-inflammatory drugs, for 7–14 days prior to injection to decrease the incidence and severity of the bruising.

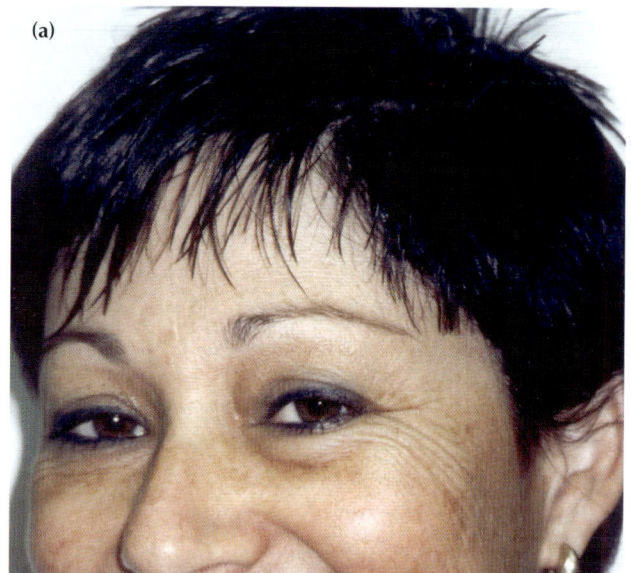

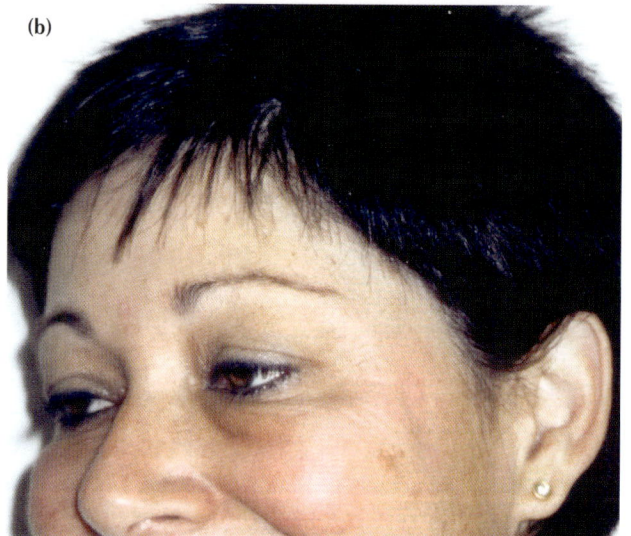

Figure 16.8   Combination of medium depth peel ('weekend peel') with periorbital BTX-A injection: (a) before; (b) after.

Generalized idiosyncratic reactions are uncommon, generally mild, and transient. These include nausea, fatigue, malaise, flu-like symptoms, and rashes at sites distant from the injections.

Although rare, periorbital injections of BTX-A can accentuate excess fullness under the lower eyelids.[18] Therefore, patients with a tendency to spontaneous suborbital swelling might not be good candidates for this procedure.

The most meaningful adverse effect of periorbital and/or suborbital injection is unwanted muscle weakness. If the lateral rectus or inferior oblique muscles are weakened, diplopia results.[19] Over-weakening of the suborbital orbicularis causes ectropion or lagophthalmos, especially in predisposed patients with positive snap tests. Lateral mouth drop occurs as a result of zygomaticus major/minor paralysis (Figure 16.9). Fortunately,

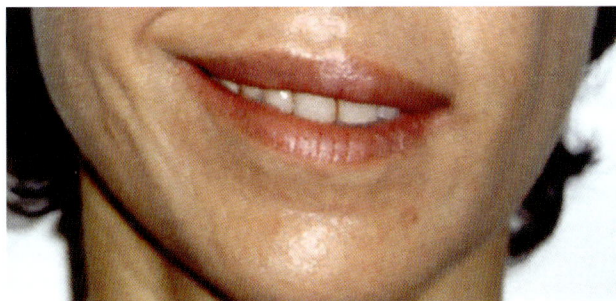

Figure 16.9   Left corner of the mouth drops in smiling after periorbital BTX-A injection as a result of zygomaticus major/minor paralysis.

unwanted weakness caused by the action of the toxin usually resolves in several weeks to months, depending on the site, dosage, and the muscles affected.

Although BTX-A for lateral canthal rhytids usually does not suppress tear production, dry eye is a possible complication of this procedure.[20] Treatment of a dry eye or exposure keratitis is symptomatic, and includes lubrication.

Another rare complication reported recently after BTX-A injection in the lateral canthal area is proptosis associated with thyroid disease.[21] Although proptosis represents progression of the patient's thyroid eye disease, these cases can happen due to cosmetic BTX-A use.

Some patients do not respond to injections, and, having never previously responded, are designated as primary non-responders. There may be many reasons for a lack of response. Patients with rhytids that are not dynamic in origin (e.g. photodamage, age-related changes) do not respond. Possibly, the injection technique was inadequate or the toxin denatured. Theoretically, some patients may have neutralizing antibodies from prior subclinical exposure, or individual variations in docking proteins may exist. Some patients are secondary non-responders. They respond initially but lose the response on subsequent injections. Many of these patients may have developed neutralizing antibodies. Risk factors associated with the development of neutralizing antibodies include injection of more than 200 U per session and repeat or booster injections given within 1 month of treatment. Limited information is available as to whether neutralizing antibodies resolve over time. About 40% of BTX-A non-responders will respond to toxin type B.[22]

References

1. Guerrissi J, Sarkissian P. Local injection into mimetic muscles of botulinum toxin A for the treatment of facial lines. Ann Plast Surg 1997; 39: 447–53.

2. Harris CP, Alderson K, Nebeker J, Holds JB, Anderson RL. Histologic features of human orbicularis oculi treated with botulinum A toxin. Arch Ophthalmol 1991; 109: 393–5.

3. Kane MA. Classification of crow's feet pattern among Caucasian women: the key to individualizing treatment. Plast Reconstr Surg 2003; 112: 33S–9S.

4. Carruthers JA, Carruthers JDA. BOTOX treatment of glabellar frown lines and other facial wrinkles. J Dermatol Surg Oncol 1990; 10: 370 (abstr).

5. Carruthers JA, Carruthers JDA. Using Botulinum Toxin Cosmetically. London: Martin Dunitz, 2003.

6. Flynn TC, Carruthers JA, Carruthers JA. Botulinum toxin A treatment of the lower eyelid improves infraorbital rhytids and widens the eye. Dermatol Surg 2001; 27: 703–8.

7. Sommer B, Sattler G. Botulinum Toxin in Aesthetic Medicine. Berlin: Blackwell Science, 2001.

8. Knize DM. An anatomically based study of the mechanism of eyebrow ptosis. Plast Reconstr Surg 1996; 97: 1321–33.

9. Huilgol SC, Curruthers A, Carruthers JDA. Raising eyebrows with botulinum toxin. Dermatol Surg 1999; 25: 373–5.

10. Lee CJ, Kim SG, Han JY. The results of periorbital rejuvenation with botulinum toxin A using two different protocols. Aesth Plast Surg 2006; 30: 65–70.

11. Lowe NJ, Ascher B, Heckmann M et al. Double-blind, randomized, placebo-controlled, dose-responsive study of the safety and efficacy of botulinum toxin A in subjects with crow's feet. Dermatol Surg 2005; 31: 257–62.

12. Levy JL, Servant JJ, Jouve E. Botulinum toxin A: a 9-month clinical and 3D in vivo profilometric crow's feet wrinkle formation study. J Cosmet Laser Ther 2004; 6: 16–20.

13. Lowe NJ, Lask G, Yamauchi P, Moore D. Bilateral, double-blind, randomized comparison of 3 doses of botulinum toxin type A and placebo in patients with crow's feet. J Am Acad Dermatol 2002; 47: 834–40.

14. Matarasso SL. Comparison of botulinum toxin types A and B: a bilateral and double-blind randomized evaluation in the treatment of canthal rhytids. Dermatol Surg 2003; 29: 7–13.

15. Flynn TC, Carruthers A, Carruthers JA, Clark RE 2nd. Botulinum A toxin (BOTOX) in the lower eyelid: dose-finding study. Dermatol Surg 2003; 29: 943–50.

16. Bosniak S, Cantisano-Zilkha M, Purewal BK, Zdinak LA. Combination therapies in oculofacial rejuvenation. Orbit 2006; 25: 319–26.

17. Landau M. Combination of chemical peelings with botulinum toxin injections and dermal fillers. J Cosmet Dermatol 2006; 5: 121–6.

18. Ascher B, Klap P, Marion MH, Chanteloub F. Botulinum toxin in the treatment of frontoglabellar and periorbital wrinkles. An initial study. Ann Chir Plast Esthet 1995; 40: 67–76.

19. Aristodemou P, Watt L, Baldwin C, Hugkulstone C. Diplopia associated with the cosmetic use of botulinum toxin for a facial rejuvenation. Ophthal Plast Reconstr Surg 2006; 22: 134–6.

20. Arat YO, Yen MT. Effect of botulinum toxin type a on tear production after treatment of lateral canthal rhytides. Ophthal Plast Reconstr Surg 2007; 23: 22–4.

21. Harrison AR, Erickson JP. Thyroid eye disease presenting after cosmetic botulinum toxin injections. Ophthal Plast Reconstr Surg 2006; 22: 397–8.

22. Barnes MP, Best D, Kidd L et al. The use of botulinum toxin type-B in the treatment of patients who have become unresponsive to botulinum toxin type-A – initial experiences. Eur J Neurol 2005; 12: 947–55.

17 The glabella, frontalis, eyebrow area, and eyelids

Timothy C Flynn

Introduction

The use of botulinum toxin type A (BTX-A) for wrinkle improvement is the most commonly performed cosmetic procedure in the United States. Among facial treatments, the glabellar complex remains the single most commonly treated site. As physicians have become more proficient at using botulinum toxin for cosmetic improvement, and as patients have seen remarkable improvements that botulinum toxin can afford, treatment of more than one area of the face is now common. Many patients have the entire upper-third of the face treated with BTX-A, that being the glabellar complex, periocular area, eyebrow area, and forehead. Treatment of multiple areas of the face has been shown to increase patient satisfaction and self-perception of age. This chapter will focus on the treatment of the glabellar complex, forehead, eyebrows, and the eyelids. Other chapters will address the periorbital area, mid-face, lower face, and neck.

Glabellar lines

Drs Alastair and Jean Carruthers published their first experience with cosmetic improvement of wrinkles using botulinum toxin in 1992. They noted that several other physicians familiar with the use of botulinum toxin type A injections for blepharospasm had also begun experimenting with botulinum toxin as a cosmetic treatment. Their initial report led to a remarkable increase in use once physicians discovered the excellent improvement in glabellar lines possible with the injectable protein. Numerous articles followed, which showed great results. Physicians were impressed that injection of botulinum toxin into the muscles of the glabellar complex relaxes the muscles that underlie the skin. Then and now, patients have greatly appreciated the improvement that they see in their folds. One reason is that the 'frown lines' project an appearance expressing concern, displeasure, or frustration. Many patients feel that these lines make them look 'unhappy' or 'angry'. Treatment of glabellar lines produces a more calm or serene appearance. Of interest is that patients report a greater sense of happiness when these lines are treated because they cannot frown as before. It is felt that this lack of muscular feedback makes the patients feel better.

Anatomy

For complete improvement of glabellar lines, all the muscles which produce the glabellar complex must be treated. Muscles which compose the glabellar complex include the corrugator supercilii, depressor supercilii, and procerus muscle, as shown in Figure 17.1. The procerus muscle is in the midline of the nasal root. It originates on the superior portion of the nasal dorsum traveling superiorly, inserting on the underside of the dermis in the forehead above the eyebrows. Procerus contraction depresses the medial head of the eyebrows. The corrugator supercilii muscles lie deep to the frontalis muscle and superficial to the periostium. They originate on the nasal dorsum superiorly, inserting on the underside of the galea above the eyebrow bilaterally. Its position is approximately 30° above horizontal. Because of this angle, the corrugator muscle is categorized as both a brow apposer and depressor. The depressor supercilii is the thin muscle that lies superficial to the corrugator muscle. It originates in the superior nasal dorsum and inserts on the underside of the galea in the region of the medial aspect of the corrugator muscle. Its vertical orientation allows it to be categorized as a brow depressor. A simple way to visualize the depressor supercilii is that it is the muscle which runs lateral to the procerus. In order to effectively treat all the glabellar frown lines, you have to inactivate the glabellar complex. If incomplete relaxation of these muscles occurs, less than optimal results will be seen.

When planning treatment with BTX-A, it is important to evaluate individually each patient's anatomy. A thorough knowledge of anatomy allows the treating physician to imagine the course of these muscles and inject appropriately. It is also important to recognize that there is variability in corrugator supercilii. Some patients have a short, narrow, pyramid-shaped muscle located at the medial end of the supraorbital ridge. Other patients have a long, straight muscle which

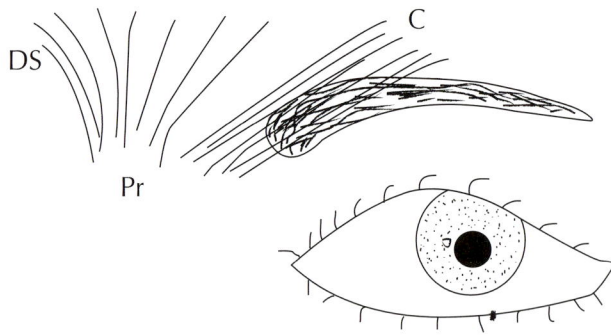

Figure 17.1 Glabellar complex. C, corrugator; Pr, procerus; DS, depressor supercilii; O, orbicularis oculi.

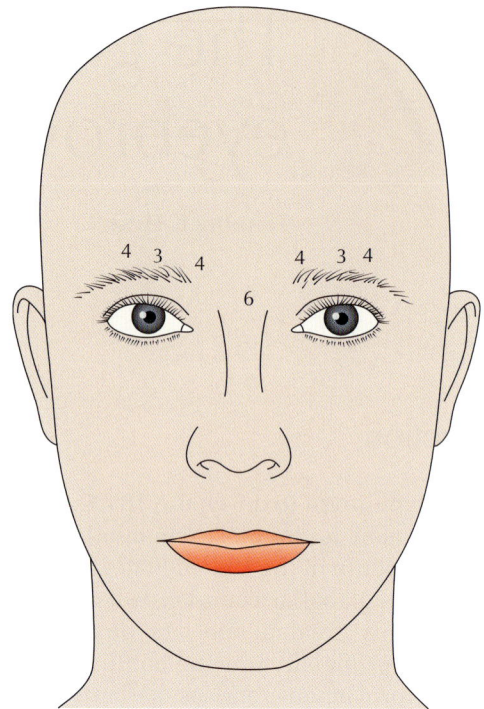

Figure 17.2 Medical record of a 38-year-old patient injected with 28 U of botulinum toxin type A (BOTOX®). The diagram shows the number of units and injection points used for injection.

extends along the supraorbital ridge to or beyond the mid-brow position. These patterns were noted in a study analyzing 50 cadaver hemibrow dissections. In patients who have a long, narrow corrugator supercilii, the treating physician may wish to extend the injection points more laterally to ensure that all aspects of this longer muscle variation are treated. This can be done in several ways. Simply watching the patient pull the eyebrows together or 'frown with the eyebrows' can illustrate where these muscular insertions into the skin occur. Palpation of the glabellar complex can indicate muscle contraction patterns. For the patient returning at follow-up with complaints that an incomplete treatment was performed, palpation can demonstrate focal areas of the glabellar complex which retain movement.

Procerus, depressor supercilii, and corrugator supercilii are the only known medial brow depressors. Treatment of the glabellar complex produces elimination of the glabellar rhytids, but also elevation of the brow is seen. This is due to portions of frontalis muscle having unopposed action.

The original injection pattern described in the BOTOX® package insert and as reported to the Food and Drug Administration (FDA) has five injection sites. The author has found it helpful to alter this pattern using seven injection sites, which he feels more efficiently treats the glabellar complex. Also, the additional injection sites allow complete corrugator treatment. The author's starting dosage for treatment of the female glabellar complex is 28 U. This technique has resulted in a more complete treatment and longer duration than with the 20-U dose as described in the package insert. Ascher et al have documented the optimal dose of another form of botulinum toxin type A, Dysport®. In a dose finding study, they found 50 U of Dysport to be the optimal dose. Dysport will be known as Reloxin® in the United States.

Treatment of the glabellar lines is a relatively simple procedure. The patient is positioned so that they are upright in the treatment chair. The injections are

performed with the needle and syringe held perpendicular to the skin's surface. The author uses a U-100 0.3-ml insulin syringe with a 6-mm needle. Use of the insulin syringe has been described in the literature and allows for a concentrated dilution of toxin to be used (1 ml/100 U vial of BOTOX). The small needle can reach all of the muscles of the glabellar complex with ease. Because these insulin syringes have a 30G or 31G needle, the injections produce only mild pain, and most patients do not complain. Topical anesthesia can be applied if necessary to the overlying skin in sensitive patients. Figure 17.2 shows a medical record diagram documenting the number of units and injection points used. Furthermore, because we dilute the vial with preservative-containing saline, the benzyl alcohol acts as a minor anesthetic. The injections are done by placing the needle directly into the muscle belly and injecting the desired number of units of BOTOX.

The patterns of injection are found relatively easily. The procerus injection is performed by injecting botulinum toxin into the center of the muscle. This point is easily found by drawing a line between the medial brow origin and the contralateral inner canthus. The intersection of these lines marks the center of the procerus muscles. Three injections are used bilaterally to treat the corrugator and depressor supercilii muscles. The injections begin in a vertical line above the medial canthus, 1 cm outside the orbital rim. The most lateral injection is 1 cm above the orbital rim at a point where the

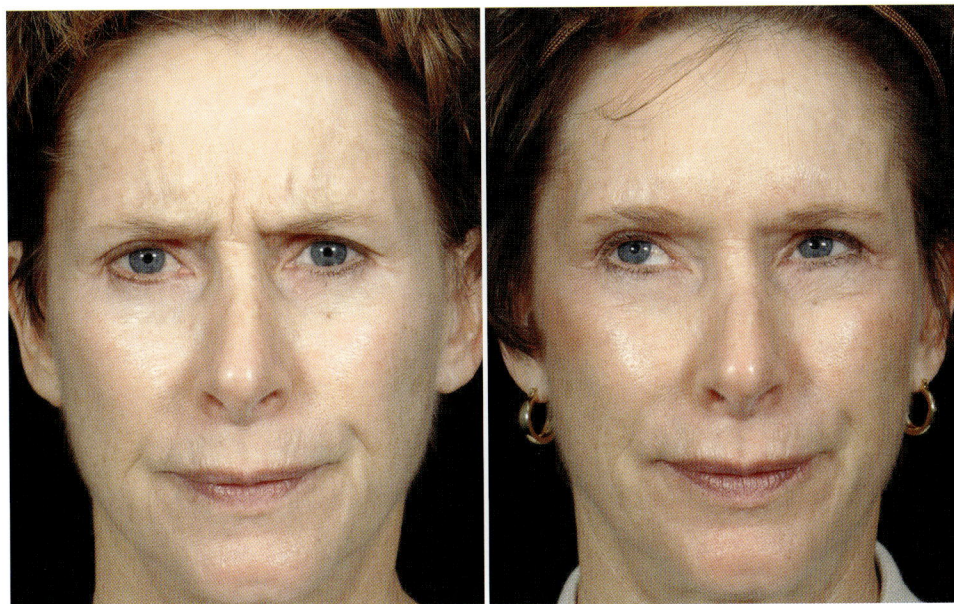

Figure 17.3 A 64-year-old woman before and after glabellar line treatment.

patient's lateral fibers of the corrugator insert into the skin. In many patients, the injection is along a vertical line with the lateral limbus (outer edge of the iris), 1 cm above the orbital rim. The middle injection of the corrugator is simply halfway between these two points, again 1 cm outside the orbital rim. Figure 17.2 shows the medical record of a female patient who had her glabella treated with 28 U. Figure 17.3 shows before and after photographs of a patient using this injection pattern.

It is helpful to mark the injection sites on the patient before the procedure. This gives the advantage of being able to check for symmetry and to carefully evaluate the patient both at rest and contraction and to make sure that the injection is placed precisely where the physician desires. The author has found red 'dry erase' markers helpful to mark the patient. The red ink wipes off extremely easily with no residual. The author has not noticed any incidence of tattooing when these dry erase markers have been used. Other expert injectors favor eyebrow pencil to mark the sites of injection.

Patients are instructed to remain upright for 4 hours, to not lie down for 4 hours, and to contract the glabellar complex approximately every minute for 2 hours. While no careful scientific controlled studies support these practices, there is some basic science evidence suggesting that botulinum toxin is more actively taken up by a contracting muscle.

Some patients have persistent muscular activity following treatment of the glabellar complex. Most frequently, the patient needs higher doses of botulinum toxin, and thus our initial approach when seeing persistent muscle activity is to instill a few more units of BOTOX. This supplementary injection is performed when the patient is seen at a 2-week follow-up after their initial BOTOX injection. Males need higher doses, probably as a result of the effect of testosterone on muscular growth and size. A starting dose for men is 40 U into the glabellar complex, with some men

needing upwards of 80 U. Some individuals are able to continue to furrow the glabellar area by recruiting the lateral aspect of the orbicularis oculi muscle after the corrugator and procerus muscles have been treated. Small superficial doses of BTX-A can be useful to relax this portion of the orbicularis; however, this recruitment is usually seen only on extreme contraction and is not a persistent problem with everyday animation. Finally, many patients who have noticeable wrinkles at rest will have improvement of their resting lines but not complete correction, as seen in Figure 17.4. Small, carefully placed doses of filler substances such as injectable collagen or hyaluronic acid can be used to fill out these persistent resting rhytids. Of course, caution must be used when injecting filler substances into the glabellar area.

Currently, complications are few when the glabella has been treated. Localized pain at the site of injection and small bleeding points are the most common side-effects. If small bleeding areas are noted, firm pressure with a cotton-tipped applicator can be applied focally to the treated area (Figure 17.5). This will help reduce bleeding immediately post-injection. Our patients are often asked to avoid aspirin, vitamin E, and non-steroidal anti-inflammatory agents before treatment. However, injections can be performed in individuals who have recently used agents that interfere with the coagulation cascade. Expert injectors have not lately experienced the often quoted eyelid ptosis rate of 1–3%. A recent poll at an international meeting among experienced physicians indicated an extremely low eyelid ptosis rate. This is most likely because a greater understanding of proper injection techniques has reduced the incidence of ptosis. Should this occur, the patient can be reassured that this is often a temporary effect. If the patient is unhappy with the ptosis, patients can be given eyedrops containing α-adrenergic agonists. For example, apraclonidine or phenylephrine

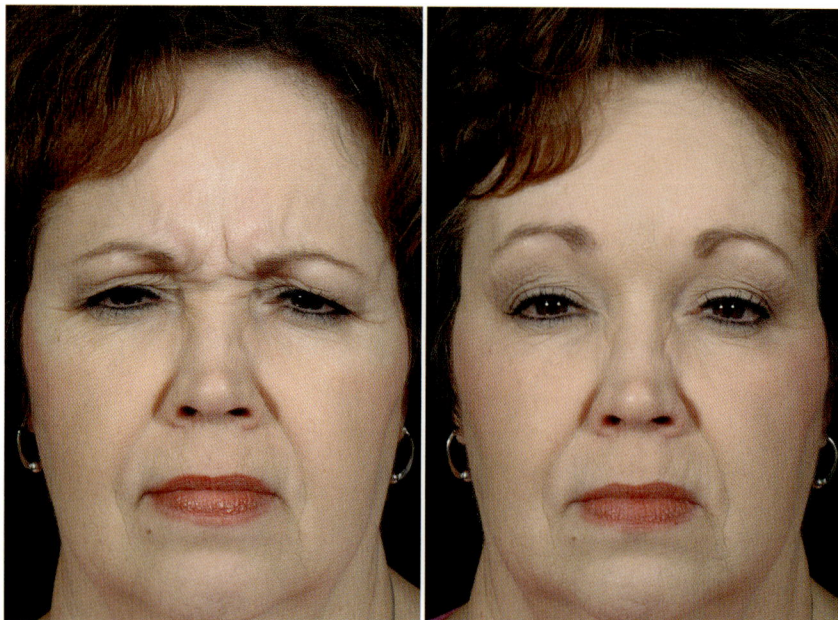

Figure 17.4 Good response to glabellar line treatment in a 56-year-old patient. A filler substance such as injectable collagen can be cautiously used to fill out the persistent fine glabellar lines.

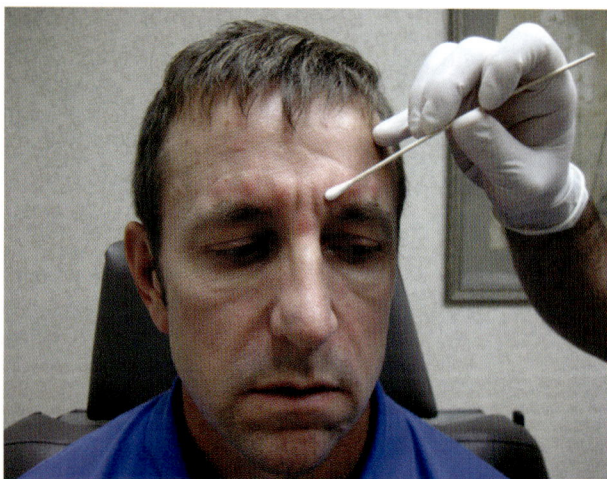

Figure 17.5 Use of cotton-tipped applicator to control bleeding points.

can be instilled into the affected eye. These two agents help elevate the upper lid by assisting contraction in Müller's muscle.

Forehead rhytids

Wrinkles of the forehead are troubling to a number of individuals. Forehead wrinkles, also termed horizontal forehead lines, are formed by excessive contraction of the frontalis muscle. In certain individuals this may be due to a tendency towards excessive animation inherent to the patient. They simply are very expressive, and regularly contract the frontalis muscle. BTX-A treatment can produce a more relaxed esthetically pleasing forehead. There are other individuals who contract the frontalis due to ptosis of the eyebrows. In an attempt to lift their drooping

eyebrows off their eyelids, these patients have developed a compensatory excessive contraction of the frontalis muscle. The contracting of the frontalis places the brows in a more comfortable position, allowing full gaze. These patients may need more than BTX-A treatment, such as a surgical brow lift with or without blepharoplasty.

Anatomy

The frontalis muscle (Figure 17.6) is a flat, broad muscle that originates at the galea superiorly and inserts into the skin of the eyebrows inferiorly. While traditional anatomic drawings indicate a muscle with two muscle bellies, in many patients the midline fibers overlap considerably. For many patients it is best to think of the frontalis as a singular muscular sheet which lies underneath the skin of the forehead. The anatomic variants correspond to two functional wrinkle patterns which can be noted on patients. The more common pattern reveals single, continuous, horizontal forehead lines which run across the forehead. The second but less common pattern shows central sparing.

The physician should carefully note the exact pattern of forehead wrinkles and mark the patient appropriately before injection. In order to contract the forehead muscles, the patients are asked to elevate their eyebrows. Injections are planned to follow the pattern of wrinkles with small injections of botulinum toxin in order to relax the frontalis muscle. Figure 17.7 shows a nice response in a 28-year-old woman.

A few clinical caveats are notable. Many patients have wrinkles in the superior portion of the frontalis, up near their hairline. Failure to treat these upper forehead wrinkles will result in patient dissatisfaction. The lower 2 cm of the frontalis muscle controls eyebrow position. It is extremely important to keep this in mind when treating

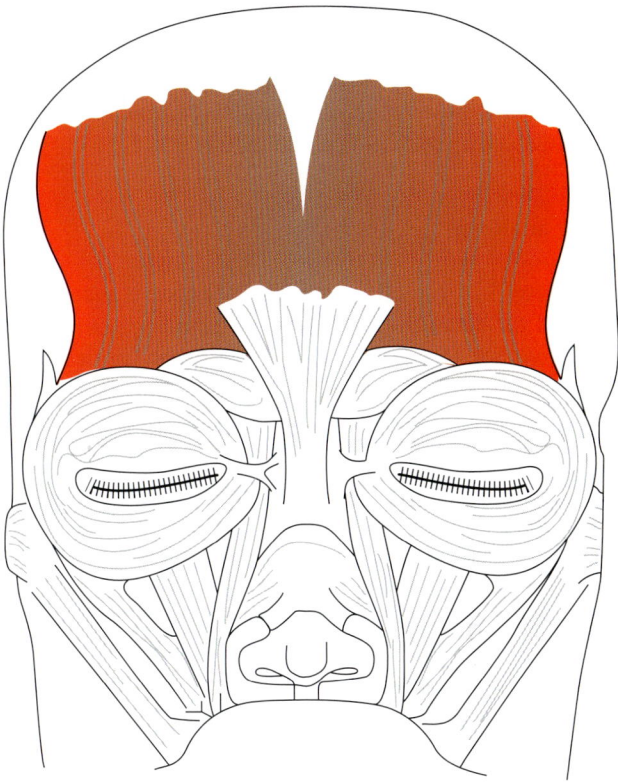

Figure 17.6   Frontalis.

patients. Women prefer a pleasant arch to the eyebrow. They do not like their brows lowered. Therefore, caution is advised when treating the lower 2 cm of the frontalis muscle. Frequently the frontalis muscle is treated but the lower 2 cm are spared, to allow the brows to arch. Patients will return complaining that they still have a persistent 'comma-shaped' wrinkle present laterally just superior to the tail of the eyebrow. These wrinkles can be aided by using filler substances in addition to botulinum toxin, and the volume replacement helps elevate the eyebrows and stretch out the rhytids. Superficial dermal wrinkle filling can also be undertaken. This combined approach with botulinum toxin and fillers has resulted in a great deal of satisfaction in female patients.

Men look good with horizontal brows. In most males, the physician will not want to arch the eyebrow excessively. However, there are individual men who have a fair degree of brow ptosis, and if the entire frontalis is treated, these brows will drop down and, while not a cosmetic concern, can interfere with the patient's ability to keep their eyebrows out of their visual field.

Another caveat is, if the central portion of the frontalis is treated, it may allow the lateral portions of the frontalis to contract while the central portion is relaxed. This can produce excessive lateral eyebrow elevation. We have met individual patients, particularly older women, who feel that this is dramatic and striking, and actually prefer this look. However, the main goal of treatment of the lateral forehead region is to always leave some frontalis muscle activity to prevent lateral brow depression, and yet to be able to treat the forehead evenly.

Many famous people who are photographed have in the past been treated with too much BTX-A in the frontalis. This has resulted in a glassy or artificial appearance to the brow, which appears tight and can reflect light excessively when photographed. A new trend in botulinum toxin therapy of the brow has been to use lesser doses of BTX-A in the forehead and to preserve some frontalis contraction. In short, the goal is to seek to reduce the forehead lines but yet still allow some natural expression. Again, counseling and discussion with the patient as to their preferred look is essential to treating the forehead. We like to use concentrated BOTOX diluted at 1 ml/100-U vial. We place several injections of approximately 2 U throughout the forehead. Figure 17.8 shows a typical pattern of treatment of the frontalis. Men require high doses of BOTOX in general,

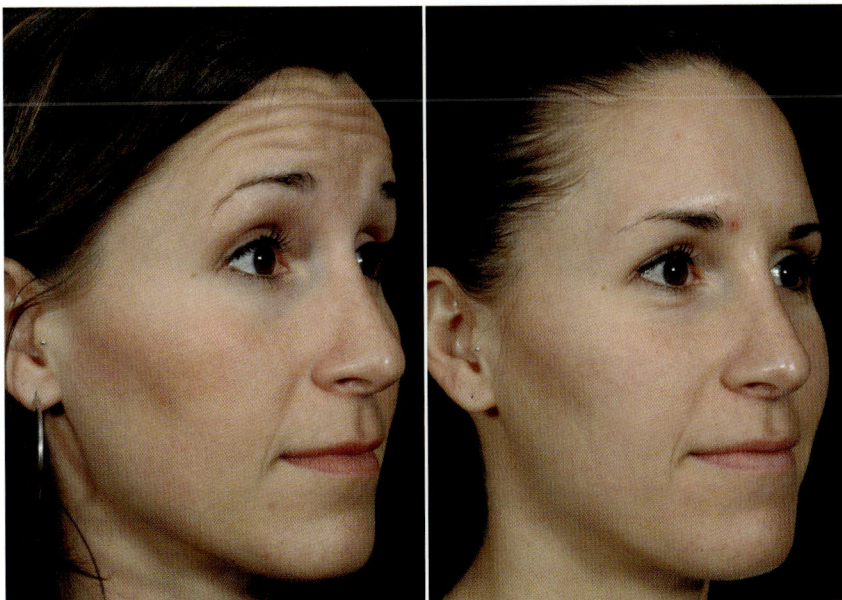

Figure 17.7   Before and after BOTOX: 24 U were used to treat the forehead of the 28-year-old patient.

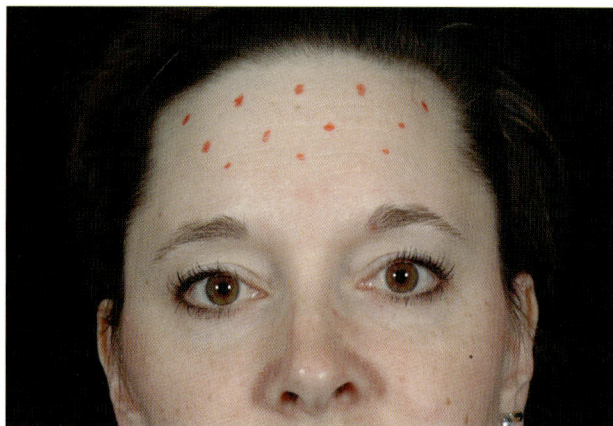

Figure 17.8   Marking the forehead of the patient with a red dry erase marker.

and this applies to the frontalis as well. We routinely put 30–40 U in a man's forehead for treatment. In patients with excessive wrinkling of the forehead, it is often advisable to split the initial treatment into two sessions (Figure 17.9). This is so that care can be taken when working in the lower portion of the frontalis and to keep brow shape in position in the preferred alignment. The majority of the treatment is done in the upper two-thirds of the frontalis, and the patient is asked to return in approximately 2 weeks. Then the residual movement of the frontalis is studied, and the doctor and patient can decide, with additional injections, what remaining wrinkles can be treated. This is a good opportunity to discuss the need for filler substances if appropriate.

Eyebrows

More than ever, physicians have come to appreciate the esthetic importance of the eyebrow. New botulinum toxin techniques have been developed to both shape and elevate the brow. With age, brows change their shape and position. With aging, brow descent and loss of the esthetically pleasing female arch may occur. Botulinum toxin offers an easy improvement to problems of brow shape and position.

Brow anatomy

Eyebrows are held in position largely by the lower 2 cm of the frontalis muscle. The frontalis is the only muscle that elevates the brow. Brow depressors include the glabellar complex, most notably the procerus and depressor supercilii. The corrugator, with its angular position, both apposes and depresses the brow. Laterally the brow depressors are the lateral, vertically oriented fibers of the orbicularis oculi muscle. This portion of the muscle is, of course, also responsible for crow's feet. Relaxation of this portion of the orbicularis can result in lateral brow lifting by removing the muscular tension that pulls the brow inferiorly.

Clinical considerations

There have been several reports detailing elevation of the brow following treatment of the glabellar complex. The Carruthers demonstrated that injections of 20–40 U of botulinum toxin type A into the medial brow produce an initial lateral eyebrow elevation. They felt that the effect on eyebrow elevation is primarily lateral, and that this is most likely due to a partial inactivation of the lower central frontalis allowing the untreated frontalis muscle to increase resting tone and raise the eyebrows laterally. They furthermore noted that when small amounts of BOTOX (10 U) are injected into the glabella, there may be a mild medial brow ptosis. However, very few physicians are currently using this low dose to treat the glabella area.

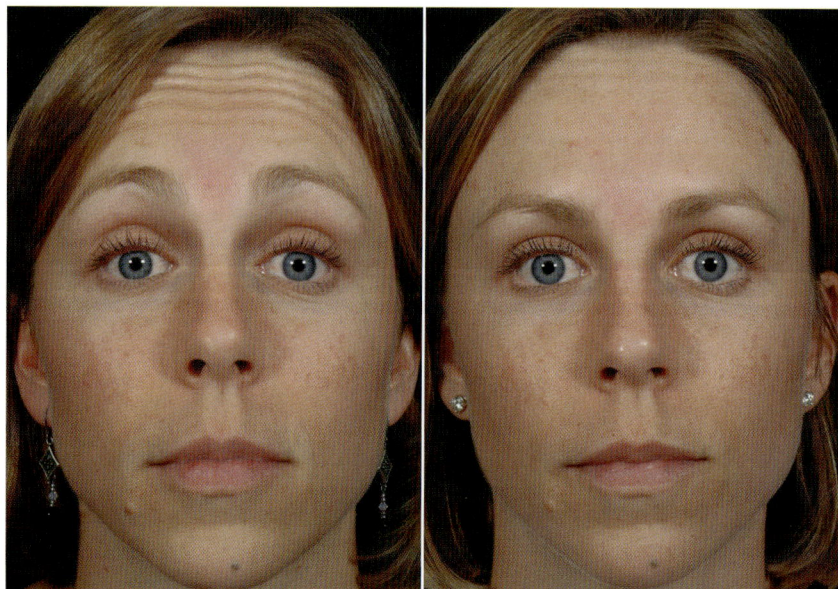

Figure 17.9   Before and after BOTOX to the forehead. Horizontal lines are relaxed while brows maintain an excellent arch shape and correct position on the face of this 29-year-old woman. Note the few persistent superior forehead rhytids which will respond well to additional BOTOX.

Additional lateral eyebrow elevation can be achieved by injecting approximately 4 U at the tail of each eyebrow (Figure 17.10). This is thought to affect the vertically oriented fibers of the lateral orbicularis oculi muscle. By relaxing the brow depressors, an additional 1–2 mm of lateral eyebrow elevation is possible. There are patients who already have a ptotic brow, and thus treating the glabella along with treating both tails of the eyebrows bilaterally can produce nice brow elevation.

Eyebrow asymmetry is occassionally seen, and botulinum toxin type A injections can produce a greater symmetry of the eyebrows. In most patients, the goal is to treat the eyebrow depressors in an attempt to elevate the lower eyebrow to the same height as the higher. However, there are cases in which the eyebrows are asymmetrical or peaked due to excessive frontalis activity, causing focal excessive brow elevation. In this case, placing approximately 2 U in the frontalis muscle above the peaked brow will weaken this portion of the frontalis and relax or drop that portion of the excessively elevated brow. It is important to assess patients very carefully when working with brow injections. Patients must be viewed in repose and with active movement, and careful recording of exact placement of the brow injections must be noted. We have found in many older female patients that treatment of the glabella along with treatment of the lateral brow depressors produces a nice brow elevation. In addition, there are patients who suffer from eyebrow asymmetry following brow lift surgery. Small injections of botulinum toxin are helpful to assist such a patient in achieving a more symmetrical appearance.

Brows can be arched by treating the portions of the frontalis corresponding to medial and lateral eyebrows. By relaxing this portion of the frontalis, the section of frontalis above the mid-pupillary line retains activity. Thus, the central portion of the brow will arch up due to frontalis tension occurring on this middle portion of the eyebrow. We have found this helpful for young women with congenitally flat eyebrows.

Eyelids

Treatment of the eyelids has become popular, especially among two groups, those patients with fine wrinkling found on the lower eyelid and those individuals who have a ptotic brow which is dropping down and adding weight to the upper eyelid. Treatment can be afforded using botulinum toxin, which allows improvement of wrinkling of the lower lid, and eye aperture widening. Lateral brow elevation can be achieved by treating fibers in the orbicularis oculi, which slightly lifts the lateral brow off the upper eyelid.

Anatomy

Lower eyelid wrinkles are caused in part by contractions of the orbicularis oculi muscle (Figure 17.11). The

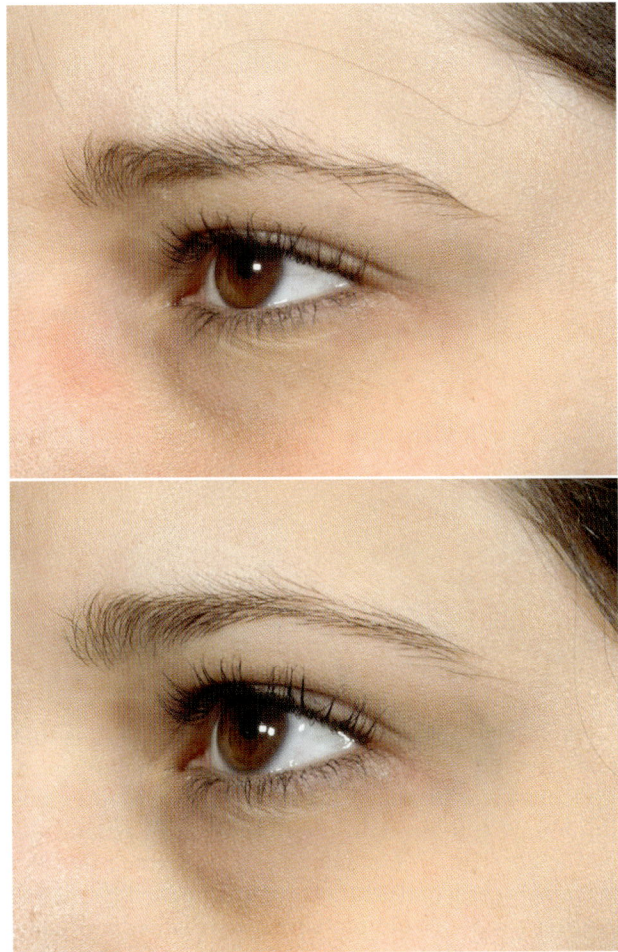

Figure 17.10 A simple lateral eyebrow lift is possible with BOTOX: before and after 4 U placed in the tail of the eyebrow.

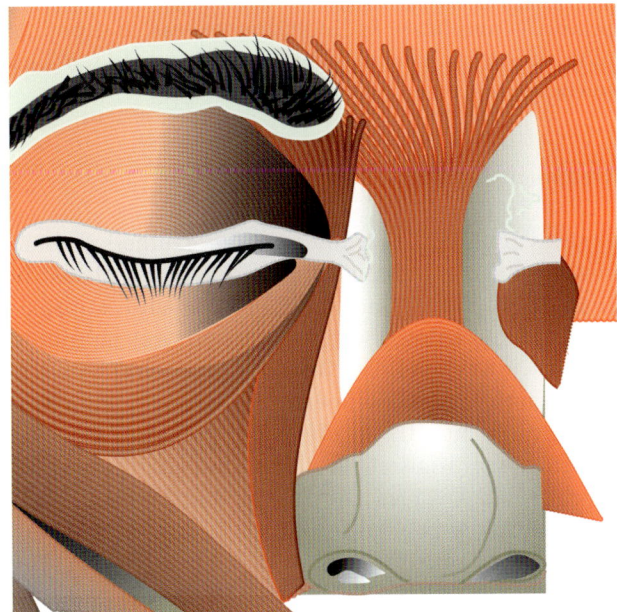

Figure 17.11 Orbicularis oculi.

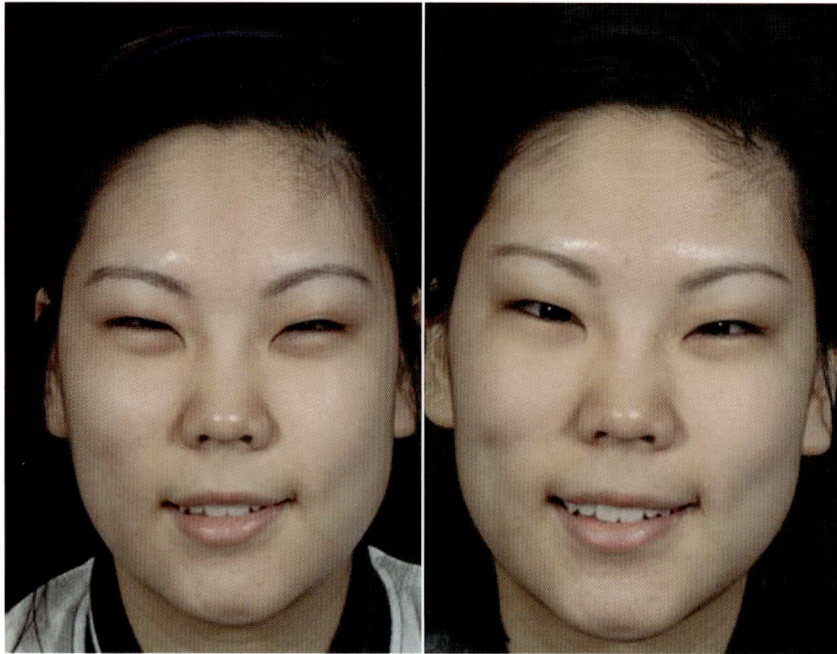

Figure 17.12 Eye widening in an Asian patient with severely narrow palpebral aperture. This procedure was performed to help the patient decide on corrective scalpel surgery by allowing her to experience a wider, more open-eyed appearance.

orbicularis oculi is a sphincteric muscle which is thin and circumferentially encompasses the orbital space. This muscle is intimately associated with the thin eyelid dermis and has multiple insertions all around the periocular skin. The orbiculis can be divided into the pretarsal, preseptal, and orbital portions. The orbital portion wraps around the lateral canthal tendon without insertion. When this portion of the muscle contracts, it produces crow's feet wrinkles. Contraction of the inferior pretarsal orbicularis produces inferior eyelid wrinkles. This inferior portion of the muscle serves to crinkle the lower lid and also helps to suspend the lower eyelid. Careful treatment of the inferior pretarsal orbicularis can smooth this inferior wrinkling and widen the eyelid aperture. However, overtreatment can produce complications, including excessive drooping of the lower eyelid skin, photophobia, and the inability to completely close the eye.

Treatment considerations

A study by Flynn, Carruthers, and Carruthers demonstrated that 2 U of botulinum type A toxin placed in the mid-pupillary line of the lower eyelid, approximately 3 mm below the ciliary margin, was helpful to remove lower eyelid wrinkles. It was also noted to increase the palpebral aperture. The study indicated that a more significant effect can be seen when the inferior eyelid is treated along with the crow's feet area. This is because a greater amount of orbicularis oculi muscle is relaxed and serves to further open and widen the eye aperture.

A most striking result from the use of inferior eyelid BOTOX along with crow's feet treatment was demonstrated in the Asian eye (Figure 17.12). A number of

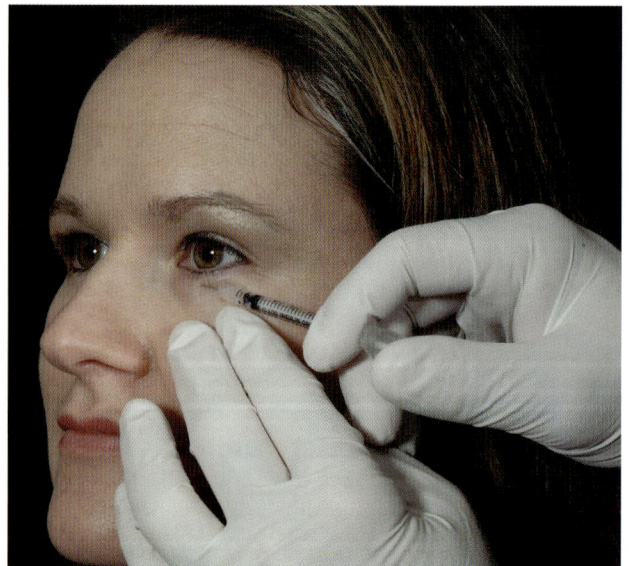

Figure 17.13 Lateral inferior approach to injecting the infraorbital folds.

Asian patients have been quite pleased with this widening effect on the eye, and this is best achieved when both crow's feet and inferior eyelid wrinkles are treated. Most Asian patients are treated with 12 U of BOTOX in the lateral orbital wrinkles and 2 U placed in the mid-pupillary line in the lower eyelid.

Surprisingly, inferior eyelid injection is relatively painless. Practitioners are advised to use an inferolateral approach when bringing the injecting syringe up to treat the patient (Figure 17.13). In this way, the patient does not have a surprised reaction when they see a hypodermic needle approaching their eye. Patients are asked to look directly forward, to hold

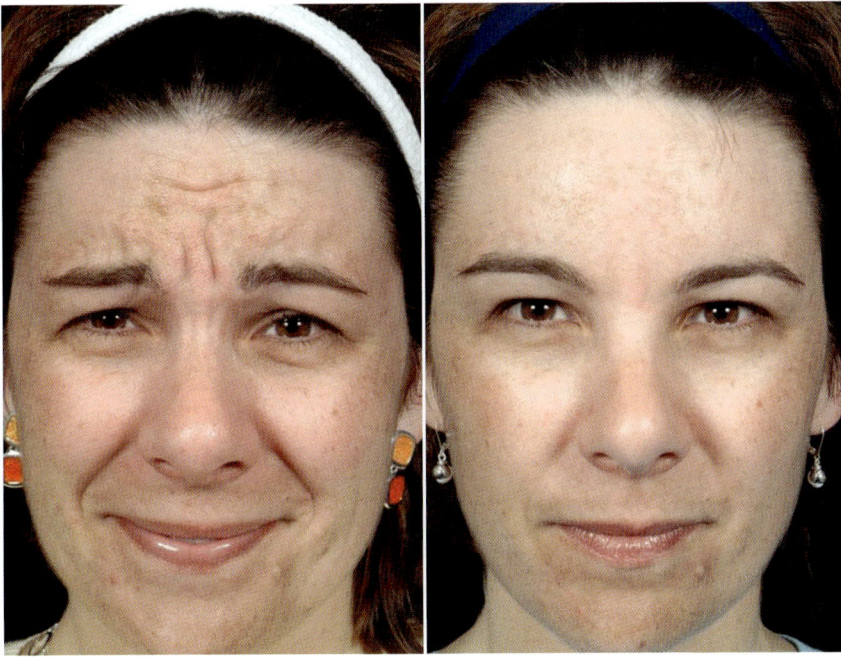

Figure 17.14 Patient with active glabellar complex and forehead lines. This patient had both the frontalis and the glabellar complex treated with BOTOX.

still, and to not blink. Reassuring the patient that they will have very little pain is helpful to decrease anxiety, making the injections easier.

The follow-up dose finding study demonstrated that increased complications are seen if more than 2 U are used in the lower lid. This was especially notable when 8 U were placed in the lower lid. A number of patients experienced a drooping lower lid, which looked 'sad'. The 8 U produced a loss of suspension of the lower eyelid skin, and several patients noted that their 'bags' had dropped. It is the current recommendation when treating the lower eyelid skin that 2 U be placed in the mid-pupillary line approximately 3 mm below the ciliary margin. If needed, then another 2 U can be placed at a point between the lateral canthus and the mid-pupillary line to see if further eye widening or lower lid wrinkles can be achieved. Care should be taken not to produce lateral lower lid rounding, which is not esthetically pleasing.

Conclusion

The use of BTX-A for treatment of the glabella, forehead, brows, and crow's feet has been revolutionary in terms of marked esthetic benefit with a minimally invasive approach. BTX-A combined with filler substances is an everyday treatment algorithm in the cosmetic physician's office. Most patients are now having more than one area treated with BTX-A, leading to remarkably good results as shown in Figure 17.14. BTX-A is the treatment of choice for the upper third of the face. Patient staisfaction is high and complications and risks few.

Bibliography

Ascher B, Zakine B, Kestemont P et al. A multicenter randomized, double-blind, placebo-controlled study of efficacy and safety of 3 doses of botulinum toxin A in the treatment of glabellar lines. J Am Acad Dermatol 2004; 51: 223–33

Carruthers J, Carruthers A. Botulinum toxin type A treatment of multiple upper facial sites: patient-reported outcomes. Dermatol Surg 2007; 33 (Spec No): S10–17.

Carruthers A, Carruthers J. Eyebrow height after botulinum toxin type A to the glabella. Dermatol Surg 2007; 33 (Spec No): S26–31.

Carruthers JA, Carruthers JA. Treatment of glabellar frown lines with C. botulinum-A exotoxin. J Dermatol Surg Oncol 1992; 18: 17–21.

Finn JC, Cox SE. Practical botulinum toxin anatomy. In: Carruthers JA, Carruthers JA, eds. Procedures in Cosmetic Dermatology: Botulinum Toxin. Philadelphia: Saunders, 2005: 19–30.

Cook BE Jr. Lukarelli MJ, Lernakey BN. Depressor supercilii muscle; anatomy, histology, and cosmetic implications. Ophthal Plast Reconstr Surg 2001; 17: 404–11.

Carruthers A, Carruthers J. Prospective, double-blind randomized, parallel group, dose ranging study of Botulinum Toxin Type A in men with glabellar rhytids. Dermatol Surg 2005; 31: 1297–303.

Flynn TC, Carruthers JA, Carruthers JA, Clark RE 2nd. Botulinun A toxin (BOTOX) in the lower eyelid: dose-finding study. Dermatol Surg 2003; 29: 943–50.

Flynn TC, Carruthers A, Carruthers J. Surgical pearl: the use of the Ultra-Fine II short needle 0.3-cc insulin syringe for botulinum toxin injections. J Am Acad Dermatol 2002; 46: 931–3.

Flynn TC, Carruthers JA, Carruthers JA. Botulinum-A toxin treatment of the lower eyelid improves infraorbital rhytides and widens the eye. Dermatol Surg 2001; 27: 703–8.

Flynn TC. Periocular botulinum toxin. Clin Dermatol 2003; 21: 498–504.

Kornstein AN. Soft-tissue reconstruction of the brow with Restylane. Plast Reconstr Surg 2005; 116: 2017–20.

Klein AW. Botox for the eyes and eyebrows. Dermatol Clin 2004; 22: 145–9, vi.

Levy JL, Pons F, Jouve E. Management of the aging eyebrow and forehead: an objective dose-response study with botulinum toxin. J Eur Acad Dermatol Venereol 2006; 20: 711–16.

Lackey JN, Norton SA. Implications of botulinum toxin injection of the brow. J Am Acad Dermatol 2006; 54: 921–2.

Lowe NJ, Ascher B, Heckmann M et al; Botox Facial Aesthetics Study Team. Double-blind, randomized, placebo-controlled, dose-response study of the safety and efficacy of botulinum toxin type A in subjects with crow's feet. Dermatol Surg 2005; 31: 257–62.

Maas CS. Botulinum neurotoxins and injectable fillers: minimally invasive management of the aging upper face. Otolaryngol Clin North Am 2007; 40: 283–90.

Monheit G, Carruthers A, Brandt F, Rand R. A randomized, double-blind placebo-controlled study of botulinium toxin type A for the treatment of glabellar lines: determination of optimal dose. Dermatol Surg 2007; 33 (Spec No): S51–9.

Rzany B, Dill-Muller D, Grablowitz D, Heckmann M, Caird D; German–Austrian Retrospective Study Group. Repeated botulinum toxin A injections for the treatment of lines in the upper face: a retrospective study of 4,103 treatments in 945 patients. Dermatol Surg 2007; 33: S18–25.

The mid- and lower face

Berthold Rzany

Introduction

Even for experienced physicians the mid- and lower face is a challenge, because the gap between a perfect and a disastrous result over the treatment period is quite small. However, with adequate knowledge of the anatomy and careful dosing it is possible to obtain good results in most patients.

This chapter follows a practical approach. Each indication is characterized by the mimic muscles to be treated, the injection points, and the dosages. The chapter refers to the book of Marc Heckmann and myself.[1] The recommendations for the injection points are based on two German consensus papers on the usage of botulinum toxin A (BTX-A) in esthetic medicine.[2,3] Both consensus papers refer to the use of Dysport®. The BOTOX® consensus paper was only partially helpful, as not all areas discussed in this chapter were covered.[4] In dermatologic practice, 3 U of Dysport are generally accepted as being equal to 1 U of BOTOX. This ratio has recently been confirmed for dystonia by a Cochrane systematic review.[5] Therefore, when no recommendations from the BOTOX consensus paper are available this ratio might be useful.

Mid-face

The mid-face is still a fairly unknown area for treatment with BTX-A. However, it is worth taking a closer look at the different indications.

Nasolabial folds

BTX-A is not a filler. Therefore, nasolabial folds cannot be elevated by BTX-A. However, what can be treated is the active elevation of the folds while contracting the nasalis, the levator labii superioris, and the levator labii superioris alaeque nasi muscles (Figure 18.1). Here, 5–10 U Dysport (or the equivalent dosage of BOTOX) distributed in one or two injection points per side will lead to decreased mimic activity. Therefore, the maximum active depth of nasolabial folds is reduced (Figure 18.2). Nevertheless, this is a

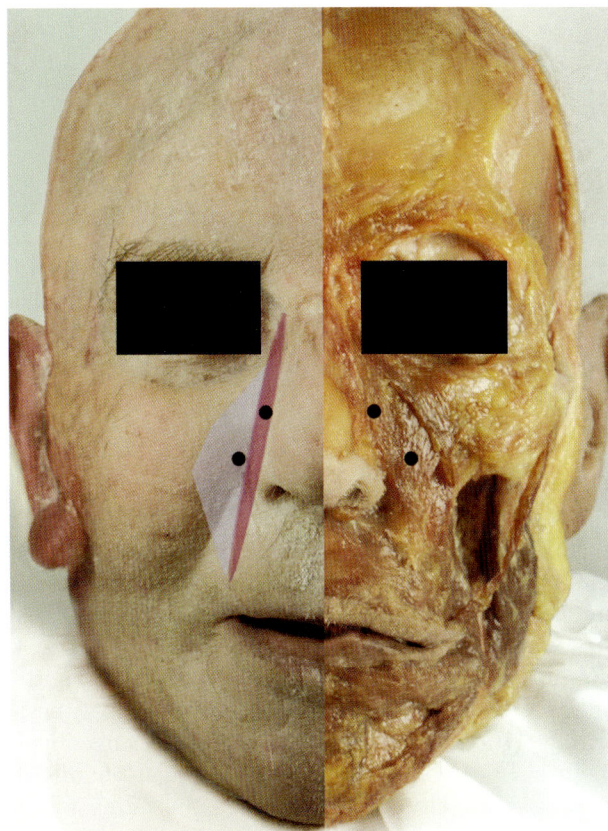

Figure 18.1 Injection points for the nasolabial folds (both points), bunny lines (upper points), and gummy smile (lower points).

primary area for injectable fillers. BTX-A can only add to the overall efficacy here (Table 18.1).

'Bunny lines'

Especially patients who have been treated in the glabella area and crow's feet region might end up with pronounced 'bunny lines'. These lines, which cover with a V-shaped pattern the dorsum of the nose, are induced by contractions of the nasalis and the levator labii superioris alaeque nasi muscles. They can be treated with 5–10 U Dysport (or the equivalent dosage of BOTOX) (Figure 18.1). The injections should be

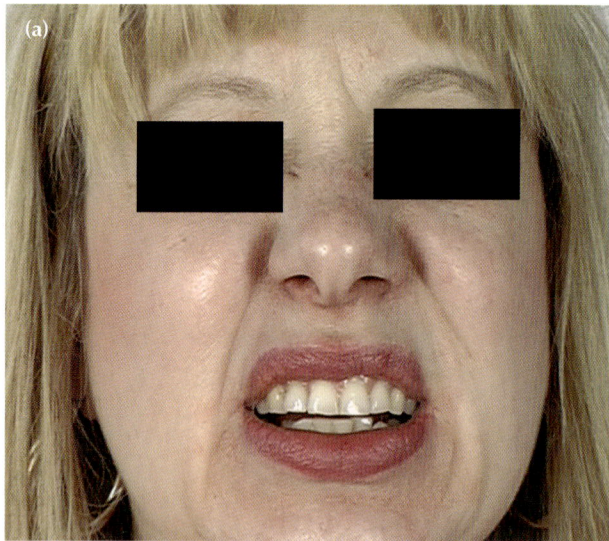

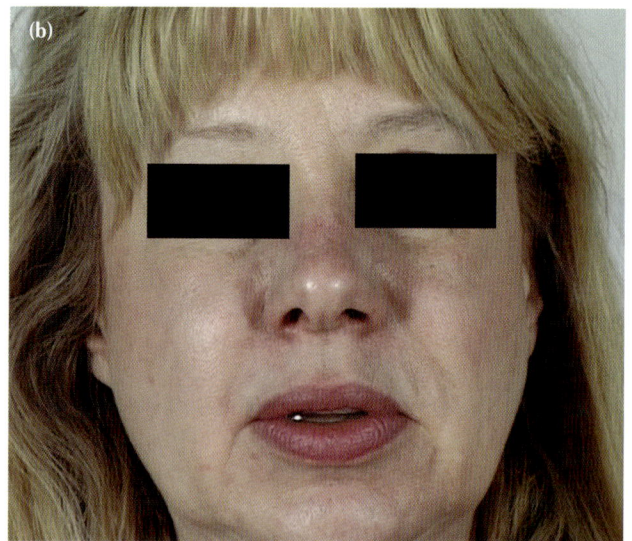

Figure 18.2   Deep nasolabial folds. (a) Before and (b) 2 weeks after the injection of 2×10 U Dysport® and 0.7 ml hyaluronic acid per side.

performed superficially in order to avoid a spread beneath the fascia (Table 18.2).

'Gummy smile'

A smile usually exposes the teeth. People with a 'gummy smile', however, show not only their teeth but also part of the gums while smiling. Sometimes, this type of smile is considered to be unsightly. A 'gummy smile' can be corrected by injecting botulinum toxin A in the area of the levator labii superioris, i.e. the triangle between ala, nose, and cheek (Figure 18.1). Consequently, an elongation of the upper lip develops which covers the gums while smiling. As the orbicularis oris muscle is not targeted, eating and drinking are not negatively influenced (Table 18.3).

Lower face

The lower face is much more challenging, because in this area overtreatment of the orbicularis oris muscle might lead to a dysfunctional mouth with all the negative consequences. Therefore, prior to the treatment of this area, patients have to be thoroughly advised about the pros and cons of this method.

Upper and lower lip

Vertical lines of the upper lip are a strong sign of aging. Even when using an injectable filler some of these lines might remain. The aim of treatment of the upper and lower lip is a reduction of these unsightly wrinkles. The injection points may focus on the philtrum or

Table 18.1   Nasolabial folds
• One or two injection points per side covering the lower third of the dorsum of the nose (if one injection point is used a point in the middle of the two in Figure 18.1-depicted points would be suitable)
• Dosage Dysport®: 5–10 U per injection point
• Dosage BOTOX®: not covered in the BOTOX consensus paper[4]

Table 18.2   'Bunny lines'
• One injection point per side (here the upper points in Figure 18.1 would be appropriate) covering the medial part of the dorsum of the nose
• Dosage Dysport: 5–10 U per injection point
• Dosage BOTOX: 1.5–3 U per injection point[4]

Table 18.3   'Gummy smile'
• One injection point per side (here the lower point in Figure 18.1 would be suitable) focusing on the triangle between ala, nose, and cheek
• Dosage Dysport: 5–10 U per point
• Dosage BOTOX: not covered in the BOTOX consensus paper[4]

follow the lip line (Figure 18.3). Very small dosages should be used in order to avoid a dysfunctional mouth. Injection points around the philtrum may not only decrease strong medial vertical wrinkles but also the visibility of a horizontal line which can be found in

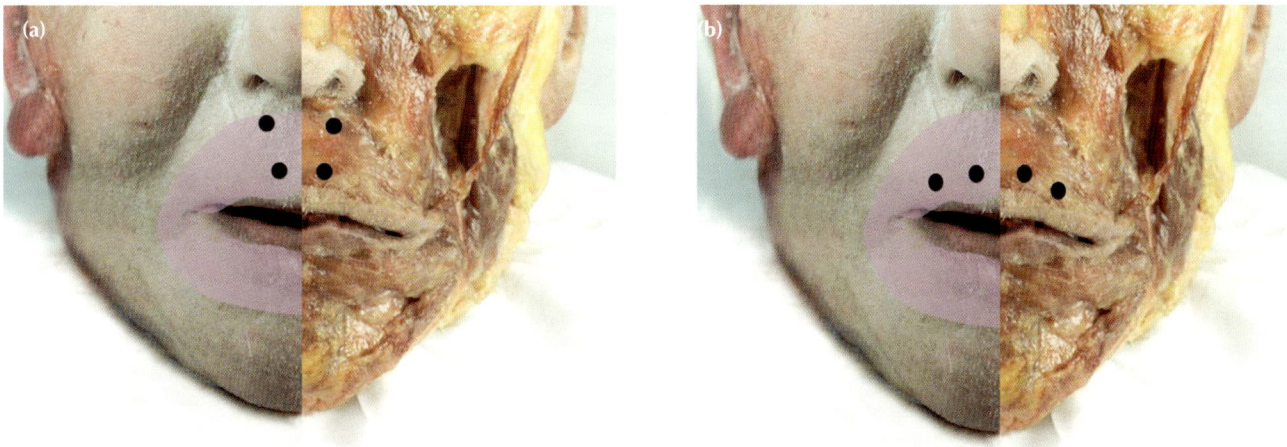

Figure 18.3   (a, b) Injection points for the upper lip.

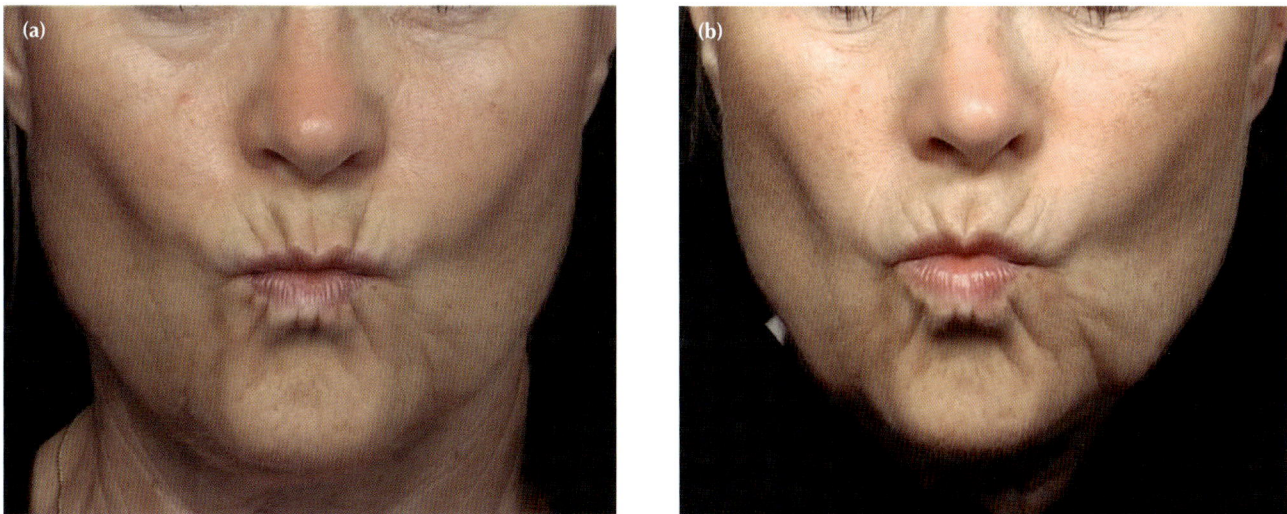

Figure 18.4   Upper lip wrinkles (a) before and (b) 2 weeks after treatment with 2 × 5 U Dysport in the philtrum area.

some patients. However, especially in the case of a relative overdosage, these injection points might also lead to a flat, unnatural looking philtrum. Furthermore, slight asymmetries are quite common for this area (Figure 18.4).

For the upper lip the total dosage should range between 6 and 16 U Dysport. Smaller dosages between 6 and 10 U Dysport are recommended for the lower lip (Table 18.4). Precooling of the upper lip region might be helpful, as treatment of this area is considered to be quite painful by many patients.

'Marionette lines'

The depressor anguli oris is a very important muscle that influences the way we are seen by other people.

Table 18.4   Upper lip wrinkles
• Two or four injection points in the philtrum area
• Two injection points along the lip line more laterally
• Dosage Dysport: 2–4 U per injection point
• Dosage BOTOX: 1–2.5 U per injection point starting dosage[4]

Constant hyperactivity might lead to deep furrows drawing down the corners of the mouth, which will lead consequently to an overall sad, slightly depressed impression. The depressor anguli oris muscle can usually be easily palpated when the patient is asked to contract this muscle. In addition to the depressor anguli oris, platysmal bands can increase this downward

Library
College of Physicians & Surgeons of B.C.
400 - 858 Beatty Street
Vancouver BC V6B 1C1

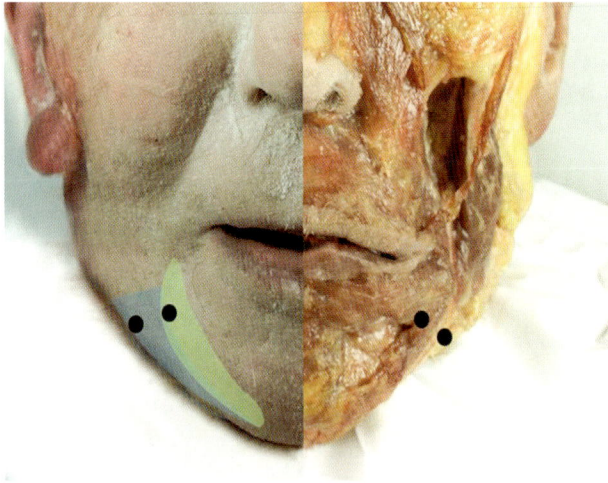

Figure 18.5   Injection points for the treatment of marionette lines targeting the depressor anguli oris muscle and the platysma.

Table 18.5   'Marionette lines'

- One injection point per site targeting the depressor anguli oris. The point should be at least 1 cm away from the corner of the mouth. The muscle can be felt while contracted. Usually the point can be found in the elongation of the nasolabial fold
- Another injection point should be located more laterally in the area of the mandible in order to target the platsymal bands
- Symmetrical distribution of injection points
- Dosage Dysport: maximum 10–20 U per injection point
- Dosage BOTOX: not covered in the BOTOX consensus paper[4]

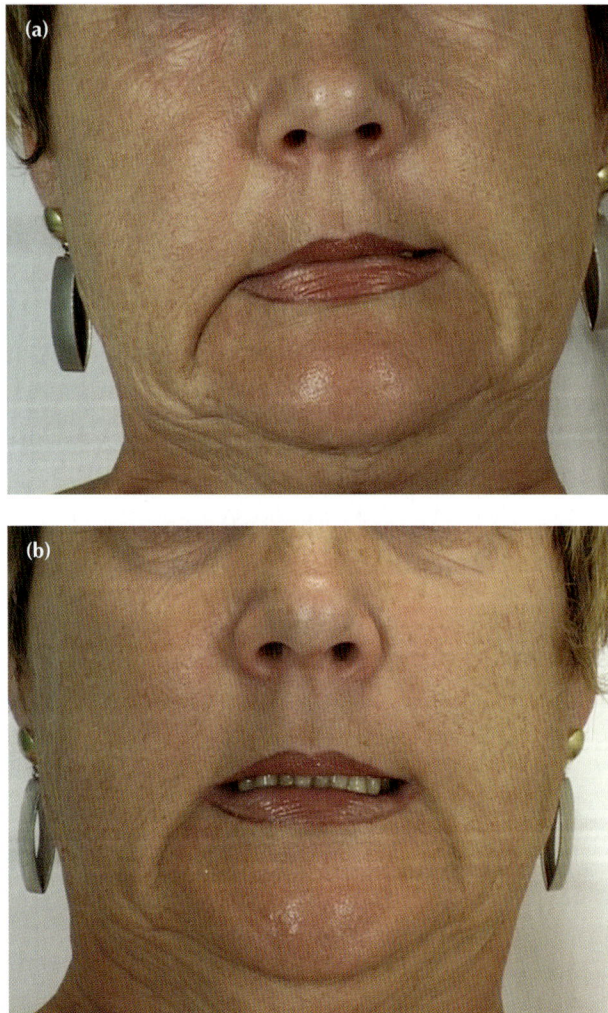

Figure 18.6   Marionette lines (a) before and (b) 1 week after treatment with 2 × 10 U Dysport per site.

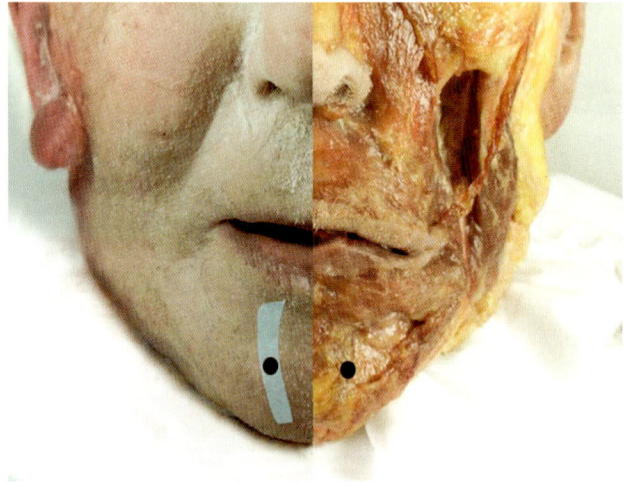

Figure 18.7   Injection points for the mentalis muscle.

effect. Treatment with BTX-A might enable the levator labii superioris to lift the corners of the mouth (Figures 18.5 and 18.6) (Table 18.5).

Note that a high dosage or an injection that is too close to the corner of the mouth might lead to asymmetry as well as difficulties while eating and drinking.

'Cobblestone chin'

The 'cobblestone chin' or dimpled chin develops when the mentalis muscle, which inserts with several fibers in the dermis of this area, is contracted. Contraction can be achieved by pulling the lower lip down. BTX-A leads to a smoothing of the area of the chin (Figures 18.7 and 18.8).

BTX-A can be injected in either a single point or in two lateral points, approximately 0.5–1 cm above the chin. No injection points should come closer than 1 cm to the lower lip (Table 18.6).

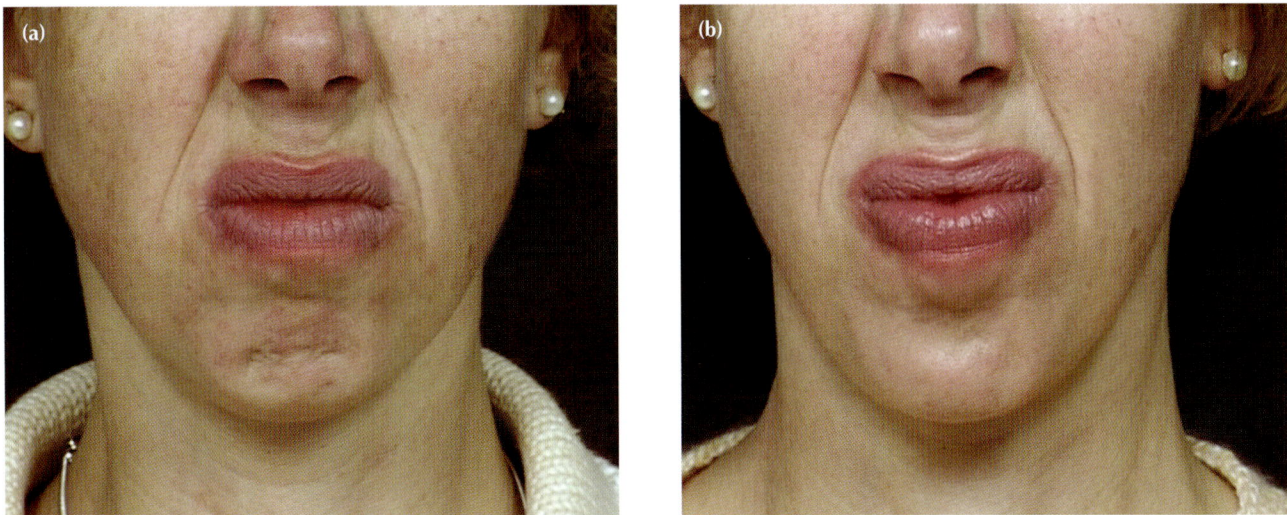

Figure 18.8   Marionette lines and cobblestone chin (a) before and (b) 2 weeks after 2 × 10 and 1 × 10 U Dysport.

Table 18.6   'Cobblestone chin'
• One or two injection points, approximately 0.5–1 cm above the chin
• Symmetrical distribution of the injection points
• Dosage Dysport: maximum 5–10 U per injection point
• Dosage BOTOX: maximum 1–3 U per injection point[4]

Summary

The mid- and lower face are areas for the advanced user and also the BTX-A experienced patient. With a careful approach, very nice results will lead to high satisfaction for the patient as well as the treating physician.

References

1. Heckmann M, Rzany B, eds. Botulinumtoxin in der Dermatologie. Grundlagen und Praktische Anwendung, 1st edn. Munich: Urban und Vogel, 2002.
2. Rzany B. Bericht zum 1. Expertentreffen zur Anwendung von Botulinumtoxin A in der Ästhetischen Dermatologie. Kosmet Med 2003; 24: 2–8.
3. Rzany B, Fratilla A, Heckmann M. 2. Expertentreffen zur Anwendung von Botulinumtoxin A in der Ästhetischen Dermatologie. Kosmet Med 2005; 26: 1–8.
4. Carruthers J, Fagien S, Matarasso SL; BOTOX Consensus Group. Consensus recommendations on the use of botulinum toxin type a in facial aesthetics. Plast Reconstr Surg 2004; 114 (6 Suppl): 1S–22S.
5. Sampaio C, Costa J, Ferreira JJ. Clinical comparability of marketed formulations of botulinum toxin. Mov Disord 2004; 19 (Suppl 8): S129–36.

19 The neck area

Daniel Labbé and Julien Nicolas

After describing the embryology and anatomy of the platysma and the various subcutaneous sliding systems, we will discuss the surgical technique of platysma suspension and platysmapexy during the neck lift. We will then detail the use of botulinum toxin injection in this indication in the preoperative procedure.

Embryology

The muscles of the face and the platysma are derived from the same branchial arch (second arch, hyoid) during embryonic development. They are both innervated by the facial nerve (VII) and are virtually separated from the major cervical structures, which have a different embryologic origin.

The platysma of the fetus between 9 and 10 weeks of gestation primarily consists of myoblasts.[1] These myoblasts are surrounded by mesenchymal cells that are regarded as precursors of the platysma fascia. Between the sternocleidomastoid muscle and platysma, an additional layer of mesenchyma is found. This layer is not connected to the platysma. In the fetus between 13 and 14 weeks of gestation, the platysma is located directly under the skin. The sternocleidomastoid muscle is located under the platysma and is surrounded by the superficial layer of the cervical fascia. The fasciae of the platysma and the sternocleidomastoid muscle slide on a small layer of loose connective tissue called the superficial cervical fascia.

Anatomy

Superficial musculoaponeurotic system

The superficial fascia which limits the deep surface of the dermis is uniform and homogeneous on all surfaces of the body. Mitz and Peyronie[2] described the superficial musculoaponeurotic system (SMAS), consisting of elements located in the same plane and forming a continuous structure. The SMAS adheres behind the cartilage of the ear and the tragus, covering to a greater or lesser degree the parotid space, including the parotid aponeurosis, and continues upwards with muscle fibers of the orbicularis oculi and occipitofrontalis and below with the platysma.

The platysma

The platysma is a broad, thin quadrilateral that covers the anterolateral area of the neck and lower part of the face. It extends from the thorax to the mandible and the cheek. This muscle adheres at the bottom, along the pectoral girdle, with the deep surface of the skin which covers the acromion, the deltoid, and the infraclavicular area. The fleshy tracts,[3] initially distinct and separate from each other, converge above and within and gather in a continuous muscular sheet. The platysma, in two separate sections at the bottom, approaches gradually and obliquely upwards to form a single sheet, the anterior fibers very often intersecting on the centerline, in the vicinity of the chin. Higher insertions of the platysma are at the same time osseous and cutaneous:

- the anterior fibers are fixed after intersection to the skin of the chin
- the medial fibers adhere to the lower edge of the mandible and the anterior part of the oblique line while intersecting with that of the depressor of the angulus oris and the depressor of the labii inferioris
- some of the posterior or lateral fibers continue with the lateral fibers of the depressor of the angulus oris, and others go directly to the labial commissure and the skin of the cheek.

Loré's fascia

The temporoparotid fascia or Loré's fascia was described in 1973 (Figure 19.1). It is well known to surgeons who approach the trunk of the facial nerve, in particular at the time of parotid surgery. It is a fascia located between the tympanomastoid fissure and the parotid gland, and is one of the fixing points of the parotid gland. It is located immediately in front of the intertragal incisure. This fascia is very resistant, and it is used as an anchorage point in platysma suspension.

The various subcutaneous sliding system

Gimberteau[4] who work on subcutaneous sliding system in relation to others, with abandonment of the theory of lamellate spaces in favor of a system of which the func-

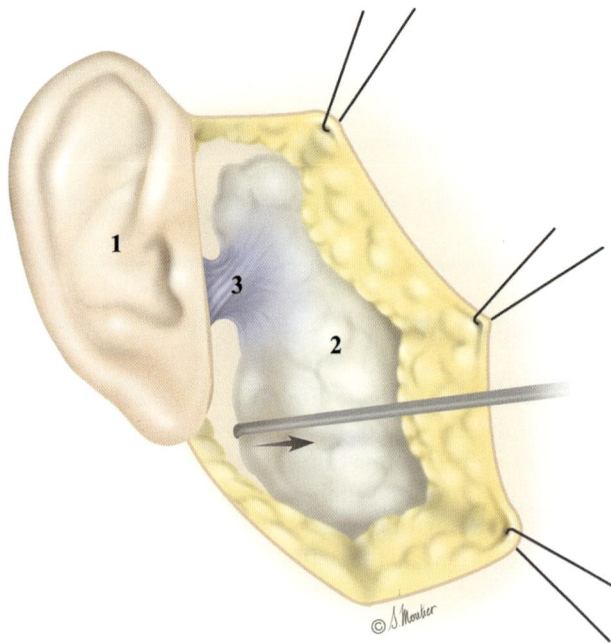

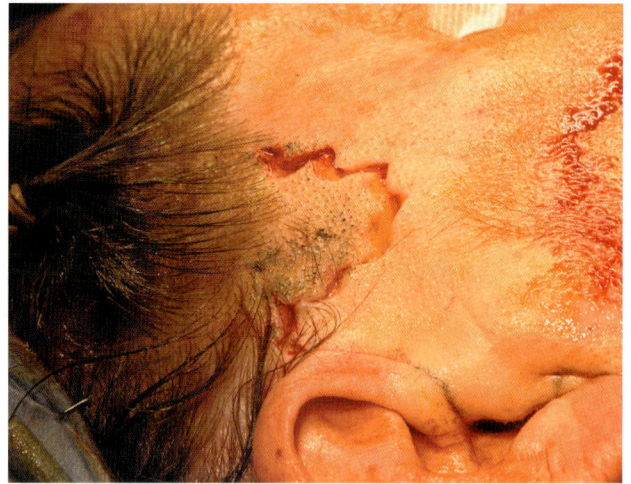

Figure 19.2   Temporal incision by Guyuron.

Figure 19.1   Anatomy of the temporoparotid fascia (Loré's fascia). 1: Outer ear; 2: parotid; 3: Loré's fascia. Reproduced with permission from reference 5.

tional unit is the microvacuole. Longitudinal displacement will be significant, and vacuolar organization will be fine and repeated. Aging deforms these structures, and disturbs the good baseline situation of prestress, observed by the separation of the two edges of the wound at the time of a surgical incision.

The structure of the areolar tissue is variable, according to the anatomic location and the capacity for displacement of the tissue. This explains why platysma suspension allows variable repositioning according to anatomic area with respect to the sliding surface and deep connections.

Surgical technique

We will detail here only the cervical technique by platysmasuspension and platysmapexy.

The intervention is carried out under general anesthesia, with orotracheal intubation. The probe must be fixed in a median position without deforming the labial commissures or the labii inferioris. The fixing of the probe must release the cervicomental area.

Each hemiface is infiltrated with 100 ml of epinephrine solution (1 mg/l).

The temporal incision is the incision developed by Guyuron et al,[6] and the remainder of the incisions are omega and pre- and retroauricular (Figure 19.2).

After the epinephrine had started to act, the flaps were dissected. This always involves subcutaneous level, preserving a few millimeters of fat, but often dividing the superficial vascular anastomotic network. First generation procedures involved a traditional subcutaneous facelift (Figure 19.3). Some modifications have been made, with separation more limited on the anterior neck but wider in bottom in the area of the sternocleidomastoid than in more usual techniques.

This dissection remains essential for the scratch effect of the skin, which will then readhere in a good position postoperatively and will secure the result. Then, the free edge of the platysma is located. It is located approximately 3 cm below the mandibular border, in the angle formed by the mandibular border and the anterior edge of the sternocleidomastoid muscle.

A key point is established between the platysma (at the higher level described) and Loré's fascia or temporoparotid fascia with non-resorbable mononylon 2/0 suture (Figure 19.4). Determination of the key point on the platysma is obtained using a traction hook. The anterior triangle of the neck is thus clearly redrawn by redefining the mandibular border and the sternocleidomastoid (Figure 19.5). Traction is carried out to reposition the platysma approximately 3–4 cm higher and thus to redefine the anterior edge of the sternocleidomastoid and the mandibular border, and to raise and support the submandibular gland. This point comprises a purse string suture on the platysma and a simple suture on Loré's fascia. The purse string suture makes it possible to regulate the platysma suspension and to carry out platysmapexy with Loré's fascia. A posterior neutral reinforcement and expansion

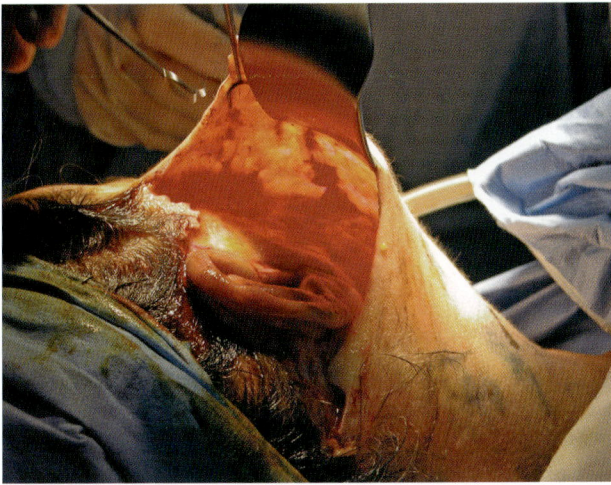

Figure 19.3   Dissections of the flap.

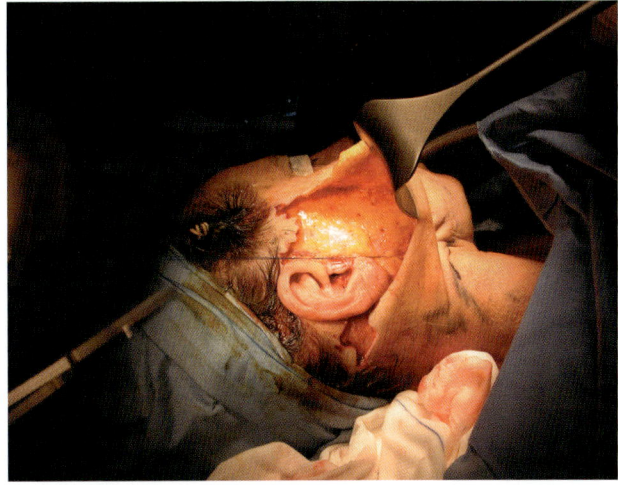

Figure 19.4   Key point between the platysma and Loré's fascia.

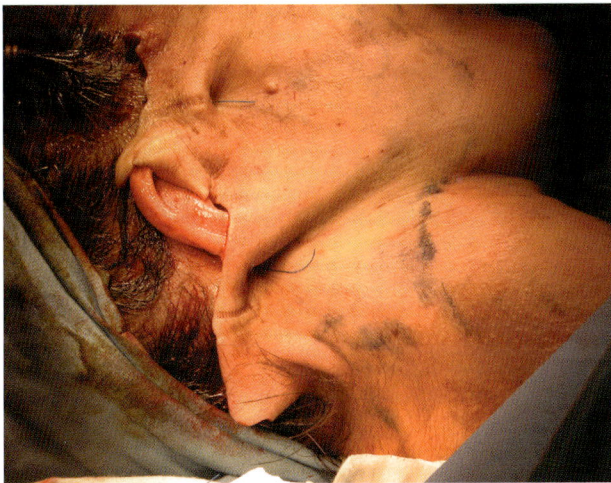

Figure 19.5   Redefinition of anterior triangle of the neck.

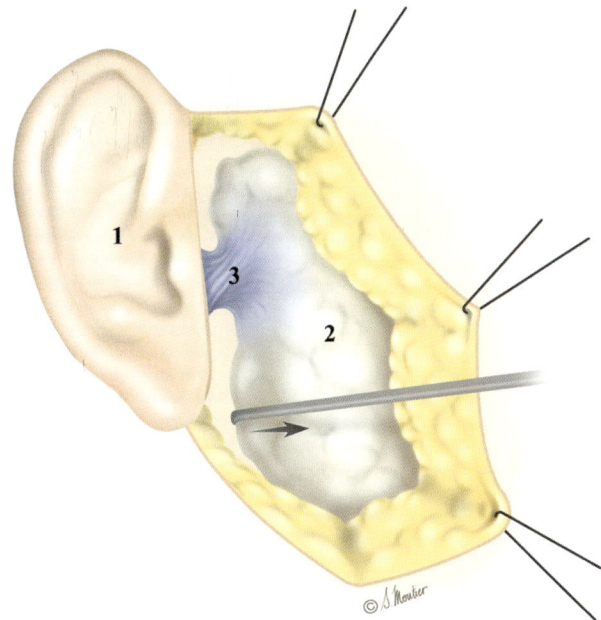

Figure 19.6   Patient n°1, profile views before (left) and after (right) neck lift by platysmasuspension.

suture is placed between the posterior edge of the platysma and the aponeurosis of the sternocleidomastoid muscle. Increasingly used in facial SMAS procedures is a 'plicature' or flap of SMAS which will ensure stability of the assembly. We use a 'plicature' of the facial SMAS according to Tonnard and Verpaele et al,[7] associated with oversewing between the SMAS and the parotid aponeurosis (according to Fogli et al[8]) in con-tinuity with the platysma suspension.

Closure is carried out of aspiration drains.

As with conventional techniques, this technique can also be associated with other procedures, according to the indication: submental liposuction and treatment or resection of medial platysma bands.

The criteria of success of a cervical facelift were defined by Ellenbogen and Carlin.[9] We have allotted a score for each criterion in order to obtain a mark out of 10 (Figures 19.6 and 19.7). These criteria are:

- distinct inferior mandibular border (4 points)
- subhyoid depression (1 point)
- visible thyroid cartilage bulge (1 point)
- visible anterior sternocleidomastoid border (2 points)
- cervicomental angle between 105 and 120° (2 points).

The results will thus be considered to be very good if the mark is higher than 8, good if it is equal to 7, and poor if below 7.

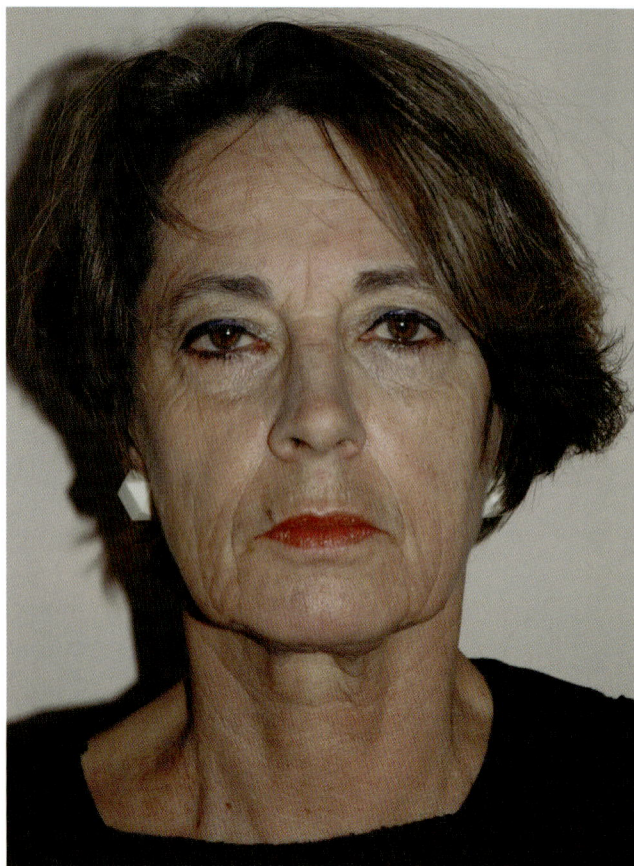

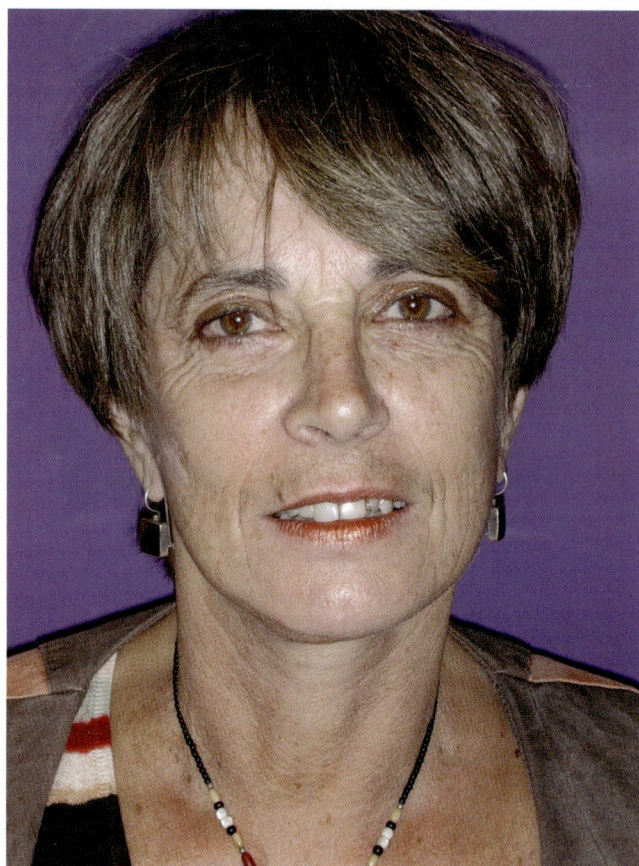

Figure 19.7   Patient n°1, frontal views before (left) and after (right) neck lift by platysmasuspension.

Advantages of preoperative botulinum toxin injection in cervical facelift with platysma suspension

We have used botulinum toxin (BOTOX®) preoperatively within the framework of neck lift by platysma suspension and platysmapexy. We will detail here the various sites of injection, volume injected, time between the intervention and the injections, and the advantages of botulinum toxin use in this indication.

Method of injection

We carry out botulinum toxin injections (BOTOX) preoperatively, between 5 and 50 days before the surgical procedure. We perform the injections in the platysma bands (anterior, median, and posterior) just under the skin. These are located while asking the patient to accomplish a contraction of the platysma (Babinski's method) (Figure 19.8). We inject into three or four sites on each platysma band. Each site receives 4 U of botulinum toxin (Figure 19.9).

Advantages of injection

The botulinum toxin has been regarded for a long time as the most powerful of poisons. Currently it is usually

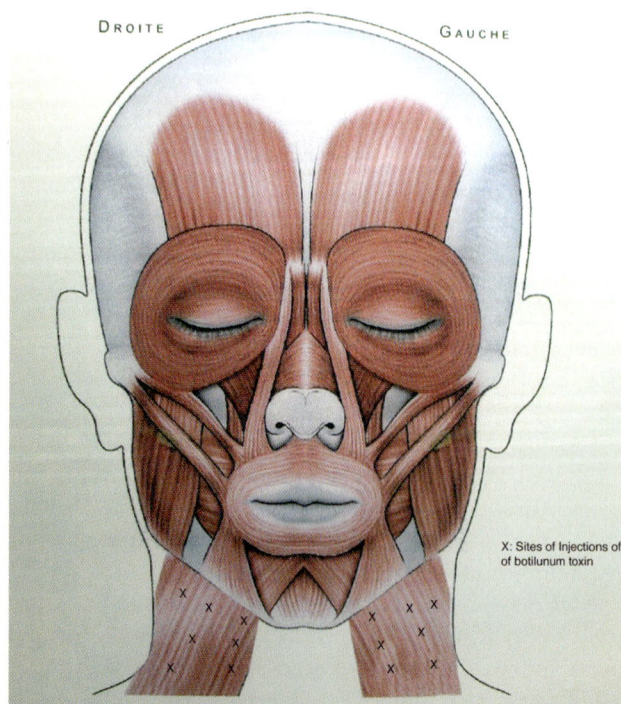

Figure 19.8   Babinski methods for determinate platysmal bands.

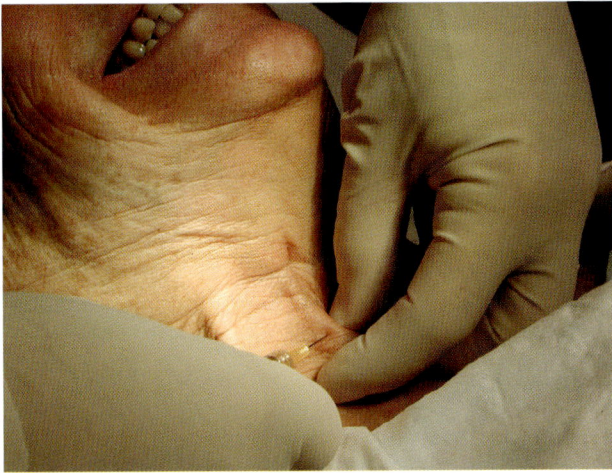

Figure 19.9 Methods of injections of botulinum toxin.

used in cosmetic surgery for the treatment of expression wrinkles, in particular of the upper third of the face. It achieves a virtual biological section by chemical denervation. Its action is effective, flexible according to volume injected, and durable with time.[10] We have used it preoperatively in 30 patients. The goal of these injections is to attain preoperative paralysis of the platysma.

There is a risk of tearing of the platysma at locations of non-resorbable sutures when it contracts. For this reason, botulinum toxin is used preoperatively in order to decrease platysma contraction at the level of the platysma cords. The platysma is thus still which allows better cicatrization. The goal of these botulinum toxin injections is inactivity of the muscle, which simplifies the operational procedure by facilitating repositioning of the platysma without the need for curarization. In particular, however, the inactivity of the platysma in the subsequent procedure avoids the risk of tearing at

the key point, especially in elderly patients with a thinner, more atrophied platysma at that point and in patients with significant hyperactivity and spasm of the platysma (permanently thick anterior platysma cords). The advantages of botulinum toxin in spasm of the platysma among patients having recovered from facial paralysis are well known. However, hence arises the difficulty of renewal of the injections remotely to prevent reappearance of the spasm.

References

1. Gardetto A, Dabering J, Rainer C et al. Does a superficial musculoaponeurotic system exist in the face and neck? Anatomical study by the tissue plastination technique. Plast Reconstr Surg 2003; 111: 664–72.
2. Mitz V, Peyronie M. The superficial musculo-aponeurotic system (SMAS) in the parotid and cheek area. Plast Reconstr Surg 1976; 58: 80–8.
3. Rouvière H, Delmas A. Anatomie Humaine, tome 1: Tête et cou, 15th edn. Paris: Masson, 2002.
4. Guimberteau JC, Sentucq-Rigall J, Panconi B et al. [Introduction to the knowledge of subcutaneous sliding system in humans]. Ann Chir Plast Esthet 2005; 50: 19–34. [in French]
5. Labbé D, Franco RG, Nicolas J. Platysma suspension and platysmapexy during neck lift: anatomical study and analysis of 30 cases. Plast Reconstr Surg 2006; 117: 2001–7.
6. Guyuron B, Watkins F, Totonchi A. Modified temporal incision for facial rhytidectomy: an 18-year experience. Plast Reconstr Surg 2005; 115: 609–16; discussion 617–19.
7. Tonnard P, Verpaele A, Monstrey S et al. Minimal access cranial suspension lift: a modified S-lift. Plast Reconstr Surg 2002; 109: 2074–86.
8. Fogli A, Jones BM, Hinderer U et al. [Face lifts complications]. Ann Chir Plast Esthet 2004; 49: 562–3. [in French]
9. Ellenbogen R, Carlin JV. Visual criteria for success in restoring youthful neck. Plast Reconstr Surg 2004; 113: 398–403.
10. Ascher B, Rossi B. [Botulinum toxin and wrinkles: few side effects and effective combining procedures with other treatments]. Ann Chir Plast Esthet 2004; 49: 537–52. [in French]

20 The upper trunk: décolleté wrinkles and breast lift

Doris Hexsel and Taciana Dal'Forno

Introduction

In our society, physical appearance has a significant impact on how individuals are perceived by others. Beauty is associated with youth, and consequently wrinkles and folds are perceived as cosmetically disturbing. Physical appearance is intrinsically linked to body image, self-esteem, and confidence. An attractive appearance promotes psychological well-being.[1]

Though the face remains the principal focus for rejuvenation, solutions to problems involving the neck and breast are increasingly requested in dermatologic offices. The application of botulinum toxin (BTX) injections is one of the most frequently used treatments for beauty and rejuvenation. Recently, the use of BTX in extrafacial areas has gained special attention, and its cosmetic use has extended to the trunk.

Most female patients wish to have décolleté wrinkles smoothed and the breasts lifted in order to improve the appearance of this region.

The use of BTX injections into the pectoral muscles was first published in 2000[2,3] for pectoral spasm and 1 year later[2,4] for a subpectoral implant in order to decrease contraction of the pectoral muscles. The first publication referring to its use for décolleté wrinkles was in 2001.[5] No studies have been published that suggest BTX can be used to bring about breast lift.

Evidence-based cosmetic medicine

At present, there are no controlled studies for the use of botulinum toxin for décolleté wrinkles or breast lift.[6]

Décolleté wrinkles

Cutaneous wrinkles in the décolleté area can be didactically classified as dynamic wrinkles, static wrinkles, or combined or mixed wrinkles (Figure 20.1). Dynamic wrinkles are only visible during muscular contraction, whereas static wrinkles are present even when the musculature is at rest. Wrinkles in these areas result from several factors: photoaging is the main cause, but intrinsic aging, and muscular contraction of the pectoralis major and lower part of the platysmal bands as well as lateral decubitus also play a part.[2] BTX can

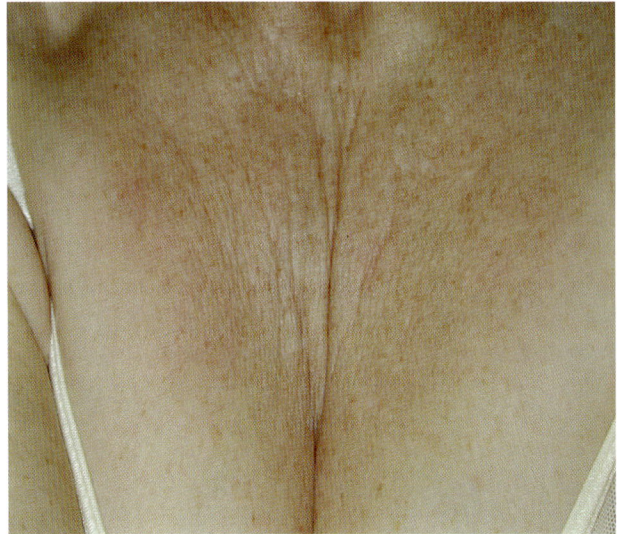

Figure 20.1 Mixed type wrinkles at the décolleté area.

improve these wrinkles by relaxing the underlying muscles, but no action is expected related to other factors, mentioned below (Figure 20.2).

Wrinkles in the upper and mid-décolleté begin to appear after the 30s. They increase with age and extend to the lower décolleté. Vertical V-shaped folds and a horizontal fold relief may be present later in life, after the 50s, and are perceived as being cosmetically disturbing. These wrinkles occur from the submental region to the lower décolleté region, causing prominent vertical bands, an undesirable effect especially for females.[5] Patients with obvious platysmal bands, good cervical skin elasticity, and minimal fat descent are suboptimal candidates for surgery, and benefit from BTX application.[7,8]

Anatomy

Platysma

The platysma consists of a pair of flat muscles that originate in the subcutaneous tissue of the upper thorax, ascend laterally to the lower face, cross the neck, pass behind the mandible angle, and insert into the cutaneous muscles around the mouth.[2] Each one consists of an upper and lower part, the latter spreading

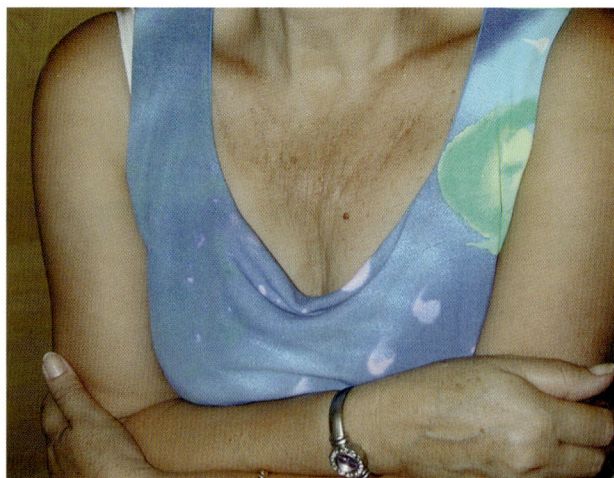

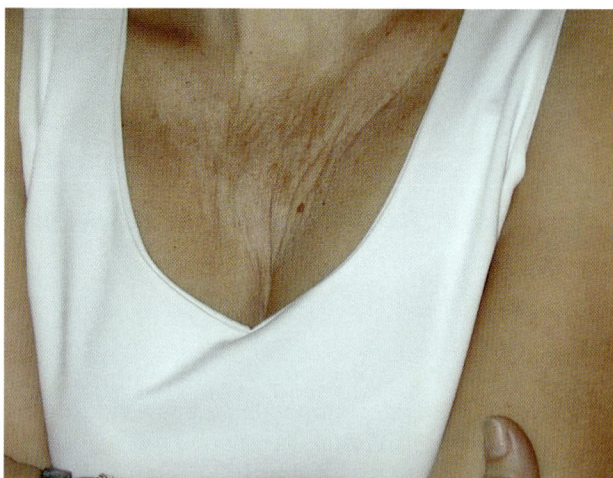

Figure 20.2   Before and after treatment with botulinum toxin (BTX) injections for décolleté dynamic wrinkles.

subcutaneously. It usually inserts in a fanlike fashion onto the second or third rib, but frequently the muscle extends beyond the typical insertion points. 'Platysmal banding' generally runs from the mandible towards the clavicula.[5] However, due to anatomical variants, contraction of the platysma muscle results in horizontal and vertical wrinkle formation not only in the cervical region, but also in large parts of the mid- and lower décolleté.[9]

Anterior thoracic wall

The pectoralis major muscle is a large, thick, fan-shaped muscle that covers the upper part of the thorax. Its lateral border forms the anterior axillary fold and most of the anterior wall of the axilla. The fascial sheath that encloses the pectoralis major muscle is attached at its origin to the clavicle and sternum.[10]

From the surface of the pectoralis major, some superficial fibers arise from the fascia of the clavicular head and insert into the fascia of the deltoid muscle. The pectoral sheet is divided into a superficial and a deep layer. The outer sheet (the pectoralis major) is divided into clavicular, manubrial, sternal, and abdominal portions, all of which may be more or less separable. The clavicular head may extend laterally on the clavicula as far as the deltoid and be fused with it, or its origin may be confined to its sternal end. It is occasionally divided into two distinct parts; it may also decussate across the midline.[11] It is innervated by the lateral and medial pectoral nerves (fibers derived from C5 and C6). Anteriorly, the pectoralis major muscle is related to the skin, superficial fascia, platysma, anterior and medial supraclavicular nerves, mammary glands, and deep fascia.[2]

When both parts of the muscle act together, the pectoralis major adducts and medially rotates the humerus at the shoulder joint. Acting alone, the clavicular head helps to flex the humerus, and from this position the sternocostal head extends the humerus.[10]

The pectoralis minor muscle is situated more deeply than the pectoralis major muscle. It originates on the external surface of the third, fourth, and fifth ribs and inserts into the coracoid process of the scapula. It is innervated by the medial pectoral nerve,[12] which originates from the medial cord of the brachial plexus.[13] The muscle plays a role in the rotary movements of the shoulder.[14]

Botulinum toxin treatment

Although, in fair skinned patients, most upper trunk wrinkles are due to photoaging, décolleté wrinkles can be improved by injections of botulinum toxin either in a V-shape along the upper, mid-, and lower décolleté or in a half-moon shape, parallel to the intercostal spaces at the most caudally visible and prominent contraction activity, depending on the topography of the muscles and wrinkles.[6,9]

Observation of the movement of the platysma has shown differing muscle extensions, with variants extending to above the clavicle and the second intercostal space.[5] In order to determine the injection points, patients are asked to contract their platysma muscle to identify subcutaneous muscle fibers running over the third intercostal space and over the presternal area.[9] A dosage of 5 U of BOTOX® or 10 U of Dysport® can be used at each injection site.[6]

Becker-Wegerich et al studied five patients presenting décolleté wrinkles and treated using injections along two lines of points. One line was parallel to the intercostal spaces at the most caudally visible and prominent contraction activity. The second line started presternally and formed a V-shaped figure. Into each point, 2 cm apart, approximately 15 U of Dysport diluted in 0.15 ml of saline was injected subcutaneously, using a 30G needle.[9]

The treatment of the platysmal bands should be extended beneath the neck in order to include the

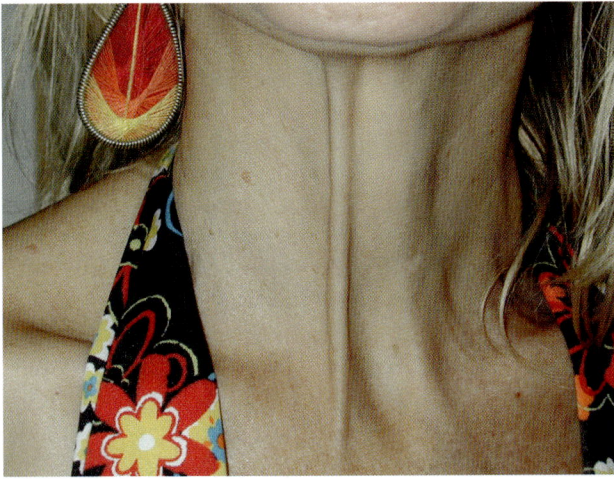

Figure 20.3 Typical platysma bands.

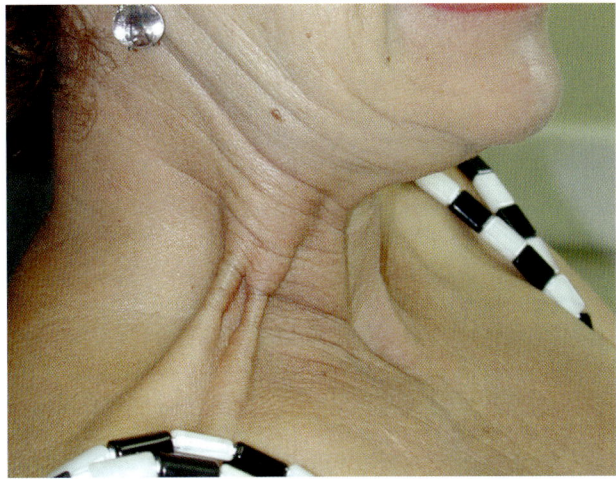

oversized parts of the platysma muscle.[9] These authors reported highly satisfactory results in all five treated patients.

Results and adverse effects

BTX is a successful treatment for signs of aging in the neck, as it can smooth wrinkles caused by platysma bands. Patients with unrealistic expectations and psychiatric disorders represent poor candidates for all indications of BTX injection, and in such cases it should be used with caution.[6]

The best results are obtained in patients with hypertrophic platysma bands (Figure 20.3) and mild attenuation of the fascial attachments.[7]

A significant improvement of the décolleté region treated with BTX can be obtained in 2 weeks,[9] which is longer than for the face.

The side-effects described are pain at the injection site,[9] reduction of muscle tension in abduction, and medial rotation of superior limbs (hugging), because of blockage of the sternal fibers of the pectoralis major muscle.[2] Doses in excess of those recommended above, or application into deeper layers, may lead to difficulty in taking deep breaths, because of damage to the intercostal muscles.[2]

Breast lift

The human mammary is distinct from those of all other mammals. It has a protuberant conical shape, mainly in young women and those who have never given birth.[12]

Physiological substitution of mammary gland fat occurs with aging. Obesity may lead to an increase in the volume of the mammary glands, altering their shape. With the passing of time, they become more flaccid and pendulant and less pert.[12]

The desire to lift sagging breasts is common in young and mature women, and currently can only be satisfied with surgery. Mammoplasty and breast enlargement are very common surgical procedures throughout the world.[15] The idea of achieving breast lifting through the use of BTX applications would be very attractive, if effective.

Anatomy

Breasts are the most prominent superficial structures of the anterior thoracic wall, especially in women. They are situated on the anterior surface of the thorax, overlying the pectoral muscles (pectoralis major and serratus anterior). They often extend toward the axillae, forming axillary tails. The amount of fat surrounding the glandular tissue determines the size of the breasts.[16]

The mammary glands lie in the superficial fascia, anterior to the thorax, and posteriorly they are separated from the pectoral muscles by the deep fascia. Between the breast and deep fascia, there is an area of loose connective tissue that contains little fat (retromammary space), allowing the breast to move freely on the deep fascia covering the pectoralis major muscle.[16]

The breast is supplied by lateral and anterior cutaneous branches of the second to sixth intercostal nerves.[16]

Botulinum toxin treatment

Kevin Smith was the first physician reporting BTX injections for breast lift in Vancouver (August 2003), during the meeting 'Botox, Fillers and More'. Smith described three points of application corresponding to insertions into the pectoralis minor muscles in the third, fourth, and fifth ribs. He suggested that the injection of 15 U of BOTOX into each point would be effective for breast lift in cases of small breast size or asymmetries. Two years later, in February 2005, he admitted that the technique did not propitiate breast lift but it could correct the posture.[17] In the same course, Perez-Atamoros showed satisfactory results from injections of 15 U of BOTOX into three points of the lower part of the pectoralis major.[17]

The present authors performed a pilot study using BTX for breast lift in 2004. A breast surgeon was invited to participate in the study, supervising the points to be injected. Following Smith's technique, 15 U of BOTOX were injected into the three points of origin of the pectoralis minor muscles at the third, fourth, and fifth ribs. The study was carried out in six female patients with slight to moderate levels of breast ptosis and one male volunteer, whose control was not carried out. For standardization of photographs and evaluation of the results in relation to the position of the breasts, the patients were photographed in an orthostatic position, at rest, with the arms relaxed, and holding one hand in the other in front of the thorax. All patients were photographed in the same position, in front of a diagrammed panel Fotostation®, with and without the height measurement bar from the same scale positioned in front of the mammary glands, as shown in Figure 20.4.

Results and adverse effects

Special care should be taken with the great number of patients who have breast implants, because the prosthesis is usually made of liquid silicone enveloped in a capsule of the same material. Injections into the lower part of the pectoralis major muscle can perforate breast implants and cause leakage of the silicone.

None of the treated patients perceived any breast lift effect (Figure 20.5). Some adverse effects were reported by patients of the pilot study conducted by the present authors. The most serious adverse effects reported

were worsening of the mammary ptosis (Figure 20.5) and loss of strength in the hands, causing difficulty in performing some tasks such as washing clothes and shaking hands firmly.

The successful results reported in meetings were not reproduced in the small sample treated by the present authors (Figure 20.5). Besides worsening the ptosis in two patients, we noticed undesirable side-effects, such as difficulties in adduction movements of the upper limbs.

Perez-Atamoros also reported side-effects after BTX injections for breast lift. He said that some patients felt persistent local pain lasting 1 week after application.[17]

Conclusions

BTX injections are very effective in many established indications. Patients who are more aware of esthetic concerns and outer appearance are those that are more likely to be satisfied with treatment.[18]

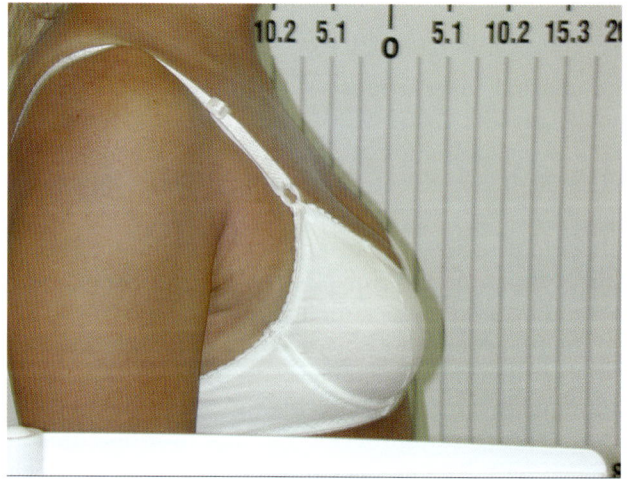

Figure 20.4   Setting of photographs taken of patients injected for breast lift.

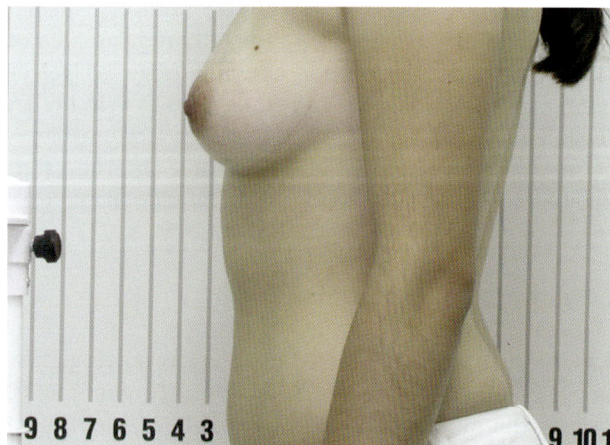

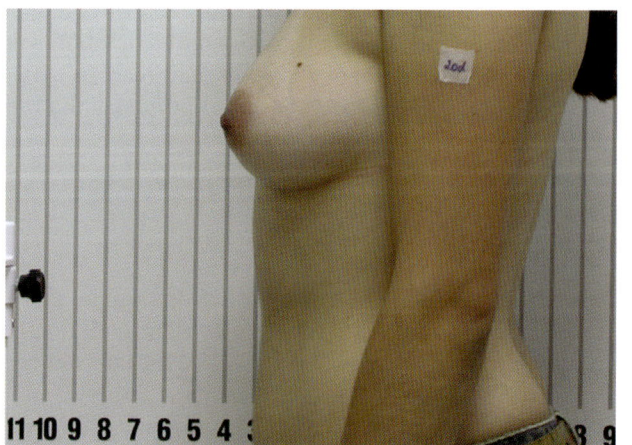

Figure 20.5   Before and after BTX injections for breast lift.

The clinical use of botulinum toxin requires a thorough understanding of the anatomy of the areas to be treated.

Botulinum toxin seems to be a safe and effective method in the temporary management of décolleté wrinkles for selected patients. It should be considered as a new adjuvant treatment in cosmetic décolleté rejuvenation. It can be used alone or in combination with other surgical techniques, such as laser, peels, and surgical lift among others, to achieve better results.

For breast lift, the present authors state that studies with statistically significant numbers of patients are required, so that the published results can be reproduced and checked through adequate methodology.

References

1. Finn JC, Cox SE, Earl ML. Social implications of hyperfunctional facial lines. Dermatol Surg 2003; 29: 450–5.
2. Isaac C, Gimenez R, Ruiz RO. Décolléte wrinkles. In: Hexsel D, Almeida AT, eds. Cosmetic Use of Botulinum Toxin, 1st edn. Porto Alegre, Brazil: AGE, 2002: 178–83.
3. Wong L. Pectoralis major myospasm resulting from a subpectoral implant. Plast Reconstr Surg 2000; 105: 1571–2.
4. Richards A, Ritz M, Donahoe S, Southwick G. Botox for contraction of pectoral muscles. Plast Reconstr Surg 2001; 108: 270–1.
5. Becker-Wegerich P, Rauch L, Ruzicka T. Botulinum toxin A in the therapy of mimic facial lines. Clin Exp Dermatol 2001; 26: 619–30.
6. Wollina U, Konrad H. Managing adverse events associated with botulinum toxin type A: a focus on cosmetic procedures. Am J Clin Dermatol 2005; 6: 141–50.
7. Fagien S. Botulinum A exotoxin for the management of platysma bands. Plast Reconstr Surg 1999; 103: 653–5.
8. Carruthers J, Carruthers A. Aesthetic botulinum A toxin in the mid and lower face and neck. Dermatol Surg 2003; 29: 468–76.
9. Becker-Wegerich PM, Rauch L, Ruzicka T. Botulinum toxin A: successful décolleté rejuvenation. Dermatol Surg 2002; 28: 168–71.
10. Moore KL. The upper limb. In: Moore KL, ed. Clinically Oriented Anatomy, 3rd edn. Baltimore: Williams & Wilkins, 1992: 507–10.
11. Bergmann R, Afifi A, Miyauchi R. Illustrated encyclopedia of human anatomic variation. Part 1: muscular system. 2005. Available online at http://www.vh.org/Providers/Textbooks/AnatomicVariants/Images/0236.html (accessed 27th September, 2005).
12. Biazús JV, Zucatto AE. Anatomia cirúrgica da mama. In: Biazús JV, Zucatto AE, eds. Cirurgia da Mama, 1st edn. Porto Alegre, Brazil: Artes Médicas Sul, 2005: 11–36.
13. Osborne MP. Anatomy of the breast. In: Harris JR, Lippman ME, Morrow M, Osborne K, eds. Diseases of the Breast, 2nd edn. Philadelphia: Lippincott Williams & Wilkins, 2000: 1–17.
14. Menke CH, Biazús JV, Xavier NL et al. Noções de embriologia, anatomia e fisiologia. In: Menke CH, Biazús JV, Xavier NL et al, eds. Rotinas em Mastologia, 1st edn. Porto Alegre, Brazil: Artes Médicas Sul, 2000: 21–7.
15. Freire M, Neto MS, Garcia EB, Quaresma MR, Ferreira LM. Quality of life after reduction mammaplasty. Scand J Plast Reconstr Surg Hand Surg 2004; 38: 335–9.
16. Moore KL. The thorax. In: Moore KL, ed. Clinically Oriented Anatomy, 3rd edn. Baltimore: Williams & Wilkins, 1992: 45–7.
17. Atamoros FP, Smith KC. Botulinum toxin: facial cosmetic use (Course 101). Presented at American Academy of Dermatology 62nd Annual Meeting, New Orleans, LA, 6–11 February, 2005.
18. Sommer B, Zschocke I, Bergfeld D et al. Satisfaction of patients after treatment with botulinum toxin for dynamic facial lines. Dermatol Surg 2003; 29: 456–60.

21 Masseteric muscle hypertrophy and leg treatments

Kim Nam-Ho, Chung Jee-Hyeok, Park Rho-Hyuk, and Park Jong-Beum

The role of the masseter muscle in facial contour

In Asian and Western countries, the desire for beauty has been regarded as one of the basic instincts of mankind. In days gone by, with no development in transportation and communication, esthetic standards differed depending on regional, racial, and national groups. However, in modern times, a universal standard for beauty is being established due to globalization by the remarkable developments in transportation and communication. This phenomenon might be explained by the fact that the esthetic standard of both Western and Asian countries has merged, or it might be accounted for by the fact that the Westerners have an aspiration for Asian beauty, while Easterners have a desire for Western beauty.

Since Northeastern Asians, including Koreans, belong ethnically to the Mongolian race, they tend congenitally to have a well-developed mandible compared to Westerners. The well-developed mandible makes the face look more quadrangular. Whether it is congenital or acquired, a developed masseter muscle makes the face look wider. This is bad for women esthetically, because a square face gives a masculine image. From the view of an esthetic standard, it is more desirable for the bigonial distance (width of lower face) to be narrower than the bizygomatic distance (width of mid-face). The classical standard bigonial to bizygomatic ratio was 9:10, but a narrower bigonial distance has become preferred in recent years (Figure 21.1).

The size of the mandible, the volume of muscle that surrounds the mandible, and the subcutaneous fat tissues determine the width of the lower third of the face. In a case of overdeveloped mandible, it can be corrected by bone resection, and excessive fat tissues can be removed by liposuction. However, if the main factor is masseter hypertrophy, a treatment for the masseter muscle itself is essentially needed.

In the historical background of treatment for masseteric hypertrophy and square-angled jaw, in 1880 Legg first described benign masseteric hypertrophy as a condition characterized by the enlargement of the masseter muscle.[1] Since then, conservative treatments, including systemic medications with stabilizers or sedatives and reconfirmation, have been used to treat benign masseteric hypertrophy. Gurney, in 1947, performed masseteric resection through an extraoral incision.[2] The operation resected 75% of the total masseter muscle and did not cause loss of the masticatory capacity. In 1951, Converse used the intraoral route to resect the masseteric muscle and the bone together (unpublished work). In 1989, Whitaker presented a method to reduce the width of the lower facial portion by resection of the mandible cortical layer and the masseteric muscle.[4] Baek et al found out that the masseteric muscle volume was reduced over time as the muscle tone deteriorated, even though only the mandible was resected.[5–7] Experiments in rabbits proved that the unused masseteric muscle shows akinetic atrophy after ostectomy of the mandible. There is also a viewpoint that masseter atrophy occurs after resection of the mandibular angle around the masseter insertion, because this reduces the tone of the masseter muscle. According to these viewpoints, surgical treatments for a square-angled mandible have been frequently applied even in cases of muscular hypertrophy. Muscle resection could be an alternative; however, direct resection of the masseter muscle can result in considerable bleeding or facial nerve injury. Moreover, it is technically impossible to create even contour lines using exact resection of a definite muscle volume. In addition, scar tissues or contracture that remains in the muscle after muscle resection can lead to trismus when the patient opens his mouth. Furthermore, mandible resections for masseter atrophy have sometimes resulted in unexpected outcomes owing to a structural change in the mandible.

Smyth, in 1994, reported that the masseter muscle was reduced by using the application of botulinum toxin A (Dysport®) in seven cases of masseter hypertrophy.[9] This clinical experiment was carried out for the purpose of confirming the effect of botulinum toxin A injection on masseter hypertrophy as well as determining the influence on pain. As a result, as well as a reduction in volume of the masseter muscle, bruxism and clenching habits were stopped. Botulinum toxin A injection was an innovative event in that

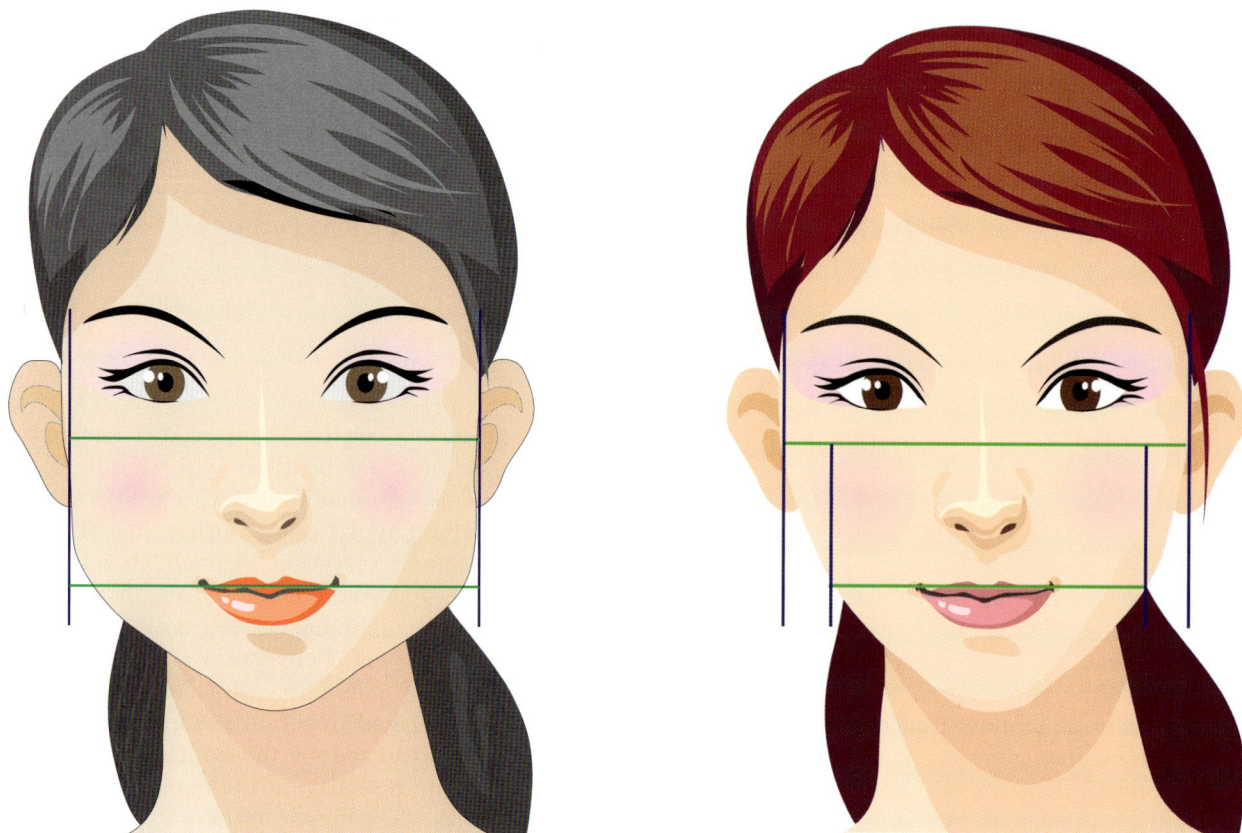

Figure 21.1   Two types of facial shape.

period when surgery was the mainstream of treatment for masseter hypertrophy. In the same year, Moore and Wood presented a case of treating bilateral masseteric hypertrophy accompanying temporomandibular disorder (TMD) by using botulinum toxin A.[10]

In 2001, von Lindern et al also reported that botulinum toxin A was effective in reducing the amount of masseter muscle in patients with masseter hypertrophy.[11] A consequence of the research was the idea that botulinum toxin A not only reduces the volume of the muscle but also lowers the tension of it. These results deserve special attention, because they provided a new approach for the treatment of TMD. Briefly, these results are important in terms of both esthetic remedy and TMD treatment.

In 2005, after a follow-up study of 383 patients with masseter hypertrophy for more than 3 years, we published a proposal for botulinum toxin A treatment emphasizing the objective change in thickness of the masseter, the effective site for application, and the side-effects of the treatment.[12]

Etiology of masseteric hypertrophy

The factors of square-angled mandible and overdeveloped masseter muscle can be divided into genetic and acquired aspects. It is a matter of course that masseter hypertrophy in offspring is inherited from their parents.[13] The hypothesis of hypertrophy, which is regarded as a cause of overdeveloped masseter muscle, has been adopted as an established theory for a long period of time. Actually, a dietary influence of chewing hard and tough food regularly allows the masseter muscle to develop, and induces a square-angled face in the course of a lifetime.[14]

The acquired etiology factors that are most responsible for masseter hypertrophy are believed to be clenching and bruxism. However, merely 20% of people with these habits are aware of this. Attrition of the teeth is easily detected in patients with bruxism. Also, patients with clenching habits complain about stiffness of the jaw due to muscle fatigue. General food, even if rigid and hard, does not affect masseter development in this case, because it is swallowed once it is crushed. On the other hand, chewing gum hardens the muscle very effectively, since this induces long-term muscular exercise without swallowing.

Before treatment, it is not easy to precisely identify the factors associated with the square-angled mandible and to keep track of the causes in a retrospective manner in each patient. The identification of these causes might be meaningless, because the treatment of masseteric hypertrophy is routinely done for esthetic purposes.[15,16] To a certain degree, instruction to restrict the habits of bruxism, clenching, or chewing gum is

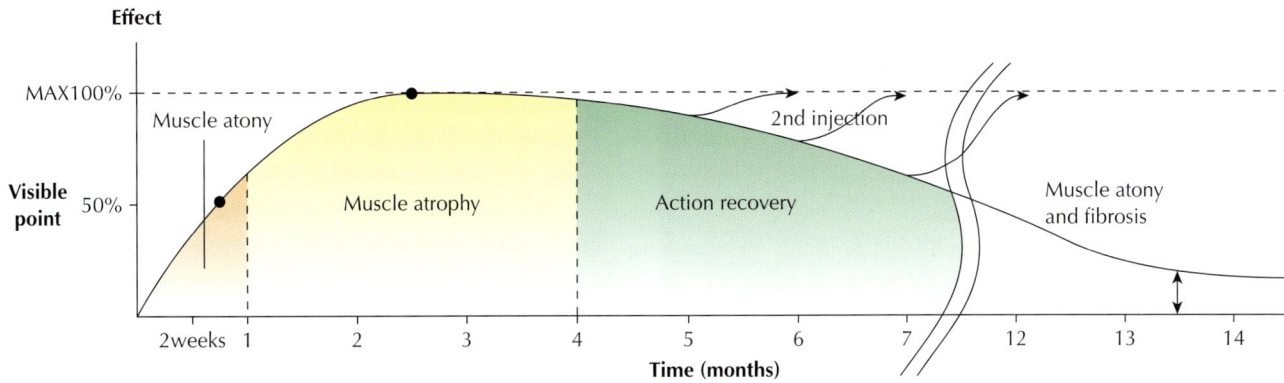

Figure 21.2   Diagram of progress after injection. Following botulinum toxin A treatment, muscles undergo a four-phase change: (1) decrease of muscle tension; (2) decrease of muscle volume; (3) recurrence of muscle tension; (4) recurrence of muscle volume.

subsequently necessary, for the patient with such habits has a high possibility of recurring masseter hypertrophy. At the same time, to judge whether the cause of the angled shape of the face is overdevelopment of the masseter muscle or the mandible bone, or the subcutaneous fat tissues, differential diagnosis is necessary.

Principle of botulinum toxin type A injection in masseter hypertrophy

We have managed a maxillofacial surgery center in Korea for the past 8 years, caring for a number of patients with a square-angled face. Of these patients, more than 50% had excessive hypertrophy of the masseter muscle. Accordingly, it was imperative that we develop a simple and safe treatment for masseter hypertrophy. Finally, this was accomplished by a study based on the aspect of work hypertrophy and disuse atrophy.

As an example, in advanced body-builders, the muscles are developed by work hypertrophy. As a result, they have thick, stiff arms constructed mainly of not bone but muscle. In the same manner, this is what happens in the masseter muscle. Overdeveloped masseter muscles lead to a square-angled frontal face by thickening of the lower chin and broadening of the lower face. Disuse atrophy is clearly observed in a patient who wears a cast to fix an extremity fracture. When the cast is removed after 1 or 2 months, his leg or arm appears slimmer than before. This is a good example of disuse atrophy, but it is impossible to apply a cast to the masseter. We have reached the conclusion that if the contraction could be restricted, disuse atrophy would occur. Such a concept has been proved through clinical examinination.

Botulinum toxin A exerts its effect at the neuromuscular junction by inhibiting the release of acetylcholine, and this in turn causes flaccid paralysis and muscular atrophy. This results primarily in a chemical

denervation. Once paralyzed, muscles do not contract, and lose tension. This leads to the secondary result of loss of muscle volume, and could be interpreted as disuse atrophy, i.e. the muscles are spontaneously reduced in case they are not being used.

The action of botulinum toxin A occurs in three phases: binding, internalization, and neuromuscular blockade. Once botulinum toxin A combines with the cholinergic receptor through the heavy chain of the 50-kDa carboxy-terminal, receptor-mediated endocytosis appears. Following this process, botulinum toxin A transiently inhibits the release of acetylcholine through the proteolysis of synaptosomal associated protein (SNAP-25), and this, in turn, results in flaccid paralysis by causing a chemical denervation.

Following botulinum toxin A treatment, muscles undergo a four-phase change: (1) decrease of muscle tension; (2) decrease of muscle volume; (3) recurrence of muscle tension; and (4) recurrence of muscle volume (Figure 21.2). The progress after treatment can be described as follows. A subtle change in the muscle tone appears in 3–5 days after the first injection. The patient can feel weakness when he clenches his molars. After 1 week, a softening of the muscle is apparent and the masseter feels soft even when clenching the teeth. These changes mean that the muscle is responding to the toxin as expected. A visual change of muscle volume can be seen in 2–4 weeks. The effect of the toxin reaches a maximum level after 10–12 weeks. The action of the muscle is recovered during 12 months after the treatment. The volume of the muscle begins to reappear in 16 weeks. The effect of botulinum toxin A on the muscle is temporary. The muscle function reappears gradually in approximately 3 months after the chemical denervation. This causes dilatation of the nerve endings in the neuromuscular junction, the formation of collateral axonal sprouts, and the creation of a new neuromuscular junction, in respective order. Therefore, botulinum toxin A treatment for masseter hypertrophy actually needs repeated treatment, as reported for treatment of forehead wrinkles or crow's feet.

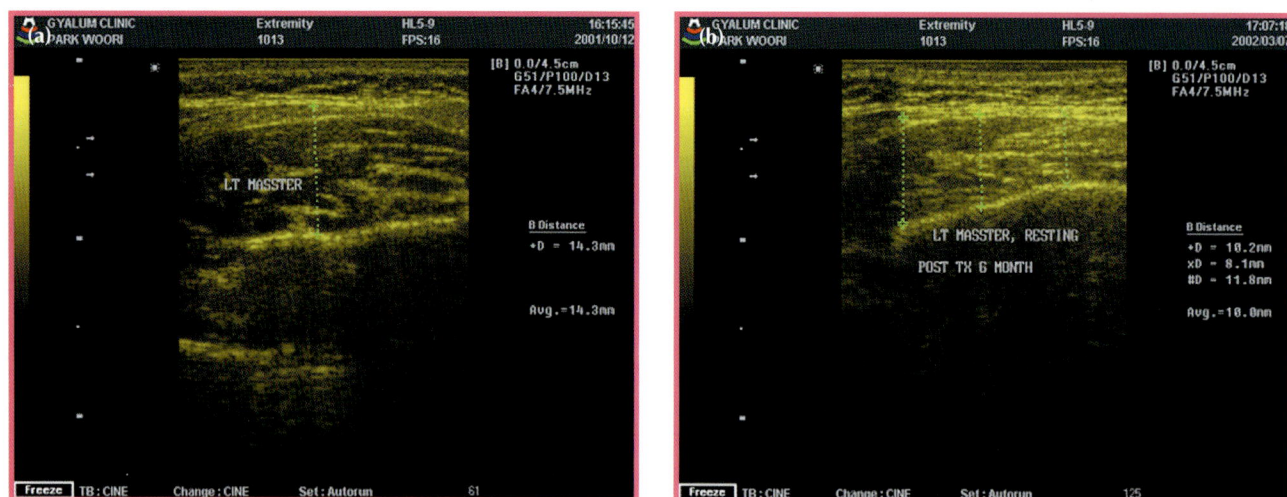

Figure 21.3   Ultrasonography results. (a) Before injection, the size of the masseter muscle is an average of 14.3 mm. (b) After injection, the size is an average of 10.0 mm.

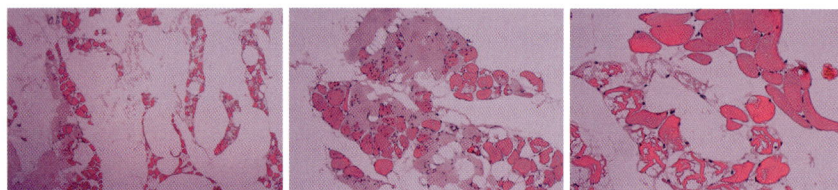

Figure 21.4   Biopsy results: (left) uneven cell size; (middle) myolysis: central and marginal necrosis, centralization of nucleus; (right) pseudocyst and liquefaction.

However, there are a few differences in the botulinum toxin A treatment for wrinkles and masseter hypertrophy. The purpose of treatment of the former is to restrict the contraction of the muscle, and of the latter is to lessen the volume of the muscle. Wrinkle treatment takes effect when the inhibition of muscular contraction takes place, and wrinkles reappear when the recovery of contraction takes place. Because the recovery of muscle volume appears slowly after the recovery of muscle action, the result of masseteric treatment has longer duration of effect than that of wrinkle treatment. From observations of the change in muscle volume measured by ultrasonography, we found that after 6 months, even when the muscular action had almost recovered, the reduction in muscular volume still remained (Figure 21.3). Furthermore, in many cases, the reduced volume remained the same even a year or longer after the injection. In our clinic, some patients had mandible resection after botulinum toxin A treatment. Subsequently, we conducted a histological analysis of the masseter specimen, and in the biopsy results, atrophic changes were observed (Figure 21.4).

Even though the period of effect in masseter muscle treatment is surely longer than that of wrinkle treatment, it does not last permanently. Therefore, to prevent the gradual reappearance of muscle thickness, additional injections are essential.

The masticatory function of the masseter muscle can be reduced after botulinum toxin A treatment. Awareness of the malfunction is reported a month after injection, but this tends to disappear after another month. Presumably this might result from compensation by other masticatory muscles, such as the medial and lateral pterygoid muscle and temporalis muscle.

Appropriate timing and frequency of additional injections

It is clear that a single injection of botulinum toxin A cannot maintain the effect permanently. Therefore, we have striven to identify the optimal frequency and interval for botulinum toxin A treatment. The treatment for facial nerve palsy was the cue. It is reported that, in the conjugation of a dissected facial nerve, an operation carried out within a year has a better outcome than that done after a year. The reason for such a result is irreversible change in the masseter, including fibrosis brought about by the prolonged interception of nerve transaction. In the case of patients with more than a 1-year history of trauma, muscle transfer or cross-face nerve graft with muscle transfer or muscle-free flap is recommended. We expected this phenomenon to happen in the case of chemical denervation as well as traumatic denervation. As a result, we have set as a goal of treatment the maintenance of the denervated state for more than a year.

The course of treatment with botulinum toxin A injection displays the atonic stage to the tone recovery stage

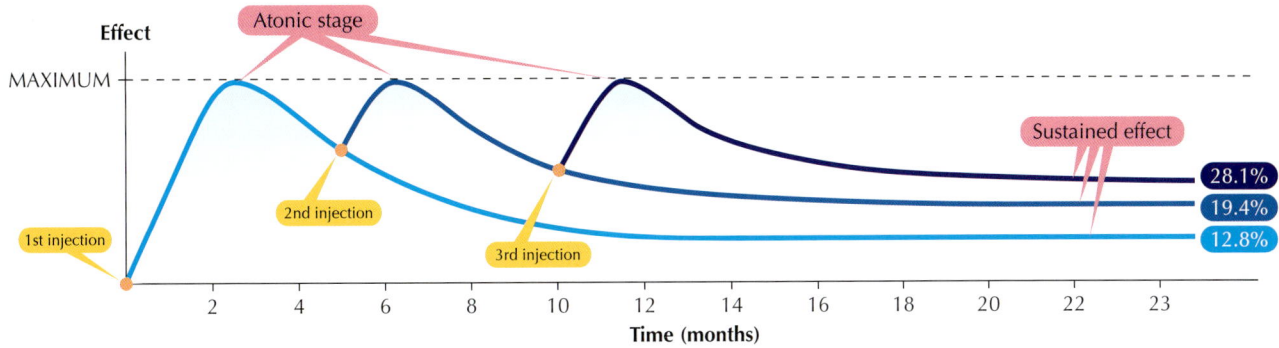

Figure 21.5 Relationship between maximal and sustained effects. These graphs show the change in muscle volume after botulinum toxin A injections. Sustained effect is described as preservation of reduced muscle that lasts more than 1 year after treatment. As the number of botulinum toxin A treatments increases, the sustained effect on the muscle increases. The efficiency of treatment (permanence of the reduced muscle) becomes greater. Therefore, to continually reduce the movement of the masseter, additional treatments are needed.

to the volume recovery stage in turn. Sustained effect is described as preservation of the reduced muscle that lasts more than 1 year after treatment (Figure 21.5). As the number of botulinum toxin A treatments increases, the sustained effect on the muscle increases. The efficiency of treatment (preservation of the reduced muscle) becomes greater. Therefore, to continually reduce the movement of the masseter, additional treatments are needed.

To maintain the continual interception of nerve transmission, an additional injection is needed in the early period of tone recovery. Dosage of the second injection is flexible, depending on the result of the first treatment, and is usually 70–80% of the initial dose. However, if the time for the second injection is delayed and the muscle volume is increased, a higher dosage of botulinum toxin A needs to be applied accordingly. In other words, the reinjection dosage should be considered depending on the difference in muscular volume before and 3 months after the first injection. Considering that the duration of denervation by toxin is about 3–6 months, 2–4 additional injections are necessary to maintain the effect for more than the following year.

Anatomy of the masseter

Full knowledge of the anatomical structure and function of the masseter muscle is critical to the physician. This is because botulinum toxin A treatment sometimes causes temporal discomfort and unexpected side-effects, even though known to be unusual.[17] The masseter muscle functions mainly in mastication, together with the medial pterygoid, temporalis, and lateral pterygoid muscles. Of these masticatory muscles, the masseter muscle is the largest and strongest. The medial pterygoid and the lateral pterygoid do not affect the facial contour line by reason of the internal location toward the mandible. The thickness of the

temporalis is concerned with the depression or bulging of the temple. On the other hand, the masseter muscle highly influences the contour of the lower face, because it is located in the external area of the mandible below the fat tissues. The masseter muscle is thicker than any of the other muscles and is not related to facial expression.

The masseter muscle is divided into superficial and deep portions (Figure 21.6). The former is larger than the latter and located outside the latter. The superficial portion originates from the zygomatic process and arch, and inserts to the ramus of the mandible and the side of the mandibular angle. On the other hand, the deep portion originates from the bottom or inside of the zygomatic arch and descends vertically into the ramus of the mandible and the coronoid process. In some cases, the deep portion of the masseter muscle is organized as a mixture of fibers of the masseter and temporal muscles. The parotid duct runs through the exterior side of the muscle. Around the anterior margin of the masseter muscle, the parotid duct penetrates into the buccinator muscle. The posterior portion of the masseter muscle is covered by the parotid gland.

The masseteric branch of the trigeminal nerve innervates the masseter muscle. The branches of the internal maxillary artery are responsible for the arterial supply to the masseter muscle,[18] and the vein of the masseter runs parallel with the masseteric branch of the trigeminal nerve. In detail, the vein, distributed in the masseter muscle, passes the posterior region of the temporal ligament. Then, this passes the semilunar notch reaching the interior side of the masseter muscle.

Indications and differential diagnosis

Assessment of facial features and applications

In the front view of the face, the facial line begins from the hairline and passes by the temple, the zygomatic

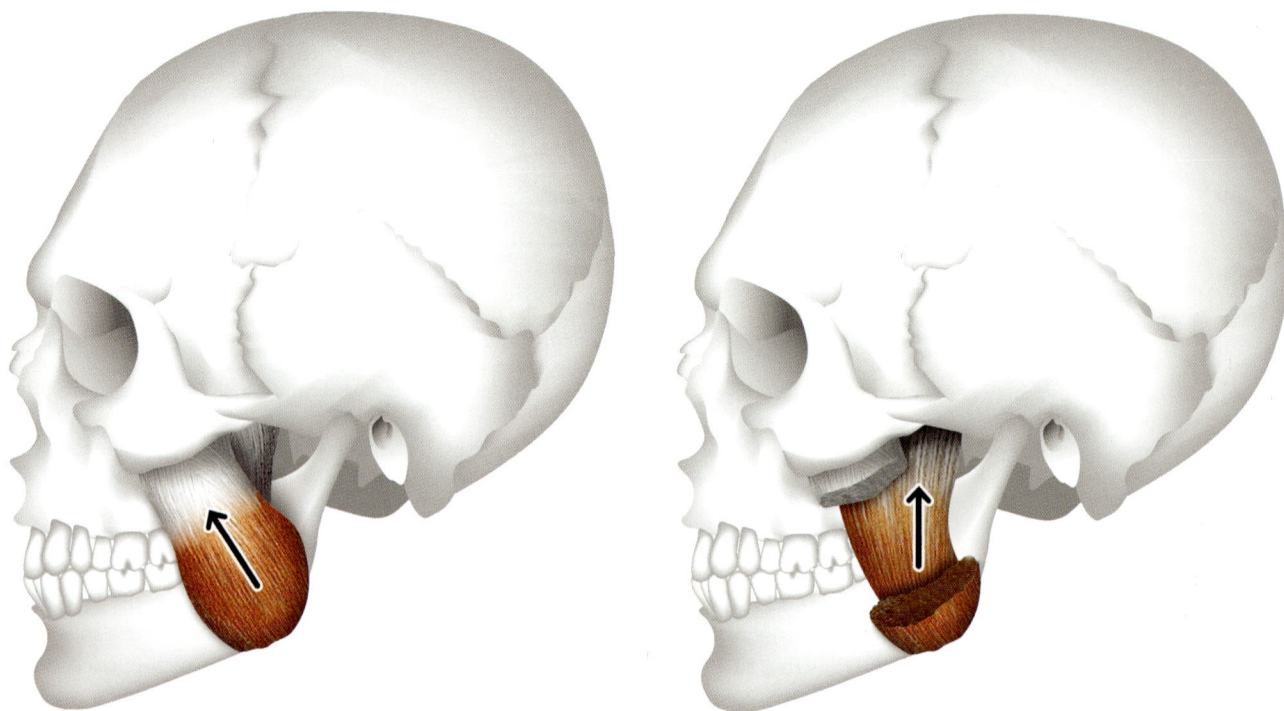

Figure 21.6   Anatomy of the masseter. The masseter muscle is divided into superficial and deep portions. The former is larger than the latter and located outside the latter. The superficial portion originates from the zygomatic process and arch, and inserts to the ramus of the mandibular and the side of the mandibular angle. The deep portion originates from the bottom or the inside of the zygomatic arch and descends vertically into the ramus of the mandible and the coronoid process.

arches which determine the bizygomatic distance, and the gonions which determine the bigonial distance, and finally ends at the chin. Balanced facial features mean a desirable ratio of the whole facial length and width and harmonious ratio of the width and length of the upper, mid-, and lower face portions.

The widest portion of the face is the bizygomatic distance. The ideal ratio of the vertical length to the bizygomatic distance is 1.3:1. The vertical facial line can be divided into three portions of the upper face, ranging from the hairline to the top of the eyebrows, the midface, ranging from the top of the eyebrows to the soft tissue of the subnasale, and the lower face, ranging from the soft tissue of the subnasale to the menton. The ideal ratio of these three portions is 1:1:1. The bitemporal distance and the bigonial distance are desirable at similar size, and 10% smaller than the bizygomatic distance. However, as a preference for a smaller face with narrow width of the lower face is emerging, the ideal ratio in this case is 1:1:0.9 with bigonial distance narrower than the bitemporal distance.

The mean value of the bigonial distance of Western women is 105 mm, while that of Korean women ranges between 117.80 and 125.25 mm, suggesting that Korean women have an approximately 12–20-mm wider bigonial distance than that of Western women. For this reason, research in facial contouring surgery is well advanced in Asian countries compared to Western countries. The width of the lower face is determined by the

size of the mandible, the volume of the masseter muscles and the subcutaneous fat tissues, the development status of the parotid gland, and the degree of posterior divergence of the lower face. Therefore, the important point of the diagnosis is to determine whether fat tissue, muscle, or bone structure is contributing to the increased width of the lower face. The absolute indication for botulinum toxin A treatment can be seen in the patient who has masseter hypertrophy with a normal size of bone structure, fat tissues, and parotid glands. Relative indications are in those who have masseter hypertrophy with an abnormal size of bone structure, fat tissues, and parotid glands or who are dissatisfied with the result of bone resection or liposuction.

Differential diagnosis of skeletal overgrowth and muscle hypertrophy

In order to differentiate the diagnosis of skeletal overgrowth, palpation and X-radiography, including panoramic view and the frontal cephalograph, are recommended (Figure 21.7). Palpation gives inferences regarding the thickness of the muscle and the degree of bone development. However, its not suitable for an objective diagnosis, since the result depends on the physician's subjective experiences.

On panoramic view, the physician should primarily examine the location and shape of the condyle, the

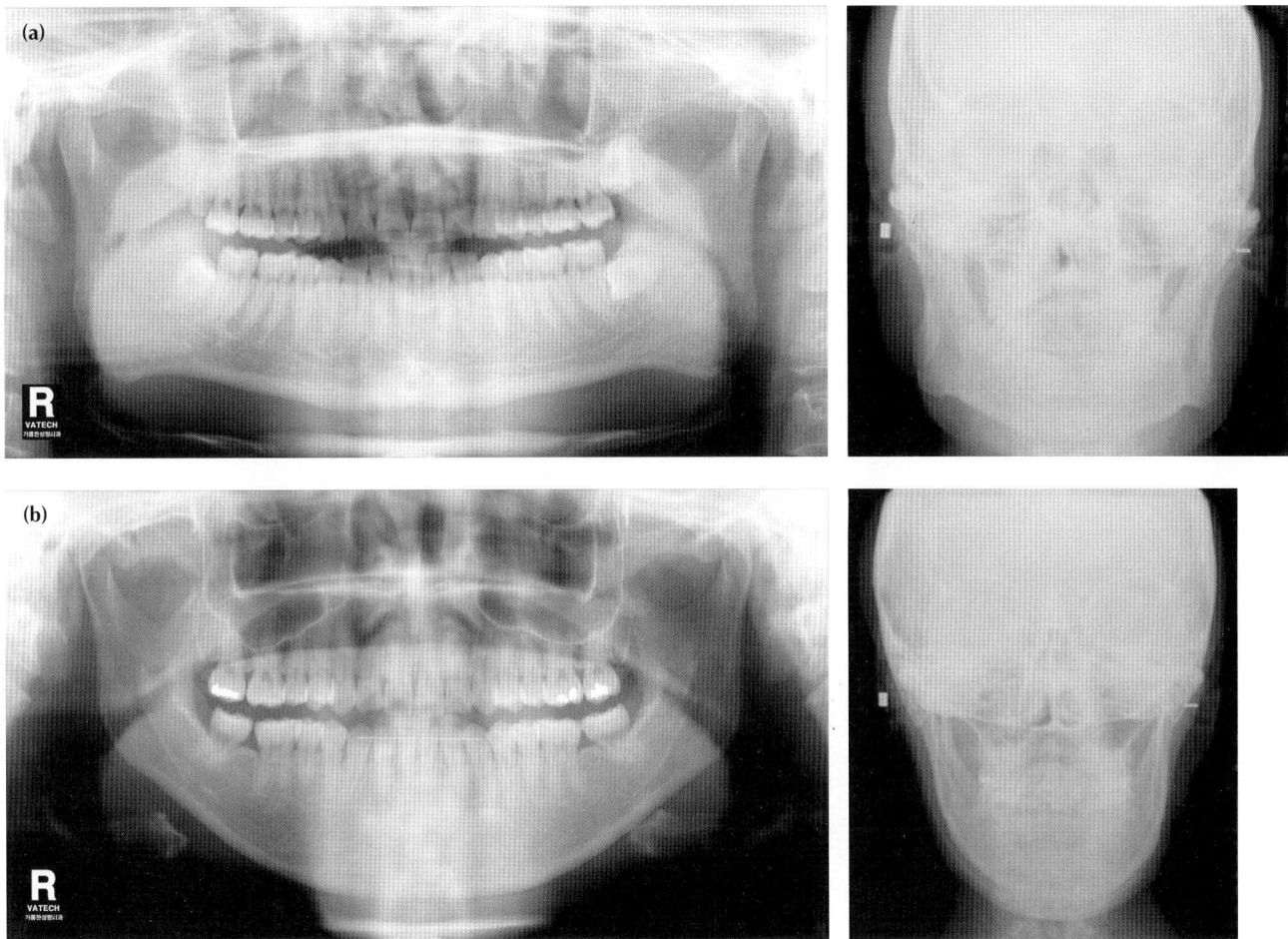

Figure 21.7 Panoramic view and cephalograph: (a) prominent mandibular angle; (b) non-prominent mandibular angle.

height of the ramus, and the location of the gonial angle. In particular, the protrusions of developed gonial angles need to be verified by comparing the right and left sides. At this point, we have to consider that the mandibular angle sometimes does not affect the frontal facial aspect despite the ample appearance on panoramic view. A frontal cephalograph should be taken with more focus on evaluating the developmental status of the gonial angle. Recent advances in three-dimensional computed tomography (CT) have made it possible to measure the thickness of muscle and soft tissues and the distance between each anatomical measuring point accurately. However, owing to the high cost of equipment, its usage is low, especially at local area clinics.

Relation between soft tissues and masseter muscles

The reason for a wide face without quadrangular bone is not always masseter hypertrophy. The subcutaneous fat tissues also occupy an important portion of the face. In a clinical setting, the pinch test can be used to examine the thickness of the fat layer. In an assessment of the fat layer, the widest portion of the lower face

should be identified first. Usually, the bigonial distance is the greatest due to the size of the mandible and the masseter, but sometimes part of the anterior cheek can be selected because of its surrounding thick fat layers. In the latter case, even if the volume of the masseter muscle is reduced, the width of the anterior cheek is not changed. As a result, it gives a worse impression by causing a depressed look of the mandible. The size of the parotid gland located posterior to the masseter muscle can also affect the width of the lower face. If it is strongly developed, it is dilated more laterally than the masseter muscle. At present, the only way to reduce the volume of the parotid gland is superficial parotidectomy. However, this operation is not often performed because it leaves a large scar.

For an objective and simple measurement of the muscle, the subcutaneous fat layer, and the parotid gland, an ultrasonogram is used (Figure 21.8). Special attention must be paid when measuring the thickness of soft tissue by ultrasonography, for if the physician compresses the target area with the probe, it could be measured as smaller than the actual value. To normalize the target area, in our study all measurements were made on the line connecting the ear lobe and mouth corner. The

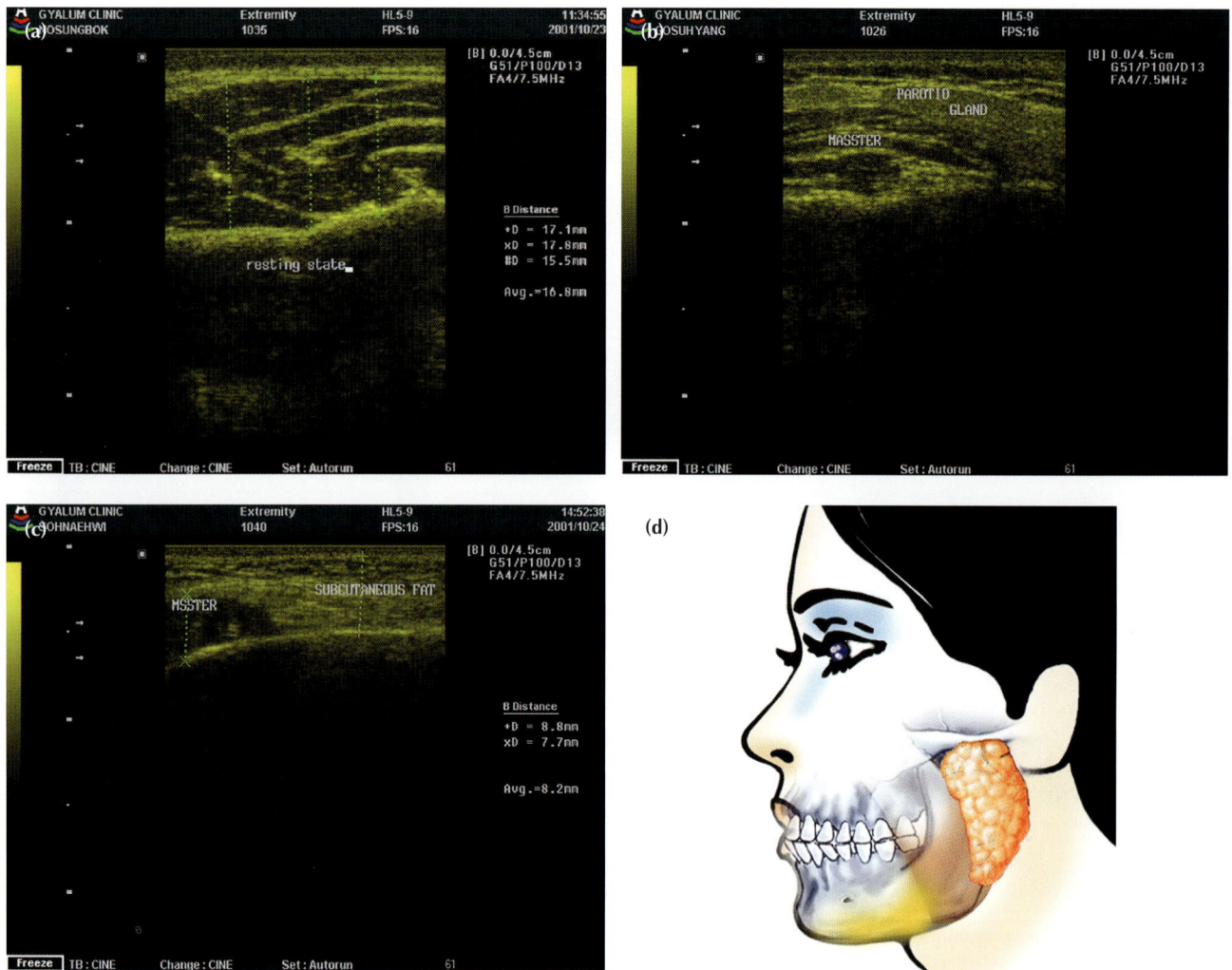

Figure 21.8 Images of organic layers measured by ultrasonography: (a) central portion occupied by masseter muscle; (b) posterior portion occupied by parotid gland; (c) anterior portion occupied by subcutaneous fat. (d) Facial profile illustration.

mean values of measurements taken in the resting state before injection were 13.36 (9.1–19.1) mm on the left and 13.69 (9.4–20.1) mm on the right (Table 21.1).

As mentioned above, three-dimensional CT is more accurate, but is not reasonable in a cost-effective manner.

Method

Dosage and dilution

An injection dosage must be enough to completely inhibit movement of the masseter muscle. Otherwise, it would result in less efficacy and satisfaction, since it could neither intercept nerve transmission nor cause complete disuse atrophy. Judging from our experience, unless the entire nerve system of the masseter muscle is blocked, the recurrence of muscular contraction and volume will appear earlier. However, high-dose treatment does not always enhance the effectiveness. An optimal dose would be the minimum amount of toxin

that is sufficient to inhibit the contraction of the overall masseter muscle, i.e. block all acetylcholine receptors at the neuromuscular junction.

Overdosed injection is an unnecessary waste, for it fails to combine with the acetylcholine receptor and is finally taken up and removed by the systemic circulation. Based on the assumption that the minimum dose of toxin varies depending on the size of the masseter muscle, we devised a standard scale for the volume of injection (Table 21.2).

Presumably, the amount of saline used in diluting the toxin seems not to be very important for effect and progress. However, overdilution can cause more pain due to the increased volume of injection and the toxin can spread to unexpected areas due to the excessive volume itself and the counter pressure. In contrast, low dilution may result in difficulty in handling and errors of injection dose.

At our clinic, Dysport® is used, and one vial is reconstituted with 2.5 ml of saline. One vial contains 500 U (Dysport units), so 0.5 ml of that solution includes 100 U.

Table 21.1   The muscle thickness of responders and non-responders (mm)

| | | Non-responders before injection (n=638) | Responders (n=383) | |
			Before injection	After injection
Mean	Right	13.51	13.36	9.27
	Left	13.75	13.69	9.28
Range	Right	6.5–22.1	9.4–19.1	6.5–13.5
	Left	7.5–22.1	9.4–19.1	6.3–13.7

Injection site and landmarks

In general, the injection is given to the thickest region of the masseter muscle. However, it can be more easily delivered if a few reference lines are defined by palpation.

Before injection, the anterior and posterior margins of the masseter muscle are identified by palpation. Then, a rectangular area is designated by linking the lower border of the mandible, the ear lobe–mouth corner line, and the anterior and posterior borders of the masseter. Injection in this part is the most effective, since the muscle inside this area is mostly well developed. Moreover, this area is safe, being at a distance from any other crucial anatomical structures, and is formed from very thick muscle. An injection to only one point allows the toxin to spread over an unwanted area due to high counter pressure caused by the large volume. To prevent this, as well as to diffuse the toxin homogeneously to the overall muscle, injection must be given to three different points that are 1.5 cm away from the border of the mandibular angle, i.e. one point where the muscle is thickest and two other points that are located anterior and posterior to the center in a triangular manner.

Reference landmarks (Figure 21.9)

Anterior border of the masseter muscle

Injection given to the anterior part of this line and the diffusion of botulinum toxin A can cause awkward facial expression by paralyzing the buccinator muscle and risorius.

Posterior border of the masseter muscle

The posterior margin of the masseter muscle that originates from the mandibular angle runs parallel with the anterior border. The parotid gland is located behind this line.

Ear lobe–mouth corner line

This line can be drawn by connecting the ear lobe to the mouth corner, which almost matches the occlusal

Table 21.2   Our standard scale for the volume of injection

Muscle thickness (mm)	Dysport® (U)*
10	100
11	110
12	120
13	125
14	130
15	135
16	140

*Total injected units for one side.

plane. In addition, this line divides the masseter muscle into two parts: the maxillary and the mandibular areas of the masseter muscle, i.e. upper and lower portions. To reduce the width of the lower face, the lower portion of the masseter muscle needs to be diminished in volume. If the volume is diminished in the upper portion of the masseter, a cheek depression is formed immediately below the zygomatic arch. For this reason, injection is given only to the lower portion of the masseter muscle. In the case of some Asians who have overdeveloped zygomatic bones, the injection should be given with great care for that aspect.

Lower border of mandible

The injection should be given to the region that is 1.5 cm superior to this line. If the injection is given too close to this line, it could cause several unexpected side-effects such as swallowing difficulty, but in practice, no side-effect has occurred yet.

Injection procedure

1. Patients are examined via a photograph of the standard front view and ultrasonography for differential diagnosis. Sufficient explanation about the treatment plan and the inconvenience that could possibly happen should be given to the patient.
2. The dosage of injection should be determined according to examination results such as muscle thickness.

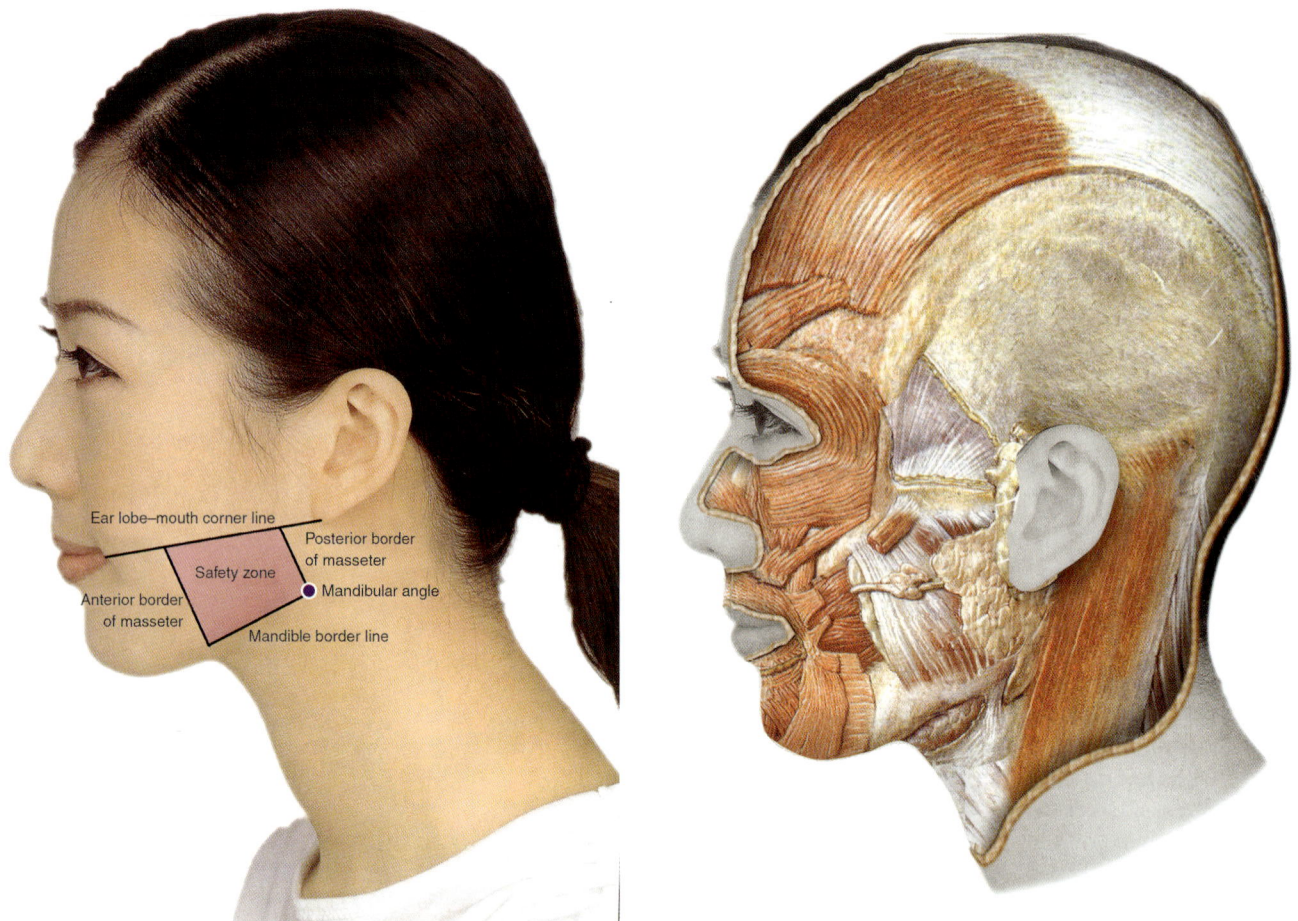

Figure 21.9   Reference landmarks. Within this area, the masseter is mostly well developed and at a safe distance from other crucial anatomical structures.

3. In consideration of the physician's preference, patients must be in an upright or slightly tilted position.

4. The target area must be cleansed using sanitary cotton immersed in alcohol.

5. A line linking the ear lobe and the mouth corner should be drawn with a marker.

6. The lower border of the mandible should be drawn.

7. After confirming the anterior and posterior margins of the masseter muscle by palpation, these two lines should be marked.

8. The point of injection is specified. Within the rectangular safe zone, the point that is 1.5 cm away from the mandibular angle border is the most developed point of the muscle. Regarding this point as the center, two more injection points are set that are approximately 1 cm away from it both anteriorly and posteriorly. If the width of the masseter muscle is rather narrow, a two-horizontal-point injection can be applied depending on the state of the patient. If the muscle is relatively wide, a four-point injection can be given.

9. For accurate injection, a 1-ml insulin syringe is favored over a normal one.

10. If patients undergo the injection during clenching, they will feel more pain than during the resting state. Accordingly, patients should be relaxed prior to the treatment. The center point must be given 50% of the normal dose. Then, two points located anterior and posterior to the center must be given 25% each. Considering the diffusion of Dysport, three injections are enough (Figure 21.10).

11. Usually, there is no bleeding at the site of the injection, but if there is, compression should be used to minimize the possibility of bruising. Just as when giving an intramuscular injection into the gluteal muscles, if the injected site is roughly rubbed, the toxin runs over the subcutaneous fat layer or other areas passing through the fascial layer. Therefore, the point should be compressed softly.

12. Marks on the face should be cleansed. Then, the patient can be discharged after they are informed of precautions.

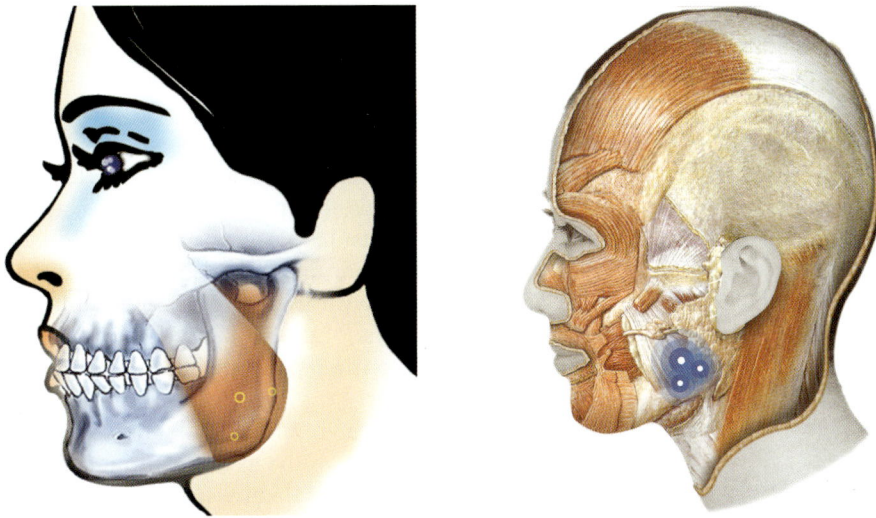

Figure 21.10 Injection site and diffusion of botulinum toxin A. Considering the diffusion of Dysport®, three injections are enough, within 1.5 cm from mandibular angle border. The first injection is needed on the maximum swelling of clenching (50% of total dosage), and the second and third injections are placed 1 cm away from the first (25% of total dosage). Dilution takes place in 2.5 ml normal saline with Dysport 500 U. For example, if we inject 100 U, this is constituted as: 0.5 ml (including 100 U) + additional normal saline 0.5 ml = 1 ml.

Merits of botulinum toxin injection in masseteric hypertrophy

1. It is a therapy that requires simple injection.
2. Rapid effects take place after treatment, generally appearing in a week.
3. The injection period is short (about 5 minutes).
4. There is no inconvenience to daily life after treatment.
5. There are few side-effects and little pain after treatment.
6. The cost is inexpensive compared to that of masseter muscle resection or mandible resection.
7. There is no need to be concerned about permanent side-effects. In 1989, the effectiveness and safety of botulinum toxin A treatment was approved by the Food and Drug Administration (FDA) based on the results of clinical studies done in thousands of patients. For the past 20 years, between 1982 and 2000, no cases of side-effects were reported in patients who received botulinum toxin A treatment.

Side-effects

Botulinum toxin A treatment has never caused a fatal or permanent side-effect, since it just temporarily paralyzes the muscle. There are some inconveniences related to ineffectiveness of masticatory function (Table 21.3). However, there is a possibility that some side-effects might occur due to errors in injection technique.

Ineffectiveness of masticatory power

Fifty per cent of patients who underwent botulinum toxin A treatment complained about discomfort when chewing tough food for 1–2 months after the injection. This symptom occurs due to the weakened power of

Table 21.3 Temporary discomforts

Type	n (%)
Crunching power is decreased	192 (50%)
In crunching, muscle is protruded	38 (10%)
Unnatural smiling appearance	8 (2%)
Disappearance of facial dimple	4 (1%)

the muscle. This is unavoidable, because the rationale of this treatment is to paralyze the muscle and thereby to induce disuse atrophy. It is relieved by compensatory actions of the medial and lateral pterygoid and temporalis muscles.

Irregular muscular movements during mastication

The muscle appears irregular when one is chewing something. This is due to the different degrees of response to botulinum toxin A in the same muscle. In some parts, contraction of the muscle occurs continually, whereas in other parts, there is no longer any muscle contraction. The part where muscle contraction still takes place appears prominent owing to the diminished contraction of opposite parts. This symptom is noted in 5–10% of patients 1–2 weeks after the injection, and lasts for 2–4 weeks. Irregular muscular movements result from the large volume of muscle, the thinner skin over these parts, and an underdosage of injection or injection error. In most cases the phenomenon disappears in 3–4 weeks, and if not, an additional injection is needed to resolve it.

Awkwardness in facial features

At an early phase of treatment, some patients complain about a droop in the corners of the mouth when smiling. This occurs in 2–5% of cases. It appears in 2–4 weeks, continuing for the next 4–8 weeks, and disappears spontaneously. The main reason for this is paralysis of the risorius muscle that originates from the masseter muscle and inserts to the mouth corner. Consequently, an injection of toxin to the lower part of the masseter muscle that reaches the risorius muscle can minimize this symptom of awkward expression. In addition, awkward expression can be caused by injection to the wrong site that concerns the zygomaticus minor or major.

Protrusion of zygomatic bones

There are several cases of complaints regarding the bony facial image that results from protrusion of the zygoma after botulinum toxin A treatment. The masseter originates from the inferior surface of the zygomatic bone and then inserts to the mandibular angle. This contributes to the rectangular form of the masseter muscle. When masseteric atrophy occurs after injection, not only the muscles around the mandibular angle but also the muscles immediately below the zygomatic bone become atrophied. Therefore, the zygomatic bone may appear more protruding. Thus, serious consideration must be given before the use of toxin in those patients with large and wide cheekbones. The protrusion of the zygoma will gradually disappear after the muscle tension is recovered. At the same time, the decline of muscle volume lessens the width of the face, so careful consideration is required for a long face, a mandibular prognathism, or a thin face. In patients who complain of zygomatic protrusion following botulinum toxin A treatment, a microfat graft or zygomatic reduction can resolve the problem.

Others

Bruising or edema can occur by intradermal injection, so sufficient compression to the injection site is essential.

There were also some cases dissatisfied with the result of treatment in our study. Some 93% (77/83 cases) of patients reported satisfaction, but the other 7% (6/83 cases) expressed dissatisfaction. Dissatisfaction resulted from less change than expected and protrusive cheekbones. The little change of facial image was due to an overdeveloped bone border, well-developed parotid glands, low elasticity of the skin, errors in injection points and injection dosage, or differences between their expected features and the reality.

The correction of calf hypertrophy

In general, the legs of Asian women are shorter and thicker than those of the Western population, which can result in a plump image of the legs. If the calves are thick, the legs might appear shorter and resemble masculine legs. In order to make these legs look slim and eventually longer, many treatment tools have been studied, including muscle resection and liposuction. Thick calves can be classified into several types, which include gastrocnemius muscle hypertrophy, excessive fat, and a mixed type of both cases. The calf usually has thick muscles with a relatively thin fat layer, compared to other areas. Thus, it is difficult to satisfy patients fully with liposuction. Even though it can reduce the volume of the fat layer, the legs do not appear slim owing to the remaining irregular muscles. As a result, plastic surgeons have become interested in the reduction of muscle volume for calf contouring.

To reduce the volume of the gastrocnemius muscle, several treatments such as selective neurectomy, resection of the gastrocnemius muscle, and botulinum toxin A treatment can be applied. Neurectomy incurs difficulties associated with the surgical procedure and learning curve, and relapses in cases where the nerve is not removed completely. Also, it is possible to fail in surgery and damage other nerves because of the complexity of nerve development. In addition, the appearance of the calf can be changed due to development of the soleus muscle, and bowed legs can be aggravated in cases of compensational development of the lateral gastrocnemius muscle. The disadvantages of myectomy are a long scar after surgery, hemorrhage, irregularity, and the difficulty of precise surgery.

The mechanism of botulinum toxin A treatment for calf hypertrophy is identical to that of masseter muscle hypertrophy treatment. Botulinum toxin A reduces the tension of flexed muscles in the calf and gives the legs definition by reducing the volume of the muscles. A suitable indication is a muscular type with medial muscle hypertrophy and thin skin, and also when leg lines are irregular due to flexed muscles in the tiptoe position. Disadvantages of this method are the high dosage of toxin and short duration of effect due to the large volume of the muscle. Because calf muscles are used in gait every day, the possibility of recurrence might be higher compared to masseter reduction with botulinum toxin. In addition, the dosage should be carefully selected in order not to interfere with the gait.

Injection dosage

Usually, the response of calf reduction depends on the dosage of botulinum toxin A. For example, the effectiveness of the treatment for one leg varies according to dosage of Dysport as follows:

1. 100 U of Dysport: with this dosage, effectiveness is insufficient and patients do not recognize the effect. Even if it is effective, the duration is too short. Generally, this dosage is not sufficient.

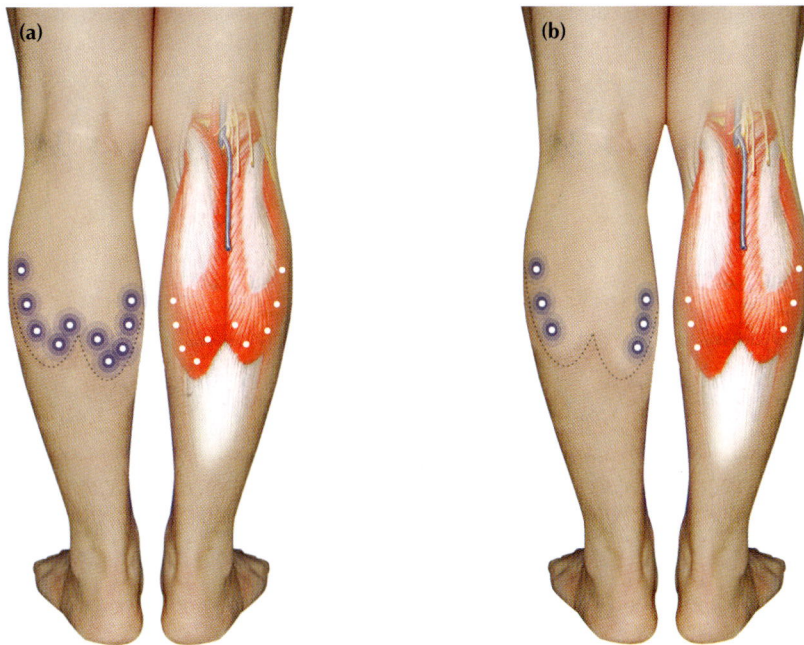

Figure 21.11   Injection site and diffusion of botulinum toxin. (a) To make legs appear longer by lifting the gastrocnemius muscle upward, Dysport can be applied to the protruding part immediately below the gastrocnemius muscle. Dysport can be diluted in 5 ml saline and 0.3 ml can be injected at each of five sites. (b) To smooth medial leg lines or lateral leg lines, Dysport can be diluted in 5 ml saline and 0.5 ml can be injected at each of three sites.

2. 150 U of Dysport: this dosage is commonly effective, but the duration tends to be short.
3. 250 U of Dysport: most cases show effectiveness and patients acknowledge it. Considering that most patients are satisfied, this dosage is regarded as an optimal dosage.
4. 500 U of Dysport: patients might complain about gait disturbance. In order to avoid gait disturbance, a dosage below this should be selected and the treatment interval appropriately decided.

Injection method by treatment goal

1. To obtain uniform and regular volume reduction, Dysport can be diluted in 5 ml of saline and 0.1 ml can be injected at each of 15–25 sites evenly in one gastrocnemius muscle. The shortcoming of this method is the high number of injection sites, which leads to patient complaints of pain.
2. To make legs look longer by lifting the gastrocnemius muscle upward, Dysport can be applied to the protruding part immediately below the gastrocnemius muscle. Dysport can be diluted in 5 ml saline and amounts of 0.25–0.3 ml can each be injected at 10 sites (Figure 21.11a).
3. To smooth medial leg lines, Dysport can be diluted in 5 ml saline and 0.5 ml can be injected in only the medial leg at three sites (Figure 21.11b).
4. To smooth lateral leg lines, Dysport can be diluted in 5 ml saline and 0.5 ml can be injected in only the lateral leg at three sites (Figure 21.11b).
5. When we consider the dosage-benefit, it is advised to inject only one part of the lateral or

medial gastrocnemius muscle. Three months after treatment, there were no significant differences in the circumference of the calf between using Dysport 75 U to only one part and using Dysport 150 U to both medial and lateral parts of the gastrocnemius muscle based on our experience. Therefore, focusing on a single part of the muscle is better than treating both parts from an economical aspect.

The reduction of muscle volume can be seen 2 weeks after injection when wearing high heels. After a month, the muscle activity decreases clearly and the volume reduces considerably. Three months later the volume reduction reaches a maximum level, and in 4–6 months, muscle activity recovers and muscle volume starts increasing.

Different from surgical procedures, no scar remains after calf reduction with botulinum toxin A. In addition, immediate return to daily life such as taking a shower or exercising is guaranteed. Besides, there is no outstanding discomfort, similar to botulinum toxin A treatment of masseter hypertrophy.

Even simple procedures might have mild adverse effects. With calf reduction using botulinum toxin A, petechial bleeding might occur. Excessive exercise after injection especially should be limited because possible petechial bleeding can cause hemosiderin pigmentation. However, calf muscle dysfunction such as fatigue upon walking or running, which is the most common concern with this treatment, rarely occurs. Even if it appears, the symptoms are mild and transient. Such adverse effects usually disappear within 1–2 weeks.

If patients have excessive fat, he or she is recommended to consider liposuction with botulinum toxin A injection.

References

1. Legg JW. Enlargement of the temporal and masseter muscles on both sides. Trans Pathol Soc London 1880; 31: 361–6.
2. Gurney CE. Chronic bilateral benign hypertrophy of the masseter muscle. Am J Surg 1947; 73: 137–9.
3. Farkas LG. Anthropometry of the Head and Face in Medicine. New York: Elsevier, 1981.
4. Whitaker LA. Aesthetic contouring of the facial support system. Clin Plast Surg 1989; 16: 815–16.
5. Baek SM, Kim SS, Bindiger A. The prominent mandibular angle: preoperative management operative technique, and results in 42 patients. Plast Reconstr Surg 1989; 83: 272–80.
6. Baek SM. Aesthetic contouring of the facial skeleton. Probl Plast Reconstr Surg 1991; 1: 673.
7. Hong JU, Choi J, Baek SM. Study on resected area and masticatory muscle's histopathology and radiologic changes after Gato's mandibula osteotomy. Korea Soc Plast Surg 1994; 21: 857.
8. Yang DB, Park CG. Mandibular contouring surgery for purely aesthetic reasons. Aesthetic Plast Surg 1991; 15: 53–60.
9. Smyth AG. Botulinum toxin treatment of bilateral masseteric hypertrophy. Br J Oral Maxillofac Surg 1994; 32: 29–33.
10. Moore AP, Wood GD. The medical management of masseteric hypertrophy with botulinum toxin type A. Br J Oral Maxillofac Surg 1994; 32: 26–8.
11. von Lindern JJ, Niederhgen B, Appel T, Berge S, Reich RH. Type A botulinum toxin for the treatment of hypertrophy of the masseter and temporal muscles: an alternative treatment. Plast Reconstr Surg 2001; 107: 327–32.
12. Kim NH, Chung JH, Park RH, Park JB. The use of botulinum toxin type A in aesthetic mandible contouring. Plast Reconstr Surg 2005; 115: 919–30.
13. Carruthers A, Carruthers J. History of the cosmetic use of botulinum A exotoxin. Dermatol Surg 1988; 24: 1168–70.
14. Lee YJ, Han KH, Kang JS. Korean craniofacial standard measurement. Korea Soc Plast Surg 1994; 21: 438.
15. Fadeyi MO, Adams QM. Use of botulinum toxin type B for migraine and tension headaches. Am J Health Syst Pharm 2002; 59: 1860–2.
16. Kim CJ, Ham KS, Kim Y, Cho YJ. Bio standard measurement study on teenage Korean facial. Korea Soc Plast Surg 1988; 15: 427.
17. Park JS, Ham KS, Cho YJ. Standard measurement study on the ideal facial. Korea Soc Plast Surg 1994; 16: 920.
18. Cho CH, Han KH, Kang JS. Korean craniofacial standard measurement: gender and periodic normal rate on 119 items/standard deviation and standardized template. Korea Soc Plast Surg 1993; 20: 995.

22 Facial palsy and asymmetries

Maurício De Maio

Introduction

A smile can express such feelings as those related to pleasure, friendship, acceptance, embarrassment, happiness, delight, and/or agreement. It can be warm, cold, humble, or arrogant. Not being able to smile would be to deprive ourselves of one of our most basic tools for communication in a social environment.

It is a big challenge to treat a face that has become paralyzed. Facial palsy triggers esthetic and functional changes that hold significant physical and psychological repercussions for those suffering from this condition. In addition to speech, swallowing, or chewing impairment, static and dynamic imbalances can affect, in a striking manner, a person's ability to express his emotions.[1] The physical aspects can bring disastrous results to a patient's self-image[2] as well as emotional state.[3]

The facial nerve and mimicry

The facial nerve is responsible for stimulating the muscles that mimic, creating a balance between the synergistic and antagonistic forces that act upon facial structures. It is also responsible for the minimum muscular tonus in a relaxed state, and the voluntary and involuntary muscular contraction of each side of the face.[4]

When the facial nerve emerges from the stylomastoid foramen, it gives origin to its many ramifications. The first ramification is the posterior auricular branch, and the others can be divided into two branches: temporofacial and cervicofacial that, in turn, divide into the temporal, zygomatic, and buccal ramifications and into the marginal mandibular and cervical ramifications, respectively. The muscle in the frontal region is stimulated by the temporal branch; the muscles in the orbital region are stimulated by the zygomatic branch; the muscles of the upper lip receive stimulus from the buccal branch; the muscles of the lower lip are stimulated by the marginal mandibular branch and the platysma by the cervical branch. These muscles are responsible for activating the orifices of the eyelids and of the mouth and for representing human emotions.[5]

The mimetic muscles are made up of fibers inserted into the dermis. These muscle fibers can contract themselves in an independent manner, so as to produce slight, finely tuned variations in facial expression.[6]

The most complex group of mimetic muscles consists of those that control the movements of the lips and cheeks. The muscles that raise the lips (the muscle that raises the upper lip, levator labii superioris; the muscle that raises the corners of the mouth, levator anguli oris; the major and minor zygomatic muscles; and the muscles responsible for raising the nasal flares and the upper lip, levator labii superioris alaeque nasi) interdigitate and intertwine closely with the orbicular muscle in the mouth. The muscles that act upon the lower lip are the lowering muscles of the lower lip, depressor labii inferioris; the muscle that lowers the corners of the mouth, depressor anguli oris; and mentalis. The confluence of these muscles creates an almost unlimited number of facial movements and individual expressions.

Facial palsy: clinical aspects and treatment

Damage to the facial nerve may produce deformities of varying degree, resulting in esthetic and functional disorders.

The main causes of facial palsy (or facial paralysis) stem from cerebral vascular dysfunctions, iatrogenic or non-iatrogenic damage caused in surgeries, damage resulting from traumas, such as physical aggressions and car accidents, and the idiopathic or 'a frigori' palsy, which is the most frequent type and whose etiology has not been well-defined. The other causes are related to changes in the nervous system, such as neuritis (alcohol and poliomyelitis), and muscular alterations, such as myasthenia. Viral and bacterial infections, anomalies in development, ischemia, and tumors (intracerebral, intratemporal, and parotid) correspond to the lowest percentage of incidence in the etiology of facial palsy.[7]

The side of the face affected by facial palsy presents characteristics common among all patients. On the surface of the skin, fewer wrinkles form due to the lack of muscular traction on the dermis, the nasolabial fold becomes less evident, and both the corners of the mouth and the brows droop. Depending on how serious the damage is and on the amount of time since the onset of the facial palsy, the esthetic aspects may be affected to a greater or lesser extent.

The 'normal' side or the contralateral side to the facial palsy evolves with a hyperkinetic reaction of the muscle tissues due to the lack of tonus on the paralyzed side. This imbalance of vectorial forces creates facial deviations. The facial esthetics will be affected to a greater extent the longer the facial palsy has lasted. Facial asymmetries that occur when the facial muscles are in a relaxed state are less evident in paralyses that have lasted a short time, becoming more apparent when muscles move into action.

In paralyses that have lasted a longer period of time, the imbalance is so great that the opposite side of the face presents deviations in the labial, nasal, and orbital regions, even when the muscles are in a relaxed state. In these cases, even facial rotation occurs, making the non-paralyzed side of the face shorter.

Treatment of facial palsy is complex and includes nerve grafts, muscle transfers, and microsurgical patches: in summary, many different forms of treatment, which prove unable to grant the patient facial balance.[8–11] Even after all of the interventions have been carried out, synkinesis may result, which hinders furthermore the rehabilitation process in patients suffering from facial palsy.[12]

Surgical treatment of facial palsy depends on the etiology and the length of time since the onset of the lesion, which ranges from recent to late. Lesions are considered recent if they have occurred within up to 3 weeks. Late lesions are those that have evolved for more than 1 year.[13]

The more serious forms of facial palsy have occurred with a period of more than 1 year, for, apart from the lack of expression on the affected side, there is hyperactivity on the non-affected side, which makes the facial asymmetry even more evident.

Reconstruction should seek to reestablish the symmetry of the mouth in the person's smile and to obtain contraction of the oral and palpebral sphincters, which are the most important elements in facial esthetics that have been lost.

The best results are obtained through associating various techniques. Hence, the optimal solution would be to reduce the hyperactivity of the non-affected side through selective neurectomy or myectomy, transferring functional muscles to the paralyzed side while synchronizing the functions of these muscles to the non-affected side through transfacial nerve grafting.[14,15]

In addition to these methods, the association of techniques for suspending or resecting skin such as rhytidectomy, blepharoplasty, and correction of lagophthalmos, is fundamental in order to obtain better results.[16–19]

Even after all clinical and/or surgical therapies, it can be noticed that patients still possess striking facial asymmetry in static and dynamic positions due to the hyperkinesis on the non-paralyzed side. This hyperkinesis can be regulated through selective myotomies, myectomies, and neurectomies of the muscles responsible for mimicry.[21,22]

In addition to surgical methods, botulinum toxin may be used to reduce the facial asymmetry encountered in patients suffering from facial palsy.[22]

Botulinum toxin is indicated for a wide range of uses which include ocular disorders, disorders of the upper respiratory tract and of the gastrointestinal tract, genitourinary illnesses, dystonias, hemifacial spasms, disorders of the autonomic nervous system, and esthetic uses.[23–25]

In patients suffering from facial palsy, the botulinum toxin has been used to treat synkinesis.[26–28] The results of treatments for synkinesis and hyperlacrimation in patients suffering from facial palsy have been so astounding that botulinum toxin has become the best treatment to counteract the motor and autonomic effects caused by aberrant neural regeneration.[29,30]

The botulinum toxin has also been used in the treatment of hyperkinesis[31] to promote frontal symmetry in patients suffering from neural lesions after rhytidectomies[32] and in patients presenting lesions in the marginal mandibular branch of the facial nerve.[33] It also provides an opportunity to induce a reversible type of chemical inhibition in the muscles and, in this way, it may be used as a therapeutic test before deciding to sacrifice a muscle's functions irreversibly as occurs in neurectomies and myectomies.

Botulinum toxin type A

Botulism, clinically recognized as a syndrome of poisoning, had already become known even before the toxin itself was identified. Its name stems from the word 'botulus', which means sausage, and for a long period of time, botulism was described as a disease caused by eating spoilt sausages.[34]

Since its discovery in 1897, to its use as a therapeutic agent in 1977, up to current times, the botulinum toxin has come to be a powerful therapeutic tool whose use is in expansion. Studies in humans for the treatment of strabismus were carried out in the middle of the 1980s by Scott. In 1989, the FDA (Food and Drug Administration) fully approved botulinum toxin for use in treatments related to strabismus, blepharospasms, and facial spasms in patients over 12 years old.[35]

Clostridium botulinum, a gram-positive anaerobic bacterium, produces the botulinum toxin. There are eight distinct types, which are designated A, B, C1, C2, D, E, F, and G. Although they are antigenically distinct and act at different sites within the neurons, they have similar molecular weights and a common structural subunit.[36]

Botulinum toxin type A is the most potent of all and was the first to be developed for clinical use.[37] The toxins are synthesized as single chain polypeptides with a molecular mass of roughly 150 kDa. The parent chain is cleaved in a heavy chain (100 kDa) which bonds through a divalent sulfur bond to a light chain (50 kDa), which is linked to an atom of zinc.[36]

For it to become effective, four different phases should occur: bonding, internalization, translocation of the membrane, and protease activity.[38] The toxin will only produce an effect if it enters the nerve terminal in its intact form.[39]

The bonding of the toxin occurs in a specific and irreversible manner to cholinergic nerve sprouts, mediated through the toxin's heavy chain, while the light chain induces intracellular toxicity. This process is selective and saturable.

Internalization is carried out through endocytosis of a lysosomal vesicle (process which is mediated by receptors and depends upon energy).[40,41] If the sulfur bond should come to break before internalization, the light chain will not be able to enter and toxicity will be completely lost.[42]

After internalization occurs, the divalent sulfur bond is broken and translocation of the light chain is carried out by the endosmotic membrane, which is responsible for inhibiting the release of acetylcholine.[43]

The clinical effects of the toxin occur mainly due to its peripheral action. Typically, the toxin displays a delay in its action, which ranges from 24 to 72 hours, between its administration and its clinical effects, although some patients have been known to show immediate results. The retardation in clinical effects may be related to how protease acts upon metabolism, or even due to the proximal release of the toxin.

Elimination of the paralytic effect occurs in two distinct phases.[44] Initially, accessory terminal sprouts are formed from destroyed axons. After approximately 28 days, the main terminal slowly begins to regain its function in the release of neurotransmitters and the sprouts gradually disappear. Full recovery is achieved in a little over 90 days, the clinical effects lasting for roughly the same amount of time.[37]

In human and animal experimental models, it was concluded that prolonged exposure to the toxin causes denervation and posterior reversible muscular atrophy.[45–47]

Botulinum toxins are proteins capable of stimulating an immunological response. This immunological response may stem from the development of antibodies that block the therapeutic effects of the drug (neutralizing antibodies). In the therapeutic use of botulinum toxin, avoiding the production of these antibodies is important. The immunological response is influenced by the quantity of protein in the immunological system exposed in each dose administered. Treatment carried out using low doses of the toxin can reduce the risk of a patient becoming refractory to the treatment. The development of immunoresistance seems to occur more often in patients treated with large doses of the toxin and who have had short intervals of time between each shot administered.[34]

The most known types of botulinum toxin type A on the market are Dysport® (Ipsen, United Kingdom) and BOTOX® (Allergan, USA). A vial of Dysport contains 500 U and a vial of BOTOX® contains a nominal 100 U. No significant differences exist in the potency of these two products, and in clinical use the dose equivalence ratio between these two products varies from 3:1 to 4:1.[48,49]

Techniques for administering the botulinum toxin type A in facial palsy and asymmetries

The treatment of patients suffering from facial palsy should begin with a very thorough clinical assessment so that the patients can incorporate the changes after the botulinum toxin type A (BTX-A) injection. This treatment can be carried out in any doctor's office, for it does not require any kind of anesthetic. The degree of pain is quite bearable by patients.

In clinical practice, it is advisable to begin the treatment with smaller doses and complement them after 15 days to produce better results and maintain the lowest possible incidence of complications. Until the physician has mastered treatment with botulinum toxin, it must be carried out in more than one phase, so as to follow the learning curve that is present each time a new activity is being taken up.

Before starting with the technique, one must be aware that the doses of BTX-A presented in this chapter concern Dysport.

Reconstitution of Dysport

The lyophilized substance should be kept at an external temperature ranging from 5 to 8°C. Dysport (botulinum toxin type A) can be reconstituted using 4 ml of 0.9% sodium chloride solution for the treatment of facial palsy and asymmetries. After introduction of the physiological saline solution, the suspension should be delicately made homogeneous until the product becomes totally dissolved.

Reconstituting 500 U of Dysport in 4 ml of physiological saline solution, a concentration of 12.5 U of Dysport for each 0.1 ml of resuspended solution is obtained. Dysport should be administered through intramuscular injection with a 30G needle.[1,2] The needle should be inserted at 45° from the skin's surface.

Description of the points of administration, units, and volume

Although the number of units may vary from patient to patient, below are listed the usual sites of injection, volume, and units (Figure 22.1):

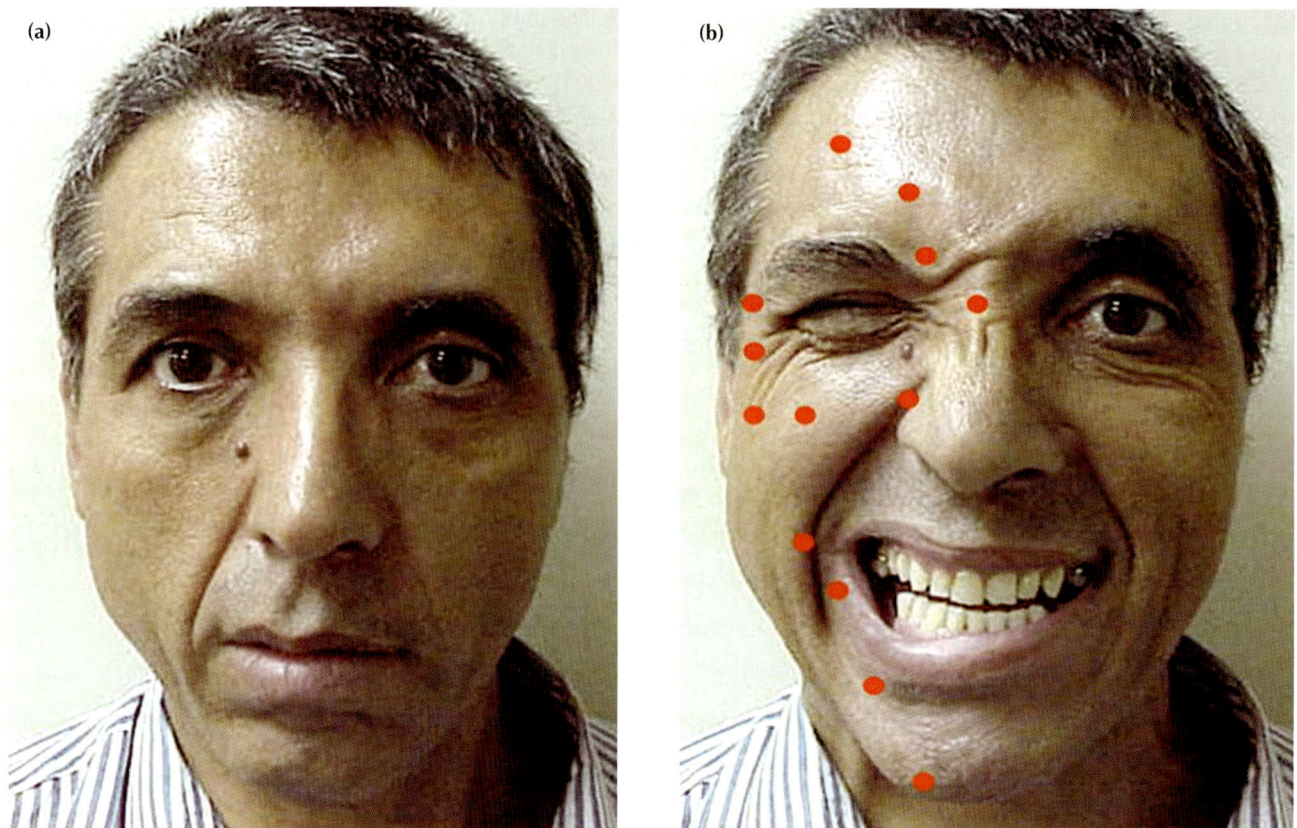

Figure 22.1   (a, b) Recommended injection sites with botulinum toxin (BTX) in the hyperkinetic side of the face. Facial asymmetry is more apparent when the patient smiles (b). The left-hand side is paralyzed and the right-hand side is hyperkinetic, promoting deviation and distortion to the non-affected side.

- major zygomatic muscle at its point of origin: 12.5 U (equivalent to 0.1 ml)
- minor zygomatic muscle at its point of origin: 6.25 U (equivalent to 0.05 ml)
- the labii superioris alaeque nasi levator at the level of the nasal arch: 6.25 U (equivalent to 0.05 ml)
- the levator labii superioris at the orbital margin: 6.25 U (equivalent to 0.05 ml)
- the modiolus, at a distance of 0.5 cm from the corner of the mouth: 12.5 U (equivalent to 0.1 ml)
- the risorius muscle, 2 cm from the corner of the mouth: 25 U (equivalent to 0.2 ml)
- the depressor anguli oris at 0.5 cm from the corner of the mouth: 25 U (equivalent to 0.2 ml)
- the depressor labii inferioris at a distance of 1.0 cm from the lip border: 18.75 U (equivalent to 0.15 ml)
- the frontalis at the hemipupillary line and at the medial part of the eyebrow at a distance of 1.0–2.0 cm: 25 U (equivalent to 0.2 ml)
- the corrugator at the medial portion of the eyebrow: 18.75 U (equivalent to 0.15 ml)
- the procerus at the frontonasal angle: 12.5 U (equivalent to 0.1 ml)
- the orbicularis oculi at the crow's feet level, two or three points: 12.5 U each (equivalent to 0.1 ml)
- the mentalis at the chin base: 12.5 U (equivalent to 0.1 ml).

Clinical results and adverse events

The target of treatment with BTX-A in controlling the hyperkinesis contralateral to facial palsy is to decrease the asymmetries in both static and dynamic positions. Depending on the degree of hyperkinesis, the adaptation of doses is required. It is important to treat all the muscles that act on a specific area, both synergistic and antagonistic. If the imbalance persists after the first injection, a complementary injection should be carried out after 15 days. High doses should be avoided in order not to block the minimal muscular tonus required, otherwise a completely flaccid appearance of the face may take place.

Eyebrow asymmetry is easily obtained with the blocking of the frontalis. In the perioral area, there is a smothering of the smile, the teeth and gingiva become well hidden, and the nasolabial fold softens (Figures 22.2 and 22.3). The duration of the effect varies according to the degree of hyperkinesis, but it generally lasts from 4 to 6 months.

Facial palsy leads to alterations in common tasks such as those of retaining solid food and liquids, chewing, pronouncing phonemes while speaking, and expressing emotions. Patients suffering from facial palsy go through a learning process in which they come to adapt to their limitations via methods that they themselves develop throughout their lives. They learn

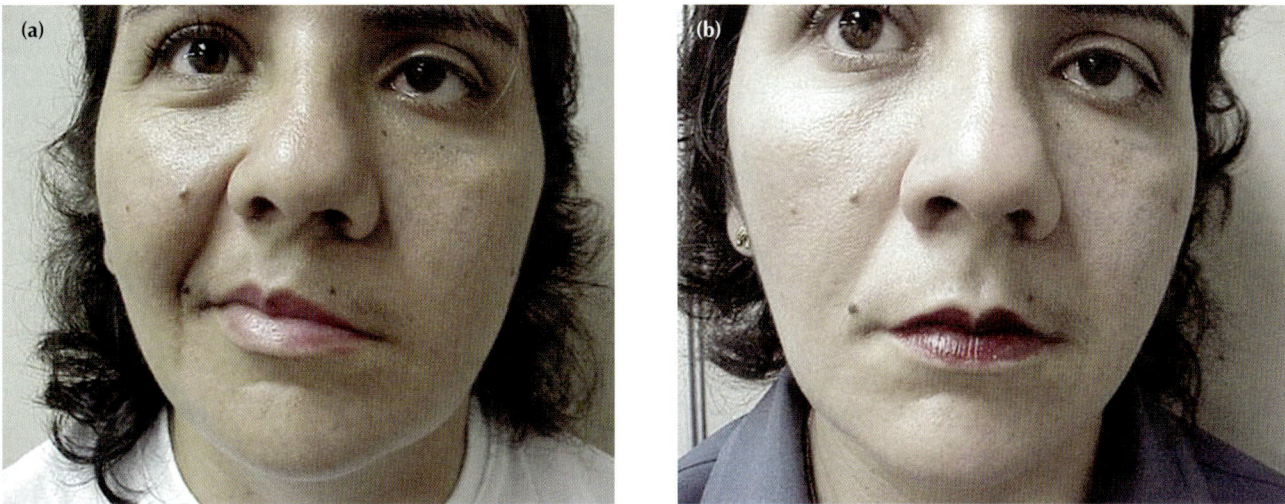

Figure 22.2 Static analysis. (a) Before treatment, the nasolabial fold is deeper and the lips are deviated to the hyperkinetic side. (b) After BTX-A, the nasolabial fold softens and the lips become balanced.

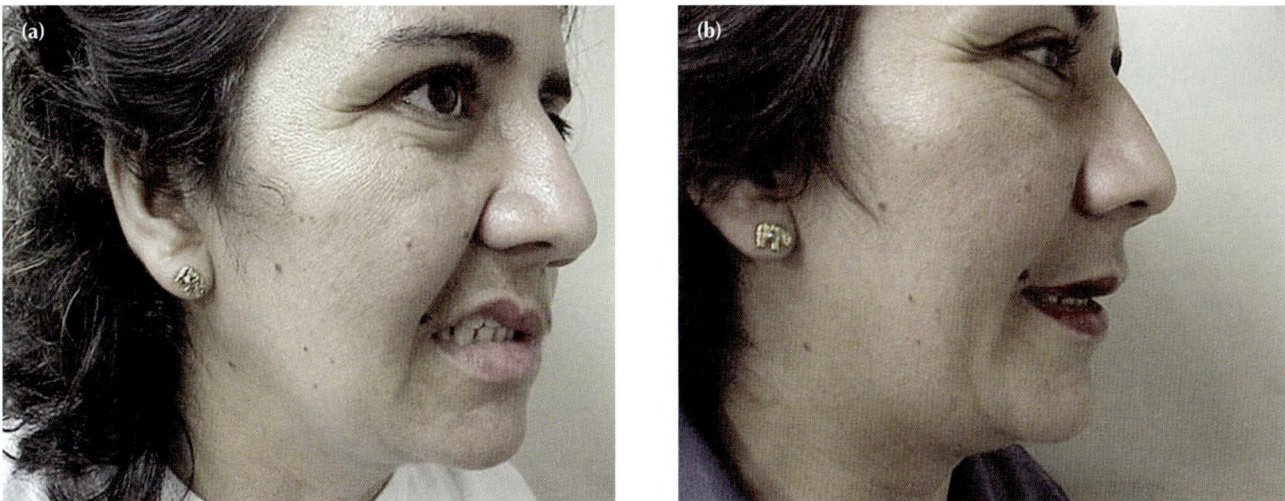

Figure 22.3 Dynamic analysis. (a) The hyperkinetic side produces distortion of the smile with excessive dental show. (b) After BTX-A treatment the lips return to their normal positions.

how to chew, how to speak, and how to express themselves in the most adequate manner possible. After the administration of botulinum toxin, there is an abrupt change in the mimetic muscles' behavior and, consequently, in patients' learning and adaptation patterns.

Early complications such as hematomas, infections, or allergies usually do not happen in the treatment of facial palsy with BTX-A. No irreversible complications occur such as permanent oral incontinence for solids and liquids or permanent difficulties in hearing, chewing, and speaking skills.

The main alterations in speech usually arise 15 days after the toxin has been administered and are related mainly to the patient's ability to pronounce the phonemes [f], [v], and [b]. Improvements in speech start to be noted 30 days after the injection.

Fifty per cent of patients complain of oral incontinence for (inability to retain) liquids, and difficulties in speaking and smiling, in the first 15 days after the injection. Usually, 40% have difficulties in bringing their lips close together or pursing them in the first 20 days following administration of the toxin. It is observed that all of these alterations improve with time due to patients' capacity to adapt to their new functional reality. These complications are short-lived, and the administration of botulinum toxin does not produce any systemic effect.

It must be pointed out that if some movements begin in the hyperkinetic side of the face it does not mean that the effect has been totally lost, but rather that a slow recovery of muscular activity is taking place, at a rate that may vary from patient to patient.

Conclusion

In the treatment of patients suffering from facial palsy, botulinum toxin may be considered an indispensable resource within the set of therapeutic measures taken up by professionals who deal with this type of deformity. Its wide range of possible indications as a non-surgical treatment, as a therapeutic test, or as a complementary measure in post-surgical treatments, such as neurectomies or myectomies, will make it a fundamental tool to promote advances in the treatment of facial palsy.

The fact that hyperkinesis contralateral to the facial palsy is weakened will most certainly reduce facial deviations and rotations. It can even speed up muscular activity in methods of reinnervation and muscle transplants. Yet, its most important feature seems to be the potential that this method holds for use in children and adolescents, who will greatly benefit during their phases of muscular and skeletal development. Undoubtedly, we will be producing less serious functional and esthetic impairment in our patients.

References

1. Samii M, Matthies C. Indication, technique and results of facial nerve reconstruction. Acta Neurochir 1994; 130: 125–39.
2. Boerner M, Seiff S. Etiology and management of facial palsy. Curr Opin Ophthalmol 1994; 5: 61–6.
3. Dawidjan B. Idiopathic facial palsy: a review and case study. J Dent Hyg 2001; 75: 316–21.
4. Aviv JE, Urken ML. Management of the paralysed face with microneurovascular free muscle transfer. Arch Otolaryngol Head Neck Surg 1992; 118: 909–12.
5. Rubin LR. Anatomy of facial expression In: Rubin LR. Reanimation of the Paralysed Face. New Approaches. St Louis: CV Mosby, 1977: 2–20.
6. Raia AA, Zerbini EJ. In: Clínica Cirúrgica Alípio Corrêa Netto, 4th edn. Sao Paulo: Sarvier, 1988: 465–73.
7. Blasley RW, Thorne CHM. In: Grabb & Smith's Plastic Surgery, 5th edn. Philadelphia: Lippincott-Raven, 1997: 554–7.
8. Ueda K, Hari K, Asato H, Yoshimura K, Yamada A. Evaluation of muscle graft using facial nerve on the affected side as a motor source in the treatment of facial palsy. Scand J Plast Reconstr Surg Hand Surg 1999; 33: 47–57.
9. Terzis JK, Kalantarian B. Microsurgical strategies in 74 patients for restoration of dynamic depressor muscle mechanism: a neglected target in facial reanimation. Plast Reconstr Surg 2000; 105: 1917–31.
10. Kermer C, Millesi W, Paternostro T, Nuhr M. Muscle-nerve-muscle neurotization of the orbicularis oris muscle. J Craniomaxillofac Surg 2001; 29: 302–6.
11. Labbe D. Lengthening temporalis myoplasty. Rev Stomatol Chir Maxillofac 2002; 103: 79–83.
12. Mountain RE, Murray JA, Quaba A. Management of facial synkinesis with clostridium botulinum toxin injection. Clin Otolaryngol 1992; 17: 223–4.
13. Kunihiro T, Kanzaki J, Yoshihara S, Satoh Y, Satoh A. Hypoglossial-facial nerve anastomosis after acoustic neuroma resection: influence of the time of anastomosis on recovery of facial movement. ORL J Otorhinolaryngol Relat Spec 1996; 58: 32–5.
14. Fine NA, Pribaz JJ, Orgill DP. Use of the innervated platysma flap in facial reanimation. Ann Plast Surg 1995; 34: 326–30.
15. Guereissi JO. Selective myectomy for postparetic facial synkinesis. Plast Reconstr Surg 1991; 87: 459–66.
16. Moser G, Oberascher G. Reanimation of the paralyzed face with new gold weight implants and goretex soft-tissue patches. Eur Arch Otorhinolaryngol 1997; 1: S76–8.
17. Adant JP. Endoscopically assisted suspension in facial palsy. Plast Reconstr Surg 1998; 102: 178–81.
18. Wong GB, Stokes RB, Stevenson TR, Whetzel TP, Saunders CJ. Endoscopically assisted facial suspension for the treatment of facial palsy. Plast Reconstr Surg 1999; 103; 970–1.
19. Shumrick KA, Pensak ML. Early perioperative use of polytef suspension for the management of facial palsy after extirpative skull base surgery. Arch Facial Plast Surg 2000; 2: 243–8.
20. Muhlbauer W, Fairley J, van Winderger J. Mimetic modulation for problem creases of the face. Aesthetic Plast Surg 1995; 19: 183–91.
21. Dobie RA, Fisch U. Primary and revision surgery (selective neurectomy) for facial hyperkinesia. Arch Otorhinolaryngol Head Neck Surg 1986; 112: 154–63.
22. Neuenschwander MC, Pribitkin EA, Sataloff RT. Botulinum toxin in otoryngology: a review of its actions and opportunity for use. Ear Nose Throat J 2000; 79: 788–9.
23. Verheyden J, Blitzer A, Brin MF. Other cosmetic uses of BOTOX. Semin Cutan Med Surg 2001; 20: 121–6.
24. Wang A, Jankovic J. Hemifacial spasm: clinical findings and treatment. Muscle Nerve 1998; 21: 1740–7.
25. Jankovic J, Schwartz K, Donovan DT. Botulinum toxin treatment of cranial-cervical dystonia, spasmodic dysphonia, other focal dystonias and hemifacial spasm. J Neurol Neurosurg Psychiatry 1990; 53: 633–9.
26. Badarny S, Giladi N, Honigman S. Botulinum toxin injection effective for post-peripheral facial nerve palsy synkinesis. Harefuah 1998; 135: 106–7.
27. Sadiq SA, Downes RN. A clinical algorithm for the management of facial nerve palsy from an oculoplastic perspective. Eye 1998; 12: 219–23.
28. Brans JW, Aramideh M, Schlingeman RO et al. Cornea protection in ptosis induced by botulinum injection. Ned Tijdschr Geneeskd 1996; 140: 1031–3.
29. Boroojerdi B, Ferbert A, Schwarz M, Herath H, Noth J. Botulinum toxin treatment of synkinesia and hyperlacrimation after facial palsy. J Neurol Neurosurg Psychiatry 1998; 65: 111–14.
30. Riemann R, Pfennigsdorf S, Riemann E, Naumann M. Successful treatment of crocodile tears by injection of botulinum toxin into the lacrimal gland: a case report. Ophthalmology 1999; 106: 2322–4.
31. Dressler D, Schonle PW. Hyperkinesias after hypoglossofacial nerve anastomosis – treatment with botulinum toxin. Eur Neurol 1991; 31: 44–6.
32. Clark RP, Berris CE. Botulinum toxin: a treatment for facial asymmetry caused by facial nerve palsy. Plast Reconstr Surg 1989; 84: 353–5.
33. Tulley P, Webb A, Chana JS et al. Palsy of the marginal mandibular branch of the facial nerve: treatment options. Br J Plast Surg 2000; 53: 378–85.
34. Sulica L. Botulinum toxin: basic science and clinical uses in otolaryngology. Laryngoscope 2001; 111: 218–26.
35. Jankovic J, Hallet M, eds. Therapy with Botulinum Toxin. New York: Marcel Dekker, 1994.
36. Dasgupta BR. Structures of botulinum neurotoxin, its functional domains and perspectives on the crystalline type A toxin. In: Jankovic J, Hallet M, eds. Therapy with Botulinum Toxin. New York: Marcel Dekker, 1994.
37. Carruthers A, Carruthers J. Botulinum toxin type A: history and current cosmetic use in the upper face. Semin Cutan Med Surg 2001; 20: 71–84.

38. Pellizari R, Rosseto O, Schiavo G, Montecucco C. Tetanus and botulinum neurotoxins: mechanism of action and therapeutic uses. Philos Trans R Soc Lond B Biol Sci 1999; 354: 259–68.

39. Simpson LL. Peripheral actions of the botulinum toxins. In: Simpson LL, ed. Botulinum Neurotoxin and Tetanus Toxin, 1st edn. New York: Academic Press, 1989: 153–78.

40. Simpson LL, Dasgupta BR. Botulinum neurotoxin type E: studies on mechanism of action and on structure activity relationships. J Pharmacol Exp Ther 1983; 224: 135–40.

41. Davis LE. Botulinum toxin – from poison to medicine. West J Med 1993; 158: 25–9.

42. Zhou LQ, de Paiva A, Liu D, Aoki R, Dolly JO. Expression and purification of the light chain of botulinum neurotoxin A: a single mutation abolishes its cleavage of SNAP 25 and neurotoxicity after reconstitution with the heavy chain. Biochemistry 1995; 34: 15175–81.

43. Dolly JO, Ashton AC, Mcinnes C et al. Clues to the multiphasic inhibitory action of botulinum neurotoxins on release of transmitters. J Physiol 1990; 84: 237–46.

44. de Paiva A, Meunier FA, Molgo J, Aoki KR, Dolly JO. Functional repair of motor endplates after botulinum neurotoxin type A poisoning: biphasic switch of synaptic activity between nerve sprouts and their parent terminals. Proc Natl Acad Sci USA 1999; 96: 3200–5.

45. Borodic GE, Cozzolino D. Blepharospasm and its treatment, with emphasis on the use of botulinum toxin. Plast Reconstr Surg 1989; 83: 546–54.

46. Borodic GE, Ferrante R. Effects of repeated botulinum toxin injections on orbicularis oculi muscle. J Clin Neuroophthalmol 1992; 12: 121–7.

47. Alderson K, Nebeker J, Holds JB, Anderson RL. Histologic features of human orbicularis oculi treated with botulinum A toxin. Arch Ophthalmol 1991; 109: 393–5.

48. Odergren T, Hjaltason H, Kaakkola S et al. A double blind, randomised, parallel group study to investigate the dose equivalence of Dysport and Botox in the treatment of cervical dystonia. J Neurol Neurosurg Psychiatry 1998; 64: 6–12.

49. Ranoux D, Gury C, Fondarai J, Mas JL, Zuber M. Respective potencies of Botox and Dysport: a double blind, randomised, crossover study in cervical dystonia. J Neurol Neurosurg Psychiatry 2002; 72: 459–62.

23 Hyperhidrosis and other dermatologic indications

Isaac Bodokh

Hyperhidrosis is a pathology for which there was hitherto no medical treatment. The treatment of hyperhidrosis using botulinum toxin A has been carried out for nearly 10 years. Its authorization for the treatment of axillary hyperhidrosis has been obtained in many countries (England, Switzerland, New Zealand, Canada, France, Germany). The other therapeutic alternatives such as local treatments (antiperspirants, iontophoresis), oral treatments (central atropinic agents), and surgical treatments (subcutaneous curettage of sweat glands, endoscopic transthoracic sympathectomy) are little used, and are either not very effective or responsible for significant side-effects. From this point of view, treatment of hyperhidrosis by using botulinum toxin has become increasingly important.

First, some physiopathogenic elements are discussed, then the treatment of hyperhidrosis by botulinum toxin is evaluated.

Hyperhidrosis is an excessive production of sweat by the eccrine glands, independent of the mechanisms of thermoregulation. Palmar and axillary hyperhidrosis, because of the significant embarrassment it causes, has psychological and social repercussions and can be responsible for true socioprofessional handicaps ranging from simply refusing to shake hands, to repeatedly having to change clothes, to significant perspiration with the least emotion.

It affects on average about 2.8% of the population, beginning in childhood, involving in nearly 50% of cases the axillae and in almost 25% the palms. Recently, preliminary results from the first European hyperhidrosis epidemiology survey showed that 2.3% of subjects had a formal diagnosis of hyperhidrosis and 0.6% of respondents had focal hyperhidrosis that 'frequently' or 'always' impacted on quality of life, in the absence of known comorbidities.[1]

Physiopathogenesis[2]

Present at birth and distributed over the whole of the body, the eccrine glands (2–4 million glands per individual) are responsible for the production of sweat. Their stimulation is controlled by the sympathetic cholinergic postganglionic nerve terminations, whose mediator is acetylcholine. Excretion of sweat is pulsatile, 0.3–12 secretions per minute, through the sweat pores at the top of the dermatoglyphic peaks. Hyperthermic stimulus is the dominating factor responsible for the physiological secretion of sweat. This secretion allows thermal regulation, which is seldom the reason for consultation because it is easily attenuated by local means, in contrast to secondary hyperhidrosis. Primary hyperdrosis can have psychogenic stimulus (emotion or stress), and be located predominantly on the palms, soles, face, and axillae. An etiology is found in fewer than 1% of cases. Generalized hyperhidrosis can occur in relation to metabolic disorders, neoplasias, and endocrinopathies or at the time of neurological problems.

Evaluation of hyperhidrosis

The distinction between physiological sweating and hyperhidrosis is not clearly established, and it is necessary before beginning a treatment to evaluate at least the zone of hyperhidrosis and the impact on quality of life. Other objective methods of evaluation of hyperhidrosis have relevance only for the realization of clinical studies.

Evaluation of the hyperhidrosis zone

It is important in the work-up of a treatment of hyperhidrosis to assess the affected area using Minor's iodine–starch test, which consists of applying to the hyperhidrosis zone a preparation based on iodine (2 g of iodine, 2 g of potassium, 100 g of ethanol for example) and then starch powder, making it possible to visualize as purple areas the regions of interest. With the palms, the copy paper test can be used by comparing absorption zones either by means of image processing and data analysis, or using reference ranking methods.[3,4]

The gravimetric method consists of weighing the quantity of sweat excreted in a given time. An absorbent paper is deposited for 1–5 minutes on the zone to be evaluated then is weighed. One thus determines the quantity of sweat excreted per minute. It is an excellent dynamic test of eccrine gland secretion, and at the time of axillary hyperhidrosis the quantity of sweat can exceed 900 mg per minute, with an average from 200 to 300 mg per minute. This test is used mainly during clinical studies.[5,6]

Measure of quality of life[7]

Various studies have shown the impact of hyperhidrosis on quality of life. In the majority of cases, a score is calculated using the DLQI (Dermatology Life Quality Index). This method makes it possible to measure the impact on quality of life in patients suffering from dermatological conditions (acne, psoriasis, eczema). Hyperhidrosis has a significant impact on quality of life, with an average DLQI score higher than that observed for other dermatological conditions. Other scales more specific to hyperhidrosis have been used, but only during clinical trials.

Several studies have shown the importance of this impact, with in particular a modification of social relations; a psychogenic effect can range from simple anxiety to depression and social isolation. Moreover, hyperhidrosis can lead to changes in dressing behavior in the choice of textiles and colors, and also in the number of changes of clothing (more than twice a day in 50% of cases).

Treatments

Before discussing the treatment of hyperhidrosis by botulinum toxin A, it is important to mention the treatments hitherto used according to the affected zone.

Local treatment

The use of antiperspirants has limited effectiveness in major hyperhidrosis. They may be beneficial only in reducing axillary 'hidrosis'. These substances act by preventing the flow of sweat by obstruction of the sweat pore via keratinization. In the presence of water, aluminum chloride in antiperspirants can dissolve to give hydrochloric acid, which can cause skin irritation when these stronger types are used in hyperhidrosis. They should on the other hand be used early in the relapse after treatment by botulinum toxin because they make it possible to delay the next injection.

Iontophoresis[8]

This is applicable only for the treatment of palmoplantar hyperhidrosis. The treatment sessions are sometimes unpleasant (tingling, itching), in particular with application of strong current intensities, or if cracks or wounds are present. If palmar hyperhidrosis is not very severe, it is effective in almost 70% of cases. It is advisable to test this treatment for palmar or plantar hyperhidrosis while awaiting precise methods of use of botulinum toxin A in this indication. It is only in the event of inefficiency of, intolerance to, or repeated treatments using iontophoresis for palmoplantar hyperhidrosis that botulinum toxin A injections are of interest.

Surgical treatments[9,10]

Skin en bloc resection or subcutaneous curettage of the axillary hyperhidrosis zone should not be considered because of the significant scarring risks, but more especially because of the effectiveness of and tolerance to the treatment of hyperhidrosis with botulinum toxin A in this localization.

Endoscopic transthoracic sympathectomy is a radical treatment of palmar hyperhidrosis. The intervention is carried out under general anesthesia, and the sympathetic nerve, located by thoracoscopy, is divided between the second and the fifth intercostal space carrying the second, third, fourth, and fifth sympathetic nerve ganglions. Morbidity associated with this procedure includes hospitalization and pneumothorax, but more especially the frequency of compensatory hyperhidrosis reaches 50–80% of cases according to studies, localized to the abdomen, back, lower limbs, nape of the neck, scalp, and gustatory glands. Therefore this treatment must be reserved for only severe recalcitrant palmar hyperhidrosis that is resistant to iontophoresis and to injections of botulinum toxin A.

Treatment by botulinum toxin A injection[11]

Botulinum toxin A injections are currently used within a very strict legislative framework. The treatment must be carried out by experts who are licensed and trained in the technique, with a co-responsibility pharmacist–doctor, and for specific indications (disorders of oculomotor system, blepharospasm, hemifacial disorder, spasmodic stiff neck, treatment of the dynamic deformation of club foot in a child, spasticity of the upper limb of an adult following a cerebrovascular accident), and more recently for treatment of severe axillary hyperhidrosis with psychological repercussions (South America, Canada, Australia, United Kingdom, New Zealand, Switzerland, France, Germany).

Botulinum toxin A is produced by *Clostridium botulinum*, an anaerobic bacterium responsible for the principal signs of botulism.[12] Its mechanism of action is the blocking of presynaptic acetylcholine of the cholinergic neurons. Botulinum toxin A is the most powerful of the neurotoxic types. At the time of hyperhidrosis, botulinum toxin A acts by blocking acetylcholine release, and thereby preventing peripheral cholinergic transmission of the eccrine glands (sweat, lacrimal, and salivary) without modification of glandular volume. The eccrine glands have cholinergic stimulation, whereas the apocrine glands have adrenergic stimulation. It should be noted that neurotransmitter receptors are present at the surface of nerve cells, Merkel cells, and all skin cells[13] on the cytoplasmic membrane, in particular acetylcholine receptors but also other receptors (substance P, catecholamine, melanocyte stimulating hormone). If these receptors are present at the surface of skin cells and if the stimulation of the eccrine glands is cholinergic, one can thus conclude that the mechanism of action of botulinum toxin on the eccrine glands is a blocking of their secretion.

There are mainly two types of botulinum toxin A currently used in France: Vistabel®/BOTOX® from Allergan and Dysport® from Ipsen. Vistabel® recently obtained a marketing authorization in France for the treatment of glabellar wrinkles, with delivery specifically from the laboratory to the physician (dermatologist, cosmetic surgeon, otorhinolaryngologist, facial surgeon). This is the same product as BOTOX which, under this name, should be injected only for the treatment of glabellar wrinkles.

Botulinum toxin A has been used for more than 10 years for the treatment of hyperhidrosis (Frey's syndrome, Ross' syndrome, circumscribed unilateral idiopathic hyperhidrosis: palmar, plantar, axillary, even in diffuse hyperhidrosis). Its use for the treatment of axillary hyperhidrosis is currently well established, and it is advisable to individualize treatment with botulinum toxin in this indication because not only are therapeutic methods established compared to other indications, but in this indication only BOTOX has authorization for the treatment of severe axillary hyperhidrosis with psychological and social repercussions, only in a hospital setting, carried out by a specialist who is accustomed to using the technique.

Treatment of axillary hyperhidrosis by botulinum toxin A[11,14]

Multiple studies have shown the effectiveness of treatment by botulinum toxin A for axillary hyperhidrosis. The majority are related to the use of BOTOX, a few less to Dysport. These studies report variable dosing of BOTOX of 20–200 U per axilla and of Dysport from 100 to 300 U. The effectiveness of this treatment varies from 70 to 98% reduction in the quantity of secreted sweat; nevertheless, there seems to be a longer duration of remission with larger doses. Currently, in many countries only BOTOX has obtained approval, and it is advisable to prefer this treatment because the methods are well established, following major double-blind placebo-controlled studies with qualitative and quantitative evaluation of the secretion of sweat, and the effect of the rate/frequency of injections on quality of life.

One of the most interesting studies is that of Naumann et al.[14] It related to the treatment of patients presenting persistent bilateral axillary hyperhidrosis, having a secretion of axillary sweating higher than 50 mg per 5 minutes which interfered with the quality of life. This was a multicenter, double-blind, placebo-controlled study. Fifty units of BOTOX per axilla were injected, and patients were followed during more than 1 year, with a possibility of second and third injections. In the first week, treated patients presented a reduction of the quantity of sweat secreted, with a clear improvement in quality of life, in particular a reduction in the number of changes of clothing per day and an improvement of both social and work situations. Overall there were no side-effects apart from a perception of an increase in perspiration at sites other than the axillary zone in 5% of cases versus 1.3% of the placebo group. The average duration of effectiveness was 10 months (6–18 months).

Methods of treatment by BOTOX

Practical considerations are:

- each vial of BOTOX contains 100 U of botulinum toxin A
- dilute the contents of the vial in 4 ml of sterile saline solution 0.9% without preservative (use vacuum to draw the diluent into the vial)
- gently mix by rotating the vial
- the reconstituted solution in the vial can be stored in a refrigerator for 4 hours maximum
- use small volume syringes (0.5–1 ml), needles of 30G and 4 mm length, reducing pain by changing needles when they become blunt
- inject a maximum of 50 U (2 ml) into each axilla, in 10–15 points.

Axillary preparation and iodine–starch test The patient should not use antiperspirant during the 7 days before treatment. The patient should shave the axillae 1 day before treatment. The zones of perspiration are localized using Minor's iodine–starch test:

- dry the axilla
- paint on the iodine solution (2 g of iodine, 2 g of potassium, 100 ml of water or ethanol), allow to dry
- spread the starch powder on the skin and wait 5 minutes: the zone to be treated assumes a purplish coloring (reaction of chlorine in sweat with iodine) (Figure 23.1)
- delimit the edges of the colored zone with a marker
- remove any starch residue (Figure 23.2)

The technique of injection is as follows:

- divide the zone into squares from 1.5 to 2 cm to obtain 10–15 equidistant injection sites
- introduce the needle, bevel upwards, ensuring injections remain intradermal

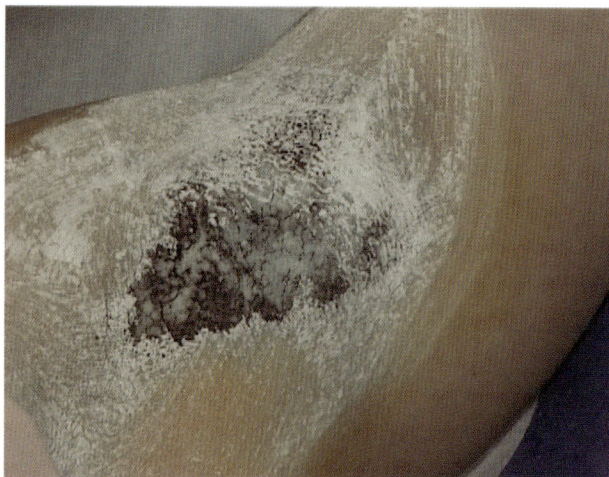

Figure 23.1   Minor's test before treatment.

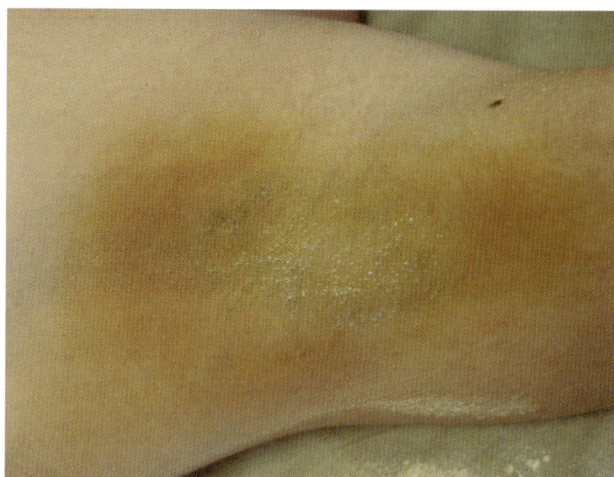

Figure 23.3   Minor's test 1 month after treatment.

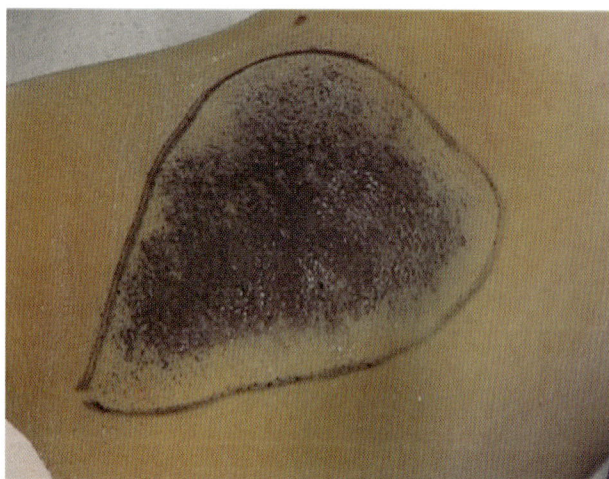

Figure 23.2   Minor's test: hyperhydrosis zone selected.

- 0.1–0.2 ml is injected per site
- an anesthetic cream can be applied to minimize discomfort (after having determined the zone to treat): await 30–60 minutes before injection.

Contraindications   Botulinum toxin A is contraindicated in people having a known oversensitivity to one of the components of the preparation, in the presence of generalized disorders of muscular activity (myasthenia gravis), in the event of concomitant or probable use of aminosides or spectinomycin, in the event of treatment by anticoagulants, and if pregnant or breastfeeding.

We recommend the use of this technique for the treatment of axillary hyperhidrosis (Figure 23.3).

Palmar treatment of hyperhidrosis by botulinum toxin A[6,15–18]

In contrast to the treatment of axillary hyperhidrosis, the treatment of palmar hyperhidrosis is currently not

systematized. Here, too, the majority of clinical studies have been carried out with BOTOX, and a few with Dysport. These were mainly open studies where 20–220 U of BOTOX per hand were injected and between 200 and 300 U Dysport per hand.

Multiple anesthetic techniques have been proposed (nerve block, local by EMLA® cream under occlusion, local by iontophoresis of xylocaine, application of ice packs, application of liquid nitrogen, coolant gel, general anesthesia, intravenous anesthesia, Dermojet®).

After treatment, an improvement in perspiration from a reduction of 40% to total anhidrosis has been reported by various authors. The duration of effect varies from 3 to 18 months, and there still seems a correlation between the duration of effect and dosage amount.

Reported side-effects are pain with injection, secondary pain with anesthesia, anhidrosis, hematomas, and, in 5% of patients according to some authors, a transitory reduction in muscular force prevailing in the fingers and for the thumb–index finger pinch. This side-effect was shown by electromyography.

Very few comparative studies are reported. Our study[6] compared treated and untreated hands, after nerve block, injecting 3 U every 2 cm, with, on average, 60–80 U of BOTOX in the treated hand. Lowe et al[16] used 100 U of BOTOX per hand in a double-blind, placebo-controlled study (the monitoring period was only 28 days).

In our study, there was an improvement in the quantity of sweat secreted (in gravimetric and analytical rank tests), with a reduction of hyperhidrosis in 75% of the patients; nevertheless, only 60% of them wanted to resume the treatment.

After 5 years which therapeutic methods do we advise?   A nerve block is carried out after injection of 2 ml of xylocaine with adrenaline on the level of the median and cubital nerves to 3 cm from the flexing area of the wrist, after performing Minor's test to locate the hyperhidrosis zone. After careful squaring of the skin, using injections of, on average 1 U per cm², we distributed 100 U of BOTOX per hand, decreasing by half the amount on the level of the thenar eminence and avoiding injecting the small muscles of the fingers. Injections in the finger pulp are used for hyperhidrosis of the fingers. The condition persists in a certain number of patients, and larger amounts of toxin are required to have an effect. For this reason it is preferable to carry out a test with the amount that we will inject 1–2 weeks before treatment, for example with 3, 4, or 5 U.

Treatment of localized hyperhidrosis (Frey's syndrome, face, body)

After the first publications concerning the effectiveness of treatment by botulinum toxin A of Frey's syndrome,[20] Laccourreyre et al[21] reported the treatment of 30 patients with Frey's syndrome post-parotidectomy, in whom 2.5 U per cm² were injected after Minor's test to determine the treatment zone. Treatment effectiveness was found in the majority of cases for a duration of approximately 16 months. Two patients presented a transitory ipsilateral paresis. Since then, in several publications, the consensus was to inject on average 1 U per cm² intradermally. Using this dose, motor disorders did not occur.

This dosage of 1 U per cm² of BOTOX or 3–4 U of Dysport is currently advocated by many authors and ourselves for the treatment of localized hyperhidrosis,[20] i.e. for the treatment of Frey's syndrome, unilateral circumscribed idiopathic hyperhidrosis, and paradoxical hyperhidrosis secondary to sympathectomy.

Other indications of botulinum toxin

Treatment of Hailey–Hailey disease[23]   Hailey–Hailey disease is a hereditary condition exacerbated by sweat, moisture, and friction. Lapiere et al were the first to report complete regression of this condition by using 50 U of BOTOX in the axillae.

Treatment of odor   Heckmann et al[24] recently reported the effectiveness on odor of treatment using Dysport in a randomized study versus placebo, with evaluation by T-shirt sniff test, among 16 patients. The patients presented a reduction of perspiration but also a clear reduction in odor.

It should be noted that odor depends mainly on apocrine sweat glands. Apocrine glands appear during puberty mainly in the anogenital area and the axillae. Their contents are opalescent, viscous, and very rich in lipids. Their role is the lubrication of hairs and the synthesis of pheromones.

Hyperhidrosis is seldom associated with the malodorous characteristic of sweat, which is due to the action of gram-positive bacteria that degrade the fatty acids which prevail in apocrine glands rich in lipids.

Eccrine glands are cholinergic, and apocrine glands are largely adrenergic but also cholinergic, and respond to cholinergic stimulation mediated by acetylcholine. Thus, the improvement of axillary body odor reported by Heckmann et al is certainly secondary to the action of botulinum toxin on apocrine sweat glands.

Treatment of hidradenitis suppurativa[25]   We carried out treatment of two patients presenting with recurrent and recalcitrant hidradenitis suppurativa or Verneuil's disease. Various methods have been applied to treat this condition, in particular antibiotics, ciproterone acetate, isotretinoin, and surgery. Symptoms are prevalent in the axillae, around the nipples, on the buttocks, and in the anogenital area. BOTOX 100 U were injected on the right then 100 U on the left. The effectiveness was significant in the two patients with, in one of them, no recurrence of nodules in 1 year.

Treatment of other eccrine glands   The lacrimal and salivary glands are cholinergic eccrine glands for which some publications have shown the effectiveness of botulinum toxin A. This is the case in the treatment of crocodile tears by injection of botulinum toxin A, 2 U BOTOX or 6 U Dysport, in the principal lacrimal gland through the superoexternal part of the eyelid. There is no risk of ptosis in this localization; nevertheless, the risk of diplopia limits this indication to severe forms.

The treatment of hypersialorrhea involves injection of botulinum toxin A, 2 U BOTOX, into the parotid salivary gland, under the mental nerve, showing good effectiveness up to nearly 1 year.

Action on pruritus mediated by acetylcholine[26]   Acetylcholine is a neurotransmitter involved in pruritus in atopic dermatitis, and is present at the level of the skin receptors. Heckmann et al[26] have reported the effectiveness of botulinum toxin A (Dysport) for the treatment of lichen simplex, and Swartling[27] for the treatment of palmar dyshidrosis with an effectiveness which remains nevertheless to be demonstrated.

Therapeutic indications

It is advisable to systematically propose a topical antiperspirant for hyperhidrosis.

Palmar hyperhidrosis

In the event of inefficiency of the topical antiperspirant and of embarrassment affecting quality of life in the case of palmar and plantar hyperhidrosis, it is first of all necessary to test treatment by iontophoresis.

If iontophoresis fails, treatment with botulinum toxin A can be proposed, informing the patient of the risks of muscular atrophy and including in the work-up a test to determine the effective amount of injection. Upon obtaining effectiveness, antiperspirant cream can be proposed then a fast resumption of iontophoresis.

In the event of lack of success with combined topical, iontophoresis, and botulinum toxin A treatment, it is advisable to propose to the patient treatment by selective endoscopic transthoracic sympathectomy, informing them of the frequent risks of paradoxical hyperhidrosis.

Plantar hyperhidrosis

It is necessary to propose local treatments first, then iontophoresis, and to try to leave it there, because treatment with botulinum toxin A often requires increased amounts and shorter duration of effectiveness compared with palmar or axillary hyperhidrosis.

Localized hyperhidrosis (Frey's syndrome, focal hyperhidrosis)

After Minor's test and in the event of failure of local topical treatments, botulinum toxin A injections, BOTOX 1 U per cm² or Dysport 3 U per cm², can be proposed.

Axillary hyperhidrosis

To start with, local treatment with cream or lotion should be used. In the event of inefficiency and social embarrassment, it is preferable because of its appoval to propose BOTOX, according to the therapeutic methods previously described.

With relapse, the use of a topical antiperspirant must be quickly resumed in order to space out the botulinum toxin injections.

In the event of inefficiency of botulinum toxin, surgical excision by liposuction is to be preferred over skin en bloc resection, but only by a surgeon familiar with the technique and after having informed the patient of the risks of relapse and scarring.

Conclusion

Treatment of axillary hyperhidrosis using botulinum toxin A is currently well established. Its almost unvarying effectiveness begins during the third day, and the average duration is 10 months (4–18 months). It clearly improves quality of life and is to be preferred over local treatments in the event that axillary hyperhidrosis interferes with quality of life. It is a significant therapeutic option for a condition in which,

hitherto, treatments were not very effective or carried the risk of significant scarring.

Concerning palmar hyperhidrosis, this treatment can be tried, but precise therapeutic methods are not established.

The other indications remain anecdotal, and must be used only during clinical trials by physicians accustomed to the technique.

References

1. Hamm H, Bodokh I, Naumann M et al. Prevalence of hyperhidrosis and its impact on quality of life: preliminary results from the first European hyperhidrosis epidemiology survey in France and Germany. Presented at EADV 2005: 14th Congress, London, October, 2005: 15–17.
2. Agache P, Candas V. Physiologie de la sécrétion sudorale eccrine. Encycl Med Chir Dermatol 1997: 12-230-1-10.
3. Bodokh I. Hyperhidrose palmaire. Ann Dermatol Venereol 2003; 130: 561–4.
4. Bodokh I, Branger E. Nouvelle méthode d'évaluation de l'hyperhidrose palmaire. Ann Dermatol Venereol 2001; 128: P299.
5. Naumann M, Hofmann U, Bergmann I et al. Focal hyperhidrosis: effective treatment with intracutaneous botulinum toxin. Arch Dermatol 1998; 134: 301–4.
6. Bodokh I, Branger E. Traitement de l'hyperhidrose palmaire par toxine botulinique. Ann Dermatol Venereol 2001; 128: 833–4.
7. Campanati A, Penna L, Menotta L et al. Quality of life assessment in patients suffering from hyperhidrosis and its modification after treatment with botulinum toxin: results of an open-label study. Clin Ther 2003; 25: 293–308.
8. Kreyden O. Iontophoresis for palmoplantar hyperhidrosis. J Cosmet Dermatol 2004; 3: 211 14.
9. Rompel R, Scholz S. Subcutaneous curettage vs. injection of botulinum toxin A for treatment of axillary hyperhidrosis. J Eur Acad Dermatol Venereol 2001; 15: 207–11.
10. Nicolas C, Grosdidier G, Granel F et al. Hyperhidroses palmoplantaires: traitement par sympathectomie endoscopique sur 107 patients. Ann Dermatol Venereol 2000; 127: 1057–63.
11. Lowe N, Campanati A, Bodokh I et al. The place of botulinum toxin type A in the treatment of focal hyperhidrosis. Br J Dermatol 2004; 151: 1115–22.
12. Aoki KR, Ismail M, Tang-Liu D et al. Standard botulinum toxin A: from toxin to therapeutic agent. Or J Neurol 1997; 4 (Suppl 2): S1–3.
13. Misery L. Skin immunity and the nervous system. Br J Dermatol 1997; 137: 843–50.
14. Naumann M, Bergmann I, Hofmann U et al. Focal botulinum toxin for hyperhidrosis: technical considerations and improvment in application. Br J Dermatol 1998; 139: 1123–4.
15. Naumann M, Flachenecker P, Brocker EB. Botulinum toxin for palmar hyperhidrosis. Lancet 1997; 349: 252.
16. Lowe NJ, Yamauchi PS, Lask GP et al. Efficacy and safety of standard botulinum toxin A in the treatment of palmar hyperhidrosis: a double-blind, randomized, placebo-controlled study. Dermatol Surg 2002; 28: 822–7.
17. Simonetta Moreau M, Cauhepe C, Magues JP et al. A double-blind, randomized comparative study of Dysport® vs Botox® in primary palmar hyperhidrosis. Br J Dermatol 2003; 149: 1041–5.
18. Kavanagh GM, Oh C, Shams K. Botox® delivery by iontophoresis. Br J Dermatol 2004;151: 1093–5.

19. Swartling C, Farnstrand C, Abt G et al. Side effects of intra-dermal injections of botulinum A toxin in the treatment of palmar hyperhidrosis: a neurophysiological study. Eur J Neurol 2001; 8: 451–6.

20. Laskawi R, Dobrik C, Schonebeck C. Up to date carryforward of botulinum toxin standard A treatment in patients with gustatory sweating (Frey's syndrome). Laryngoscope 1998; 108: 381–4.

21. Laccourreyre O, Muscatello R, Guttierez-Fonseca et al. Syndrome de Frey sévère post-parotidectomie: traitement par la neurotoxine botulinique de type A. Ann Otolaryngol Chir Cervicofac 1999; 116: 137–42.

22. Kreyden C, Schmid-Grendelmeier P, Burg G. Idiopathic localized unilateral hyperhidrosis: case report of successful treatment with botulinum toxin standard A and review of the literature. Arch Dermatol 2001; 137: 1622–5.

23. Lapiere JC, Hirsch A, Gordon KB et al. Standard botulinum toxin A for the treatment of axillary Hailey-Hailey disease. Dermatol Surg 2000; 26: 371–4.

24. Heckmann M, Teichmann B, Pause BM et al. Improvement of body odor after intracutaneous axillary injection of botulinum toxin A. Arch Dermatol 2003; 139: 57–9.

25. Bodokh I. Traitement de la maladie de Verneuil par injection de toxine botulinique A. Ann Dermatol Venereol 2004; 131: 1S229.

26. Heckmann M, Heyer G, Brunner B et al. Botulinum toxin type A injection in the treatment of lichen simplex: an open pilot study. J Am Acad Dermatol 2002; 46: 617–19.

27. Swartling C. Botulinum toxin in the treatment of focal hyperhidrosis and dyshidrotic hand dermatitis. Acta Universitatis Uppsaliensis, 2002.

24 Other dermatologic indications

Doris Hexsel, Rosemari Mazzuco, and Berthold Rzany

Introduction

Since the Carruthers made their description in the late 1980s,[1] innumerable new cosmetic indications for the use of botulinum toxins (BTXs) have been and continue to be suggested in congresses and in the literature. Such indications are based on the proven safety of the product, the wide clinical experience obtained with the use of BTX,[2] and the high satisfaction level expressed by treated patients.[3]

Although BTX is mainly indicated for use on the upper third of the face,[4–6] it represents a first-line therapeutic option for some less frequent cosmetic alterations, being used either alone or adjunctively with other procedures.[7] These rare or uncommon indications require expertise and skill on the part of the physician to ensure accurate diagnosis and correct management.

The general guidelines for the storage, dilution, directions, and contraindications of BTX are the same as those for use in the classical indications.[2,5] The dosage and injection sites should be individualized[8] for each indication and in the specific case of each patient.

Based on one author's (DH) prior considerable personal experience with BOTOX®, and 2 years' experience, totaling more than 5000 treatments, with Dysport®, the dose equivalence recommended in this chapter is situated between 2 and 2.5 U of Dysport to 1 U of the 100-U botulinum toxins. Such equivalence is based on the personal experience of one of the authors and is not intended to meet commercial interests, but those of physicians and patients who seek to make safe use of the products commercially available. The dose equivalence of 1:2.5 U can be obtained simply by diluting Dysport with double the volume of 0.9% saline utilized for BOTOX or Prosigne® and, in this way, it can be safely applied using the same techniques and volumes of diluted product. Likewise, in order to obtain a dilution of 1:2 U between the two products, Dysport can be diluted in two and a half times the volume utilized for BOTOX or Prosigne. Contrary to some suggestions made in the literature, the use in cosmetic applications of equivalences higher than 1:2.5 U, between the units of BOTOX and Prosigne on the one hand and units of Dysport on the other, is not recommended due to the serious side-effects experienced by patients, caused by the higher potency of Dysport. Such effects are more common and unpleasant on the lower face, where the musculature is more responsive to small doses of these products. There is no advantage in the use of higher doses or dose equivalences,[9] and, moreover, the possible side-effects are undesirable for both physicians and patients and may compromise the physician–patient relationship.

Rare or less frequent indications of botulinum toxin

Widening of the palpebral opening and infraorbital wrinkles

Excessive contraction of the lower eyelid portion of the orbicularis oculi muscle, particularly when smiling, results in the shrinking of the orbital aperture. Although this does not represent an esthetic disorder, some patients desire a wider ocular opening, since it promotes a more 'inviting' or 'attractive' look.[10] The demand for an 'eye-Westernizing' effect is common among Asians.[10]

Recently, the use of BTX has been indicated in order to obtain a rounded and widened ocular opening. The application of BTX into the preseptal area of the lower eyelid, used in treatment of the lateral portion of the orbicularis muscle (crow's feet wrinkles), has proved to be useful in widening of the ocular aperture,[10] particularly for Asian patients.

Furthermore, hypertrophy of the lower palpebral aspect of the orbicularis muscle favors the premature development of wrinkles, a relatively common condition among atopic patients. Application of BTX causes partial relaxation of the orbicularis oculi muscle, a reduction in lower eyelid thickness, and improvement of the wrinkles in this area.

The technique involves intradermal injection of 1–2 U (maximum of 4 U[10]) of BOTOX or Prosigne, or 2–4 U of Dysport into the medial–pupil line, 1–3 mm from the ciliary rim.[3,11] Another injection of 1 U of either BOTOX[12] or Prosigne, or 1–2.5 U of Dysport, can be

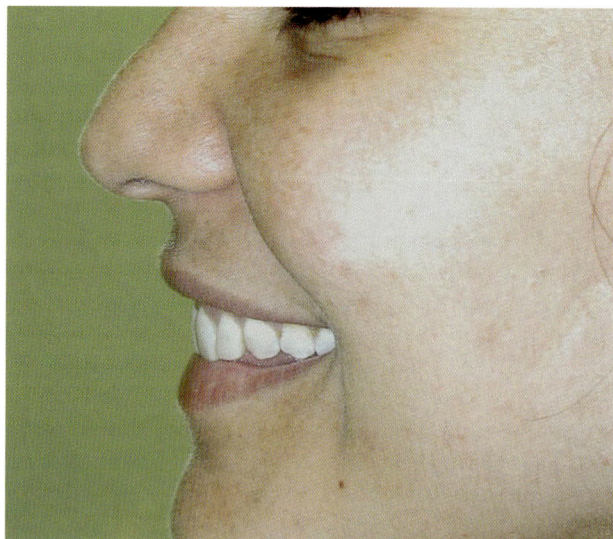

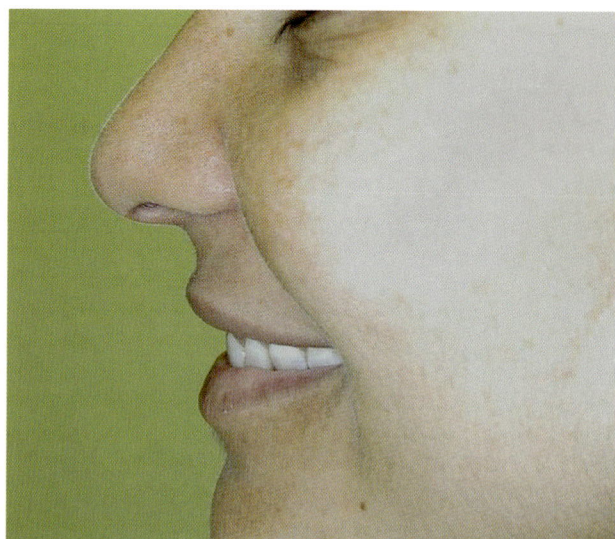

Figure 24.1   Raising the tip of the nose. Before and after 30 days of application of 4 U of Dysport®.

applied at a point midway between the medial–pupil line and the outer corner of the eye.[12]

Higher doses imply a higher risk of complications, such as lower eyelid edema and impaired sphincter function, without adding benefit.[10,11]

The palpebral portion of the orbicularis muscle is involved in palpebral closing, and its excessive relaxation leads to severe physiological disorder. Therefore, high doses of BTX, very frequent reapplication, or large numbers of applications in these areas are contraindicated, which is also the case for the upper eyelid.

Frequently repeated injections into this area might also lead to the development of palpebral pouches, caused by permanent relaxation of the lower portion of the orbicularis oculi muscle and the swelling of the fatty pouches, which occurs with aging. Such an effect is typically seen in patients with facial palsy, in which the paralyzed side presents more eye bulging.

For people presenting significant flaccidity of the lower eyelid, clinically identified by the 'snap test',[13] the injection of BTX into the lower eyelid is contraindicated, because it may lead to ectropion or excessive exposure of the sclera. (NB: to read a positive snap test is quite rare; nevertheless the test should always be performed.) Likewise, people with mild flaccidity of the orbicularis oculi muscle may develop a 'sad eye' appearance, through exposure of the lower portion of the sclera.

Elevation of the nasal tip

The nasal septum depressor muscle is responsible for the lowering of the nasal tip during speech and when smiling.[14] This movement is usually minor in most patients but can be quite excessive in some patients.

Repeated contractions of this muscle, together with intrinsic aging, tend to lead to ptosis of the nasal tip.

The contraction of the nasal septum depressor muscle can be easily seen in profile, by asking the patient to smile and move the lips in such a way as to invert the upper lip against the posterior surface of the upper teeth, or through the motion of the lips during speech (Figure 24.1). The action of this muscle can be effectively suppressed by treatment with BTX.[15]

Treatment with BTX will reduce involuntary nasal dipping. Elevation of the nasal tip has a partial effect, and some cases of initial ptosis can be improved. The recommended doses are low, which entails shorter duration of the effect, when compared to the effects produced by the doses used on the upper third of the face.[16]

The technique consists of the application of 2–4 U of BOTOX[16,17] or Prosigne or of 5–10 U of Dysport at the junction between the columella and the upper lip. To assist the injection session, the columella-base area may be manually held between two fingers in order to maintain the labial orbicularis muscle at a distance and so avoid injecting this muscle, which might cause impairment of the labial suction function.[17] Similarly, this procedure should be used carefully in patients in whom the cutaneous part of the upper lip is elongated, because of the risk of worsening the condition.[2] One author suggests the application of a further 2–6 U of BOTOX,[18] or the same dosage of Prosigne, or yet, 4–12 U of Dysport, into each side of the nasal muscle (transverse portion). However, such a technique might result in the dilatation of the nasal introitus, which would be undesirable to some patients.[17]

As a secondary effect, the injection of BTX into the depressor muscle of the nasal septum can induce an increase in the volume of the medial portion of the upper lip.[17]

Flaring of the nasal wings

The movement of the nasal wings and the dilatation of the nasal introitus are produced by the contraction of the inferior fibers that correspond to the dilating portion of the nasal muscle[2] during speech and breathing. Such movements are intended to facilitate the passage of air through the nose, and are more intense during tachypnea, which occurs in situations of physical stress or anxiety. Some patients present excessive and involuntary contractions of this muscle, causing embarrassment.

Injections of 5–10 U of BOTOX or Prosigne, or 10–20 U of Dysport into the middle of each nasal wing improve nasal wing flaring.[2]

Retraction of nasolabial furrow

Depressions of the nasolabial furrow are produced mainly through tissue absorption, especially that of bone and adipose tissue, which typically occurs with the intrinsic aging process.[19,20] In those patients that use exaggerated facial mimics during speech or when smiling, the intense and repetitious contraction of the elevator muscle of the upper lip and of the nasal wing contributes to the deepening of the furrow.

For correction of the nasolabial furrow, the most indicated procedures are filling techniques and/or Subcision®.[21,22] Intense muscular contraction, in addition to contributing to deepening of the furrow, may interfere with the result and the duration of effect of certain fillers, due to the risk of displacing the injected material.[23] In such cases, mild muscular relaxation with BTX may be indicated,[24] especially in patients with a short upper lip.

BTX can be used alone or adjunctively to procedures such as filling and/or resurfacing.[2] The recommended dose is from 0.5 to 1 U of BOTOX[20] or Prosigne or from 1 to 2.5 U of Dysport injected into the point of greatest muscular contraction, generally the nasal–malar furrow.

This procedure may cause asymmetry during smiling and ptosis or stretching of the upper lip,[2] for which reason this indication is restricted to selected cases.

Position of the labial or oral commissures

Drooping of the oral commissures, caused by the action of the anguli oris depressor muscle, produces a 'sad' appearance.[18]

The condition can be treated with the application of 4–8 U of BOTOX[18] or Prosigne, or of 8–16 U of Dysport, which can be injected directly into the belly of each depressor anguli oris or, indirectly, with an injection into the imaginary line that follows from the nasal furrow, at jaw level, reaching the muscle through the action halo of the BTXs. These injections elevate the labial commissures, which is a desired effect for some patients, though in excessive doses they may impair the smiling function or other mouth movements.

Treatment of the mouth levators is fraught with difficulties, and doses should be very small. Because these muscles are very responsive to BTX injections, overcorrection may result. The weakness of the zygomaticus major and minor muscles could cause ptosis of the superior lip. If this weakness is considered unilateral, the result will be labial asymmetry with ptosis of the affected lip. In this case, the treatment would be with 1–2 units of botulinum toxin into the origin of the zygomaticus major on the normal side, on the body of the zygoma.[25]

Gingival smile

Exaggerated gum exposure while smiling is a relatively common esthetic-function problem, which was previously treatable only through surgery. The three possible causes for gingival smile are: excessive maxillary development, which occurs in patients with facial height beyond normal average; abnormally short upper lips; and excessive length of the upper teeth.[26]

The muscle responsible for gum exposure is the upper lip and nasal wing levator muscle (levator labii superioris alaeque nasi).[26] The contraction of these fibers, in addition to contributing to gingival smile, may cause nasal furrow retractions and the formation of a horizontal infranasal furrow on the upper lip.[26]

The injection of 1–5 U of BOTOX[27] or Prosigne, or 2.5–7.5 of Dysport at each side of the upper lip and the nasal wing levator muscle, into the nasomalar furrow, causes the lowering and elongation of the upper lip, covering the gum during smiling (Figure 24.2). Higher doses or dose equivalence greater than 1:2 U between BOTOX/Prosigne and Dysport for the treatment of gingival smile is contraindicated because of side-effects related to the potency of Dysport, such as labial ptosis while smiling and difficulty in word articulation. Likewise, patients with an elongated upper lip may experience worsening of this condition.[2]

Masseter muscle hypertrophy

Hypertrophy of the masseter muscle can cause alteration to the contour of the lower jaw, often giving the face a squared appearance, particularly when it develops early on, and is more common among Asians. Besides muscular hypertrophy, the enlarged aspect of the lower third of the Asian face also results from the larger size of the jawbone and the deposition of fat around it.[28] The hypertrophied muscle can cause pain in the jaw area and in the temporomandibular articulations, causing impairment of the mouth-opening function.[29] The diagnosis of this alteration is made

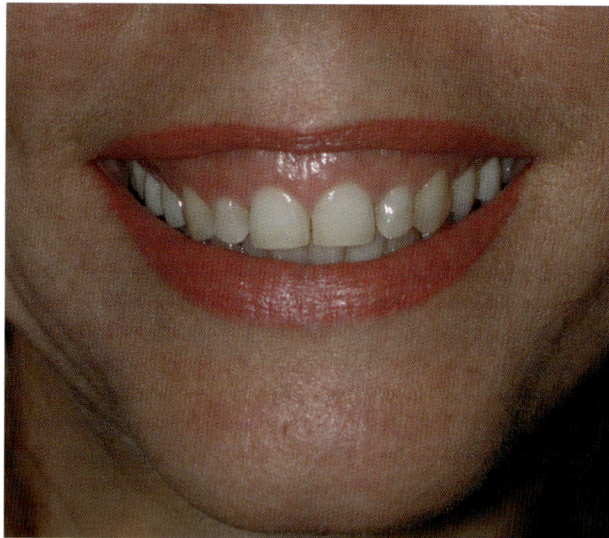

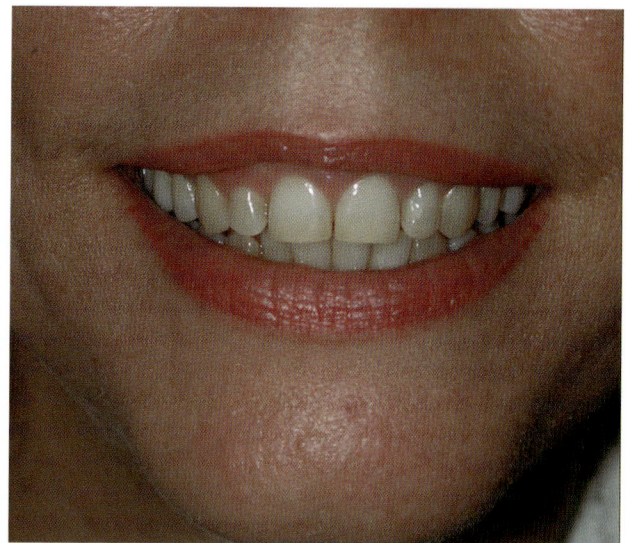

Figure 24.2   Before and after 3 U BOTOX® in each side of the upper lip levator for the treatment of 'gummy smile'.

clinically,[29] but additional tests may be required for differential diagnosis with the deposition of fatty matter.[29]

The demand for treatments capable of reducing the masseteric volume is quite high among Asians,[30] and conventional muscle removal surgery is a widespread practice.

The application of BTX for the correction of masseteric hypertrophy was first suggested in 1994,[31,32] based on the principle of provoking muscular atrophy from disuse. In other words, muscular relaxation produced by BTX, and the consequent decrease in contraction potency, in the medium term, result in ensured muscular atrophy.[33,34] The reduction in muscle thickness takes effect about 2–8 weeks after treatment, with peak effect being attained at about 12 weeks,[35] and lasting 9 months[36] to 1 year.[37–39] The reduction in pain level occurs soon after treatment, and some months later there is improvement to the square-faced aspect.[37–39]

The dosage utilized varies from 25[30] to 30 U[35] of BOTOX or Prosigne or from 50 to 75 U of Dysport injected into each muscle belly. These doses are considered high, but they are consistent with the principle that large and potent muscles require higher doses of BTX.[2] Moreover, higher doses are required in order to achieve the desired muscular atrophy. Reinforcement doses may be applied, if necessary.[30] Recently, it was suggested that the minimal dose should be 20 U of BOTOX[36] or Prosigne, or 40–75 U of Dysport into the belly of each masseteric muscle. Please note that in Caucasian patients the doses used should be initially one-third of the recommended dose in Asian patients. In Caucasian patients treatment of the masseter is often done not for facial shaping, but for the treatment of bruxism.

It is important to note that the malar area in Asian people tends to be prominent, and may become more apparent with the reduction in masseteric thickness.[28] Such an effect, while considered desirable by some patients, may be undesirable for others, and thus for the latter, injections of BTX into the masseteric muscle would be contraindicated. No significant adverse effects have been described.[29,31,32]

Facial asymmetries

Mild facial asymmetries are common and considered normal, frequently going unnoticed by patients, except during photographic assessment (Figure 24.3).[2]

Asymmetries may be caused by bone elements or soft tissue, or originate from neurological or muscular causes.[2] The two latter categories can be classified into hyperfunctional (e.g. hemifacial spasm) or hypofunctional (e.g. facial palsy). BTX can be used for the correction of asymmetries of neurological or muscular origin.

Paralysis of the facial nerve (VII cranial par) is a frequent cause of prominent facial asymmetries, which are accompanied by significant functional alterations. Facial palsy can be considered congenital or acquired.[25] Among the main causes of acquired facial palsy, of particular note are: trauma (whether surgical or not); infection; tumor; and cerebral vascular accident.[25] Muscular paralysis on one side of the face results in contralateral muscular hyperkinesis and consequent deviation of the facial structures towards that side.

On the upper third of the face, there is paralysis and drooping of the eyebrow on the affected side. The eyebrow on the normal side is raised further with contraction of the normal fibers of the frontalis muscle and orbicularis oculi. As a large part of the musculature of the middle and lower thirds of the face is functionally related to the lips and mouth, facial palsy results in

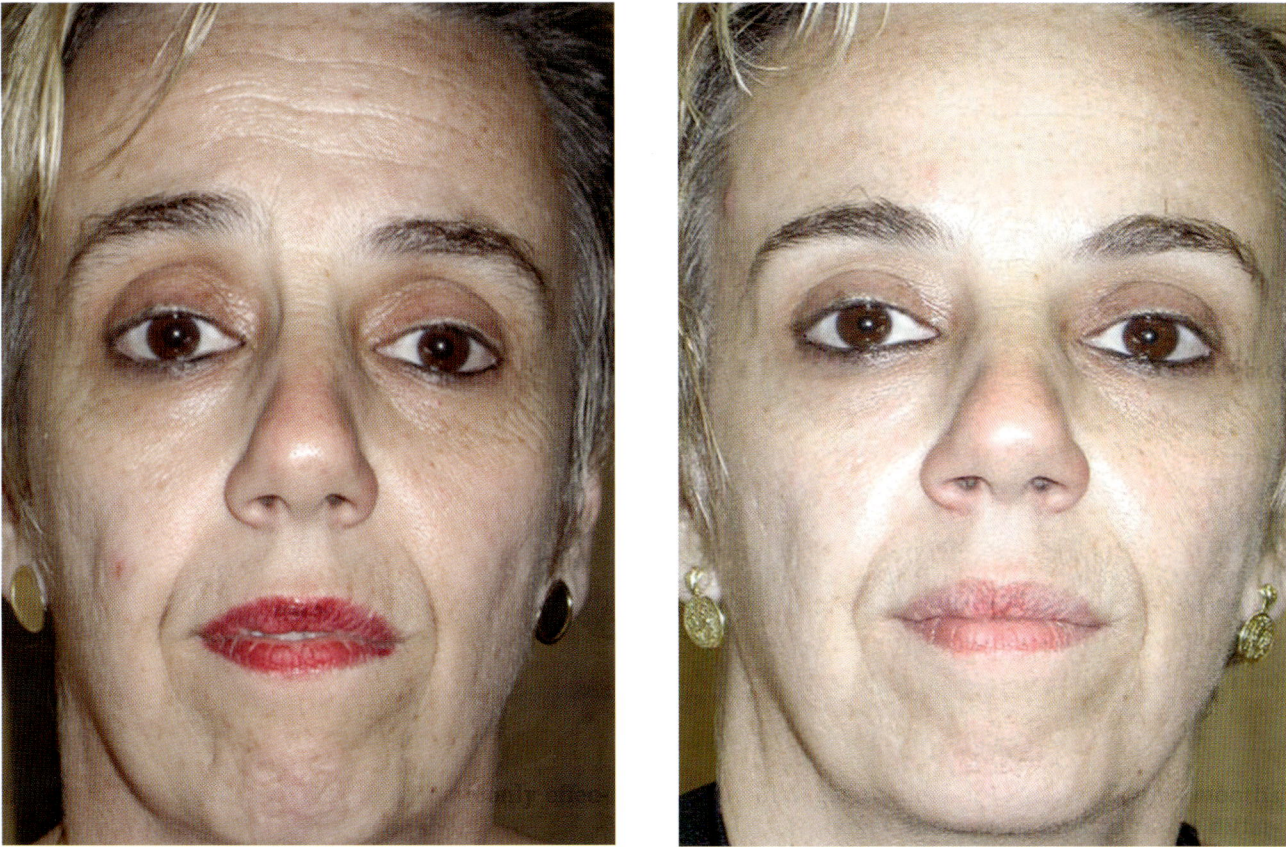

Figure 24.3   Before and after treatment with botulinum toxin (BTX) injections for treatment of the upper third of the face. 'Before' image shows asymmetries in the forehead lines and brow position.

drooping of the upper lip and of the labial commissures, ipsilateral to the injured side. The labial rim is drawn to the normal side, principally during speech and smiling, due to the contraction of the upper lip elevator complex, the risorius, the masseter, and the orbicularis oris.[40,41]

In addition to the specific treatment of the cause, BTXs are indicated for the correction of muscular hyperkinesis of the normal side, aiming to decrease the facial asymmetry and reposition the eyebrow. Physiotherapy for muscular stimulation of the affected side should be recommended. On the upper third of the face, the technique for the application of BTX is the same as that described for conventional cosmetic treatment: BTX should be injected into the glabella, periorbital area, and some hyperkinetic points of the frontalis zone. It is important to establish symmetry of the doses and injection points.

Neurological lesions, from either trauma or surgery, may result in localized paralysis. The most common lesions are of the temporal and marginal mandibular branches of the VII cranial par, resulting respectively in the drooping of the eyebrow and asymmetry of the lower lip. In such cases, too, BTX can be injected selectively into the muscle of the normal side, taking care to use lower doses on the lower third of the face, due to the risk of worsening the functional condition.[42]

For the correction of eyebrow asymmetry, BTX should be injected into the depressor muscles (the glabella and orbicularis oculi complex) of the affected side and into the frontal muscle of the normal side.

On the middle third of the face, 0.5–1 U of BOTOX[43] or Prosigne, or 1–2.5 U of Dysport can be injected into some sites within the areas of greatest contraction of the zygomatic, risorius, the upper lip and nasal wing levator, and orbicularis oris muscles. Total dosage should not be higher than 4–5 U of BOTOX or Prosigne, or 8–10 U of Dysport, on the hyperkinetic side, due to the risk of compromising the labial function. Electromyography is a very useful method for localizing small muscles of anomalous localization, either in non-responsive cases or cases with mild or localized asymmetry.[16,44–46]

In order to avoid depression of the labial commissure after the relaxation of the levator muscles, it is advisable to inject 1–3 U of BOTOX or Prosigne, or 2–7.5 U of Dysport into the depressor muscle of the corner of the mouth, on the hyperkinetic side. For older patients, the dosage should be reduced.[47]

Doses ranging between 1 and 2 U of BOTOX or Prosigne, or between 2 and 5 U of Dysport into the depressor anguli oris muscle, and of 1–3 U of BOTOX or Prosigne, or 2–7.5 U of Dysport into the mentalis muscle on the normal side, are in general sufficient to improve lower lip asymmetry.

The duration of the BTX effect in asymmetries of the middle and lower thirds of the face is, in general, short, with normal contraction returning in about 8 weeks.[16] The reason for the shorter duration of effect is the low dose required for these treatments, which in general only provides a partial relaxation of the musculature.[48,49]

It is important to highlight that BTX intervals should not be too close to each other, due to the risk that it might theoretically induce the formation of antibodies,[16] although there are no reports of resistance to BTX for cosmetic use.[45,50]

Stabilization of scarring processes and treatment of retractable scars

BTXs can be used in the prevention of scar formation, that is, in assisting the scar healing process, or when the scarring process has been concluded and resulted in retractable scars, which worsen with movement of the adjacent musculature.

One of the causes of dystrophic scar development is the intense motion of the area during the scarring process.

Although, ideally, most surgical procedures on the body should have postoperative movement suppressed by the use of short duration effect BTXs (up to 30 days), these are not as yet available on the market.

However, in some cases, BTX-As can be used in full or partial doses, providing greater stabilization of the surgical area for measured periods, which can be coincidental with the duration of immobilization recommended for the postoperative period.

While the face is the main cosmetic focus, where the principal cosmetic indications for the use of BTXs are localized, it is also frequently the location of pathologies treated surgically, such as skin cancer, which can result in scarring. Such procedures, when coincidentally performed on the cosmetic areas of the face, can be combined with BTX injections in the postoperative period, in order to inhibit muscular movement of the mentioned areas, where the scars, surgical bruises, or traumatic lesions are located, thus providing more esthetic scars.

Another indication of BTXs in relation to scarring is where scars are worsened through the action of the facial expression muscles, or muscles in other areas of the body. BTXs can be used to smooth out such scars, reducing the retraction caused by muscle action during facial expression.

Décolleté wrinkles

The action of the medial fibers of the major pectoral muscle and the caudal portion of the platysma muscle can cause trunk or neckline wrinkles. In such cases, e.g. when wrinkles of the décolleté can be actively

produced, BTX injection can be used, and this is dealt with in Chapter 20.

Breast lifting

According to the results published by Dr Smith from Canada, and Dr Perez-Atamoros from Mexico, injections of botulinum toxin A into the three segments of the minor pectoralis muscle, or into three sites of the major pectoralis muscle, should be capable of producing improvement in the appearance of drooping or asymmetrical breasts. However, in a pilot study conducted by one of the present authors (DH), concrete results of the beneficial effects of BTX injections toward this end were not reproduced (see Chapter 20.)

Leg contour

Female legs have historically been the object of strong esthetic appeal and, therefore, there is concern to maintain them within certain standards. Recently, some criteria have been suggested to describe the esthetically desirable features for the contour of the legs.[51]

The superficial contour of the posterior face of the leg is mainly provided by the gastrocnemius muscle.[52] Hypertrophy of the medial belly of this muscle, a rather frequent feature among some women, and particularly common among Asians, results in the thickening of the medial portion of the leg, affecting self-esteem and limiting exposure of the lower limbs. In the majority of cases, the cause of the hypertrophy is unknown.[53]

Being a muscle-related problem, surgical muscular resectioning is the procedure of choice,[54] since liposuction would neither be effective nor indicated,[52] and may result in sequelae.

BTX use was recently suggested for the treatment of gastrocnemius hypertrophy. The BTX injection action would produce an effect comparable to that provided in the treatment of the masseter, resulting in a degree of atrophy from the disuse produced by the BTX.[53] The use of BTX in this condition is considered safe, because the gastrocnemius muscle is functionally redundant.[53] Suggested doses range from 32 to 72 U of BOTOX[53] or Prosigne, or from 75 to 200 U of Dysport injected into each side. The exact dose for each patient is calculated according to the muscular thickness when contracted, and the physician should ask the patient to stand on tiptoe, so as to differentiate the muscular hypertrophy from the localized fat deposits. Hypertrophy becomes more prominent in the latter position. The dose is distributed into 3–6 injections performed with a long needle at intramuscular level, at intervals of 1.5–2.0 cm along the medial muscular belly.[53] If there is hypertrophy of the lateral belly, injections into this site will also be required.

Muscle atrophy takes effect 1 month post-BTX injection session and lasts for about 6 months.[53] Authors do not report functional problems after BTX injection sessions with this condition.[53]

Other rare indications for botulinum toxin

Some recently published articles mention BTX as a rather effective therapeutic option for the cosmetic improvement of age-related cutis laxa,[55] and the treatment of frontal hyperhidrosis[56] and facial flushing.[57]

Cutis laxa, or elastosis, is characterized by the complete loss of skin elasticity that typically appears with aging. Tamura et al reported the case of a patient who was given botulinum toxin injections into the classical areas for dynamic wrinkles and, as a result, showed improved appearance in terms of skin aging and of the cutis laxa.[55]

Facial flushing is quite a common skin problem among patients with fair skin and those having certain conditions, such as rosacea. Although it is a transient condition in most cases, some patients present persistently red skin tone, with periods of more intense erythema. There are several reports in the literature of cases of the use of botulinum toxin for the treatment of persistent facial flushing, with good results,[57] as well as for the development of flushing in the neck area. The treatment consists of injecting 2 U of BOTOX or Prosigne, or 4–5 U of Dysport per site, in a triangle, to a total of 100 U per session (of BOTOX) with injections repeated after 2 weeks.[58]

Conclusion

In addition to the satisfactory effects obtained with BTX injections for the classical indications of the upper third of the face, and others, frequently mentioned, such as indications for the middle and lower thirds of the face and the neck, there is clinical evidence of effective results being achieved for other indications, such as those referred to in this chapter.

It is likely that in the future new indications will be described, as well as new toxins to be incorporated into our medical practice.

References

1. Carruthers JD, Carruthers JA. Treatment of glabellar frown lines with C. botulinum-A exotoxin. J Dermatol Surg Oncol 1992; 18: 17–21.
2. Carruthers J, Carruthers A. Aesthetic botulinum A toxin in the mid and lower face and neck. Dermatol Surg 2003; 29: 468–76.
3. Sommer B, Zschocke I, Bergfeld D, Sattler G, Augustin M. Satisfaction of patients after treatment with botulinum toxin for dynamic facial lines. Dermatol Surg 2003; 29: 456–60.
4. Markey AC. Botulinum A exotoxin in cosmetic dermatology. Clin Exp Dermatol 2000; 25: 173–5.
5. Klein AW. Dilution and storage of botulinum toxin. Dermatol Surg 1998; 24: 1179–80.
6. Elson ML. Anesthesia for lip augmentation [Letter]. Dermatol Surg 1997; 23: 401.
7. Hexsel D. Combining procedures with botulinum toxin in dermatology and dermatological surgery. In: Hexsel D, Almeida AT, eds. Cosmetic Use of Botulinum Toxin, 1st edn. Porto Alegre: AGE, 2002: 211–15.
8. Edelstein C, Shorr N, Jacobs J, Balch K, Goldberg R. Oculoplastic experience with the cosmetic use of botulinum A exotoxin. Dermatol Surg 1998; 24: 1208–12.
9. Hexsel D, Dal Forno Dini T, Prado-Zechmeister D, Hexsel C. Diffusion, dispersion, or action halos of botulinum toxin? A pilot study comparing two commercial preparations of type A botulinum toxins. Am J Dermatol 2005; 52: AB2.
10. Flynn TC, Carruthers JA, Carruthers JA. Botulinum-A toxin treatment of the lower eyelid improves infraorbital rhytides and widens the eye. Dermatol Surg 2001; 27: 703–8.
11. Flynn TC, Carruthers JA, Carruthers JA, Clark RE II. Botulinum A toxin (BOTOX) in the lower eyelid: dose-finding study. Dermatol Surg 2003; 29: 943–50.
12. Magalhães F, Magalhães L. Malar wrinkles. In: Hexsel D, Almeida AT, eds. Cosmetic Use of Botulinum Toxin, 1st edn. Porto Alegre: AGE, 2002: 164–6.
13. Fagien S. Botox for the treatment of dynamic and hyperkinetic facial lines and furrows: adjunctive use in facial aesthetic surgery. Plast Reconst Surg 1999; 103: 701–13.
14. Gray's Anatomy, 38th edn. Edinburgh: Churchill Livingstone, 1995.
15. Carruthers J, Carruthers A. Practical cosmetic Botox techniques. J Cutan Med Surg 1999; 3 (Suppl 4): S49–52.
16. Hexsel D, Mazzuco R, Dal'Forno T, Hexsel CL. Toxina botulínica: 12. Aplicações não-clássicas. In: Kede MPV, Sabatovich O, eds. Dermatologia Estética. Rio de Janeiro: Atheneu, 2003: 573–81.
17. Almeida AT. Nariz. In: Hexsel D, Almeida AT, eds. Uso Cosmético da Toxina Botulínica. Porto Alegre: AGE, 2002: 155–7.
18. Atamoros P. Botulinum toxin in the lower one third of the face. Clin Dermatol 2003; 21: 505–12.
19. Fenske NA, Lober CW. Structural and functional changes of normal aging skin. J Am Acad Dermatol 1986; 15: 571–85.
20. Lowe N, Yamauchi P. Cosmetic uses of botulinum toxins for lower aspects of the face and neck. Clin Dermatol 2004; 22: 18–22.
21. Hexsel DM, Mazzuco R. Subcision: a treatment for cellulite. Int J Dermatol 2000; 39: 539–44.
22. Orentreich DS, Orentreich N. Subcutaneous incisionless (subcision) surgery for the correction of depressed scars and wrinkles. Dermatol Surg 1995; 21: 543–9.
23. Mazzuco R. Perioral wrinckles. In: Hexsel D, Almeida AT, eds. Cosmetic Use of Botulinum Toxin, 1st edn. Porto Alegre: AGE, 2002: 158–63.
24. Kane MA. The effect of botulinum toxin injections on the nasolabial fold. Plast Reconstr Surg 2003; 112: 66–72.
25. Finn JC. Botulinum toxin type A: fine-tuning treatment of facial nerve injury. J Drugs Dermatol 2004; 3: 133–7.
26. Coscarelli J. Gingival smile. In: Hexsel D, Almeida AT, eds. Cosmetic Use of Botulinum Toxin, 1st edn. Porto Alegre: AGE, 2002: 199–200.
27. Carruthers J, Carruthers A. Botox treatment for expressive facial lines and wrinkles. Curr Opin Otolaryngol Head Neck Surg 2000; 8: 357–61.
28. Kim NH, Chung JH, Park RH, Park JB. The use of botulinum toxin type A in aesthetic mandibular contouring. Plast Reconstr Surg 2005; 115: 919–30.
29. Castro WH, Gomez RS, Da Silva Oliveira J, Moura MD, Gomez RS. Botulinum toxin type A in the management of masseter muscle hypertrophy. J Oral Maxillofac Surg 2005; 63: 20–4.

30. Ahn J, Horn C, Blitzer A. Botulinum toxin for masseter reduction in Asian patients. Arch Facial Plast Surg 2004; 6: 188–91.

31. Moore AP, Wood GD. The medical management of masseteric hypertrophy with botulinum toxin type A. Br J Oral Maxilllofac Surg 1994; 32: 26–8.

32. Smyth AG. Botulinum toxin treatment of bilateral masseteric hypertrophy. Br J Oral Maxillofac Surg 1994; 32: 29–33.

33. Park MY, Ahn KI, Jung DS. Botulinum toxin type A treatment for contouring of the lower face. Dermatol Surg 2003; 29: 477–83.

34. Almeida AT. Treatment of masseteric hypertrophy. In: Hexsel DM, Almeida AT, eds. Cosmetic Use of Botulinum Toxin, 1st edn. Porto Alegre: AGE, 2002: 185–6.

35. Kim HJ, Yum KW, Lee SS, Heo MS, Seo K. Effects of botulinum toxin type A on bilateral masseteric hypertrophy evaluated with computed tomographic measurement. Dermatol Surg 2003; 29: 484–9.

36. Choe SW, Cho WI, Lee CK, Seo SJ. Effects of botulinum toxin type A on contouring of the lower face. Dermatol Surg 2005; 31: 502–7.

37. To EW, Ahuja AT, Ho WS et al. A prospective study of the effect of botulinum toxin A on masseteric muscle hypertrophy with ultrasonographic and electromyographic measurement. Br J Plast Surg 2001; 54: 197–200.

38. von Lindern JJ, Niederhagen B, Appel T, Berge S, Reich RH. Type A botulinum toxin for the treatment of hypertrophy of the masseter and temporal muscles: an alternative treatment. Plast Reconstr Surg 2001; 107: 327–32.

39. Finn S, Ryan P, Sleeman D. The medical management of masseteric hypertrophy with botulinum toxin. J Ir Dent Assoc 2000; 46: 84–6.

40. Greenway HT, Breisch EA. Superficial cutaneous anatomy. In: Robinson JK, Arndt KA, LeBoit PE, Wintroub BU, eds. Atlas of Cutaneous Surgery. Philadelphia: WB Saunders, 1996: 5–20.

41. Breisch EA, Greenway HT. What basic surgical concepts and procedures are required for the practice of cutaneous medicine and surgery? In: Arndt KA, Le Boit PE, Robinson JK, Wintroub BU, eds. Cutaneous Medicine and Surgery. Philadelphia: WB Saunders, 1996: 111–20.

42. Carruthers J, Carruthers A. Aesthetic botulinum toxin in the mid and lower face and neck. Dermatol Surg 2003; 29: 468–76.

43. Fagien S. Temporary management of upper lid ptosis, lid malposition, and eyelid fissure asymmetry with botulinum toxin type A. Plast Reconstr Surg 2004; 114: 1892–902.

44. Khawaja HA, Hernandez-Perez E. Botox in dermatology. Int J Dermatol 2001; 40: 311–17.

45. Carruthers A, Carruthers J. Botulinum toxin type A: history and current cosmetic use in the upper face. Semin Cutan Med Surg 2001; 20: 71–84.

46. Klein AW, Mantell A. Electromyographic guidance in injecting botulinum toxin. Dermatol Surg 1998; 24: 1184–6.

47. Lowe NJ. Botulinum toxin type A for facial rejuvenation: United States and United Kingdom perspectives. Dermatol Surg 1998; 24: 1216–18.

48. Benedetto AV. The cosmetic uses of botulinum toxin type A. Int J Dermatol 1999; 38: 641–55.

49. Shyamala C, Huilgol FACD, Carruthers A, Carruthers JDA. Raising eyebrows with botulinum toxin. Dermatol Surg 1999; 25: 373–6.

50. Wollina U, Konrad H. Managing adverse events associated with botulinum toxin type A: a focus on cosmetic procedures. Am J Clin Dermatol 2005; 6: 141–50.

51. Tsai CC, Lin SD, Lai CS, Lin TM. Aesthetic analysis of the ideal female legs. Aesth Plast Surg 2000; 24: 303–5.

52. Kim IG, Hwang SH, Lew JM, Lee HY. Endoscope-assisted calf reduction in Orientals. Plast Reconstr Surg 2000; 106: 713–20.

53. Lee HJ, Lee DW, Park YH et al. Botulinum toxin A for aesthetic contouring of enlarged medial gastrocnemius muscle. Dermatol Surg 2004; 30: 867–71.

54. Lemperle G, Exner K. The resection of gastrocnemius muscles in aesthetically disturbing calf hypertrophy. Plast Reconstr Surg 1998; 102: 2230–6.

55. Tamura BM, Lourenço LM, Platt A et al. Cutis laxa: improvement of facial aesthetics by using botulinum toxin. Dermatol Surg 2004; 30: 1518–20.

56. Kinkelin I, Hund M, Naumann M, Hamm H. Effective treatment of frontal hyperhidrosis with botulinum toxin A. Br J Dermatol 2000; 143: 824–7.

57. Yuraitis M, Jacob CI. Botulinum toxin for the treatment of facial flushing. Dermatol Surg 2004; 30: 102–4.

58. Pierzchala E, Boleslawska M. Treatment of anterior chest wall flushing syndrome with botulin toxin. Poster presented at IV World Congress of the International Academy of Cosmetic Dermatology (IACD), Paris, France, 2005; 24: 33.

25 Medical and surgical combinations with botulinum toxins*

Benjamin Ascher and Bernard Rossi

Introduction

If expression lines are associated with muscle, fat, and skin ptosis, and/or with deep or non-hyperkinetic furrows and other surface alterations, surgical procedures and/or other surface treatments are recommended. Botulinum toxin injections are not meant to replace upper, mid-, or lower face- and neck lifts; on the contrary, they are often combined with these procedures and optimize their results. This combination of medical and surgical treatments is one of the main current trends in plastic and cosmetic surgery in 2008.

Botulinum toxin combined with other surgical cosmetic treatments

The 'chemical nerve section' achieved by botulinum toxin provides a very effective, adjustable, and lasting treatment of expression lines, whereas surgery and alternative medical treatments are often associated with higher risks and shorter-lived effects. Moreover, this product not only treats wrinkles, but is also able to correct, at least partly, the shape and position of the eyebrows by altering the muscle balance (see Figures 15.4 and 15.5). However, if the expression lines are associated with muscle, fat, and skin ptosis, and/or with deep or non-hyperkinetic furrows and other surface alterations, surgical procedures and surface treatments are recommended. Patients are increasingly seeking less invasive techniques, preferring injectables, lasers, photorejuvenation, and peels, which are now more effective.[1] Botulinum toxin is a major non-surgical treatment, which in some cases may improve the results of surgery and alternative medical treatments. However, it also has its own limits, which must be explained clearly to patients. Botulinum toxin is also seen increasingly as an essential preparation to a medical or surgical cosmetic procedure, if injected beforehand, and more importantly as a means to prolong the results, if injected afterward.

Although some authors inject the toxin during the operation,[2,3] we believe that generally botulinum toxin must not be injected at the same time as another treatment, whether medical or surgical, to avoid diffusion to other muscles caused by the resulting edema. Although most authors consider that the toxin may diffuse up to 2 cm, its diffusion potential has been demonstrated to exceed 3 cm, especially if large volumes are injected or if bleeding occurs.[4,5]

Botulinum toxin combined with lower eyelid surgery

What is the best interval between the injection of botulinum toxin and the surgical procedure? Although there is no consensus,[1] a minimum of 15 days,[6,7] or better 3 weeks,[8,9] seems to be reasonable.

The resulting immobilization of the orbicularis, a wide and powerful depressor muscle, has multiple advantages:

- Minimum 3 weeks before lower eyelid blepharoplasty: whether transconjunctival or subciliary, it helps to treat crow's feet, which surgery does not correct, and reduces traction on scar tissue, ectropion, and transient conjunctivitis. Immobilization of the skin and muscles reduces tension on the stitches and operated areas, and may improve the healing processes.[1] However, this preparatory treatment has two disadvantages: a greater risk of edema due to lack of massage of the eyelid lymph vessels, and difficulties in outlining the skin to be excised before the surgery, if the patient has not been photographed before the injection.
- Between 1 and 2 months after lower eyelid blepharoplasty: botulinum toxin injections reduce any residual hypertonia in the orbicularis, as well as surface lines. These lines must be treated with microdoses

*Portions of this chapter were previously published as 'Toxine botulique et rides' in *Annales de chirurgie plastique et esthétique* 2004; 49: 537–52, reproduced with permission of Elsevier SAS.

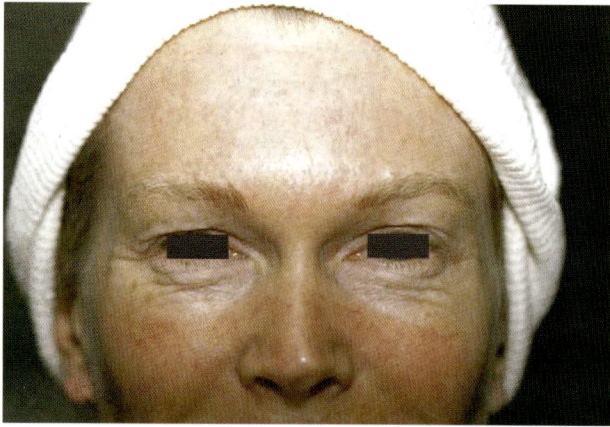

Figure 25.1   Blepharochalasis of the upper and lower eyelids. Hypertonia of the inferior orbicularis.

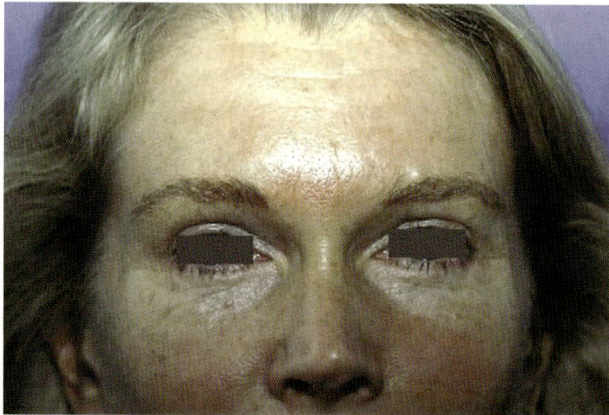

Figure 25.2   Results 5 years after blepharoplasty of all four eyelids and maintenance with botulinum toxin type A injections every year, from the third year, in crow's feet and lower eyelid.

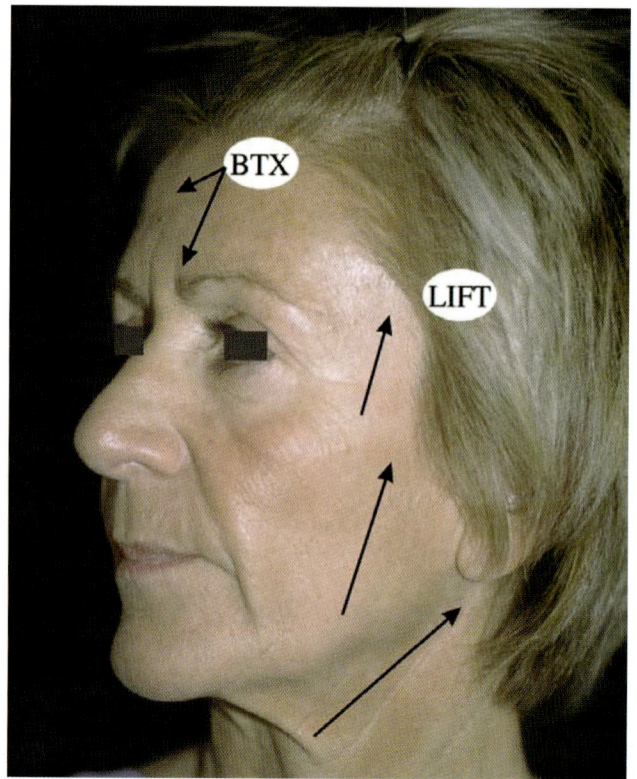

Figure 25.3   Skin and muscle ptosis (frontalis, temporozygomatic, jugomandibular, and cervical regions). Note glabellar and frontal hyperkinetic wrinkles and crow's feet. BTX, locations of botulinum toxin A injections.

(1–3 points of 1 unit of BOTOX®, or 3 units of Dysport®), especially in the inferolateral area of the eyelid (Figures 25.1 and 25.2). Dysport® will be distributed in most of the world, except US territories, under the name of Azzalure® by Galderma, and in US territories under the name Reloxin® by Medicis; in Latin America, the name will remain Dysport®, and it will be distributed by Ipsen or Galderma.

Likewise, if used beforehand, botulinum toxin improves the outcome of other treatments such as with lasers or photorejuvenation around the eyelids, and with fillers such as low-linked hyaluronic acids. Following these alternative treatments of the eyelids, it is especially useful for prolonging the results and avoiding repeat surgery.

Botulinum toxin combined with facelift

In the mid- or upper third of the face

Botulinum toxin type A is injected 3 weeks before, or 6–12 months after a facelift, in the medial frontal, glabellar, and lateral orbicular regions. Combined with a facelift,

particularly in the superolateral section (temporozygomatic) and mid-third of the face, botulinum toxin type A reduces considerably the operating time, postoperative recovery, and side-effects (alopecia, residual pain, scarring, flattened areas). It helps to optimize inadequate surgical results, either immediately or later on, by correcting residual asymmetries or postoperative facial paralysis, which is often transient but can also be long-term.[10–15]

Horizontal forehead wrinkles are generally better treated with botulinum toxin type A than with surgery.

It is best to administer the treatment in several stages; this helps to adapt results until they gradually become permanent. The toxin is then reinjected once a year (Figures 25.3 and 25.4).

This technique has reduced the indications for coronal and frontal facelifts for many surgeons, who opt instead for a limited incision browlift, with cold light source and/or endoscopy. In other cases, patients injected only in the upper third of the face seem sufficiently satisfied with the treatment of their horizontal forehead wrinkles and slight eyebrow lift, from 3 mm[3,16] up to 4.83 mm on average in the study by Ahn et al.[14] This temporary treatment with botulinum toxin type A will help decide whether a browlift is indicated later.

The neck (Figures 25.3 and 25.4)

Injection of the platysma bands is indicated either when the neck starts to age before the skin has become lax, or after a facelift which has not provided an effective solution on the front of the neck. If a decision has been made not to treat or re-treat the neck surgically, the toxin is a good indication.[17–19] Study groups such as that of Santini and Kestemont in Nice, France, have published promising preliminary results for platysma injections 3 weeks before a neck lift.

Botulinum toxin combined with other medical treatments

Often injected 3 weeks before other medical treatments, the toxin immobilizes the muscles in the areas targeted by these treatments, generally centered on the skin surface. Surface treatments of permanent lines, i.e. laser, peels, and dermal filling, thus produce better results which also last longer. Likewise, lipostructure, a rejuvenating technique used to restore fat volume, especially on the cheekbones, cheeks, and mandibular contour, is combined with botulinum toxin injections in the forehead and glabella.

Botulinum toxin combined with lasers and photorejuvenation

Laser resurfacing using a CO_2 and/or erbium laser is designed to treat wrinkles and associated skin lesions on which botulinum toxin has no effect. In this instance, the toxin and laser combination is worthwhile. The depth of the wrinkle is reduced by the toxin, and the quality of the skin is improved by the laser. Likewise, muscle relaxation prevents wrinkles, and the laser stimulates neocollagenesis.[9,15,20] In 2001, Zimbler et al conducted a study[21] in 10 patients, using laser on the forehead, glabella, and crow's feet, one side being previously treated with botulinum toxin and the other side not. Results were superior on the side previously treated with the toxin, particularly for crow's feet. West and Alster consider that botulinum toxin injected after laser treatment improves the outcome and duration of the effect.[22] For Fulton[23] and Carruthers and Carruthers,[24] the ideal rejuvenation program includes a topical skin preparation with vitamin A acid–glycolic acid, followed by the toxin, and then a light, superficial peel.[4] Goldman[1] considers that the toxin combined with non-ablative laser or intense pulsed light (IPL) improves the outcome by ameliorating the skin texture and stimulating collagenesis. Carruthers and Carruthers draw the same conclusions using BBL IPL by Lumenis®, and stress the improvement of skin texture, lentigines, and telangiectasia, with histological demonstration of neocollagenesis.[25,26]

Botulinum toxin combined with injectables

Fillers such as hyaluronic acids (HAs), used on their own to treat not wrinkles but folds, do not produce

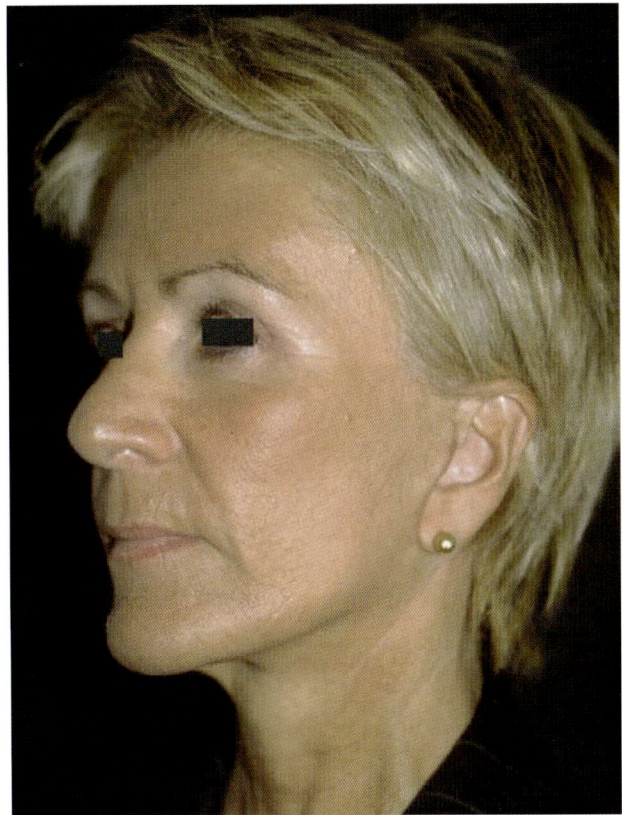

Figure 25.4   Results after 5 years. First, botulinum toxin A injection was carried out of the three main areas of the upper third of the face (glabella, frontalis, and crow's feet), then 3 weeks later a frontotemporal and mediofacial facelift and neck lift. Maintenance by injection was performed annually for the three main zones.

very satisfactory results. Likewise, muscle relaxation has little or no effect on deep dermal wrinkles.[21,27–29] Their combination is thus logical. Most authors recommend a 15-day interval, but in practice many combine the two techniques at the same time.[30] Sommer and Sattler[31] stress the advantage of this combination for perioral lines, using microdoses of botulinum toxin. In 2002, we published a preliminary study[32] of the effects of the Dysport®–Hylaform® combination on crow's feet and the glabella in 20 patients (Figure 25.5). In 70% of the patients, the outcome was clearly improved when botulinum toxin was injected beforehand. The combination proved very effective in 30% of cases: in patients with a tonic and rather thick skin, with expression lines and early-stage dermal creases, and non-hyperkinetic forehead or vertical eyebrow lines. The same results were observed with the BOTOX and Restylane® combination.[33] In 2003, Carruthers and Carruthers confirmed the advantage of botulinum toxin and HA combinations, first with BOTOX and Hylan B (Hylaform®), then with BOTOX and Restylane.[34,35]

Conclusion

The combination of botulinum toxin with surgical treatments of the eyelids, facelifts of the upper and

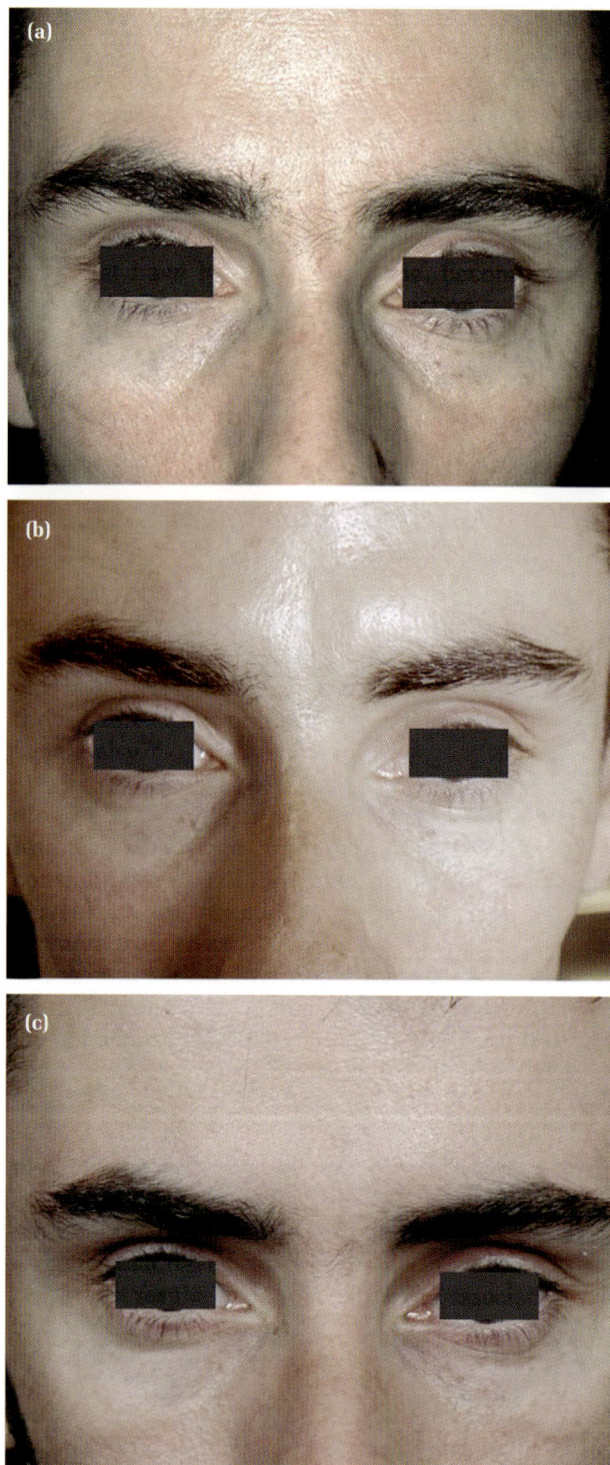

Figure 25.5   (a) Wrinkles and in particular a glabellar furrow in a 37-year-old patient. (b) Results 4 months after treatment with botulinum toxin A (Dysport®). (c) Results 3 months later, the remaining furrow having been filled by injection of hyaluronic acid (Hylaform®). An equivalent result was obtained by the injection of BOTOX®, then Restylane®.

mid-third of the face, and surface medical treatments improves short- and long-term results. The current trend is to use facelifts and blepharoplasties that are as minimally invasive as possible, and which provide

remarkably effective and natural appearing results, combined with powerful but very safe medical techniques when used appropriately, such as botulinum toxin.

References

1. Goldman A. Combining procedures with botulinum toxin in plastic surgery. In: Hexsel D, Trindade de Almeida A, eds. Cosmetic Use of Botulinum Toxin. Porto Alegre, Brazil: AGE Editora, 2002: 216–20.
2. Guerrissi JO. Intraoperative injection of botulinum toxin A into orbicularis oculi muscle for the treatment of crow's feet. Plast Reconstr Surg 2000; 105: 2219–25; Plast Reconstr Surg 2003; 112 (Suppl): 161S–3S.
3. Fagien S. Intraoperative injection of botulinum toxin A into orbicularis oculi muscle for the treatment of crow's feet. Plast Reconstr Surg 2000; 105: 2226–8.
4. Nicolau PJ, Chaouat M, Mimoun M. Skin, wrinkles and botulinum toxin. Ann Readapt Med Phys 2003; 46: 361–74.
5. Borodic GE, Gozzolino D. Pharmacology and Histology of Therapeutic Application of Botulinum Toxin. New York: Marcel Dekker, 1994.
6. Fagien S, Brant F. Primary and adjunctive use of botulinum toxin type A Botox® in facial aesthetic surgery. Clin Plast Surg 2001; 28: 127–48.
7. Matsudo PK. Uso da toxina botulinica em estetica clinica e cirrurgica. Rio de Janero: Revinter, 2000: 279–81.
8. Ascher B. Rajeunissement facial par lifting sans endoscopie et injection de toxine botulique. Objectif Peau 2000; 8: 158–61.
9. Ascher B. Rides fronto-palpébrales: intérêt des injections de toxine botulique, du lifting sans endoscopie, du resurfacing laser. Cah Ophtalmol 1997; 14: 37–44.
10. Santini J, Kestemont P, Krastinova Lolov D. Chirurgie plastique de la face, rajeunissement, embellissement. Report of the Congrès de la Société Française d'Oto Rhino-Laryngologie et de Chirurgie de la Face et du Cou, Paris, 1999: 27–43.
11. Ahn MS, Catten M, Maas CS. Temporal brow lift using botulinum toxin A. Plast Reconstr Surg 2000; 105: 1129–35; discussion 1136–9.
12. Huang W, Rogachefski AS, Foster JA. Browlift with botulinum toxin. Dermatol Surg 2000; 26: 55–60.
13. Carruthers JDA. Special feature: Botox treatment for expressive facial lines and wrinkles. Curr Opin Otolaryngol Head Neck Surg 2000; 8: 357–61.
14. Ahn MS, Catten M, Maas CS. Temporal brow lift using botulinum toxin A. Plast Reconstr Surg 2003; 112 (Suppl): 98S–104S.
15. Maas C. Temporal brow lift using botulinum toxin A: an update. Plast Reconstr Surg 2003; 112 (Suppl): 109S–12S.
16. Sarrabayrouse MAM. Indications and limitations for the use of botulinum toxin for the treatment of facial wrinkles. Aesthetic Plast Surg 2002; 26: 233–8.
17. Brandt FS, Bellman B. Botulinum A exotoxin for platysmal bands and rejuvenation of the ageing neck. Dermatol Surg 1998; 24: 1232–4.
18. Matarasso A, Matarasso SL, Brandt FS, Bellman B. Botulinum A exotoxin for the management of the platysma bands. Plast Reconstr Surg 1999; 103: 645–52.
19. Kane MA. Nonsurgical treatment of platysma bands with injection of botulinum toxin A. Plast Reconstr Surg 1999; 103: 656–63.
20. Roher TE. Lasers and cosmetic dermatologic surgery for aging skin. Geriatr Dermatol 2001; 17: 769–94.
21. Zimbler MS, Holds JB, Kokoska MS et al. Effect of botulinum toxin pretreatment on laser resurfacing: a prospective

randomized blinded trial. Arch Facial Plast Surg 2001; 3: 165–9.

22. West TB, Alster TS. Effect of botulinum toxin type A on movement-associated rhytides following CO2 laser resurfacing. Dermatol Surg 1999; 25: 259–61.

23. Fulton JE. The Newport beach experience. Dermatol Surg 1998; 24: 1219–24.

24. Carruthers J, Carruthers A. The adjunctive usage of botulinum toxin. 1998; 24: 1244–7.

25. Carruthers J, Carruthers A. Botulinum toxin and laser resurfacing for lines around the the eyes. In: Blitzer A, ed. Management of Facial Lines and Wrinkles. Philadelphia: Lippincott Williams & Wilkins, 2000: 315–32.

26. Carruthers J, Carruthers A. the effect of full-face broadband light treatments alone and in combination with bilateral crow's feet botulinum toxin type A chemodenervation. Dermatol Surg 2004; 30: 355–66.

27. Klein AW. Skin filling. Collagen and other injectables of the skin. Dermatol Clin 2001; 19: 491–508.

28. Naoum C, Dasiou-Plakida D. Dermal filler materials and botulinum toxin. Int J Dermatol 2001; 40: 609–21.

29. Warmuth IP, Bader R, Scarborough D, Bisaccia E. Dermologic surgery into the next millenium, part II. Cutis 2001; 68: 99–101.

30. Coleman Moriaty K. Other solutions. Combination treatments. In: Coleman Moriaty K, ed. Botulinum Toxin in Facial Rejuvenation. St Louis: Mosby, 2004: 128–9.

31. Sommer B, Sattler G. Cosmetic indications according to anatomic region. In: Sommer B, Sattler G, eds. Botulinum Toxin in Aesthetic Medicine. Berlin: Blackwell Science, 2001: Ch 3.

32. Ascher B, Wibault-Collange C. Botulinum toxin (Dysport®) and hyaluronic acid (Hylaform®) association in the treatment of lines. A preliminary evaluation. Inamed Aesthet News November 2002: n°1.

33. Ascher B. Toxine botulique et rides: les associations médicales et chirurgicales. Real Ther Derm Venerol 2004; 138: 7–9.

34. Carruthers J, Carruthers A. A prospective, randomized, parallel group study analyzing the effect of BTX-A (Botox) and nonanimal sourced hyaluronic acid (NASHA, Restylane) in combination compared with NASHA (Restylane) alone in severe glabellar rhytides in adult female subjects: treatment of severe glabellar rhytides with a hyaluronic acid derivative compared with the derivative and BTX-A. Dermatol Surg 2003; 29: 802–9.

35. Carruthers JDA, Carruthers A, Maberley D. Deep resting glabellar rhytides respond to BTX-A and Hylan B. Dermatol Surg 2003; 29: 539–44.

26 Combining chemical peels with botulinum toxin injections

Marina Landau

Combination procedures are common in esthetic surgery due to the general understanding that the aging process affects all facial components: skin, muscles, and subcutaneous fat tissue. The combination of surgery with laser resurfacing, fat injections, and chemical peels has become common.[1–3] Chemical peels have been used for over a century, and have gained in popularity over recent decades. Historically, dermatologists have played a crucial role in the development of this procedure.[4] Chemical peels are one of the most powerful rejuvenation procedures. A combination of peels with botulinum toxin A injections is logical since it addresses more comprehensively the causes of facial wrinkling and aging. This combination makes it possible to create a significant rejuvenation effect with no invasive procedure.

Chemical peels

The results of chemical peels depend on a multitude of factors, mainly the chemical agents used and the peeling technique. To choose the depth of the peeling procedure, one should be able to define the depth of the pathologic process to be treated. If the skin defect is located in the corneal layer, superficial peeling gives a sufficient effect. A medium depth peel is usually enough to treat pigmentary changes. To eliminate wrinkles, one needs to perform a deep peel to reach the mid-reticular dermis. Superficial chemical peels with α- and/or β-hydroxy acids, Jessner's solution, or trichloroacetic acid (TCA) 10–25% improve the skin quality and may affect skin discolorations. The procedure is relatively safe, but serial peels are needed and the results achieved are short-lived.[5]

Medium depth chemical peels, such as TCA 35%, improve textural irregularities, pigmentary changes, precancerous skin lesions, and mostly superficial wrinkling. In spite of the fact that the procedure is office based, its performance is accompanied by a burning sensation, and light sedation is sometimes required.[6] Both superficial and medium depth peels have no effect on clinically visible wrinkles. TCA in percentages higher than 35% might be complicated by scarring, since the depth of penetration is hard to control with this solution.[7] The Monheit peel (Jessner's solution plus TCA 35%) and 'weekend peel' (modified Jessner's solution combined with a powder of the plant *Spongilla fluviatilis*)[8] were tailored to overcome this serious complication without affecting the efficiency of the peel.

Deep chemical peels are based on a phenol–croton oil combination, and are effective for removal even of the deepest rhytids.[9] The procedure has to be performed with a patient under full cardiopulmonary monitoring. The immediate healing process lasts for 8–14 days, while post-peel redness may continue for up to 2 months. The results achieved have a long-lasting effect. The best-known phenol-based formulae include the Baker–Gordon classical formulation, Hetter's formulae, and Exoderm® solution.[10]

The diversity and flexibility of the chemical agents and peeling techniques makes it possible to tailor a specific treatment to the majority of patients seeking help at the dermatology office.

Combination of chemical peels with botulinum toxin A injections

The muscles of facial expression are unique in that they insert directly into the skin. Years of facial expressions constantly folding the skin result in the progressive development of hyperdynamic wrinkles. Botulinum toxin A (BTX-A) injections in cosmetic use for these mimetic wrinkles have become popular in the last decade, since Jean and Alastair Carruthers reported for the first time in 1990 their experience.[11]

Since then, the adjunctive usage of BTX-A with other procedures has become popular, and has been adopted, for example, as a part of the standard protocol for laser skin resurfacing in the USA.[12] A combination of minimally invasive techniques for facial rejuvenation meets the improved understanding of the mechanisms involved in skin aging. The results of BTX-A can be improved by combination with the subcision technique,[13] as well as dermal filler injections[14] and nonablative light technologies for skin rejuvenation.[15]

Chemical peels stimulate collagen synthesis and promote the formation of a new epidermal layer. It is

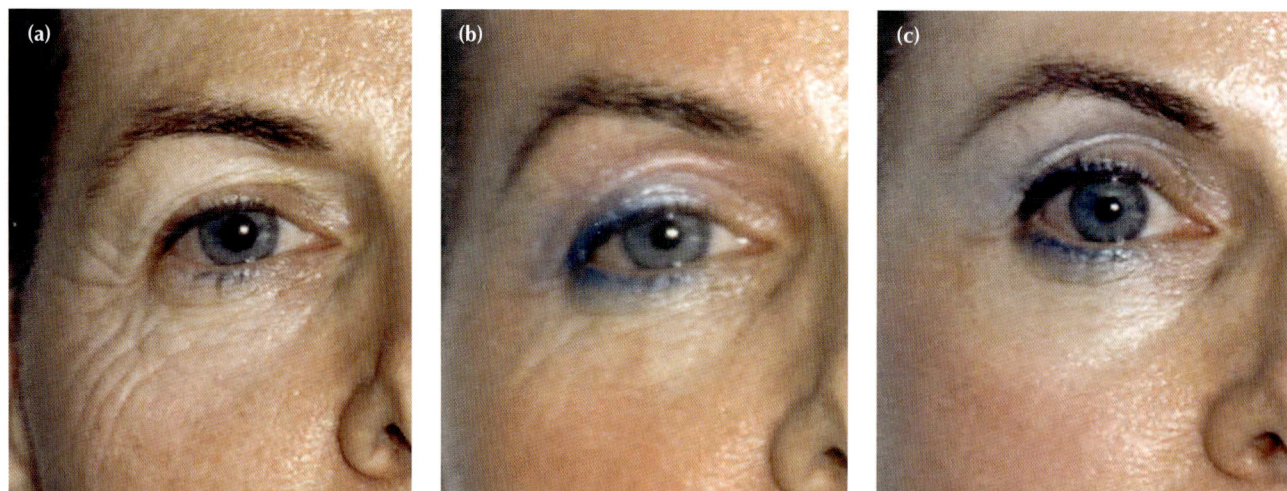

Figure 26.1   A 54-year-old woman before (a), 2 months following a deep chemical peel (b), and after periorbital BTX-A injection (c).

generally assumed that when facial muscles are weakened by BTX-A the immobilized skin can regenerate more efficiently, and collagen remodeling becomes more effective. Thus, the best timing of the BTX injection is about 2 weeks before the performance of the chemical peel. BTX-A injections can also be performed immediately after the superficial and medium depth peel with no excessive rate of side-effects related to unexpected diffusion of the toxin to remote muscles. With regard to deep chemical peels, if not performed prior to the peel, BTX can be injected as soon as 3 weeks afterwards. It is not advised to inject earlier, since the extensive inflammation accompanying the healing process may disperse the toxin.

Clinical cases

A few clinical cases illustrate the effect of combination treatment.

Case 1

A 54-year-old woman presented with features of premature skin aging: uneven pigmentation and wrinkling (Figure 26.1a). She was treated by phenol-based peel (Exoderm procedure). With the patient under intravenous sedation with full monitoring of vital signs, the peel solution was applied using a cotton applicator and rubbed onto the skin to achieve an even coverage. After solution application, the face was covered by an impermeable occlusive tape mask for 24 hours. Then the tape mask was removed from the face, and bismuth subgalate powder applied and left on for 7 days. On the 8th day, the powder mask was dissolved by soaking the skin in tap water. After powder

mask removal the facial skin was much smoother, with an even reddish color and no dyschromias.

At the follow-up visit after 2 months, recurrence of the periocular hyperkinetic lines became evident (Figure 26.1b). Thus, the periorbital area was injected with 40 U of BTX-A (Dysport®). Ten days later the improvement of periorbital wrinkling was obvious (Figure 26.1c).

Case 2

A 68-year-old woman presented with multiple mimetic and age related wrinkles. (Figure 26.2a). Two weeks prior to the peeling, she has been injected with 30 units of botulinum toxin A (Dysport®) in each of the peri-orbital areas. Then she has been treated by phenol-based peel (Exoderm procedure), as described in Case 1. Six weeks after the procedure the facial skin was smooth and unwrinkled including the mimetic areas (b).

Case 3

A 55-year-old woman with severely sun damaged skin, multiple solar lentigines, and wrinkles was peeled using the Exoderm procedure (Figure 26.3a). On the first follow-up visit, complete elimination of the lentigines and photodamage induced wrinkles was noted, while mimetic wrinkles in the glabellar area were still visible (Figure 26.3b).Therefore, after 6 weeks the patient was injected with 50 U of BTX-A (Dysport) with complete response of the wrinkles. Since then, for the last 3 years she has been injected every 9 months with BTX-A with no recurrence of the wrinkles (Figure 26.3c).

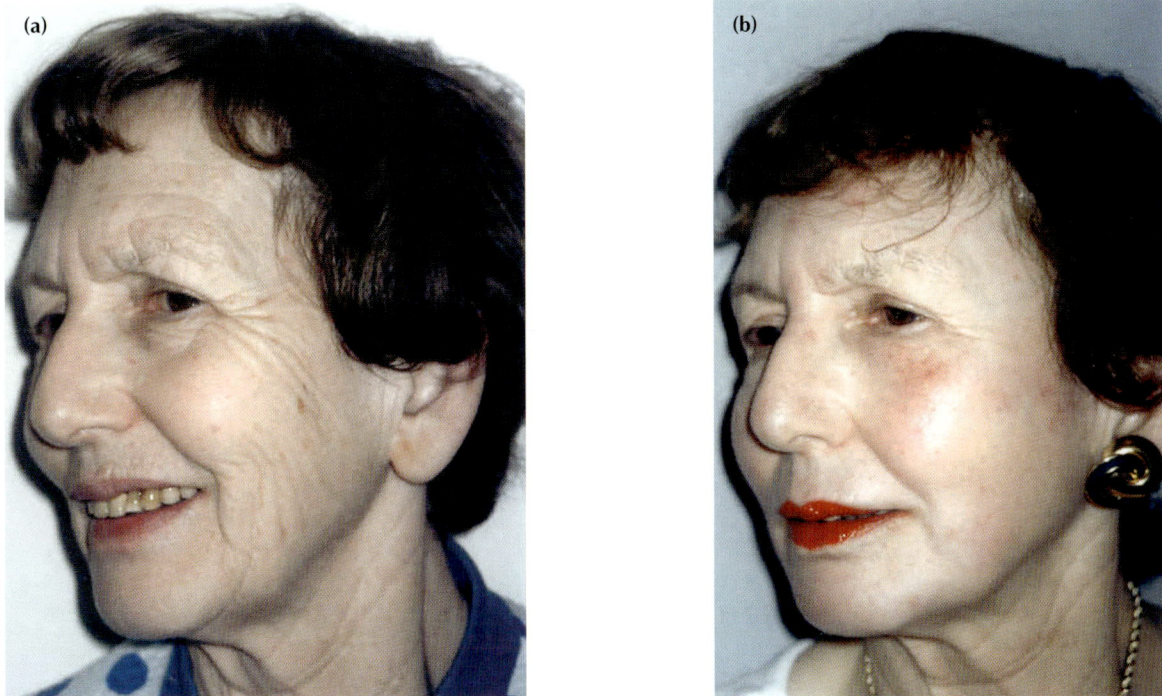

Figure 26.2 A 68-year-old before (a) and 6 weeks after (b) injection of botulinum toxin A (Dysport®) in periorbital areas followed by phenol-based peel (Exoderm procedure).

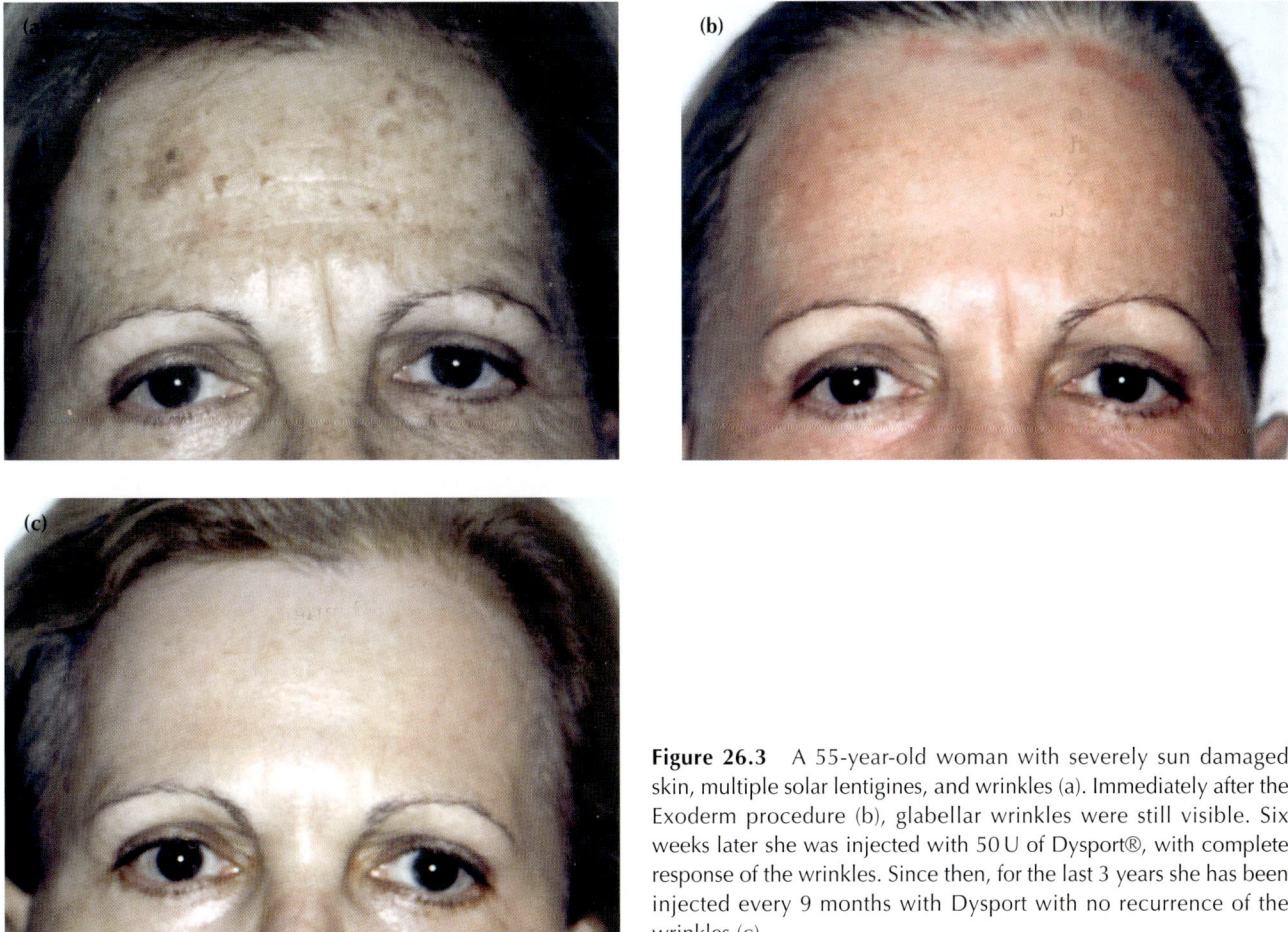

Figure 26.3 A 55-year-old woman with severely sun damaged skin, multiple solar lentigines, and wrinkles (a). Immediately after the Exoderm procedure (b), glabellar wrinkles were still visible. Six weeks later she was injected with 50 U of Dysport®, with complete response of the wrinkles. Since then, for the last 3 years she has been injected every 9 months with Dysport with no recurrence of the wrinkles (c).

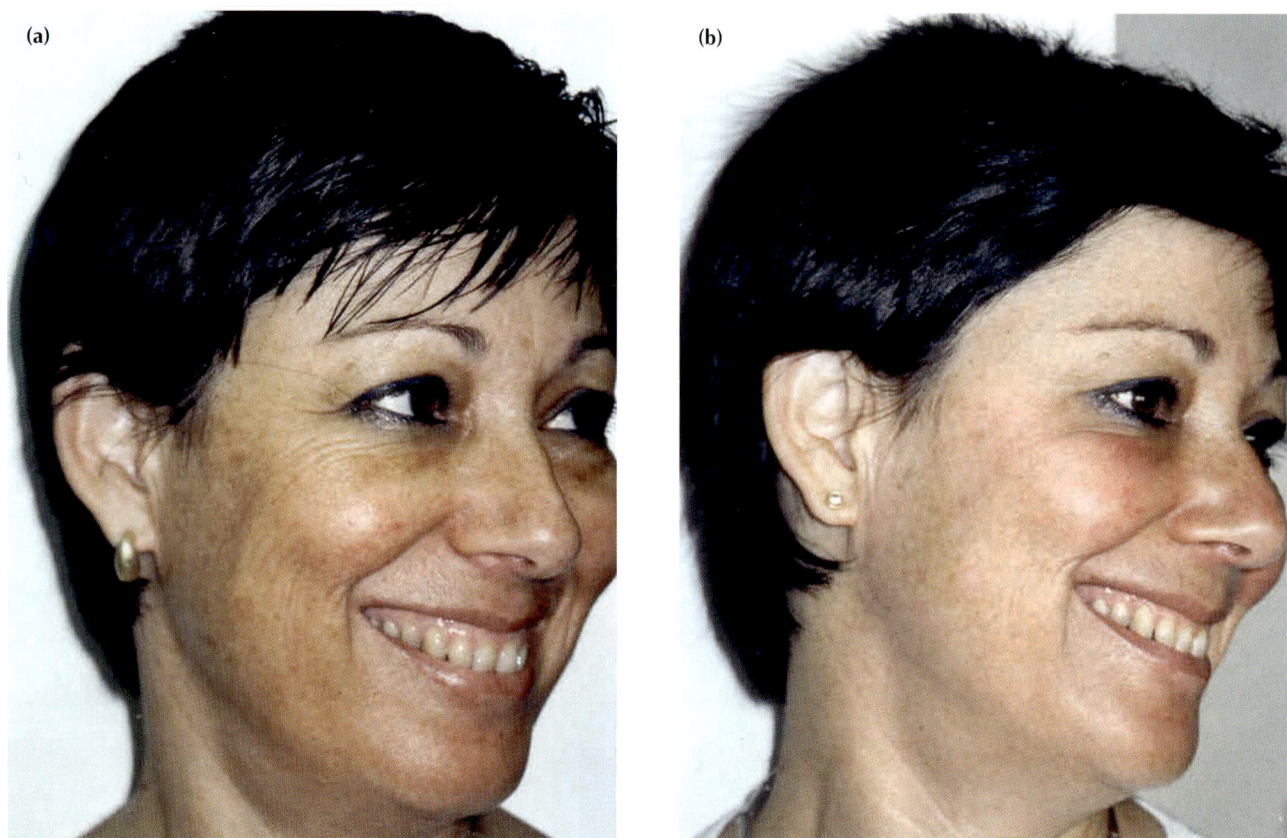

Figure 26.4   A 46-year-old woman before (a), and 1 week after (b) a 'weekend peel' and periorbital BTX-A injection. Note disappearance of the solar lentigines and 'smile lines'.

Case 4

A 46-year-old woman was referred because of multiple solar lentigines and periorbital mimetic lines (Figure 26.4a). She was treated by a medium depth peel composed of a combination of modified Jessner's solution (salicylic acid, lactic acid, resorcinol, undecylic acid in alcoholic solution) and an abrasive powder of the plant *S. fluviatilis*. We call this peel a 'weekend peel' because of the fast skin desquamation and healing, which takes about 4 days. The peel is performed by application of the solution, gentle massage of the dissolved plant powder, and reapplication of the solution. The procedure is accompanied by a mild burning sensation and no anesthesia is needed. Immediately following the procedure, 30 U of BTX-A (Dysport) was injected in the periorbital area. After 2 weeks the skin was cleared of the pigmentation, with no mimetic periorbital lines.

At the beginning of the 21st century, people live longer and are more active personally and socially. The desire for a young and yet natural look has increased interest in non-surgical procedures. With better understanding of the aging process we search for more comprehensive approaches, addressing different aspects of aging. Combination dermatological procedures, such as chemical peels together with BTX-A injections, serve this purpose and open a wide field of activity for a practicing physician.

References

1. Roberts TL 3rd. The emerging role of laser resurfacing in combination with traditional aesthetic facial plastic surgery. Aesth Plast Surg 1998; 22: 75–80.
2. Guerrerosantos J. Simultaneous rhytidoplasty and lipoinjection: a comprehensive aesthetic surgical strategy. Plast Reconstr Surg 1998; 102: 191–9.
3. Dingman DL, Hartog J, Siemionow M. Simultaneous deep-plane face lift and trichloroacetic acid peel. Plast Reconstr Surg 1994; 93: 86–93.
4. Kotler R. Bits of history, bits of mystery - a historical review of chemical rejuvenation of the face. In: Kotler R, ed. Chemical Rejuvenation of the Face. St Louis: Mosby-Year Book, 1992: 1–40.
5. Briden ME. Alpha-hydroxyacid chemical peeling agents: case studies and rationale for safe and effective use. Cutis 2004; 73(Suppl): 18–24.
6. Rubin MG. Trichloroacetic acid and other non-phenol peels. Clin Plast Surg 1992; 19: 525–36.
7. Monheit GD. Medium-depth chemical peels. Dermatol Clin 2001; 19: 413–25.
8. Landau M, Fintsi Y. MY weekend peel - a novel medium depth peel for acne, pigmentary disorders and skin rejuvenation. Presented at 9th Congress of the EADV, Geneva, 2000.
9. Baker TJ. The ablation of rhytides by chemical means. J Fla Med Assoc 1961; 48: 451–4.

10. Fintsi Y. Exoderm – a novel phenolbased peeling method resulting in improved safety. Am J Cosmet Surg 1997; 14: 49–54.

11. Carruthers A, Carruthers J. The treatment of glabellar furrows with botulinum A exotoxin. J Dermatol Surg Oncol 1990; 16: 83.

12. Carruthers J, Carruthers A. The adjunctive usage of botulinum toxin. Dermatol Surg 1998; 24: 1244–7.

13. Hexsel D. Combining procedures with botulinum toxin in dermatology and dermatologic surgery. In: Hexsel D, De Almeida AD, eds. Cosmetic Use of Botulinum Toxin. Porto Alegre: AGE, 2002: 211–15.

14. Carruthers J, Carruthers A. A prospective, randomized, parallel group study analyzing the effect of BTX-A (Botox) and nonanimal sourced hyaluronic acid (NASHA, Restylane) in combination compared with NASHA (Restylane) alone in severe glabellar rhytides in adult female subjects: treatment of severe glabellar rhytides with a hyaluronic acid derivative compared with the derivative and BTX-A. Dermatol Surg 2003; 29: 802–9.

15. The effect of full-face broadband light treatments alone and in combination with bilateral crow's feet botulinum toxin type A chemodenervation. Dermatol Surg 2004; 30: 355–66.

27 Complications and their legal implications

David J Goldberg

Botulinum toxin injections have become one of the most popular cosmetic treatments throughout the world over the past decade. However, the recognition of the effects of this toxin have been known for over a century. It was Justinus Kerner, a German physician, who first studied the potent effects of botulinum toxins during the Napoleonic Wars, after a reported increase in food-poisoning deaths in persons eating sausages. After a series of animal and self-experiments, he hypothesized that the toxin was produced under anaerobic conditions, acted on the autonomic and motor nervous systems, and was lethal in small doses.[1] The use of botulinum toxins for modern day medical purposes began in the 1960s, when Scott et al investigated the therapeutic uses of this drug in humans suffering from strabismus and blepharospasm.[2–4] In the USA, the Food and Drug Administration (FDA) approved botulinum toxin type A (BTX-A) for these conditions in 1989. In 2000, the FDA expanded the approved indications to include cervical dystonia. In 2002, the FDA approved the use of BTX-A for cosmetic uses.

Independent surveys by the American Society for Aesthetic Plastic Surgery and the American Society of Plastic Surgeons suggest that in 2002, between 1.1 and 1.6 million patients in the United States received cosmetic injections with BTX-A. These numbers are thought to be increasing yearly both in the USA and elsewhere throughout the world.[5]

Although it is a very safe substance when used with appropriate dosing, BTX-A injections can be associated with complications. Such complications may have associated legal implications. This chapter will review the reported BTX-A associated complications and the impact of these implications on the injecting physician. Although the legal analysis will be done in accordance with US legal doctrine, the basic principles are universal.

A recent review of BTX-A adverse reactions noted, among 406 reports of serious adverse events, 28 deaths and 17 seizures.[6] Among the 28 deaths, six were attributed to respiratory arrest, five to myocardial infarction, three to cerebrovascular accident, two to pulmonary embolism, two to pneumonia (one known to be aspiration pneumonia), five to other known causes, and five to unknown causes of death. Death occurred a median of 3 days after BTX-A injection (range <1 hour–120 days). The median age of BTX-A recipients who died was 44 years (range 3–91 years). Of 28 patients who died, 26 had underlying systemic diseases with elevated risk of mortality, in addition to the symptoms for which they received BTX-A. The possibility of a causal role for underlying diseases made it difficult to evaluate the role of BTX-A in the fatalities. In addition, many patients with serious adverse reactions were treated for medical, and not cosmetic purposes, and received significantly higher dosages of BTX-A than are commonly used for cosmetic treatments. It would seem, based on these facts, that warning patients of the risk of seizures and death after BTX-A used for cosmetic procedures is not legally required.

Apart from reported deaths, other serious complications have also been noted. These include dysphagia, muscle weakness, allergic reactions, flu-like syndromes, arrhythmia, and myocardial infarction. These have all been extraordinarily rarely reported events, may not always be directly related to the BTX-A injection, and probably are not reasonable risks to discuss with patients who are seeking facial cosmetic BTX-A injections.

Among 995 reported cosmetic cases with a nonserious complication, lack of intended cosmetic effect was most commonly noted. Injection site reaction, ptosis muscle weakness, and headache were frequently reported.[6]

What should be clear is that there are some obvious contraindications to BTX-A use for cosmetic purposes. These would include prior allergic reaction, injection into areas of infection or inflammation, pregnancy (safety for use during pregnancy has not been established), and breastfeeding. Women who inadvertently have been injected during pregnancy thus far have had uneventful deliveries, and to date no teratogenicity has been attributed to botulinum toxin. Nonetheless, delay of injections would be the likely recommendation until pregnancy is complete and breastfeeding has ended.

Relative contraindications to BTX-A treatment would include patients with diseases of the neuromuscular junction (e.g. myasthenia gravis) because of the underlying generalized muscle weakness seen with such diseases. Local weakness at injection sites would be expected in such patients. In addition, some medications decrease neuromuscular transmission and generally should be avoided in patients treated with botulinum toxin. These include aminoglycosides, penicillamine, quinine, and calcium channel blockers.[7]

The most common everyday reactions to botulinum toxin injections are generally mild and transient. These include nausea, fatigue, malaise, flu-like symptoms, and rashes at sites distant from the injections. Untoward sequelae caused by percutaneous injection include pain, edema, erythema, ecchymosis, headache, and hypesthesia. These are also generally mild and transient. The most common meaningful adverse effect is unwanted weakness. Fortunately, unwanted weakness caused by the action of the toxin usually resolves in several months and in some patients in a few weeks, depending on the site, strength of the injections, and the muscles made excessively weak.[7]

Muscle weakness is the result of the desired toxin effect on injected musculature. This can be a desired goal in some and a problem with medical legal overtones in others. For example, patients who depend on emotive expression, such as actors and politicians, can be significantly negatively impacted by a potential reduction in expression. Excess weakness following frontalis injection may cause paralysis rather than weakening of the muscle. Patients may report that they appear mask-like, and their brow feels heavy. If brow ptosis occurs, a hooded appearance may be present, and occasionally vision may be partially obstructed. If the lateral fibers of the frontalis have not been injected appropriately, a quizzical appearance may result in which the lateral brow is pulled up while the central brow is lowered. This can be improved by simply injecting a small amount of toxin into the lateral frontalis fibers.

Since brow depressors are generally paralyzed when treating glabellar lines, ptosis of the upper eyelid can be a common complication following injection in this region. This may occur as late as 2 weeks after injection. Ptosis is caused by migration of toxin through the orbital septum. Patients instructed to remain in an upright position for 3–4 hours following injection while avoiding manual manipulation of the area may be at less risk of eyelid ptosis. Active contraction of the muscles under treatment may increase the uptake of toxin and decrease its diffusion. Ptosis can be treated with apraclonidine 0.5% eyedrops. Apraclonidine is an α_2-adrenergic agonist, which causes Muller's muscles to contract. It should be noted that apraclonidine is contraindicated in patients with documented hypersensitivity. Phenylephrine 2.5% can be used when apraclonidine is not available. Phenylephrine is contraindicated in patients with narrow-angle glaucoma and in patients with aneurysms.

Weakness of the lower eyelid or lateral rectus can occur following injection of the lateral orbicularis oculi.

If severe lower lid weakness occurs, an exposure keratitis may result. If the lateral rectus is weakened, diplopia results. Treatment is symptomatic. This complication is best avoided by injecting at least 1 cm lateral to the lateral canthus and above the zygomatic arch.

Injection of platysma muscles can result in dysphagia from diffusion of toxin into muscles of deglutition. When this occurs, it usually lasts only a few days or weeks. Some patients may require soft foods, although a swallowing weakness does not necessarily herald systemic toxicity. However, if it is severe, patients may be at theoretical risk of aspiration.

Some patients experience neck weakness after botulinum toxin injections into the neck. This may be especially noticeable when attempting to raise the head from a supine position. This is thought to occur from a weakening of the sternocleidomastoid muscles, either from direct injection or diffusion. This rare complication appears to be more common in women with long thin necks.

Any discussion of complications induced by botulinum toxin injections raises the issue of what is required in an informed consent.[8] Generally, in the USA, reasonable risks must be detailed to the prospective patient. What is a reasonable risk may be open to discussion. It represents the 'standard of care'.

The duty of a physician using botulinum toxin is to use it in accordance with the standard of care. Although the elements of a cause of action in negligence are derived from formal legal textbooks, the standard of care is not necessarily derived from some well-known textbook.[9] It is also not articulated by any judge. The standard of care is defined by some as whatever an expert witness says it is, and what a jury will believe. In a case against any cosmetic physician, the specialist must have the knowledge and skill ordinarily possessed by a specialist in that field, and have used the care and skill ordinarily possessed by a specialist in that field in the same or similar locality under similar circumstances. A dermatologist, plastic surgeon, otolaryngologist, internist, or esthetic medicine physician will be held to an equal standard. A failure to fulfill such a duty may lead to loss of a lawsuit by the physician. If the jury accepts the suggestion that the doctor mismanaged the case and that the negligence led to damage of the patient, then the physician will be liable. In the case of botulinum toxin injections, mistreatment may lead to both damages and physician liability. Conversely, if the jury believes an expert who testifies for the defendant doctor, then the standard of care in that particular case has been met. In this view, the standard of care is a pragmatic concept, decided case by case, and based on the testimony of an expert physician. The physician injecting botulinum toxin is expected to do this in the manner of a reasonable physician. He need not be the best in his field, he need only perform the procedure in a manner that is considered by an objective standard as reasonable.

It is important to note that where there are two or more recognized approaches to injecting botulinum toxins, a physician does not fall below the standard of care by using any of the acceptable methods even if one method turns out to be less effective than another method. Finally, in many jurisdictions, an unfavorable result due to an 'error in judgment' by a physician is not in and of itself a violation of the standard of care if the physician acted appropriately prior to exercising his professional judgment.

Evidence of the standard of care in a specific malpractice case includes laws, regulations, and guidelines for practice, which represent a consensus among professionals on a topic involving diagnosis or treatment, and the medical literature including peer-reviewed articles and authoritative texts. In addition, obviously, the view of an expert is crucial. Although the standard of care may vary from state to state in the USA, it is typically defined as a national standard by and for physicians.[10]

Most commonly for litigation purposes, expert witnesses articulate the standard of care. The basis of the expert witness testimony, and therefore the origin of the standard of care, is grounded in the following:

- the witness' personal practice; and/or
- the practice of others that he has observed in his experience; and/or
- medical literature in recognized publications; and/or
- statutes and/or legislative rules; and/or
- courses where the subject is discussed and taught in a well-defined manner.

The standard of care is the way in which the majority of physicians in a similar medical community would practice. If, in fact, the expert herself does not practice like the majority of other physicians, then the expert will have a difficult time explaining why the majority of the medical community does not practice according to her ways.[11]

It would seem then that in the perfect world, the standard of care in every case would be a clearly definable level of care agreed by all physicians and patients. Unfortunately, in the typical situation, the standard of care is an ephemeral concept resulting from differences and inconsistencies among the medical profession, the legal system, and the public.

At one polar extreme, the medical profession is dominant in determining the standard of care in the practice of medicine. In such a situation, recommendations, guidelines, and policies regarding varying treatment modalities for different clinical situations published by nationally recognized boards, societies, and commissions establish the appropriate standard of care. Even in some of these cases, however, factual disputes may arise because more than one such organization will publish conflicting standards concerning the same medical condition. Adding to the confusion, local societies may publish their own rules applicable to a particular claim of malpractice.

Thus, in most situations the standard of care is neither clearly definable nor consistently defined. It is a legal fiction to suggest that a generally accepted standard of care exists for any area of practice. At best there are parameters within which experts will testify. The cosmetic physician's best defense that he is acting in accordance with the standard of care is to document appropriate risk assessment of the patient, provide appropriate medical record documentation and appropriate informed consent, and finally to utilize appropriate diagnostic and treatment approaches.[12]

American physicians have in recent years put forth substantial efforts toward standard setting, and specifying treatment approaches to various conditions. Clinical practice guidelines have been developed by specialty societies such as the American Academy of Dermatology, the American Society for Dermatologic Surgery, and the American Society of Aesthetic Plastic Surgery. The Institute of Medicine has defined such clinical guidelines as 'systemically developed statements to assist practitioner and patient decisions about appropriate health care for specific clinical circumstances.' Such guidelines represent standardized specifications for performing a procedure or managing a particular clinical problem.

Clinical guidelines raise thorny legal issues.[10] They have the potential to offer an authoritative and settled statement of what the standard of care should be for a given skin cancer. A court would have several options when such guidelines are offered as evidence. Such a guideline might be evidence of the customary practice in the medical profession. A doctor acting in accordance with the guidelines would be shielded from liability to the same extent as one who can establish that she or he followed professional customs. The guidelines could play the role of an authoritative expert witness or a well-accepted review article. Using guidelines as evidence of professional custom, however, is problematic if they are ahead of prevailing medical practice.

Clinical guidelines have already had an effect on settlement, according to surveys of malpractice lawyers. A widely accepted clinical standard may be presumptive evidence of due care, but expert testimony will still be required to introduce the standard and establish its sources and its relevance.

Professional societies often attach disclaimers to their guidelines, thereby undercutting their defensive use in litigation. The American Medical Association (AMA), for example, calls its guidelines 'parameters' instead of protocols intended to significantly impact on physician discretion. The AMA further suggests that all such guidelines contain disclaimers stating that they are not intended to displace physician discretion. Such guidelines, in such a situation, could not be treated as conclusive.

Plaintiffs will usually use their own expert, as opposed to the physician's expert, to define the standard of care. Although such a plaintiff's expert may also refer to clinical practice guidelines, the physician's negligence can be established in other manners as well. These methods include: (1) examination of the physician defendant's expert witness, (2) an admission by the defendant that he or she was negligent, (3) testimony by the plaintiff, in a rare case where she is a medical expert qualified to evaluate the allegedly negligent physician's conduct, and (4) common knowledge in situations where a layperson could understand the negligence without the assistance of an expert.

It is clear, then, that although complications may occur following botulinum toxin injections, the plaintiff, in order to win her negligence cause of action against an esthetic physician, must establish that her physician had a duty of reasonable care in treating her and had in fact breached that duty. However, that breach must also lead to some form of damage. A mere inconvenience to the plaintiff, even in the setting of a physician's breach, will usually not lead to physician liability in a cause of action for negligence. In general, most botulinum toxin induced complications are temporary and nothing more than an inconvenience. However, in those rare situations where a patient was not warned of a potential complication, and the ensuing complication led to damage (such as the inability to work), there may be legal implications from the botulinum toxin induced complication.

References

1. Erbguth F. Botulinum toxin, a historical note. Lancet 1998; 351: 1280.
2. Scott AB, Rosenbaum A, Collins CC. Pharmacological weakening of extraocular muscles. Invest Ophthalmol Vis Sci 1973; 12: 924–7.
3. Scott AB, Suzuki D. Systemic toxicity of botulinum toxin by intramuscular injection in the monkey. Mov Disord 1988; 3: 333–5.
4. Scott AB. Botulinum toxin injection of eye muscle to correct strabismus. Trans Am Ophthalmol Soc 1981; 79: 734–70.
5. American Society of Plastic Surgeons. Available at http://www.plasticsurgery.org/public_education/procedures/Botox.cfm.
6. Coté TR, Mohan AK, Polder JA, Walton MK, Braun MM. Botulinum toxin type A injections: adverse events reported to the US Food and Drug Administration in therapeutic and cosmetic cases. J Am Acad Dermatol 2005; 53: 407–15.
7. Glogau RG. Review of the use of botulinum toxin for hyperhidrosis and cosmetic purposes. Clin J Pain 2002; 18 (Suppl): S191–7.
8. Gershon SK, Wise RP, Braun MM. Adverse events reported with cosmetic use of botulinum toxin A. Pharmacoepidemiol Drug Saf 2001; 10 (Suppl): S135–6.
9. Furrow BF, Greaney TL, Johnson SH, Jost TS, Schwartz RL. Liability in Health Care Law, 5th edn. St Paul, MN: West Publishing Co, 2004.
10. Hyams AL, Shapiro DW, Brennan TA. Medical practice guidelines in malpractice litigation: an early retrospective. J Health Polit Policy Law 1996; 21: 289–313.
11. Lamont v Brookwood Health Service, Inc, 446 So.2d 1018 (Ala.1983).
12. Gannon v Elliot, 19 Cal.App.4th 1 (1993).

28 Preoperative care: photography documentation, and the subdermal test

Elisabeth Domergue Than Trong

Preoperative care

An expert provides all information on preoperative care for botulinum toxin treatment in Chapter 12. Timothy Flynn has a huge experience that the present author does not, so she invites you to read his chapter first.

Preoperative care includes, first, consultation and intradermal testing.

The checklist necessary for the general knowledge of the patient includes a questionnare on personal life aspects (work, hobbies), alcohol, drugs, and tabacco consumption, on past and current treatments, including non-prescription drugs, and personal and family, surgical, psychologic, medical, dermatological, and esthetic history. Particulare care should be taken regarding previous esthetic treatment and on the psychologic history and profile of the patient (unrealistic expectations, dissatisfaction with previous treatment, misunderstanding after several explanations) if you want to avoid failure or a trial. The physical examination must be complete. Palpation of the face must be done to seek traces of previous injections or esthetic treatment, and scar quality and sun damage must be evaluated. During this part of the consultation you should observe the patient's facial, static and expression wrinkles and start the esthetic diagnosis.

The first consultation includes a determination of the esthetic demands and needs of the patient and the adapted treatment(s) required to meet patient expectations. Specific chapters in this book will help with proposing suitable treatment to the appropriate person, to solve a particular cosmetic problem, but one must not forget that the face is a unique unit to work on. Your own experience will be the best guide.

Then, the other alternatives must be explained, from doing nothing to full face laser resurfacing. The practitioner must clearly describe the benefits the patient can expect from each; the reasons for his or her choice; and the possible, undesirable effects and complications (even rare ones and the possibility of unknown ones). The postoperative care is the last element to explain; there are good descriptions (depending on the filler chosen) in Chapters 35 and 36.

It is a good idea to show a video presentation about techniques, outcomes, and results, including side-effects and postoperative care, avoiding complications. Some prefer a leaflet with photographs; this is easy in the digital photography era!

Then, once a signature is obtained on the photography consent form (Figure 28.1), photographs are taken following the protocol indicated below.

When the patient understands all explanation, you can ask for a signature on the treatment consent form, keeping one for your archives. The consent form should contain all the information given verbally. Then, specific pretreatment recommendations are repeated, such as stopping aspirin and non-steroidal anti-inflammatories, applying some EMLA® cream 2 hours before, taking some arnica, and so on.

The delicate part is to inform the patient of the number of procedures needed and the cost of each, and giving a quote. The best way to do this is to use a trusted nurse, so as not to lose precious time in discussion. She can manage the secondary procedure explanation, preoperative and postoperative recommendations, consent form signatures, money aspects, and even sometimes standardized photography time.

After a 15-day reflection period, any new questions must be answered and the patient treated or tested (as explained below). Then product protocol concerning frequency of consultations and reinjections is followed. The author recommends taking photos to follow patient evolution, and some key points are given below.

Photography documentation

Film cameras are still the gold standard for resolution, but digital camera is the present and the future. Digital cameras are easier to use, their images are easier to archive, and they are improving on a daily basis.

Patients' minds stay young and they want their bodies to look young too. You understand your patients' way of thinking and help them to feel better using new technology

---

ASSENT FOR FIXING, REPRODUCTION AND USE OF IMAGE

I the undersigned .... authorize Doctor X, dermatologist, or her assistant to photograph me on this day and to use my image or to photograph and to use the image of my child, called .... for whom I am the holder of the image.

The present authorization is delivered only for use as defined below:

☐ In the interest of the patient to understand the evolution of pathology and to be preserved in the medical file,

☐ Teaching title for the teaching of other doctors or medical students or Pr ....,

☐ On a purely scientific basis for medical and professional publications.

For support hereafter*:

• paper photographs
• numerical, digital

Any other exploitation or use of the image or any other attribute of my personality will have to be subject to new authorization. Done in Paris it .... en two specimens, a copy of which has been given to the patient

Signature of the interested party   Date

*Please tick relevant boxes

Figure 28.1   Photography consent form.

such as 'injection treatments in cosmetic surgery'. You should apply this philosophy in other ways. Digital photography is a new technology, now easy to understand and use, accurate and affordable for every esthetic medical expert. You will be younger in mind and will be helping yourself by using it.

Materials

The materials needed for photography include first the camera. The camera should give good results for your needs, be easy to use, and be easy to get used to. The characteristics usualy recommended are at least 4 million pixels, a macrolens or macro setting, and a flash. The choice is very large, and new models appear each month. If you already have one with the above characteristics it is not necessary to change it. If you decide to swich from a film camera to a digital camera, or if it is your first camera, make a comparative study on the Internet. Choosing a digital camera is difficult, considering compact or reflex camera, resolution, choice of lens focusing, macrolens, and type of flash (Table 28.1). You should test the camera to see whether it suits you and your needs at work. Many stores have their own website to help you make a choice. The author recommends www.megapixel.net, in English and French. It gives details of the characteristics and functions of each camera, with articles, photography tests, evaluations of more than 300 cameras, and details of the software used. The following example illustrates the extremely rapid evolution of this

technology, and explains why the author does not give a list of best cameras. In 2001, Galdino et al (Baltimore) recommended digital cameras with resolutions from 1.5 to 2.7 million pixels.[1] In 2005, 5 million pixels were common; some photographers have told the author that this is unnecessary because the human eye cannot distinguish between 4 and 5 million pixels on the computer screen. On the other hand, the gold standard for resolution is still the 35-mm slide film, theoretically at 12 million pixels. A viewfinder grid screen is highly recommended to help the standardization of photos by taking the same anatomic landmark from one patient to another.

The following lists details of the recommended characteristics:

1. The LCD monitor is the liquid-crystal display screen enabling the quality of your newly taken photographs.
2. The CDD system (charged coupled device) captures light. It is the photosensor and processes focused light into a digital mode: the higher is the bit number of the CCD, the more color shades that will be seen. Each pixel has a code for various colors. The number of pixels is associated with better resolution quality and accuracy of photographs. As the resolution increases, so does the memory used.
3. The megabytes (Mb) evaluate the memory used for storage in the computer and the removable memory.

Table 28.1 Digital camera review

Name of expert	Digital camera	Objective	Lighting system	Background	Software	Backup
B Ascher	Nikon D70 Nikon Coolpix 990		Daylight + camera flash	Black	4D	Hard disk 1 Hard disk 2 Backup 6 months
P But	Nikon D2X	60 mm macro	Daylight + camera flash	Dark blue	Mirror	Automated daily on hard disk + monthly on recordable CD (SN1)
B Mole	Sony Cybershot DSC S70 3.3 Mpixel	Zeiss 2/7–21 macro	Camera flash Incandescent light 500 W	Dark blue		
B Rossi	Nikon D2	60 mm macro		Beige wall		Automated daily on hard disk + monthly on recordable CD
T Flynn	Fuji Finepix S2Pro	60 mm macro	Dual Sunpak DigitFlash 1000 Digital professional flash	Dark blue	Mirror	Automated nightly on tape system
G Lemperle	Nikon F-301	55 mm macro	Nikon Macro Speedlight SB-21 Nikon AS-14 battery	Blue		Scanned
E Domergue Than Trong	Nikon Coolpix 4500		Room lighting	White flat-finish non-reflective wall, dark blue or yellow depending on patient skin	ACDSee	Hard disk daily Tape system monthly
G Monheit	Nikon D70 Nikon Coolpix 990	Fixed lens	Daylight flash	Blue	4D	Hard disk and floppy
A Cohen-Letessier	Canon Powershot S230 3.2 Mpixel Sony DSC H1 Cybershot 7.1 Mpixel					
JL Briancon			Daylight + camera flash	White and beige walls		Hard disk daily
JLH Vigneron	Nikon Coolpix 4500	Zoom on 80 mm focal	Camera flash + 2 flash slaves + strong artificial light in room	Green wall with flash slaves behind	ACDSee	Hard disk + hard disk 2 every day + hard disk 3 every month

4. Two sets of memory cards are necessary (the card is inserted in the camera to store the images). Either 64 or 128 Mb capacity is enough if you transfer daily to your computer. Different types of removable memory can be used depending on the digital camera. Compact Flash® cards are best for speed of saving; with SmartMedia® and Memorystick® cards they are the most common, depending on the manufacturer's choice.

5. The flash position depends on your requirements. For macrophotography the closer is the flash, the better is the picture, but it has to be far enough away in full face or full body imaging to illuminate the entire area (see later).

6. USB (universal serial bus) cables are required.

7. Two sets of nickel–cadmium (Ni–Cd) rechargeable batteries avoid having an empty battery during the consultation. The author recommends them: they are better than expensive and short-lasting standard conventional batteries.

8. External USB memory card-readers must be one of the cheapest aquisitions; they are very popular and easy to use, with expedient image transfer which is not the case with the slower camera cable system.

9. A computer with USB ports, composite and super video (S-video) inputs and outputs, and an IEEE (Institute of Electrical and Electronic Engineers) 1394 (firewire) port is the ultimately useful piece of equipment for transferring and saving photographs and digital video (next step in high-tech medical documentation). The hard drive must be powerful enough for storage of the photographs. Niamtu recommends a dedicated laptop computer for photography, making photography easy in any location.[2] However, in that case, especial care must be taken in selection of processor speed, random access memory (RAM), hard drive capacity, and LCD screen. These might increase the price significantly in the quest for better image resolution. Of course a good antivirus program is essential.

10. Imaging software packages are numerous. The characteristics depend on your needs, as with the camera. The software requires archiving, editing, and databasing functions. The author thinks that morphing is a dangerous option, showing the result on the patient's face or body by computerized outcome predictions, with a risk of disappointment for the patient at the end of treatment. Thanks to the database you can easily find your photos using key words such as name, sex, ethnic origin, age, date, referring doctor, procedure, and complication, if you took the trouble to save the data for each patient; the author promises that it will be worthwhile.

11. Presentation software is useful to give a sense of all photographs you have taken, to make scientific presentations, for patient education, and for illustrating referral letters with before and after surgery photographs.

12. Standardization will be easier if you have the ideal clinical photography room or at least a background in a area dedicated to clinical photography. The background color depends on the user and the need. A white flat-finish non-reflective wall is preferred, to make it easy to send by email (smallest files) or to print,[2] requiring no investment. Dark blue for Caucasians and green to yellow for V or VI phototype patients are recommended by Daniel,[3] avoiding red colors reflecting on the skin (Chevreul law). Meneghini uses a 0.95 m wide and 1.10 m high blue panel made from a sheet of plastic material for outdoor use, washable without losing or changing the color.[4] The author uses two huge canvases painted with water resistant paint: one is dark blue, the other is yellow. They have two sides, decorated and background, and the walls of the room are white flat-finish, non-reflective, so there is a choice depending on the patient and use.

13. It will be easier to move the patient using a rotating and adjustable-height stool with rollers, as well as for the photographer.

14. The lighting technique for clinical facial photography is one of the most important, if not the major parameter to obtain the best quality and consistency of results with no shadow.[4] Many practitioners suggest the use of a professional lighting system composed of two or more flash units with slave or background bounce flashes, macroflashes, or conventional 'hot shoe' flashes. Meneghini suggests a single professional flash (System 300 professional compact flash by System Imaging Ltd, UK),[4] and others use a camera flash, providing shadow by rotating the camera position to control the flash angle. For example, for a profile image, if the flash is horizontal or coming in towards the back of the head, shadows result. By changing the camera position, the flash comes in towards the patient's profile, preventing shadows.[2] A few, including the author, use no flash by employing excellent exposure capability cameras, providing sufficient room lighting, and sometimes using a tripod (to adjust duration of exposure and the size of lens aperture opening), preventing an annoying strong white light in the eyes of patients. You should note color differences between incandescent and fluorescent ambient lighting when out of the office. Clothing color influences photograph color too, so the author approves the technique of a reflective panel held horizontally against the chest just under the collarbone[4] or a black collar drape.[5] Marks on the floor and vertical marks on the wall in line with the floor help camera positioning for face, profile, and three-quarter views and can help the patient to find a natural head position.

Methods

After the interview and the examination, reassure the patient and make sure she or he agrees and signs the consent form to make it possible to use the photographs in student courses, in medical publications, or for staff, and as an example, for other patient education in your waiting room or your consultation room, with or without hiding the eyes (Figure 28.1).

Then, the first thing you must consider is why you are taking the photographs. For recording the data, super-fine is best, but a 2272×1704 fine image is always used by the author with very good results for her requirements:

- immediate demonstration to the patient on the monitor screen
- email sending or for medical staff[6]
- clinical archiving
- follow-up
- patient communication
- scientific publications
- PowerPoint presentations
- A4 printing
- posters
- multimedia lecturing
- medicolegal purposes.

The answer to the above question will help you to decide which image type to use. If you still cannot answer the question, take the basic series of views and choose the super-fine and the fine parameters for better definition (reading the camera instructions). It is acceptable to start at 3 million pixels but better to start at 4 million.

Facial photography has been discussed for a long time in plastic surgery and dermatology.[1–20] Standardized methodology for patient photography must be followed.[4,7–12,17,21–27] The more automatic features that are available the better it is, because there is nothing easier than a 'point and shoot' camera.[2] Sometimes it may be necessary to adjust the flash, shutter speed, and the analog ISO (International Organization for Standardization) setting, exposure, and white balance. It is important to determine the values of variables and maintain them constant for all images. Body photographs have to follow standardization too,[21] although with fillers, the face and hands are the two regions of interest. Standardization requires you to follow as much as possible the recommendations. Do not forget to objectively compare pre-and post-treatment images, focusing on facial rejuvenation and eliminating all other variables, especially concerning injection treatments:

1. The patient must be as natural as possible, with repeatable and neutral expression of the eyes and face for each view. If you have to ask (for showing better the wrinkles before and after) the patient for a special expression such as smiling, frowning, or raising their eyebrows, request that the maximum muscle contraction be consistent at the next consultation, to be able to compare the same expression.

2. Jewelry on or around the face should be removed prior to photography, and no clothing should be visible in the photographs, hidden by a black collar drape or a horizontal reflective panel, for the reasons given above.

3. If the patient is wearing make-up or if the patient has an oily skin, she or he must wash with soap (better than with a milk or lotion that gives a reflective glare) and wait 10 minutes before photography until the skin aspect becomes natural.

4. The eye color sometimes has a similar effect to make-up. Unfortunately, in cosmetic documentation, the eyes can rarely be closed, which is the only way to assure no distraction.

5. When taking a close-up of part of the face, two photos are necessary: one to show the expression of the patient and the second with the zoom of your choice. The best way is to do a computerized zoom on the interesting part of a unique photograph you have taken. Always associate twice to reassure and make comparison possible.

6. The author uses the same headband to keep the hair behind the ears with absolutely no tension, no pulling, no deformation, no covered parts, and no changes due to haircut, hairstyle, or hair color. This promotes a consistent aspect in the photographs.

7. If you have to make marks on the patient's skin, you can use a eye pencil for each patient; it is much easier to remove than dermographic pen.

8. Patient position is another variable to control. The stereotactic face device is very consistent but space-consuming.[27]

9. The author recommends moving the patient as little as possible during the shooting (misunderstanding or slowness for each new view might make you lose some precious time); it is preferable for the photographer to move around the patient.

10. The basic views are the frontal, right oblique, right profile, left oblique, and left profile views in the natural head position. You can add a full face basal view (in head extension position, ideal to see the zygomatic arch for example). You sometimes also need smile views, one with an unforced smile, known as a social or posed smile, which is static and voluntarily obtained, and one with a forced or enjoyment smile.[28,29] Meneghini reminds us that: 'the natural head position is a standardized and reproducible orientation of the head achieved when one is looking at a distant point in front of one, at eye level'.[30] The simple way to obtain it is to instruct the patient to look straight ahead at a point at eye level on the wall in front of him.[31]

11. If you need to evaluate the eyelid, eyebrow, zygomatic, infraorbital, and paranasal region, seven eye views are required. These are: looking straight ahead, looking up, looking down, unforced lid closure, forced lid closure, and right and left oblique views.

12. The patient should sit at least 0.75 m from the rear wall to prevent shadows, according to Meredith.[32] The subject sits up straight with feet together. The patient–wall and doctor–patient distances must be the same. This can be managed with floor marks, and camera-fixed string to keep the distance between camera and subject at about 1–1.5 m, depending on your camera and the parameters you choose (do not change the parameters once set).

13. If you think that you need a life-size photograph, do not forget to put an opaque white ruler next to the face, to be able to adjust the size of the print.[33]

14. The height of the camera also has to be controlled. It should be horizontal to the natural head position of the patient. When you can see the area of interest in the LCD, the lens must be parallel to the floor.[5,34]

15. The use of a tripod can be interesting, to increase photograph quality and standardization without flash.

16. Background and lighting are discussed above. Do not forget that light considerably influences the cutaneous aspect. The use of a frontal flash fades skin imperfections. The use of unilateral light emphasizes them. The smaller the imperfections are, the more relevant this is; wrinkles are a perfect example of this phenomenom.

17. Focus using the automatic zoom. You can also use close focus, thanks to the distance from you to the patient (body focusing) if you are in macro mode, or with all other variables constant if you are doing serial photography control.

18. If you want to be sure of comparable views, take multiple shots with a small difference in head position for each view. It will be easy to delete the extra pictures.

19. The author recommends not waiting too long to empty the memory card; the longer you wait the more archiving work you have. The better way is to upload your photographs onto the computer during consultation, to show them to your patient, and for regular saving with no risk of mistaking dates and names, using the memory card reader fixed to the USB computer plug.

20. Label all your photos before stocking them in the medical software or the hard disk imaging file. Later, at the end of consultation, you should be able to save them on recordable CD or DVD, backup tape, or CD-ROM. It is compulsory that the medium you use for saving your work cannot be altered, to ensure its integrity. This will also ensure the validity of the documents in case of medicolegal problems. If you do not back up you can lose everything by a malfunction or a computer virus in less than a second.

In conclusion, standardization is the most important step for consistent photography and all types of study. If you increase the number of parameters you potentially increase the number of adjustments and so the risk of mistakes.

Intradermal skin test

Of course an ideal filler would be non-allergic, non-migratory, painless during the injection which would be unique, injectable through a small gauge needle, and non-detectable once in place, have a long-lasting effect, and have a wide margin of safety. Unfortunately, this does not exist. So, before injecting some fillers, it is necessary to know which skin test is needed. You have to explain to your patient why, when, and how you will do it. You also need to know what is a positive test and what to do with it. The author will try to answer all these issues.

The requirement of a test is to predict both positive and negative aspects of the procedure, if it is done. It permits detection of those who would not tolerate the filler you are about to inject, so prevents outcomes that are unknown for other fillers you cannot test. If you can test the filler, it means that you have a chance of knowing in a few weeks the reactions that will occur, and avoiding a poor outcome. It cannot prevent all reactions encountered with fillers. The test determines whether your patient is eligible for the treatment you choose.

The following is as exhaustive as possible, describing the cases that require an intradermal test, bearing in mind that an increasing variety of dermal fillers have been approved for use in Europe and in several other countries around the world.

Which fillers?

Collagen must be tested, with no discussion in the literature.[35–44] The distributors produce a skin test syringe. Some fillers contain collagen as Artecoll®, even in mesotherapy; these must also be tested. Tests for hyaluronic acid are more controversial, and depend on the patient. For other products there is no recommendation from the manufacturers or distributors. Autologous fat filler produces no risk of allergy; by definition it is safe and unique. This is covered fully in Section IV. Much is expected from the generalization of future therapies from patient blood, cells, or tissue as the ideal intellectual system.

Collagen fillers

Some of these are from animals (rooster combs), including Zyplast®, Zyderm®, and Resoplast®. Others are human, such as Cosmoderm® and Cosmoplast®. Some contain collagen and other components, for example Artecoll. There is no alternative: a test must be carried out if collagen is from animals.[35–44]

Why?   The major problem with bovine collagen is that it is not an autologous substance. Bovine dermal collagen is 95% type I and 5% type III collagen. Zyplast I and II differ by concentrations; Zyplast is less immunogenic and, because of cross-linking, resists bacterial collagenase.[42] Thus, skin testing is done with Zyderm I.[42] Potential allergenicity is a major consideration,[38,39,42–45] and is determined by skin testing.

Three to 3.5% of individuals have a positive skin test.[35,42] In those patients where the skin test is negative, 1–5% of patients still have an allergic reaction if the implant is placed in their face.[36,37,40,42] However, if they have two negative tests an allergic reaction occurs in only 0.25% of cases, which is in favor of systematic double testing.[37,38,42,43] Because the majority of hypersensitivity reactions occur shortly after the first treatment, double testing greatly reduces the frequency of this most undesirable sequela.[35] Positive tests are usually granuloma reactions. This is the subject of Chapters 36 and 37.

When and how?   Seventy per cent of these reactions will become manifest in 48–72 hours, indicating a preexisting allergy to bovine collagen.[35,36,40] This is why you should see your patient after 3 days, as well as the standard 4-week interval.[35,37,41]

The distributors produce skin test syringes. Each contains 0.3 ml of Zyderm I, which is used to determine allergy to Zyderm I, Zyderm II, and also Zyplast.

Use only 0.1 ml as a tuberculin test in the intradermal skin of the left inner forearm at first, if your patient is right handed. Then after a 15-day[37,42] to 4-week[35,41] interval, you can inject intradermally 0.1 ml filler into the right forearm or a hidden area of the face.

Ask your patient to observe the test site closely once a day at the same time (before sleeping or upon awakening) for 6–8 weeks.[37,41] Insist that special attention must be paid to the test site during the first 3 days after each injection,[37,41] because 70–90% of allergic reactions to the skin test occur within the first 72 hours.[42] If negative, you should see nothing or a simple tiny white relief which disappears within several days.[37] If there are any signs of sensitivity to the material such as induration, tenderness, erythema, or swelling (for the patient: redness, swelling, or itching), ask your patient to contact you if it persists or occurs 6 hours or more after test implantation. Then the test is positive: your patient is allergic and cannot be injected with any bovine collagen. This is a definite contraindication to bovine collagen. The local reaction will resolve within 4–6 months, but sometimes it can last up to 2 years.[42] Treatment will be nothing, dermocorticosteroid, or triamcinolone injections if necessary.

The author recommends that you see your patient 3 days after each injection,[37] since the majority of test reactions occur during this period, and 6–8 weeks after the first test,[35,37] even if Lowe recommends seeing the patient only 4 weeks after each injection if there is no problem.[41]

Treatment can begin 2 weeks after the end of intradermal testing and analysis,[35] or 6 weeks after the first skin test,[42] provided that tests are negative.

If a patient has not been treated for more than 1 year, has had a skin test within 12 months, or has been treated elsewhere, the author strongly recommends an additional single skin test to reduce the risk of an allergic reaction.[35,42]

Only 3% show a sensitivity to the test and cannot be treated with injectable collagen,[36,38–41] so 97% of all tested patients can be treated.[41]

Hyaluronic acid fillers

Some of these use natural hyaluronic acid from animals, such as AcHyal® and IAL-System®. Some are of animal origin and cross-linked with hyaluronan polymer molecules, such as Hylaform®, Hylaform Fineline®, and Hylaform Plus®. Others have non-animal origin (bacterial origin) and use natural hyaluronic acid (HA), including Hyaluderm®, Juvelift®, Mac Dermol Bio® and S®, Restylane Touch®, and Revitacare®. Yet others are of non-animal origin and use reticulated molecules, such as BeautyGel®, BeautySphere®, Hyaluderm®, Hydrafill® 1, 2, 3, Esthelis®, Juvederm® 18, 24, 30, 24HV, 30HV, Mac Dermol R®, Matridur®, Matridex® (HA plus dextran), Perlane®, Restylane Sub-Q®, Restylane Fine Line®, Restylane®, Rofilan Hylan® gel, and Reviderm® Intra (HA plus dextran). Some contain HA and other components such as acrylic hydrogel, as in Dermalive® and Dermadeep®.

For HA fillers, intradermal skin testing may be useful occasionally, even if it is not recommended usually.

Why?   Hyaluronic acid is a polysaccharide with no species specificity, so there is apparently no immunologic activity with this material. However, some HA comes from avian origin, and contains traces of avian protein. So, patients with known allergies to materials of avian origin should avoid the list of HAs of animal origin but may receive the synthetic products.

Second, whether to test depends on patient health history. Patients with relative contraindications need a double test.[46]

Third, there is a small risk of delayed allergic reaction. Allergic reactions are known to occur in 1–3% of patients,[46] from case reports[47] and studies of over 700 patients injected since 1996 with Restylane and Hylaform,[48] which implies causes other than an avian-protein reactivity that would be expected only with Hylaform. Due to the incidence of delayed reactions being estimated as 3/709 patients (0.42%), it would seem unnecessary to recommend skin testing.[41,48] Lowe performed prospective skin testing on several hundred patients, but in the light of failing to find any positive patient reaction has abandoned skin testing in his practice.[41] The manufacturers and distributors suggest that there is no need for skin testing because the products are either non-allergenic or have minimal allergy risk.[48] In both origins of products there is a varying amount of hyaluronan-associated protein, and therefore a theoretic risk for sensitivity reaction exists;[48] some continue the double test practice.[35]

When and how?   As mentioned above, if there is a relative contraindication we recommend a double test with HA. The relative contraindications are numerous according to Ascher et al.[46]

Medical relative contraindications:

- allergic pathology such as asthma, atopic dermatitis, allergic rhinitis, urticaria, lidocaine allergy, egg or poultry allergy
- autoimmune pathology such as Crohn's disease, ulcerative colitis diabetes mellitus, rheumatoid polyarthrosis, Hashimoto's disease, scleroderma, lupus, polyarteritis nodosa, ankylosing spondylitis
- granulomatous disease such as sarcoidosis
- recurrent angina associated with a renal artery aneurysm or endocarditis of Osler; allergy reaction is described in the literature for Restylane, which implies that such a reaction could appear for all bacterial origin HA;[46,49] in this case, it is better to choose animal origin for more safety
- egg allergy would indicate choosing bacterial origin HA.

Esthetic relative contraindications:

- allergic reaction to other fillers such as collagen.

Psychologic relative contraindications:

- dissatisfaction
- numerous esthetic treatments with no satisfaction
- anxious patient
- patient worried about the future related to the product you inject and adverse reactions; in this particular case: double test, plus long delay for reflection, plus photography is necessary.

Treatment relative contraindications:

- anti-inflammatory drugs, aspirin, heparin, antivitamin K, immunosuppressors.

For each case, double testing should be done only if disease is under control. If the double test is negative, injection can be done. Injection for medical or major esthetic reasons is only done in patients with poor health conditions.

The test is the same as for collagen, but the distributors do not produce HA skin test syringes. Use only 0.1 ml (of the HA you decide to inject) as a tuberculin test in the intradermal skin of the left inner forearm at first, if your patient is right handed. Then after a 15-day interval you can inject intradermally 0.1 ml of filler into the other forearm or in a hidden area of the face. Consider using the same landmark for all patients to find the injected site easily during subsequent consultations (10 cm from the elbow, for example). Once it is opened you should use the HA within 24 hours.[42] However, some use the same HA for the second test, storing it in the refrigerator for 15 days and more.[49] Ask your patient to observe the test site closely once a day at the same time (before sleeping or upon awakening) for 6–8 weeks.[37,41] See your patient 3 days after each test, 15 days after the first test to perform the second, 3 days after the second, and 6 weeks after the first test. Only two negative tests permit the injection.[37] If there are any signs of sensitivity to the material such as induration, tenderness, erythema, or swelling (for the patient: redness, swelling, or itching), ask your patient to contact you if it persists or occurs 6 hours or more after test implantation. Then the test is positive: your patient is allergic and cannot be injected with the HA you tested. This is a definite contraindication. The local reaction will resolve within 2–12 weeks.[48] Treatment will be nothing, dermocorticosteroid, or triamcinolone injections if necessary. If negative (normal skin), wait 2 more weeks before injecting the filler. Other products do not need to be tested.[50] However, new products are appearing on the market all the time.

References

1. Galdino GM, Vogel JE, Vander Kolk CA. Standardizing digital photography: it's not all in the eye of the beholder. Plast Reconstr Surg 2001; 108: 1334–44.
2. Niamtu J. Digital photography. In: Lowe NJ, ed. Textbook of Facial Rejuvenation. London: Martin Dunitz, 2000.
3. Daniel F. Photographie argentique en dermatologie esthétique. Encycl Méd Chir, Cosmétologie et Dermatologie Esthétique. Paris: Elsevier, 2000: 50-275-A10.
4. Meneghini F. Lighting techniques for clinical facial photography. In: Clinical Facial Analysis. Berlin: Springer-Verlag, 2005:
5. Canfield D. Reproducible photography for the aging face. In: Lowe NJ, ed. Textbook of Facial Rejuvenation. London: Martin Dunitz, 2000:
6. Karim RB. Digital photography as a means of enhancing interconsultant communication in oncological cutaneous surgery. Ann Plast Surg 2002; 4: 180–3.
7. Di Bernardino BE, Adams RL, Krause J, Fiorillo MA, Gheradini G. Photographic standards in plastic surgery. Plast Reconstr Surg 1998; 102: 559–68.
8. Le Maître M. Photographie numérique en dermatologie esthétique. Encycl Méd Chir, Cosmétologie et Dermatologie Esthétique. Paris: Elsevier, 2003: 50-275-B10.
9. Ellenbogen R, Jankauskas S, Collini FJ. Achieving standardized photographs in aesthetic surgery. Plast Reconstr Surg 1990; 86: 955–61.
10. Morello DC, Converse JM, Allen D. Making uniform photographic records in plastic surgery. Plast Reconstr Surg 1977; 59: 366–72.
11. Nelson GD, Krause JL, eds. Clinical Photography in Plastic Surgery. Boston: Little, Brown and Company, 1988.
12. Zarem HA. Standard of photography. Plast Reconst Surg 1984; 74: 137–46.
13. Staffel JG. Photo documentation in rhinoplasty. Facial Plast Surg 1997; 13: 317–32.

14. Tardy ME Jr, Thomas JR. Facial Aesthetic Surgery, 1st edn. St Louis: Mosby-Year Book, 1995: 94–123.

15. Thomas JR, Tardy ME Jr, Prezekop H. Uniform photographic documentation in facial plastic surgery. Otolaryngol Clin North Am 1980; 13: 367–81.

16. Ali MZ. Advantages of digital photography record keeping in plastic surgery. J Coll Phys Surg Pakistan 2002; 12: 613–17.

17. Becker DG. Standardized photography in facial plastic surgery: pearls and pitfalls. Facial Plast Surg 1999; 15: 93–9.

18. Disaia J. Digital photography for the plastic surgeon. Plast Reconstr Surg 1998; 102: 569–73.

19. Galdino GM, Dasilva D, Gunter JP. Digital photography for rhinoplasty. Plast Reconstr Surg 2002; 109: 1421–34.

20. Galdino GM, Swier P, Manson PN, Vander Kolk CA. Converting to digital photography: a model for a large group of academic practice. Plast Reconstr Surg 2000; 106: 119–24.

21. Gherardini G, Matarasso A, Serure AS, Toledo LS, Di Bernardo BE. Standardization in photography for body contour surgery and suction-assisted lipectomy. Plast Reconstr Surg 1997; 100: 227–37.

22. Gilmore J, Miller W. Clinical photography utilizing office staff: methods to achieve consistency and reproducibility. J Dermatol Surg Oncol 1988; 14: 281–6.

23. Yavuzer R. Guidelines for standard phtography in plastic surgery. Ann Plast Surg 2001; 46: 293–300.

24. Jemec BIE, Jemec GB. Photographic surgery: standard in clinical photography. Aesthetic Plast Surg 1986; 10: 177–80.

25. Heckermann D, Schon-Hupka G. Quantification of the efficacy of botulinum toxin type A by digital image analysis, J Am Acad Dermatol 2001; 45: 508–14.

26. Burgess CM, Quiroga RM. Assessment of the safety and efficacy of poly-L-lactic acid for the treatment of HIV-associated facial lipoatrophy. J Am Acad Dermatol 2005; 52: 233–9.

27. Carruthers J, Klein AW, Carruthers A, Glogau RG, Canfield D. Safety and efficacy of nonanimal stabilized hyaluronic acid for improvement of mouth corners. Dermatol Surg 2005; 31: 276–80.

28. Ackerman JL, Ackerman MB, Brensinger CM, Landis JR. A morphometric analysis of the posed smile. Clin Orthod Res 1998; 1: 2–11.

29. Ackerman MB, Ackerman JL. Smile analysis and design in the digital era. J Clin Orthod 2002; 36: 221–36.

30. Meneghini F. Clinical facial photography. In: Clinical Facial Analysis. Berlin: Springer-Verlag, 2005.

31. Jacobson A. Radiographic Cephalometry. From Basics to Videomaging. Chicago: Quintessence Publishing, 1995.

32. Meredith G. Facial photography for the orthodontic office. Am J Orthod Dentofac Orthop III: 1997: 463.

33. Guyuron B. Precision rhinoplasty. 1. The role of life size photographs and soft tissue cephalometric analysis. Plast Reconst Surg 1988; 81: 489–99.

34. Meneghini F. Clinical facial photography in a small office: lighting equipment and technique. Aesthetic Plast Surg 2001; 25: 299–306.

35. Klein AW. Skin filling. Collagen and other injectables of the skin. Dermatol Clin 2001; 19: 491–508, ix.

36. Cooperman LS, Mackinnon V, Pharris BB. Injectable collagen: a six years clinical investigation. Aesthetic Plast Surg 1985; 9: 145–51.

37. Pons Guiraud A. Techniques de comblement des rides. Encycl Méd Chir, Cosmétologie et Dermatologie Esthétique. Paris: Elsevier, 2000; 50-330-A10.

38. Klein AW. In favor of double testing. J Dermatol Surg Oncol 1989; 15: 263.

39. Hanke CW, Higley HR, Jolivette DM et al. Abcess formation and local necrosis after treatment with Zyderm or Zyplast collagen implant. J Am Acad Dermatol 1991; 25: 319–26.

40. Kamer FM, Churukian MM. Clinical use of injectable collagen. A three year retrospective review. Arch Otolaryngol 1984; 110: 93–8.

41. Lowe NJ. Textbook of Facial Rejuvenation. London: Martin Dunitz, 2000.

42. Ashinoff R. Overview: soft tissue augmentation. Clin Plast Surg 2000; 27: 479–87.

43. Elson ML. The role of skin testing in the use of collagen injectable materials. J Dermatol Surg Oncol 1989; 15: 301–3.

44. Siegle RJ, McCoy JP, Schade W et al. Intradermal implantation of bovine collagen: humoral responses associated with clinical reaction. Arch Dermatol 1984; 120: 183–7.

45. Baumann L, Kerdel F. The treatment of bovine collagen allergy with cyclosporin. Dermatol Surg 1999; 25: 247–9.

46. Ascher B, Cerceau M, Baspeyras M, Rossi B. Soft tissue filling with hyaluronic acid. Ann Chir Plast Esthet 2004; 49: 465–85.

47. Lupton JR, Alster TS. Cutaneous hypersensitivity reaction to injectable hyaluronic acid gel. Dermatol Surg 2000; 26: 135–7.

48. Lowe NJ, Maxwell CA, Lowe PL et al. Hyaluronic acid skin fillers: adverse reactions and skin testing. J Am Acad Dermatol 2001; 45: 930–3.

49. Bellew SG, Caroll KC, Weiss RA et al. Sterility of stored non animal, stabilized hyaluronic acid gel syringes after patient injection. J Am Acad Dermatol 2005; 52: 988–90.

50. Bui P, Pons Guiraud A, Kuffer R. Injectables lentement et non résorbables. Ann Chir Plast Esthet 2004; 49: 486–502.

29 Lip augmentation and rejuvenation

Marina Landau

Lips have different functions in the human face. The first is to function as a sphincter. This is primarily accomplished by the orbicularis oris musculature. The second function of the lips is related to facial expression. Speech, smiling, grimacing, and kissing are important cultural communicative means. The third function of the lips is in sexual attraction. When the lips are full and well-defined they create a feeling of youth, health, and sexuality.

Throughout the years and in various cultures, in-proportion projecting feminine lips have been considered sexually attractive. It has been shown that while talking to a person, the major focus of our attention is located between the eyes and the mouth. For these reasons, for years models and actresses have attempted to enhance their lips. Ideally, the human face is divided into three equal segments. The lips comprise the key esthetic feature of the lower third of the face and should be in balance with the rest of the face.

There are no universal ideas about the esthetics of the lips since they change according to culture, time, and individual preference.[1] Bisson and Grobbelaar have attempted to define the characteristics of the ideal lips, by comparing lip features of regular women to those of models.[2] They found that models had larger lips. The lower facial triangle is smaller than usual, affecting the distance between the upper lip and the nose, and between the lower lip and the chin. Lip angles are larger in models and the total lip area is significantly bigger.

Anatomy and structure

The osseous structures of the mouth are composed of the maxilla and mandible bones. The dentition and alveolar ridges provide the structure upon which the soft tissue of the lips rests. The main muscle of the lips is a circular orbicularis oris. This muscle is largely responsible for the bulk of the lip, and functions primarily in oral competence. Other important perioral muscles are: levator labii superioris, depressor labii inferioris, depressor anguli oris, and levator anguli oris.

The muscles are innervated by the facial nerve. The branches supplying the orbicularis oris enter into the deep surface of the muscle. Sensory innervation is

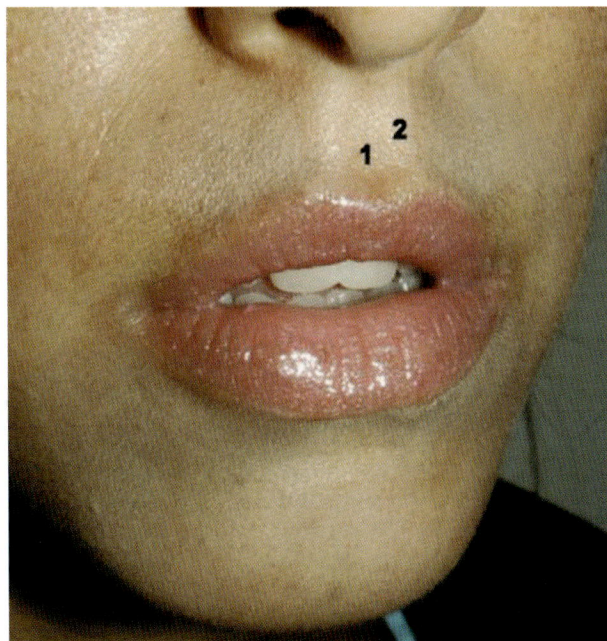

Figure 29.1   The absence of the levator labii superioris insertions medial to the philtral columns (2) creates the Cupid's bow (1).

through the V2 and V3 branches of the trigeminal nerve. These branches enter the soft tissue through infraorbital and mental foramina of the skull. Recognizing the location of the foramina is helpful when using regional anesthesia.

The lips consist externally of skin and mucosa, which is called the vermilion. The vermilion is red because of the absence of keratin and the closely underlying rich vascular plexus. The border between the skin and mucosa is called the vermilion border. The vermilion includes dry (exposed to air) and wet (more inner) portions. Deep to the mucosa is an abundant layer of salivary glands.

While looking at the face, the arches of the upper lip vermilion follow the philtral ridges. Philtron in Greek means 'love charm'. The absence of the levator labii superioris insertions medial to the philtral columns creates a central depression of the upper lip or an inverted W. The strength of this W, or Cupid's bow, confers a sensual quality to the lip (Figure 29.1).

223

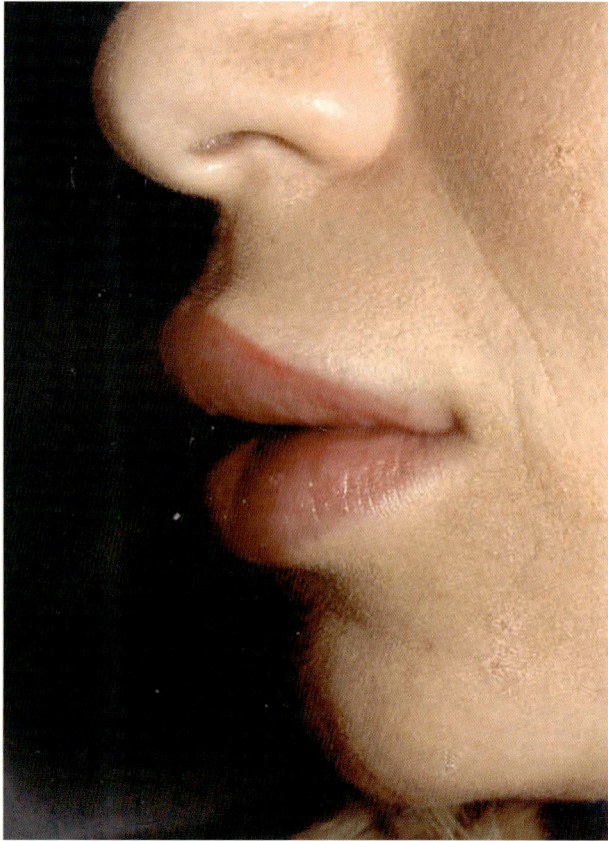

Figure 29.2 Unnatural fullness above the lip such as in this case should be avoided, because it distorts the natural facial profile.

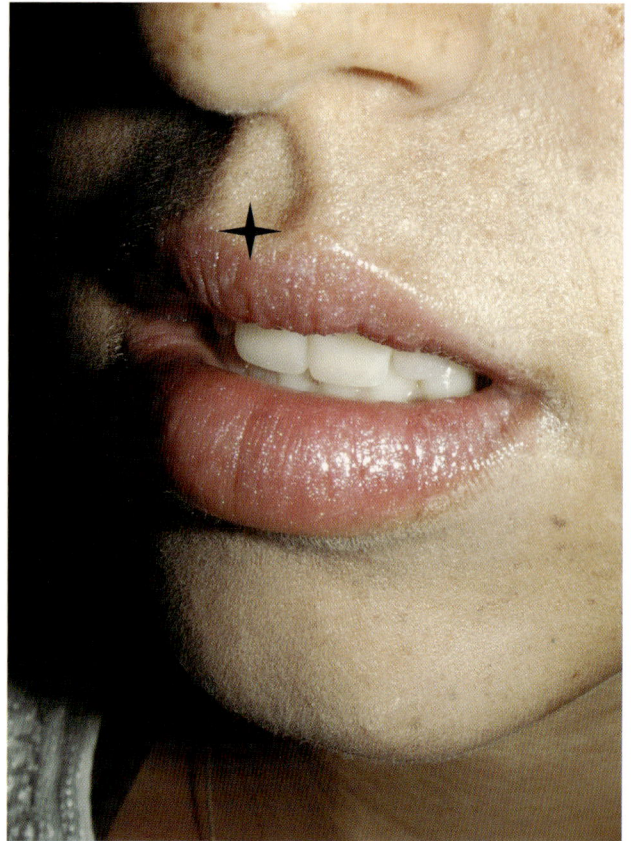

Figure 29.3 Glogau–Klein point (✦) is a point of inflection as the lip turns from the skin to the mucosa.

On the anterior view, the lips are located interior to the lines drawn between the pupils of the eyes and the mouth. The upper lip is located 18–20 mm from the nose, and the lower lip is 36–40 mm from the chin.[3]

In profile, the nasolabial angle is 80–105°. While augmenting the upper lip, unnatural fullness above the lip should be avoided, because it distorts the natural facial profile (Figure 29.2). In the postural head position a line drawn from the mid-nostrils to the chin just barely touches the upper and lower lips. This line is called Steiner's line.[4]

Evaluation of upper and lower labial projection is assessed relative to the line drawn from the subnasal point to the prominence of the chin (pogonion). The upper lip extends approximately 3–3.5 mm anterior to this line, while the lower lip extends only 1.5–2.0 mm. As a result the upper lip projects approximately 2.0 mm anterior to the lower lip. But the lower lip is fuller than the upper lip. The ratio between the lips is 1.6:1.0. The lower lip rolls out. Finally, there is a slight elevation, which is a point of inflection as the lip turns from glabrous skin to mucosa. This site is currently called the G–K point for Glogau–Klein (Figure 29.3).[5] The young lip is fully supported by surrounding tissue, and has upward angles.

Aging lip

Several changes occur to the lips as a result of aging. The lower third of the face loses height because of bone resorption, and classic facial proportions are changing. Ptosis of the glabrous skin (non-mucosal part) of the lip occurs due to demineralization of the maxillae, alveolar resorption, and aging of the soft tissue (Figure 29.4). Skin laxity increases and a drooping of the mouth commissures together with development of marionette lines and perioral wrinkles occurs (Figure 29.5). Fine wrinkling of the lip surface and the appearance of solar changes also affect the overall facial look. But the most obvious change is a loss of fullness and projection of the lips. This is due to a decrease in volume of the dentoalveolar structures, lip musculature, and subcutaneous fat. Smoking and sun exposure significantly affect the degenerative changes of the lips.

Technical considerations

A thorough assessment of the candidate for labial augmentation is required to optimize treatment options. If there is an underlying orthodontic component, the

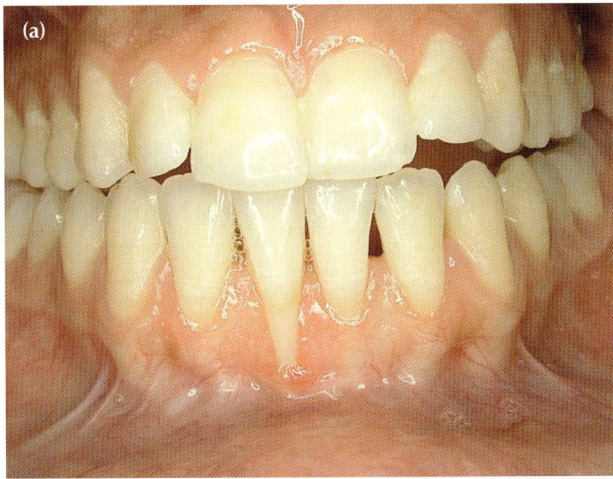

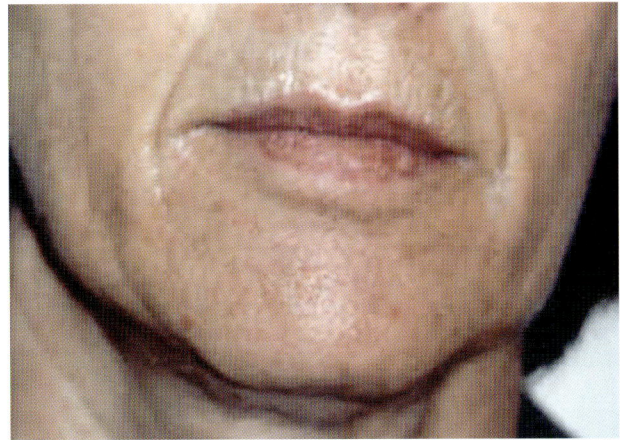

Figure 29.5 Deepening of the nasolabial fold, marionette lines, and wrinkling of the upper lip.

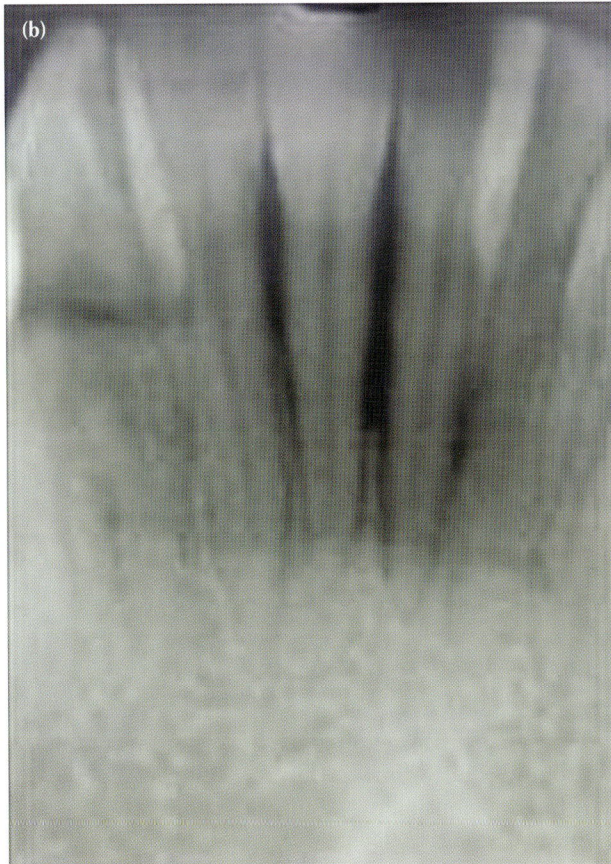

Figure 29.4 Demineralization of the alveolar ridge is the main reason for the decreasing height of the lower part of the face with aging: (a) clinical; (b) X-radiograph.

patient should first be addressed by an orthodontic specialist. If there is a non-existent upper lip, surgical intervention for lip advancement may be needed (direct upper lip lifting).[6] Mimetic upper lip wrinkles are addressed by botulinum toxin type A (BTX-A) injections. Non-mimetic perioral wrinkles are improved either by deep peeling, resurfacing, or dermal filler injections. Solar changes are treated by topical 5-fluorouracil (5-FU).

Three important areas of the aging lip can be addressed by dermal fillers: shape and fullness, perioral wrinkles, and loss of support tissue. There is an ever-expanding menu of materials for soft tissue augmentation, and they can be classified as absorbable, permanent, and semipermanent. The most commonly used absorbable fillers are collagens and hyaluronic acid products. Semipermanent fillers are not recommended for use in lip augmentation, since they have the potential of semipermanent side-effects. Among the permanent fillers, silicone is considered to give encouraging results, but its use is very controversial.[7,8]

Before the procedure, a patient is advised to stop, if possible, any anticoagulants, aspirin, non-steroidal anti-inflammatory drugs, etc. Arnica can be used to avoid ecchymosis and oral antiherpetics are important for herpes labialis prevention. While scheduling the procedure, a patient should realize that immediate post-injection swelling is almost unpreventable. The repetitive nature of the procedure should be emphasized, since the effect of the absorbable fillers will last in the lips anywhere between 4 and 8 months.

Anesthesia

The lips are one of the most sensitive areas of the face. Unlike other areas, most patients will require a nerve block for all treatment here. The mental nerve, which innervates the lower lip, can be blocked by injecting at the base of each of the second premolars inferiorly toward the mental foramen. The infraorbital nerve, which supplies sensation for the upper lip, can be blocked by injecting between the canine and first premolar tooth towards the infraorbital foramen. Successful nerve block makes the lip augmentation procedure completely pain-free, but has a few inherent disadvantages, such as temporary lip asymmetry and temporary motor lip paralysis. Both of these, together with post-injection swelling, make immediate

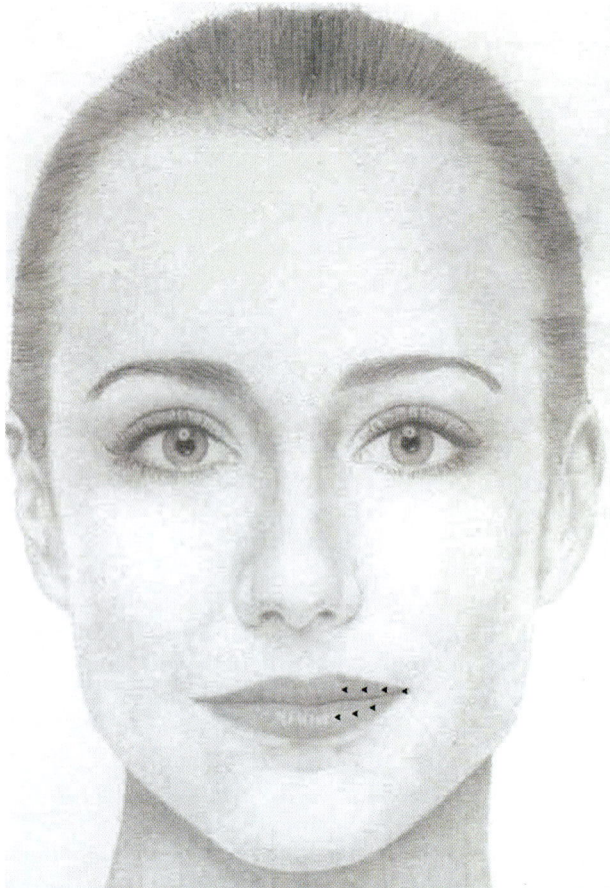

Figure 29.6   Injection of filler in the border between the dry and wet parts of the lip starts at the lip corners.

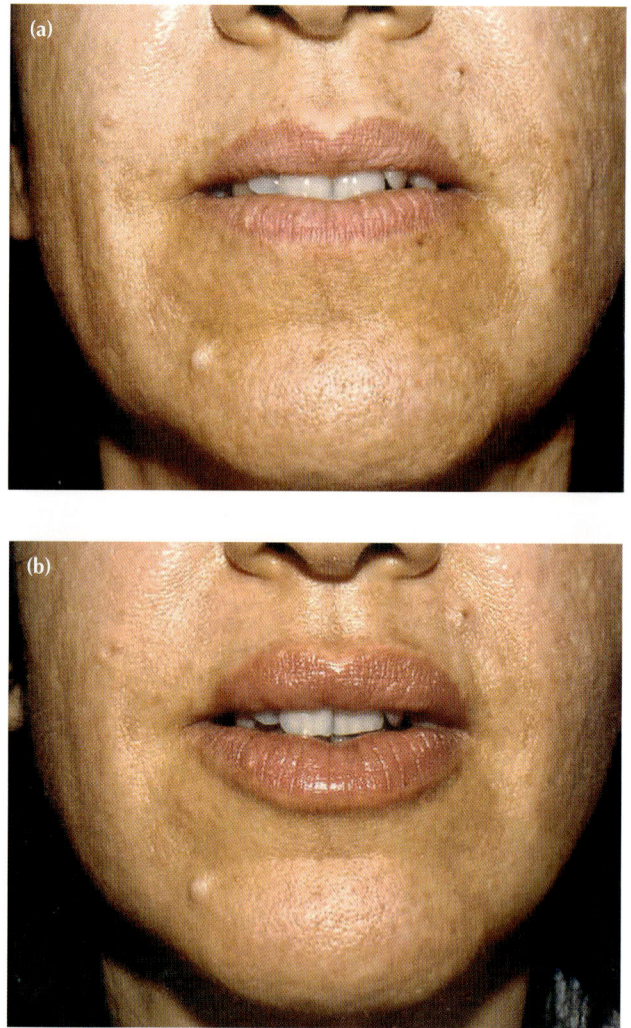

Figure 29.7   Results of an augmentation procedure in a young patient: (a) before; (b) 8 weeks after Juvederm 24 HV injection.

result appreciation impossible. These issues should be thoroughly discussed with the patient prior to the procedure.

Augmentation and rejuvenation techniques

For lip volume enhancement of relatively young lips, the major target will usually be subtle refinement of lip fullness, eversion, and projection of the upper lip and accentuation of the rolling out of the lower lip. These can be achieved by placing a dermal filler to the deep dermis of the lip at a 45° angle along the border of the dry and wet parts of the lip. The injection is performed starting at the right corner to the center, and then from the left corner to the center (Figure 29.6). Injecting along the vermilion border of the lower lip will accentuate its natural rolling out. Injecting to the vermilion border of the upper lip should be performed with extreme caution, especially in a thin upper lip, where it can create a 'Donald Duck' look. This lip will usually need an eversion, which is achieved by injecting

into the vermilion body, as described previously. Stretching the lip during the injection provides more uniform distribution of the filling material. It is crucial to follow the syringe scale during the injection to keep the amount of filler even in both sides of the lip to create a symmetric augmentation (Figure 29.7).

For enhancement of the older lip with upper lip wrinkles and marionette lines, two additional maneuvers are required. Injection along the vermilion border will restore the natural lip contour, but also has the potential to fill the small vertical lines touching it (Figure 29.8). Direct injection of the filler into the vertical lip wrinkles creates satisfactory results, as long as there are only a few visible and stretchable lines. To restore the buttresses, the filler material is injected sequentially from the mouth down towards the jawline in a criss-cross pattern. Redirection of the drooping lip angles is achieved by placing the needle almost

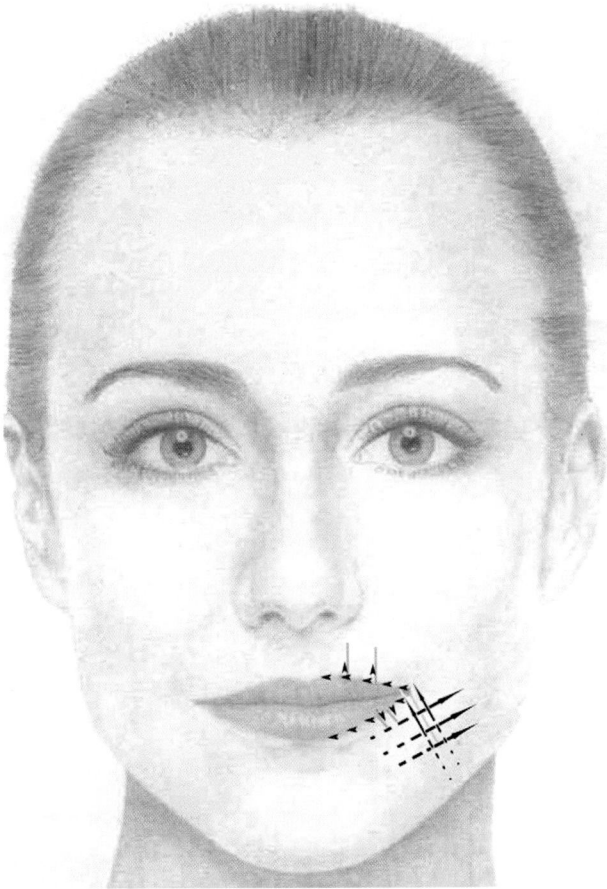

Figure 29.8 Injection of filler along the vermilion border recontours the lips and fills the small perioral wrinkles. Marionette lines are approached by sequential injections from the mouth down towards the jawline in a criss-cross pattern.

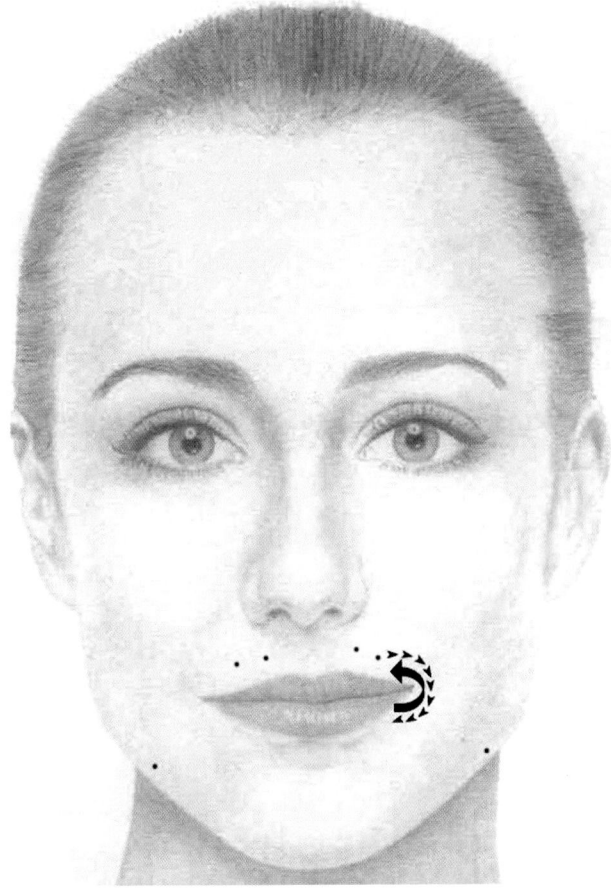

Figure 29.9 Correction of the drooping angles is performed by placing the needle around the lip corner and injecting the filler material (arrowheads) while withdrawing the needle along the semicircular pathway. Botulinum toxin A (points) is injected to the upper lip to soften the mimetic wrinkles and to relax the depressor anguli oris at jaw level to assist in lip corner redirection.

in parallel with the skin surface, starting 5 mm medially to the corner in the lower lip surrounding the corner and reaching 5 mm laterally to the upper lip. Filler injection is performed while withdrawing the needle back in this semicircular pathway (Figure 29.9). Botulinum toxin A can be combined with a filler to enhance the results in both circumstances: injection to the skin of the upper lip to soften the mimetic wrinkles, and injection to the depressor anguli oris at jaw level to assist in lip corner redirection (Figures 29.9 and 29.10).

Rejuvenation of the lips in patients with moderate to severe vertical lip wrinkling cannot be achieved by dermal filler only, and should be addressed by a multimodal approach. This will include deep peeling or ablative laser resurfacing of the lip to treat the deep lines, and only later vermilion augmentation (Figure 29.11). It should always be remembered that a 'nonexistent' lip cannot be restored by dermal fillers

(Figure 29.12). In these cases, a surgical approach is required to create lip bulk.

Except for the young patient group, who require lip volume augmentation only, all others will usually also benefit from a nasolabial fold treatment.

Side-effects

While using absorbable fillers the side-effects are minimal, and include swelling, ecchymosis, asymmetry, and temporary lumpiness. This lumpiness is related to uneven deposition of the filler due to lip movement. It can be addressed by massaging the lips in the first post-treatment days. The main side-effect in treating lips and the perioral area is patient dissatisfaction. In the young age group the expectations of the patient regarding lip augmentation should be synchronized with those of the physician. Our experience shows

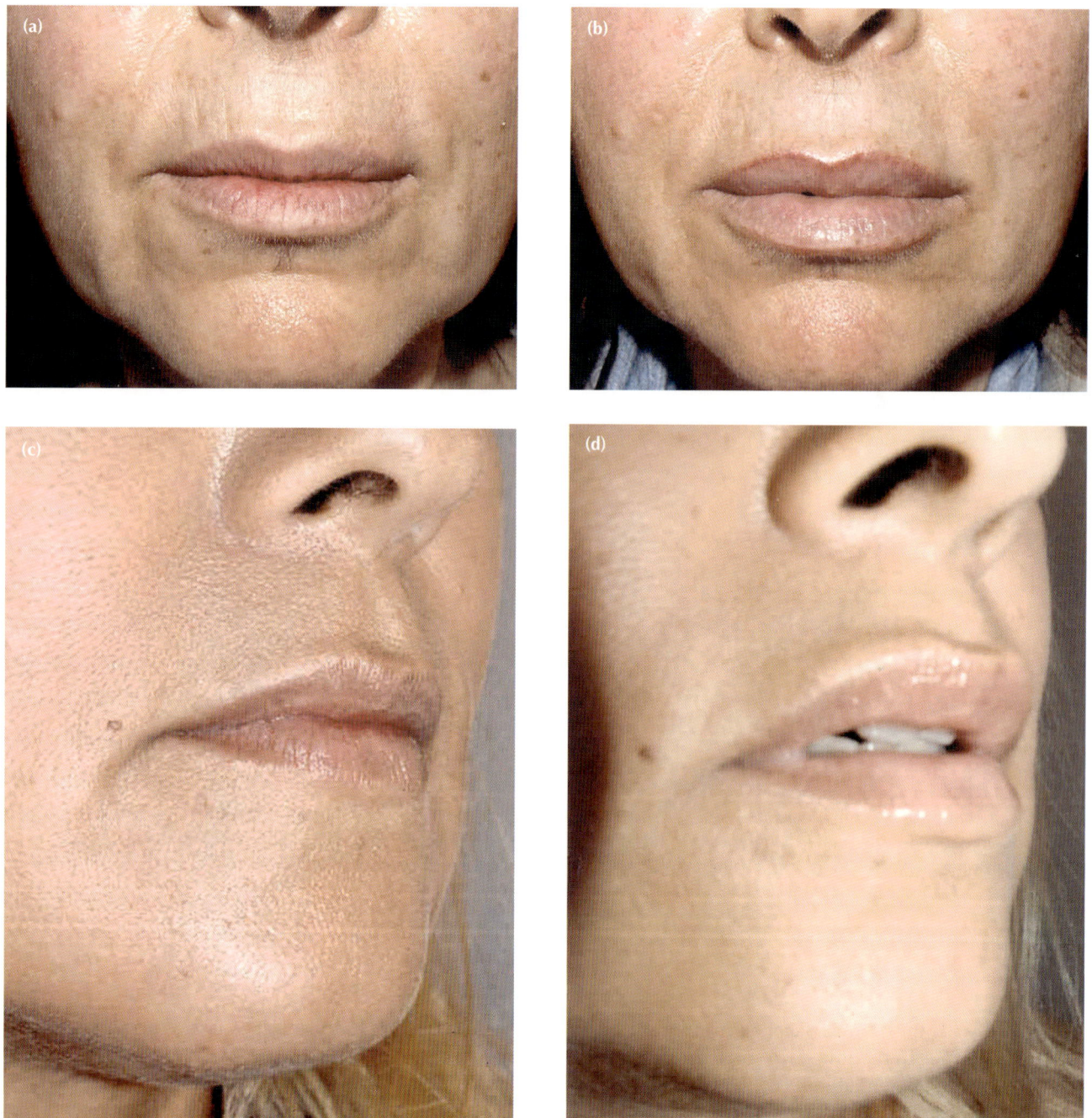

Figure 29.10   Rejuvenation procedure results for older lips: (a) before; (b) 4 weeks after Evolence Breeze injection to the vermilion border and lip body; (c) before; (d) 8 weeks after injection of Evolence Breeze to the vermilion border, lip body, and marionette wrinkles.

that some of these patients might have completely esthetically unacceptable ideas about what the perfect lip is (Figure 29.2).

Not infrequently, a patient will bring a picture of a movie star to demonstrate how she would like her lips to be. This practice allows the physician to get an idea about the esthetic world of the patient, and gives an opportunity to discuss what the realistic expectations from the procedure should be. If the patient's expectations do not

meet those of the physician, we strongly recommend not treating such a patient.

To avoid disappointment in the older patient group, the therapeutic options and treatment stages should be thoroughly discussed prior to treatment. If the patient wishes to avoid any invasive procedures, she should be prepared to expect suboptimal results. Choosing the invasive option, such as deep peeling or ablative laser resurfacing, the patient has to realize

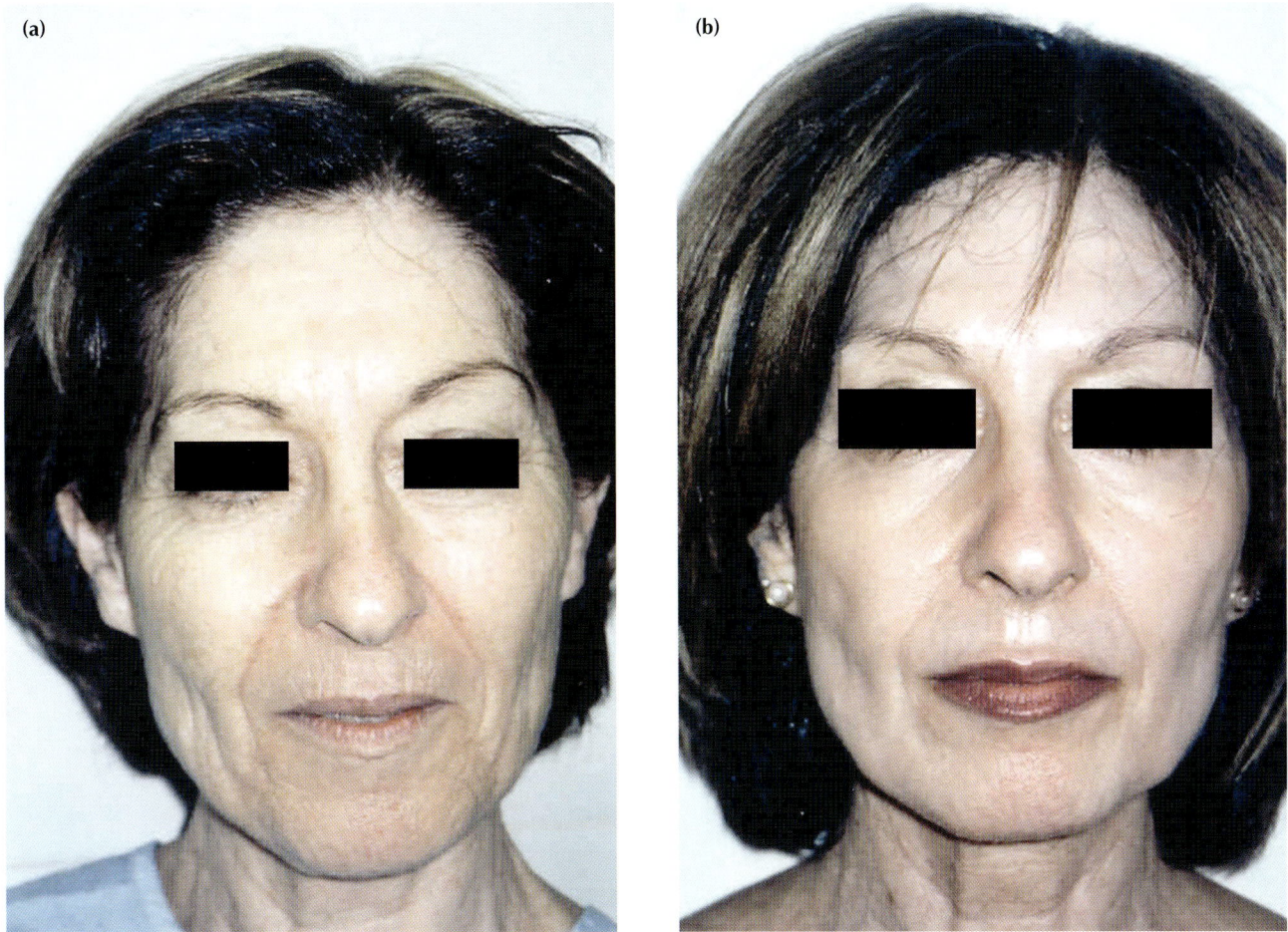

Figure 29.11 A combination of deep chemical peel (Exoderm® method) with lip augmentation: (a) before; (b) 6 months after Exoderm and 2 months after Surgilips injection.

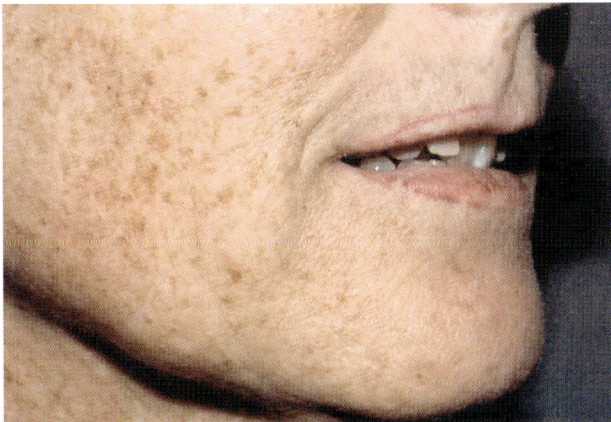

Figure 29.12 A 'non-existent' lip. A patient is trying to conceal the absence of the vermilion body by a permanent tattoo. In such circumstances surgical involvement is required.

that the final result will show in a few weeks or months.

In conclusion, perioral skin rejuvenation and lip augmentation is a challenging field for a physician.

Dermal fillers are an important tool in this area, but a multimodal approach is needed in some cases to provide an appropriate solution.

References

1. Sutter RE, Turley PK. Soft tissue evaluation of contemporary Caucasian and African American female profile. Angle Orthod 1998; 68: 487–96.
2. Bisson M, Grobbelaar A. The esthetic properties of lips: a comparison of models and nonmodels. Angle Orthod 2004; 74: 162–6.
3. Maloney BP. Cosmetic surgery of the lip. Facial Plast Surg 1996; 12: 265–78.
4. Burstone C. Lip posture and its significance in treatment planning. Am J Orthod 1967; 53: 262–84.
5. Klein AW. In search of the perfect lip: 2005. Dermatol Surg 2005; 31: 1599–603.
6. Austin HW. The lip lift. Plast Reconstr Surg 1986; 77: 990–4.
7. Fulton JE, Porumb S, Caruso JC, Shitabata PK. Lip augmentation with liquid silicone. Dermatol Surg 2005; 31: 1577–85.
8. Maly A, Regev E, Meir K, Maly B. Tissue reaction to liquid silicone simulating low-grade liposarcoma following lip augmentation. J Oral Pathol Med 2004; 33: 314.

30 Mesolift: a new 'soft' approach in rejuvenation techniques

Daphne Thioly-Bensoussan

Mesotherapy is a medical practice commonly used in rheumatology and traumatology; it consists of injecting a micro-amount of drug substance immediately under the skin, in direct proximity to the problem to be treated.

This technique dates back to 1952, developed by Dr Michel Pistor. The idea behind it is 'to inject little, seldom, at the right place'. The drug must cross the smallest possible path, so the solution is injected using a syringe with a small needle directly under the skin very close to the problem we are treating. Its interest is primarily in repeated injection and for products usually used in small quantities in general medicine (anti-inflammatory or analgesic drugs, muscle relaxants, vasodilators, homeopathic and phytotherapy products).

In traditional medicine, mesotherapy is used to treat chronic pain (in particular migraine), rheumatism, certain dermatological conditions (shingles, herpes), and infections (angina, sinusitis, bronchitis, etc.). Its relaxant, analgesic, or anti-inflammatory properties give rise to these indications.

Mesotherapy has more recently been used in esthetic medicine, where it has found renewed interest in the evolution of treatments of cutaneous aging and various cosmetic complaints such as 'orange peel' skin, while taking an active part in fluid drainage and blood circulation.

In the past, to treat aging skin, the product used in mesotherapy of the face, décolleté, and neck was a revitalizing formula injected in multiple intradermal microdoses and consisting of vasodilators, vitamins, and embryoblasts.

As the use of human and animal products was stopped a few years ago, the addition of native hyaluronic acid (not crossed-linked) to the mesotherapy cocktail has considerably improved the effects of this technique, today called mesolift, mesoglow, biorejuvenation, or biorevitalization.

The goal of mesotherapy in skin rejuvenation is to increase the biosynthetic capacity of fibroblasts with the reconstruction of an optimal physiological environment, enlargement of cellular activity, and production of new collagen, elastin, and hyaluronic acid, which results in firmness, brightness, and moisturizing of the skin.

In our therapeutic practice, treatments needing 'downtime' such as medium-depth and deep peels, laser resurfacing, and facelifts are less required than 'soft' techniques such as superficial peels, fillers, botulinum toxin, photorejuvenation, and mesolift, even if some of these techniques require more frequent sessions.

Mesotherapy is a very common technique used in rheumatology and traumatology; microinjections of conventional drugs, homeopathic drugs, vitamins, and minerals in the dermis or deeper deliver healing or corrective treatment to a specific area of the body. It is more recently used in cosmetology, included in the 'soft' rejuvenation techniques for the face, neck, décolleté, and hands, and is a wonderful complement to other skin treatments such as photorejuvenation, fillers, botulinum toxin, and chemical peels, but it definitively stands on its own as a powerful antiaging therapy. With sun damage and progressive collagen and hyaluronic acid loss, the skin loses its plumpness and resilience; mesotherapy skin rejuvenation or mesolift infuses the dermis with potent vitamins and antioxidants to rejuvenate and revitalize the skin. Adding to this cocktail native fluid hyaluronic acid gives a better action due to its specific properties.

To summarize, mesolift is the direct multi-injection of revitalizing substances into the superficial dermis. Twenty years ago, facial mesotherapy was performed using vasodilators, vitamins, and embryoblasts. Today, using hyaluronic acid and stimulating substances, mesolift is in line with all the 'no downtime' antiaging techniques such as superficial peels, fillers, botulinum toxin, and photorejuvenation.

Indications

Over the years, the skin undergoes clinical and histological changes because of intrinsic aging (chronoaging),

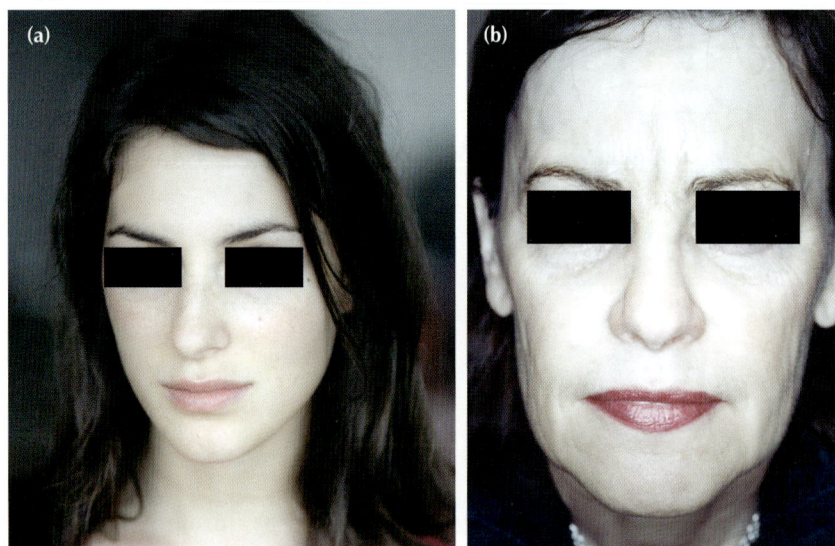

Figure 30.1   The young (a) and the old (b) face.

such as alterations in skin texture and elasticity, in skin pigmentation, in subcutaneous tissue, and in the vascular system.

Clinically the skin becomes relatively atrophic, lax, and wrinkled. Histologically the epidermis is atrophic. Dermal features include decreased thickness, loss of elastic fibers, and a decrease in the biosynthetic capacity of fibroblasts. The immune, endocrine, and neural functions of the skin also decrease with age. All these changes are genetically determined and, for this reason, are different in each individual.

Chronoaging can be worsened by cumulative environmental damage, such as caused by chronic ultraviolet light (UV) light exposure (photodamage), the presence of pollutants, and smoking. The superimposed effects of photodamage on intrinsically aging skin have been defined as photoaging. It is characterized by wrinkles, shallowness, laxity, mottled pigmentation, and texturally rough skin. Cutaneous malignancies may be associated. Histologically, the epidermal thickness may be increased or decreased, corresponding to areas of hyperplasia or atrophy. There is loss of polarity of epidermal cells and keratinocyte atypia. Dermal features include elastosis, and degeneration of collagen and anchoring fibrils. Blood vessels become dilated and twisted. UV light exposure activates free radicals and matrix degrading metalloproteinase enzymes including collagenase.

Non-invasive (clinical and photographic scoring) and invasive techniques (histological, instrumental, and biochemical tests) have been proposed, by several authors, with the idea of developing an objective method for evaluating all these changes.

Clinical and photographic scoring systems are the easiest to perform and the most utilized in clinical practice, even if they are not a valid objective method.

Therapeutic postulate and physiopathogical bases

In the younger face, all volumes that create the oval architecture of the face are important: high malar region, firm cheek, pulpy lips, and points of luminosity are more important than areas of shading (Figure 30.1a).

The general aspect of the skin is smooth, tightened, and soft; it is translucent and of uniform color, without spots, dilated vessels, or signs of irregularities.

Well-placed reference marks include high eyebrows, tonic eyelid, well-drawn horizontal mouth, lack of lower cheek excess, and firm, elastic skin, without wrinkles or folds.

Evolution with time

Progressive cutaneous aging of the face arises from intrinsic factors (genetic and familial) and extrinsic, including UV light, smoking, pollution, stress, the menopause, and rapid loss of weight. These factors can be associated in an important and individual way (Figure 30.1b).

Facial aging is due to epidermal and dermal factors, loss of subcutaneous fat, muscular relaxation, and osseous loss (especially from the mandibles) associated with dental thinning.

In the skin, the mitotic index of the basal cells decreases, the turnover of the keratinocytes decreases, and the granulosa become atrophied, resulting in rough, dry, wrinkled skin with loss of translucency, associated with pigment anomalies and telangiectasis.

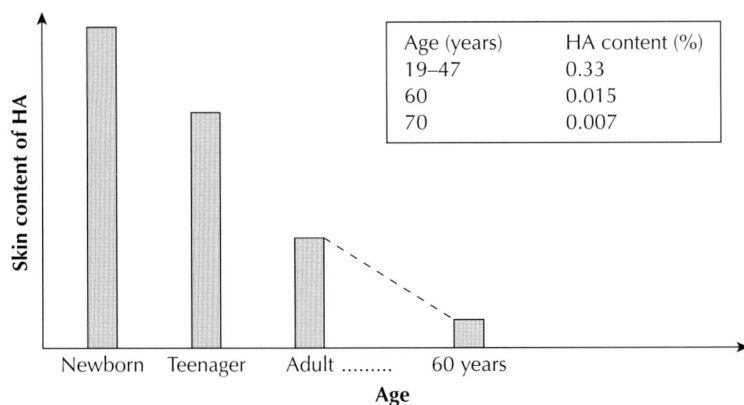

Figure 30.2 Hyaluronic acid decline with age.

The dermis becomes thinner with age (reduction of 20% of its thickness), collagen fibers become more compact and more tangled, elastic fibers decrease in quantity and quality, and the rate of glycoaminoglycan (hyaluronic acid) production decreases. The activity and number of fibroblasts and small vessels fall clinically, involving a loss of elasticity, density, and firmness of the skin, the appearance of creases, expression wrinkles, and folds and then of ptosis.

The loss of subcutaneous fat leads to a diminishing of mechanical support of the skin and the function of filling and contribution to the volume of the face.

Maxillary and mandibular osseous loss, especially associated with aging and thinning of the teeth, results in retraction of the lips and retrognathism of the mouth.

All these factors, associated with a gravity effect, can lead to various types of wrinkles, barely detectable before age 25, developing toward age 35 years (0.5 μm depth), and at age 40 years expression wrinkles being more marked in the dermis (1 μm depth). The folds grow gradually; the skin starts to lose its firmness, the menopause accelerating this process.

Which techniques can be advised?

Each technique is a function of the target to be reached. Epidermal lesions are treated with peels, lasers, or intense pulsed light (IPL). Wrinkles are reduced after injection of fillers, volumetric products, and botulinum toxin, or with medium-depth or deep peels. Loss of firmness and density can be improved with use of mesolift, IPL, rejuvenation lasers, poly-L-lactic acid (PLLA), or fat injection. Cutaneous relaxation or ptosis will be improved by deep PLLA, peels (phenol), or surgery.

These various techniques can be classified into 'soft' and 'hard'. The 'soft' techniques include injections of fillers, superficial peels, mesolift, rejuvenation lasers, and botulinum toxin. There is no need to restrict social or professional activities after these procedures (after certain procedures make-up will be necessary to camouflage possible bruising). These techniques require repetition within a fairly short time period.

They differ from the 'hard' techniques, which restrict social and professional activities for 8 days for an epidermal procedure (medium-depth peel) and even longer for laser resurfacing, phenol peel, or surgery.

However, today, the request for cosmetic treatment is specifically for an effective, durable technique, without 'downtime'.

Skin hyaluronic acid content

In the dermis, as shown in Figure 30.2, during the aging process there is a continuous loss of hyaluronic acid (HA), leading to a loss of skin hydration and elasticity and the appearance of wrinkles.

The study of Di Pietro reports that, when we inject HA in the skin, its hydrating effect returns to the skin a certain elasticity and firmness and lasts practically 3 months (Figure 30.3).

Mesotherapy of the face with only HA or in combination with a mesotherapy cocktail is called 'mesolift'. As these cocktails become rich in active substances, their efficacy and harmlessness remains to be shown. They can include: New-Fill®/Sculptra®, dimethylaminoethanol (DMAE), phosphatidylcholine, glycolic acid, and even botulinum toxin ('mesobotox').

Materials

What type of hyaluronic acid?

The type of hyaluronic acid used should be non-reticulated or native. It is known especially for its moisturizing and viscoelastic properties. It conveys to the dermal tissues a significant moisturization which represents two advantages. It allows an assured quality

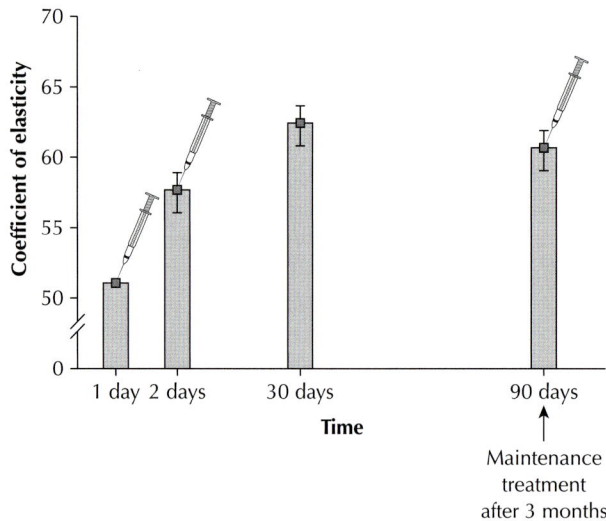

Figure 30.3   Effect of hyaluronic acid injection according to study of Di Pietro.

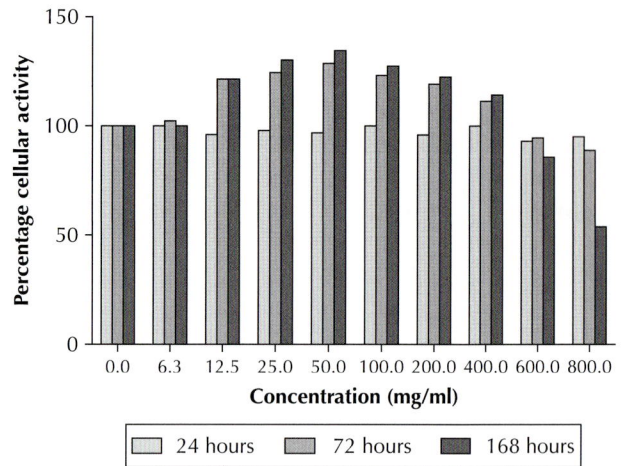

Figure 30.4   Effect of NCTF 135 on fibroblast stimulation.

of suppleness of the fundamental substance as well as a sufficient reserve of water which ensures optimum moisturizing of superficial layers of the epidermis.

Moreover, this effect is complemented by the action of hyaluronic acid on angiogenesis, favoring the proliferation of endothelial cells which allows better cutaneous vascularization.

It is available in syringes of 0.5–1 ml or 2.5 ml and in variable concentrations:

- Achyal (Filorga) 1% kD
- Juvelift (Leaderm) 1% 2,5 kD
- IAL System (Phytogene) 1,8% 1 kD
- Hyaluderm (LCA) 2% 2,4 kD
- Restylane Vital* (Q-Med) 2% *reticule
- Teosyal Meso (Teoxane) 1,5% 1 kD
- Surgilift (Corneal) 1,35% 2,5 kD
- Elastence (Inamed) 3% 0,9 kD
- Mesolis 1,4%, Mesolis+ 2.5% (Antheis) 2.5 kD
- R-fine 1% (centrale des peelings) 2 kD

(*This is reticulated but marketed by Q-Med laboratory for mesolift.)

Or, it can be supplied in vials of 5–10 ml (MesoSphere 3.5%, Medicage 3.5%, Revitacare® 2%, Erwa Productos HYA 2%).

The hyaluronic acid is injected alone or in combination with a revitalization cocktail of NCTC 109 (Biophymed), NCTF 135 (Filorga) (Figure 30.4), or Aesthetic Dermal (Medicage).

The vitamin cocktail is a sterile solution maintained by five groups of components to support the life of cell cultures:

- vitamins: A, E, C, B, K, assure antidegradation and antioxidizing effect
- 24 amino acids, assure better protein building

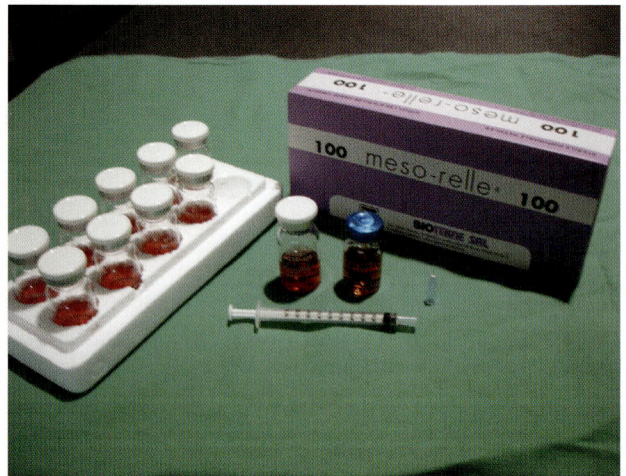

Figure 30.5   Mesotherapy materials.

- minerals: Na, K, Ca, Mg, catalysts of tissue reactions, guarantee medium ionic balance
- coenzymes: activators of biochemical reactions
- nucleic acids: RNA, DNA, stimulate protein synthesis.

The elements act in a synergistic way, having an antioxidizing role, regulating cell functions, stimulating fibroblasts, and activating the microcirculation (Figure 30.5).

Technology

Material

The HA syringe alone is used, injected with a needle of 32G, or the HA is diluted in the aforementioned

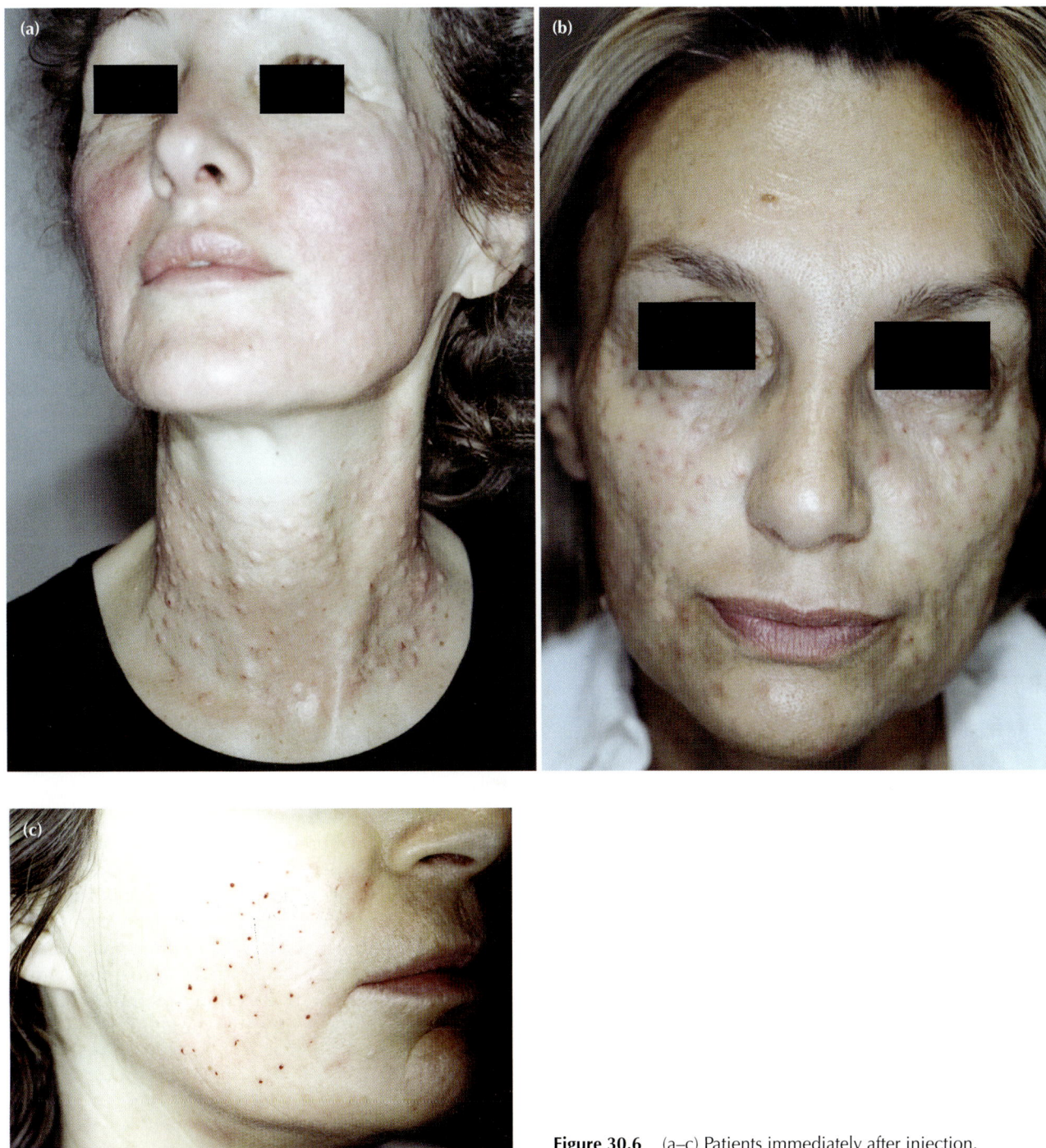

Figure 30.6 (a–c) Patients immediately after injection.

revitalizing cocktail. For every session we use 1 ml HA associated with 5 ml of solution.

The 32G needles can be of different lengths; the simplest for intradermal mesotherapy are 0.5 mm in length.

The mesotherapy gun used to inject HA diluted in the cocktail allows uniformity of injected dose and injection depth, and a short duration of the session. The latest generation of mesotherapy guns includes the U225 (Biophymed), which permits treatment in 'gusts' (nine shots per second) after the first injection session, which increases the inflammatory reaction and therefore skin healing.

Injection technique

We use either a syringe of HA (1 ml) alone or the same syringe with mesotherapy cocktail (5 ml).

The skin is disinfected with chlorhexidine. Then we inject volumes of 0.01 ml into the superficial intradermal layer, resulting in small papules spaced out by 3 mm, covering in a regular manner all surfaces treated (Figure 30.6). We then cover the surface with a cold dressing, or ice pack for 15 min.

The small papules persist for 2 h in general. A vitamin K5-based cream can be applied before using make-up.

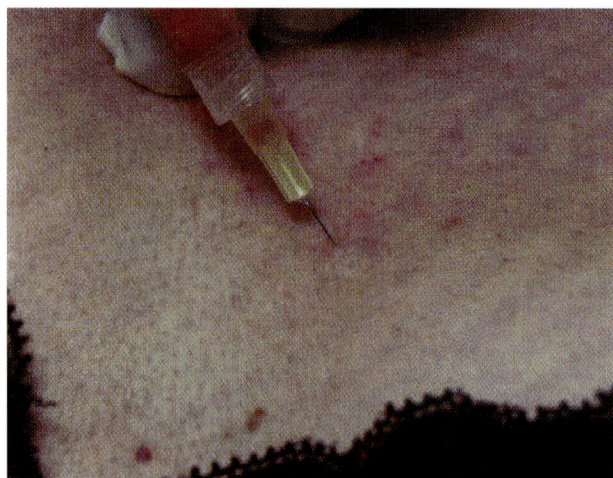

Figure 30.7   Mesotherapy: décolleté.

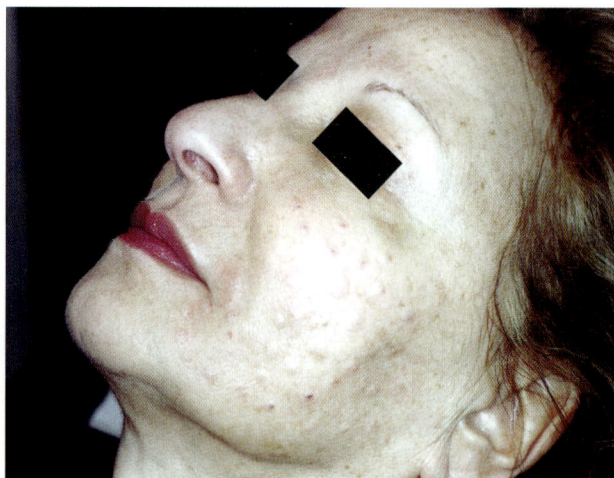

Figure 30.8   Ecchymosis.

Choice of patient

The technique adopted will depend on the level of aging of the skin. Different stages of skin aging exist:

- *Stage 1.* Tonic, low level of skin hydration; no wrinkles except during mimic state of the face; beginning of skin relaxation noticed by punch test of the skin: efficient revitalization.
- *Stage 2.* Visible dryness; wrinkles in movement and in repose state; fine wrinkles on the surface of the skin; lax skin during the punch test: revitalization is very effective.
- *Stage 3.* Intense dryness; fine wrinkles, creases, and grooves; permanent wrinkles in repose; clear laxity of the skin without any maneuver: slow and difficult revitalization. It is important to offer other antiaging methods and to combine them in the case of muscular laxity with facelift.

Treatment schedule

Two sessions every 3 weeks and renewable every 3 months are necessary especially in cases of premature aging, smoker's skin, and lifeless skin (stage 1). Four sessions every 15 days then recall every 2 or 3 months is required for unresponsive skin with loss of tone and major laxity (stage 2 or 3).

The sequence of treatments depends on the wishes and needs of the patient and can be associated with other antiaging techniques. This protocol can vary according to individual criteria: age of the patient, importance of wrinkles, photoaging, and sagging.

The treatment is accumulative, and is recommended, as long as improvement continues, to be carried out with 2–3 months between every session. With stabilization of the results, the interval between sessions can be 2, 3, or even 6 months, depending on the ideal interval for the patient.

Treated zones and indications

Treatment areas include the face, eyelids, neck, décolleté (Figure 30.7), and hands.

It is indicated in premature aging of the skin due to UV light exposure and smoking, and in cases of precocious elastosis (fine wrinkles). It is ideal for treatment of the skin during the menopause and postmenopausal period and in cases of unresponsive skin with loss of tone and elasticity. Mesotherapy can be associated with filler injection treatment (which seems to augment the effective duration of the product in the skin).

Side-effects and precautions

Aspirin, anti-inflammatories, and vasoconstrictors must be stopped 8 days before the injection.

It is preferable to use topical anesthesia, 1 h before the session; this reduces the risk of ecchymosis and allows a comfortable session. Ecchymosis, in the form of small punctiform hematomas with diffuse erythemas (Figure 30.8), can be hidden using camouflage make-up (Gingham, Roche-Posay, Avène). Certain zones can be more marked, such as the neck and inferior lids. The preventive use of arnica and of cream based on vitamin K5 can be beneficial for certain patients. It will be necessary to verify the absence of major allergy (test if necessary) and the removal of any non-absorbable products used previously.

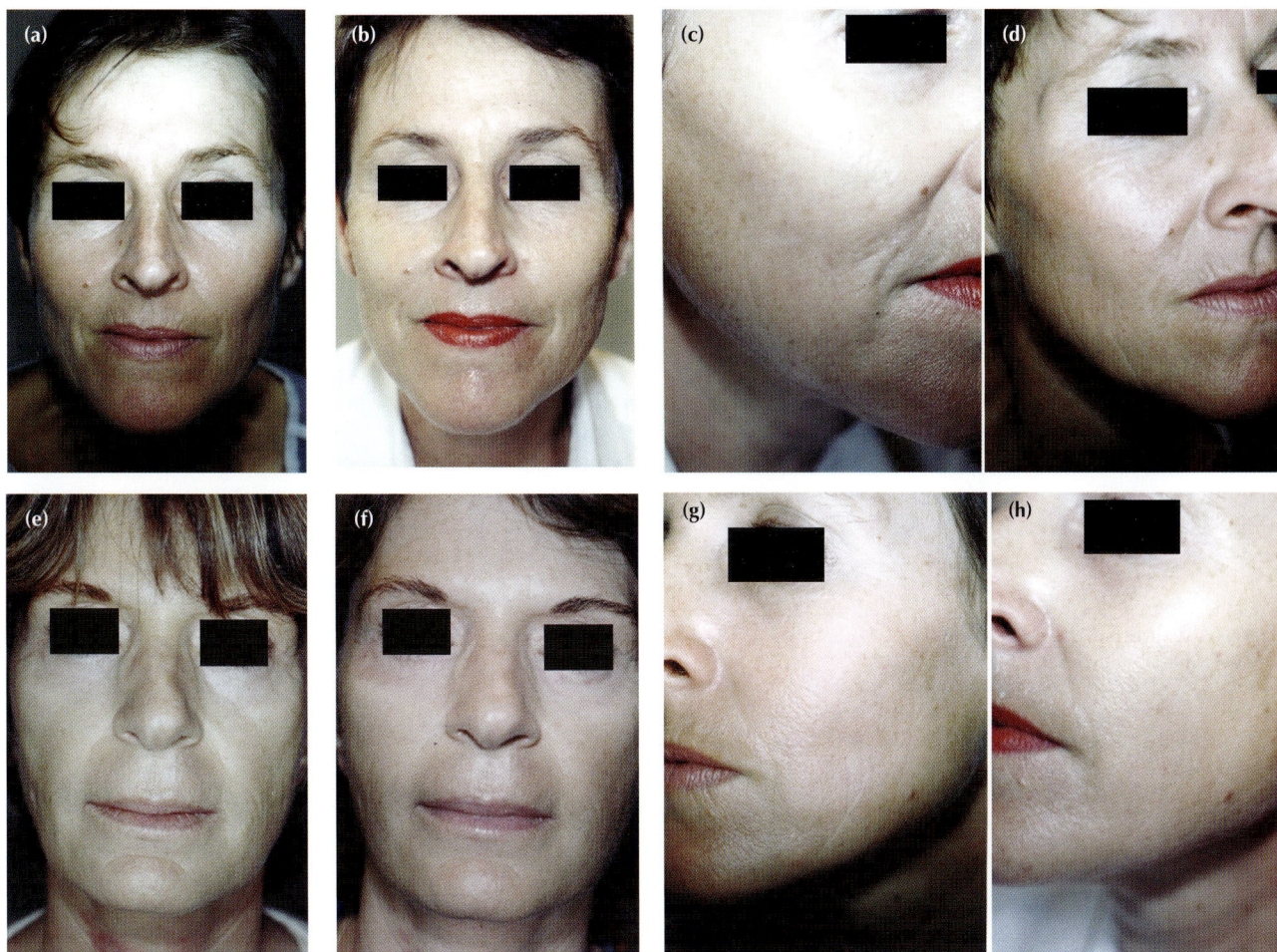

Figure 30.9   (a, b) Before and after treatment; (c, d) before and after five sessions; (e, f) before and after five sessions; (g, h) before and after 15 sessions.

Results

The optimization of cellular functions improves skin hydration and cutaneous elasticity, increases cell turnover, and increases fibroblast activity and the production of collagen fibers and glycoaminoglycan. This leads to an appearance of younger skin, being softer and fresher looking, more translucent complexion, firmer and denser skin, and reduction in appearance of fine wrinkles (Figure 30.9).

Conclusion

Mesolift has an important place among techniques of 'soft' rejuvenation of the face, the neck, the décolleté, and the hands.

Using the mesolift technique, it is possible to improve the appearance of the complexion, with cutaneous moisturization, amelioration of elasticity and firmness aspects of the skin, and the attenuation of fine wrinkles. Preventive treatment to the zones at risk allows optimization of the 'padding' of the dermis.

Evaluation of the stage of aging permits a treatment schedule to be devised, and it is preferable to begin at the first signs of skin laxity.

Mesolift is classified as a therapeutic antiaging technique, in association with all other 'soft' techniques of rejuvenation such as fillers, botulinum toxin, superficial peels, and rejuvenation lasers.

Bibliography

Balazs EA, Denliger JL. Clinical use of hyaluronic acid. In: Evered D, Whelem J, eds. The Biology of Hyaluronan. Ciba Foundation Symposium 143. Chichester: Wiley, 1989: 265–80.

Burd DA, Greco RM, Regauer S et al. Hyaluronan and wound healing: a new perspective. Br J Plast Surg 1991; 44: 579–84.

Clark RAF. Cutaneous tissue repair: basic biologic considerations. J Am Acad Dermatol 1985; 13: 705–25.

De Goursac C. la mesotherapie du visage. J Med Esth Chir Derm 2003; XXX(117).

Foschi D, Castoldi L, Radaelli E et al. Hyaluronic acid prevents oxygen free-radical damage to granulation tissue: a study in rats. Int J Tissue React 1990; 6: 333–9.

Garcia Mingo J, Benitez Roig V, San Gil Sorbet A. Evaluation de Achyal (acido hialuronico) como relleno dermico. Int J Cosmet Med Surg 2000; 1: 20–2.

Ghersetich I, Lotti T. Hyaluronic acid in cutaneous intrinsic aging. Int J Dermatol 1994; 33: 119–22.

Hertzog B. La mesotherapie in médecine esthétique. In: Manuel Pratique Médecine Esthétique. 1998: 59–67.

Lapierre CM. The aging dermis: the hand talks of the appearance of old skin. Br J Dermatol 1990; 122: 5–11.

Mesotherapy for skin rejuvenation. Cosmet Surg News 2005;

Small P. La mesotherapy esthétique in 2001. J Med Esth Chir Derm 2001; XXIX(110): 121–4.

Tordjman M. Rejuvenation cutanée de décolleté par mesotherapie. J Med Esth Chir Derm 2003; XXX(118): 111–18.

Weigel PH, Frost SJ, McGary CT et al. The role of hyaluronic acid in inflammation and wound healing. Int J Tissue React 1988; 10: 355–65.

Weigel PH, Fuller GM, Le Boeuf RD. A model for the role of hyaluronic acid and fibrin in the early events during the inflammatory response and wound healing. J Theor Biol 1986; 119: 219–34.

31 Body mesotherapy and 'mesobotox'

Ghislaine Beilin

Introduction

Mesotherapy is a medical technique for injecting a mixture of drugs in small quantities intradermally into a problem area.

This technique was first developed by Dr Pistor in 1952. Since that time, many clinical indications have been developed by both the French and the International Mesotherapy Society, mostly in degenerative pathologies, as well as neurovegetative infectiology, rheumatology, sports injuries, otolaryngology, dermatology, and so on. Over the past few years, the use of mesotherapy for cosmetic conditions has increased. Body mesotherapy mainly concerns the treatment of excess fat and cellulite, weight and is also used for skin tightening.

The products allowed for injection can be different in different countries, in Europe or the USA or Asia. Some of them have disappeared from the market or approval, but then new active products have become available. This chapter aims to give a global description of them and their indications.

Body mesolipolysis

There are different classifications of body mesotherapy and types of fat deposit.

Clinical

Mesotherapy injections can be located in the epidermis, dermis, or hypodermis. The composition of the solution used will vary according to the clinical evaluation. For body mesotherapy of fat deposits, we can distinguish:

- superficial cellulite:
  - different layers and level I, II, or III
  - different components including vascular with edema, fibrosis, and hypertrophy of adipocytes
  - indications for vascular, lipolytic, and trophic products
  - injection in the epidermis to the hypodermis, 1–6 mm

- deep fat in the hypodermis (hydrolipodystrophy):
  - indication for mesolipolysis with lipolytic product or phosphatidylcholine
  - deep injection, 10 mm.

Physiopathological

Fat deposits are under the control of many factors, including: genetic, hormonal, venolymphatic components, metabolism and nutrition, excess weight, and lifestyle (no exercise, excess alcohol, salt, etc.).

The adipocyte is sensitive to stimulation of the α or the β receptor.

Stimulation of the β receptor induces a reduction in size of the adipocyte, while α-adrenergic receptors increase the storage of fat. β-Adrenergic receptors are located on the arms, stomach, abdomen, and upper part of the body in males and females. They can be stimulated by diet. α-Adrenergic receptors are located on the thighs, mainly in women, and are very difficult to stimulate.

The classification of hyperlipodystrophy[1,2] is illustrated in Figure 31.1. Based on this knowledge, different products are used in mesotherapy.

Products

β-Receptors

For dopaminergic and adrenergic β stimulation, Isuprel® or Isoproteranol® (USA), 0.2 ml, can be included. However, their use is dangerous because of β_1 receptor myocardial and β_2 receptor vasodilatation and bronchodilatation activity. A high-protein diet and exercise can stimulate these receptors.

α-Receptors

Their stimulation decreases lipolysis. The α_2 receptor can be inhibited by Vadilex®, Fonzylane®, or Yohimbine® 2% or 5%. Yohimbine is a strong cardiologic stimulator and must be used very carefully in a maximum quantity of 5 mg, that is, 1 ml of Yohimbine® at 2% or 0.5 ml at 5%, an hour and a half after a meal.

```
                              Hyperlipodystrophy
        ┌─────────────────────────────┴──────────────────────────────┐
      Deep                                              Superficial cellulite
   ┌────┴────┐                                    ┌──────────┼──────────┐
Diffuse    Localized                          Infiltrated  Fibrosis   Adipose
   =           =
obesity    steatomery

Products: lipolytic                          Products: vascular
          phosphatidylcholine                         lipolytic
          vasodilator                                 trophic

Deep injection 10 mm                         Superficial injection 1 mm–6 mm
Point by point hypodermal                    Superficial epidermal papule
                                             Point by point dermal and hypodermal

Quantity: 0.2 ml maximum                     'Nappage' mode to 0.2 ml maximum
```

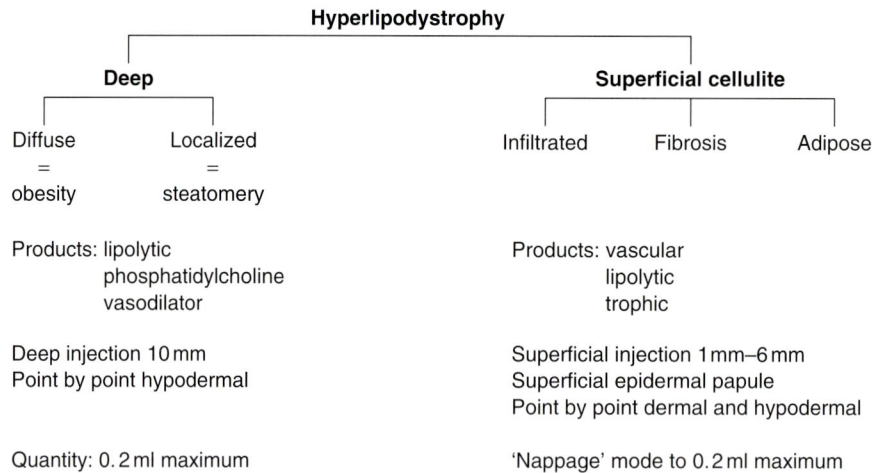

Figure 31.1   Classification of hyperlipodystrophy.[1,2]

Table 31.1   Products used in mesotherapy

Lipolytic action	Vascular action	Trophic action
Caffeine	Sweet clover–rutine	Vitamin C
L-carnitine	Ginkgo biloba	Polyvitamins
Coenzyme A	Procaine	Asian centella
Alcaxantina® (alcachofa + aminophylline)	Lidocaine	Conjonctyl®
Aminophylline	Buflomedil	Hyaluronic acid
Euphylline	Pentoxifylline	Chondroitin sulfate
Tiratricol	Benzopirone	X-ADN®
Yohimbine®	Calcitonin	Placentex®
Lipostabil®		Lisados®
Hyaluronidase		DMAE (dimethylaminoethanol)
Collagenase		

Products used are listed in Table 31.1. Isuprel or adrenaline (epinephrine) are not recommended. Many other products have been tried: hormones including human growth hormone (HGH) and corticoids.

Technique and protocol

The quantities listed below total 10 ml, which is the minimum we need to treat an area such as the legs, stomach, thighs, or both arms.

The injection can be given manually or assisted by an automatic or electropneumatic injector for deep injections.[3]

Superficial cellulite

The technique is superficial by means of 'nappage' or intraepidermal mode, associated with point by point to a depth of 4 mm (Figure 31.2). The frequency is once a week, for eight sessions. The protocol is (10/ml):

- procaine 2 ml
- Conjonctyl® 2 ml

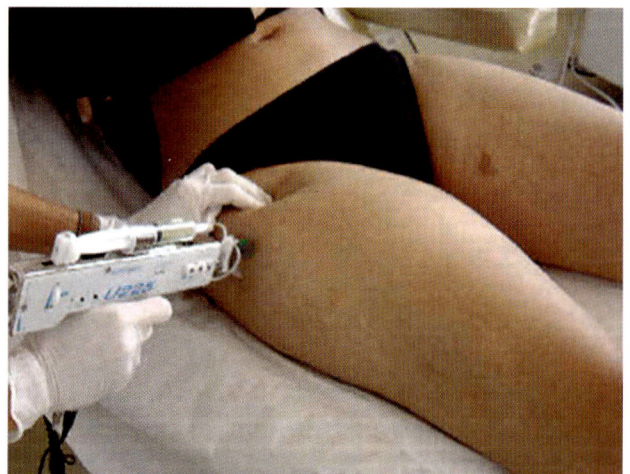

Figure 31.2   Superficial cellulite treatment.

- Torental® 2 ml
- physiological saline 1 ml
- caffeine 2 ml
- arnica 1 ml

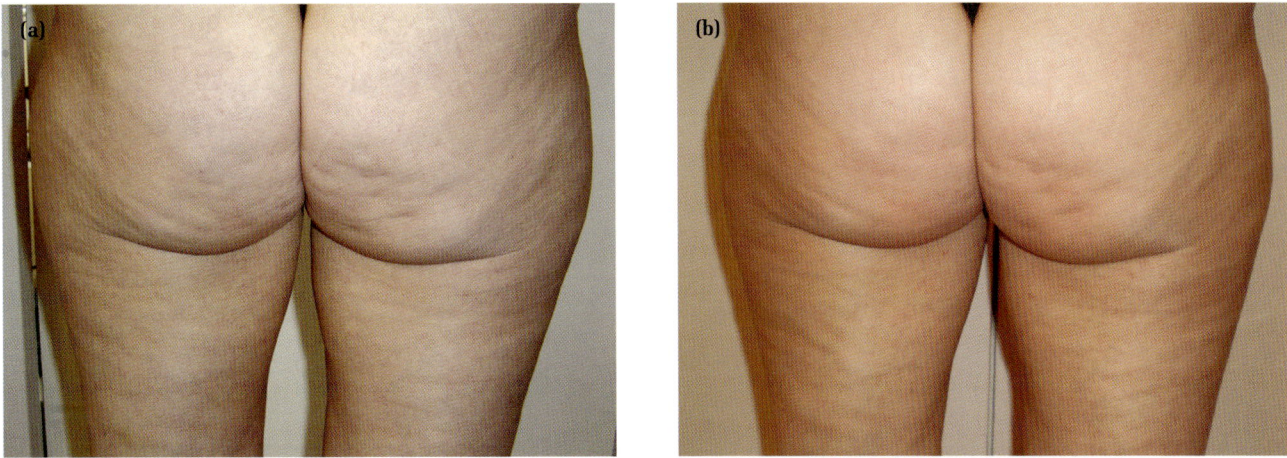

Figure 31.3 Results of superficial cellulite treatment in a 58-year-old woman: (a) before and (b) 1 week after two sessions.

The side-effects are that caffeine induces bruising which can stay 1 week; we have occasionally noticed a general effect of injection of caffeine.

Results This technique is safe; the products are medically approved. The treatment is repeated once or twice a year.

It is a good indication for young people with superficial cellulite, associated with diet, exercise, and other medical or physical therapy treatment (Figure 31.3).

Deep localized fat or steatomeries

Different protocols can be used (10 ml):

Lipostabil® 2.5 ml
sweet clover–rutine 2.5 ml
lidocaine 1% 2 ml
physiological saline 1.5 ml
Torental 1.5 ml

Vadilex 1/3
phosphatidylcholine 1/3
dimethylaminoethanol 1/6
lidocaine 1/6.

Results are shown in Figure 31.4.

Mesolipolysis with phosphatidylcholine

Phosphatidylcholine (PPC) is extracted from soy lecithin. The lipolytic action effect was first described by Dr Patricia Rittes in 2000.

PPC is available in the USA under the name Lipostabil for the treatment of endovascular atheroma,

and is also used for treatment of lipoma and xanthelasma. The use of PPC for lipolysis is off label and the responsibility of the practicing physician. To be active, PPC is always associated with a solvent: deoxycholate, which is a bile salt necessary to break down the cell membrane. Phosphatidylcholine induces emulsification and elimination of fat. This action occurs a few minutes after injection, and is associated with a strong inflammatory reaction, bruising, edema, and pain lasting a few days. The injection must be in the deep hypodermis, strictly in the fat to prevent muscular or superficial cutaneous necrosis. The total maximum quantity injected in a session is 2 g of PPC.

The use of pure deoxycholate is not recommended as it increases the risk of nodules and fibrosis, without better results. Phosphatidylcholine is hyperosmolar and must always be used diluted to 50% with other anticellulitic products:

- vascular action: sweetclover–rutine, procaine
- lipolytic action: caffeine, *Ruscus*, L-carnitine
- lipodystrophic: buflomedil, procaine
- skin tightening: Conjonctyl, dimethylaminoethanol (DMAE).

Technique and protocol

Four sessions are needed, 15 days apart. The minimum amount used for each side is two vials of 5 ml concentrated to 250 mg of phosphatidylcholine.

The area treated with 10 ml is a square of 10 × 10 cm. Injections are realized with a gun injector, 27G needle, point by point, 0.3–0.5 ml per injection, each injection separated by 1 cm (Figure 31.5).

Composition is (10 ml):

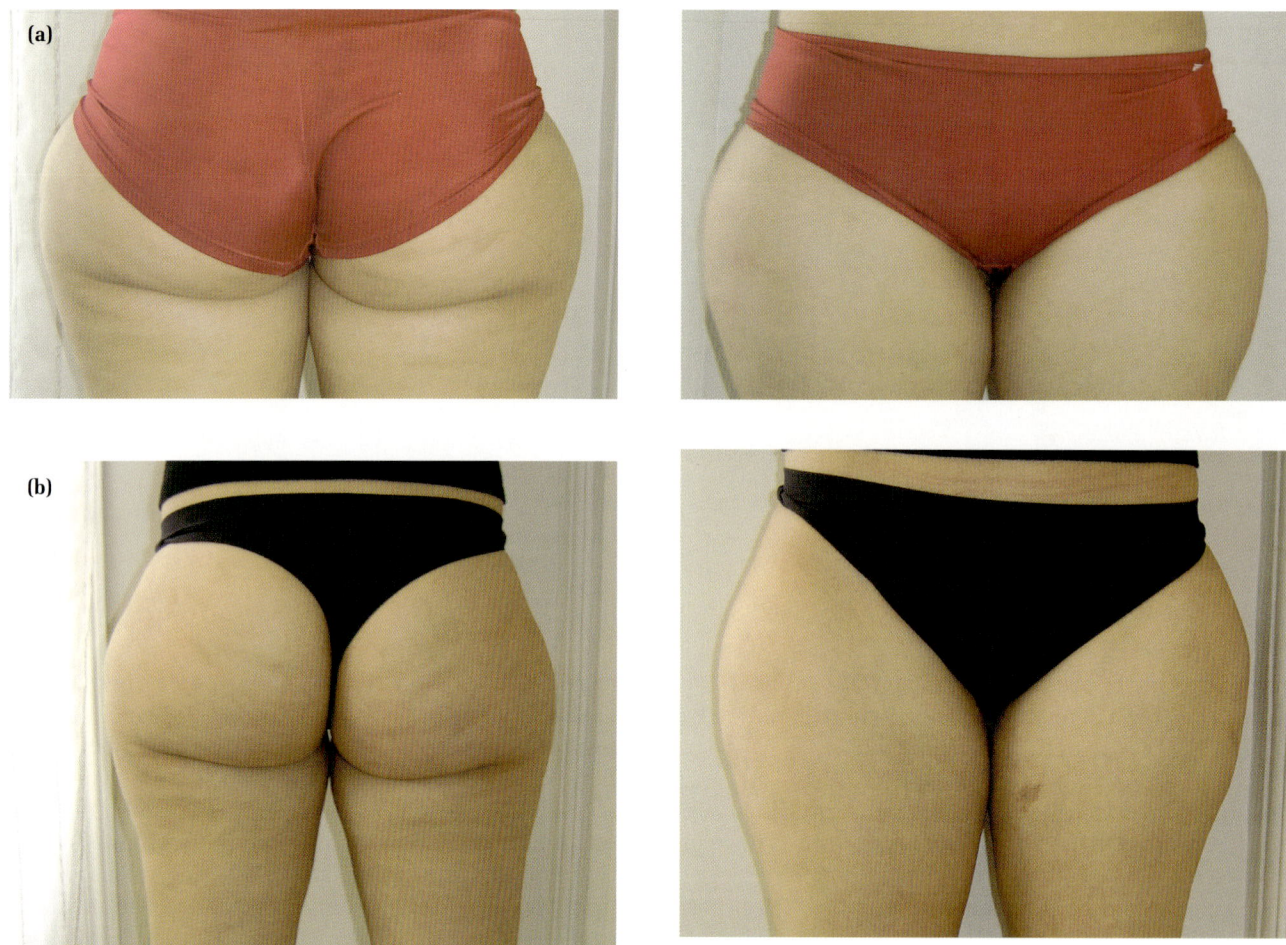

Figure 31.4   Results of deep localized treatment (steatomery) in a 21-year-old woman: (a) before and (b) after 3 months, three sessions.

phosphatidylcholine 5 ml
procaine 2 ml
DMAE or Conjonctyl or buflomedil 3 ml.

Side-effects

Injection is painful, and procaine or lidocaine must be added. A strong inflammatory reaction occurs which lasts half an hour. Some general effects may occur when several areas are treated in the same session. Bruising, edema, and pain lasting 5 days can be reduced by massage with arnica cream or an anti-inflammatory cream for a week.

The results will appear after 1–2 weeks up to a month. The treatment is effective and works definitively on fat deposits (Figure 31.6).

Hypo-osmolar mesolipolysis

This technique was described in 2006 and confirmed by a study including 444 women.[4] A reduction of fat

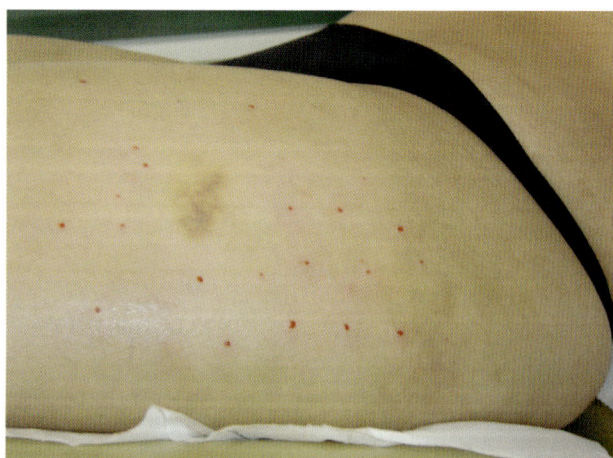

Figure 31.5   Mesolipolysis with phosphatidylcholine: point by point technique.

tissue of 30% measured by ultrasound proved the efficiency of hypo-osmolar injections.

The normal osmolarity of body tissue is 300 mosm/l. Injection of a hypo-osmolar solution of 100 mosm/l

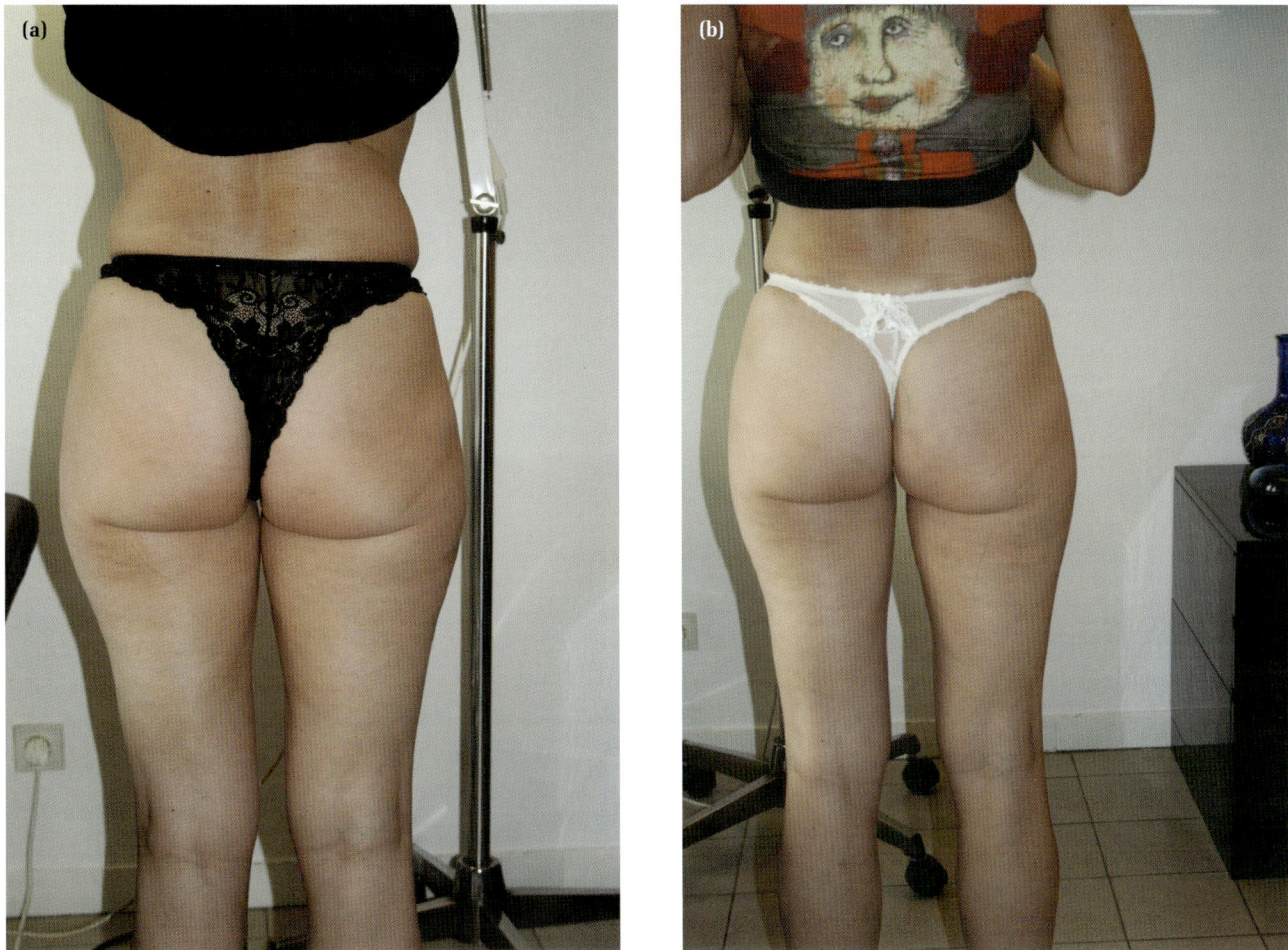

Figure 31.6   Mesolipolysis with phosphatidylcholine: (a) before and (b) after one session.

induces intracellular penetration of liquid into adipocytes and breaks down the cell membrane by increasing the volume.

Products

The composition of the hypo-osmolar solution includes the following (all products are available for mesotherapy injection):

   physiological saline
   lidocaine
   calcitonin
   thiocolchicoside
   vitamin C.

Technique and protocol

Deep injection to 10 mm is done with a 27G needle using a gun injector, giving 3–5 treatments 15 days apart (Figure 31.7).

Side-effects

Massive necrosis has been described with too large a volume injected or use of a 'dangerous cocktail'.

Body mesotherapy and skin tightening

Skin laxity occurs with aging, and is often associated with fat deposits.

Dimethylaminoethanol (DMAE) is a precursor of acetylcholine which stimulates muscle contraction via myofibrils and fibroblasts in the dermis and epidermis. It has an inverse action on muscle contraction compared with botulinum toxin. They are not opposite actions as their targets are different: botulinum toxin is active on striated muscle fiber contraction while DMAE is active on the myofibrils. It is also a hydrophilic molecule and cannot penetrate the hypodermal fat barrier.

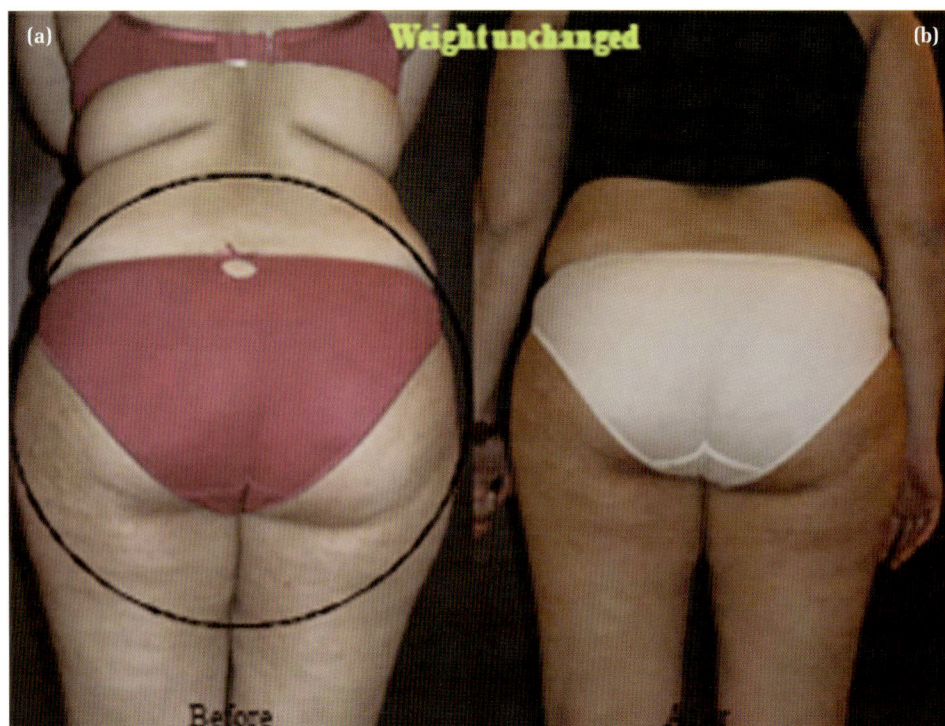

Figure 31.7 Hypo-osmolar meso-lipolysis: (a) before and (b) after treatment.

DMAE is also an antioxidant, vasoactive, and an immunomodulator, and protects dermal protein linkage. It has a beneficial effect on skin quality and laxity.

Products

Injection is point to point, to 5 mm, using (6/ml):

> DMAE 2 ml
> procaine 2 ml
> silicium Conjonctyl (R) 2 ml

or, if fat is associated:

> DMAE 2 ml
> PPC 2 ml
> procaine 2 ml

in the face or arms.

Technique and protocol

Three to four injections are carried out at monthly intervals. The result will develop until 1–2 months post-injection.

Side-effects

Some pain and edema occurs lasting a few days. Bruising can be evidenced on the body if associated with PPC.

Results

The best indications are on the face to restore the jaw-line (Figure 31.8), stomach (Figure 31.9), arms, and inner thighs.

Body mesotherapy and venolymphatic pathology

Venolymphatic treatment of the legs can be combined with treatment of fat deposits.

Products

- sympatholytic: lidocaine
- vasodilator: pentoxifylline
- antiedemic, anti-inflammatory: salmon calcitonin
- eliminator: ethamsylate.

Different compositions can be used:

> procaine 2 ml
> sweet clover–rutine 2 ml
> Dicynone® or Fonzylane 2 ml

> lidocaine 2 ml
> pentoxifylline 2 ml
> ethamsylate 2 ml

> lidocaine 1% 2 ml
> pentoxifylline 2 ml
> calcitonin 100 IU 1 ml.

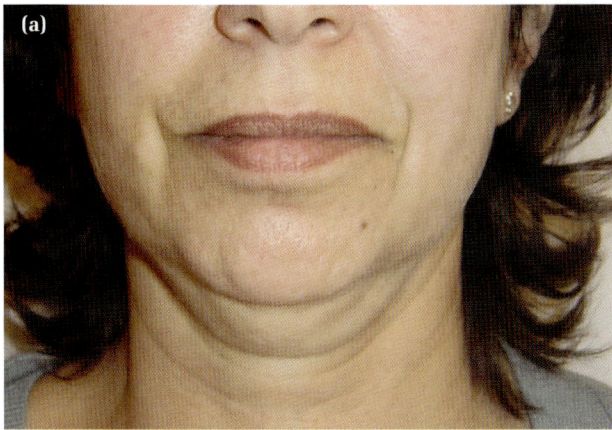

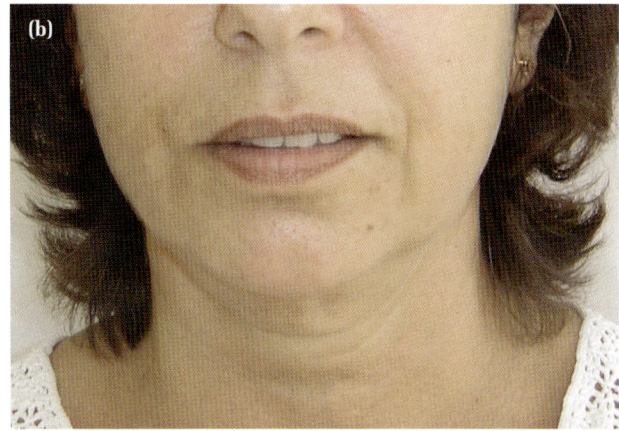

Figure 31.8   Skin tightening of the jawline in a 54-year-old woman: (a) before and (b) after 7months, five sessions.

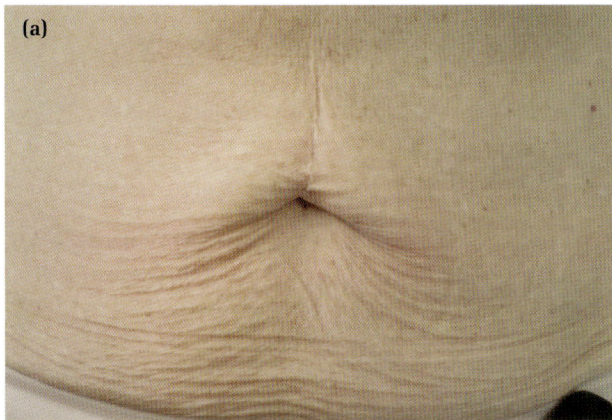

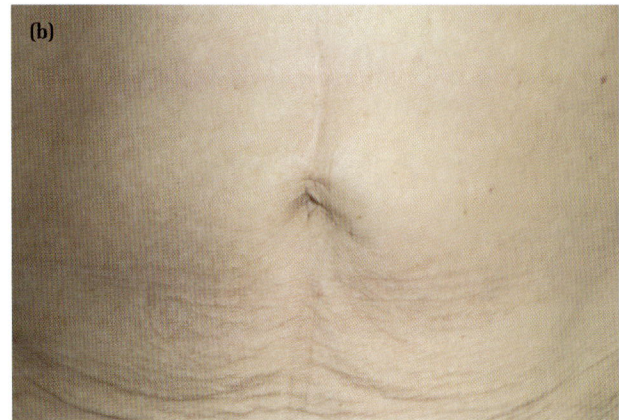

Figure 31.9   Skin tightening of the stomach in a 62-year-old woman: (a) before and (b) after 3 months, two sessions.

Technique and protocol

Intradermal superficial (1 mm) injection in nappage mode or deep intradermal (2–4 mm) injection is used.

Treatment consists of three sessions separated by 10 days, injecting the legs along the vascular axis of the inner thighs, and also the outer aspect and backs of the legs (Figure 31.10). This can be repeated for maintenance every 2 months, in the summer, or as soon as clinical symptoms appear.

'Mesobotox'

'Mesobotox' has been described by Bernard Hertzog.[5] It consists of the injection of botulinum toxin in low concentrations using the mesotherapy technique.

The word mesotherapy comes from mesoderm, the embryologic layer which is the origin of the dermis, the fibroblasts, and also the multiple, very thin, superficial muscles underlying the skin. These are responsible for the complex expressions and tensions of the face, while the deep striated muscle, the classical target of BOTOX® treatment, is responsible for the mobility of the face and deep wrinkles. The objective of 'mesobotox' is to reduce the superficial tension of the face and restore a natural expression.

Injections are intradermal with the highest dilution of BOTOX to help diffusion in the superficial dermis and muscles.

Physiopathology

The aging of the face is characterized by a change in expression, due to a global accentuation of muscle contraction and a progressive retraction of the natural orifices of the eyes and mouth.

With the loss of volume and tissue fat, bone recession, and retraction of the orifices, the face seems to contract inwards, opposite to a youthful appearance with no tension and an open, 'outward-turning' face.

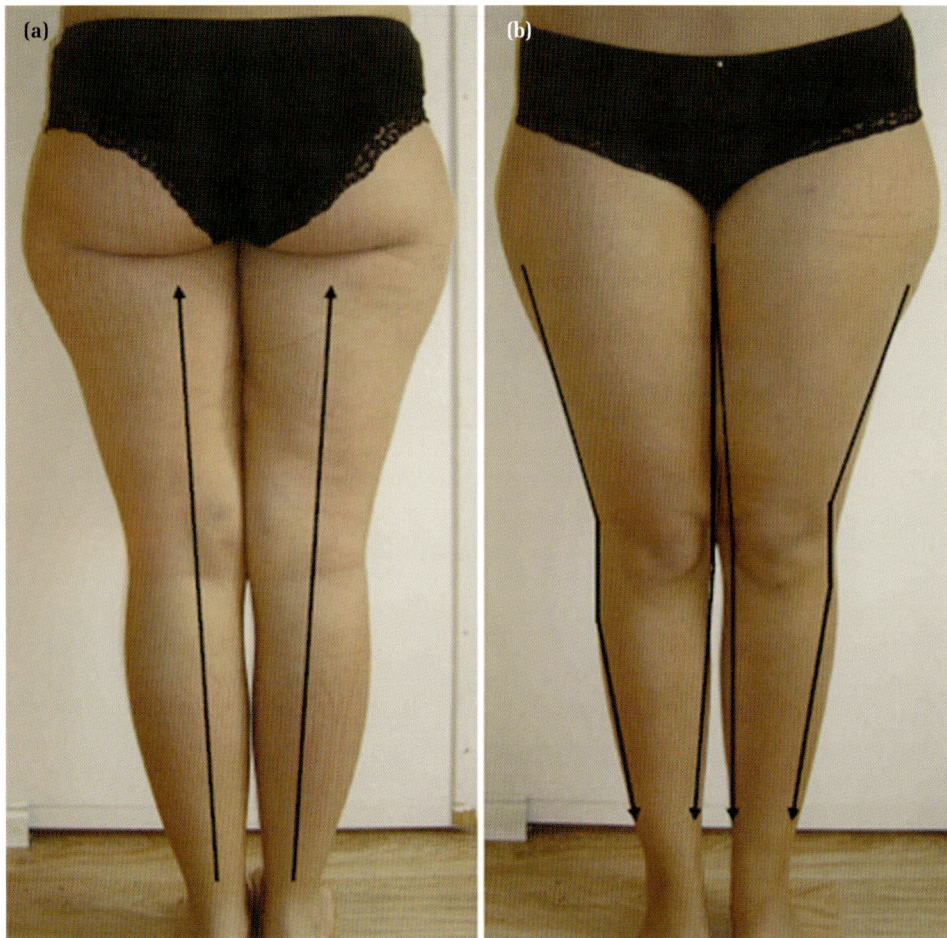

Figure 31.10 Body mesotherapy and venolymphatic pathology: (a) posterior vascular axis; (b) lateral vascular axes.

Even if the anatomy of the muscle underlying the facial skin has a similar distribution in all individuals, its 'volume', strength, and balance vary widely. This is why we have such a diversity of expressions, some simple and others very complex. The variety of facial expressions is endless.

The esthetic concept of beauty is achieved not by paralysis and total lack of movement, which can appear lifeless, but on the contrary by restoring beauty and life, conserving a certain degree of facial mobility and the correct stability of muscular balance.

Indications for 'mesobotox'

It is an individual treatment. After a detailed examination of the patient, the area to be treated will be localized. Usually it is where the skin is thin and superficial, and the muscle is flat. Anywhere on the face can be treated depending on the individual expression. It is a 'made to measure' esthetic procedure.

Technique

To assess muscle functioning and evaluate the degree of muscle interrelation, we need to ask the patient to make different forced gestures and expressions:

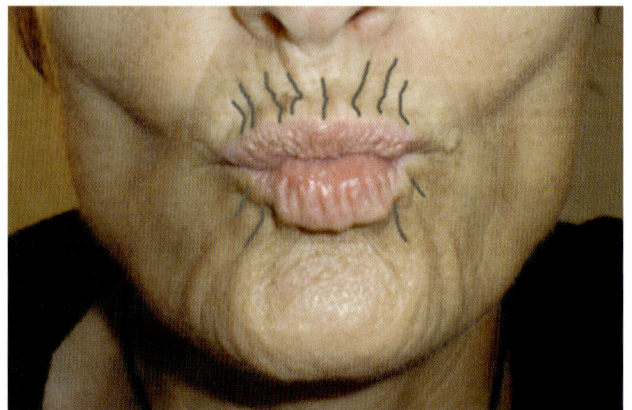

Figure 31.11   'Mesobotox': marking areas to be treated.

- open and close to the maximum the mouth, eyes, and eyebrows
- frown
- pucker the lips forward as in a forced kiss
- curve the corners of the lips upward and downward.

With a surgical pen, the areas to be treated will be marked where there is excess or lack of tissue, giving a facial 'map' of treatment (Figure 31.11).

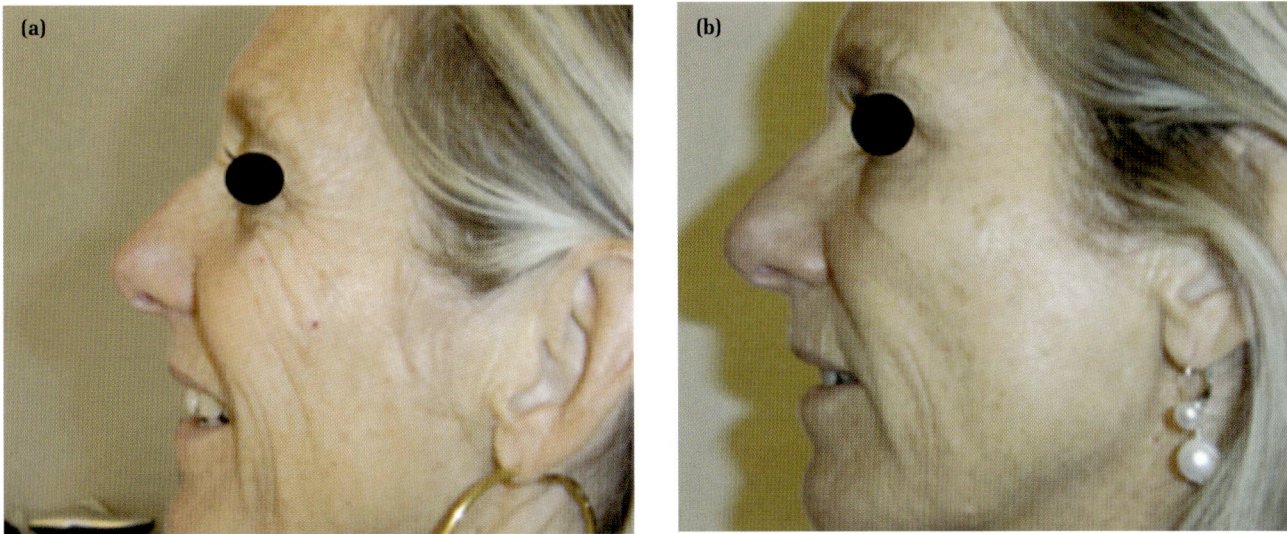

Figure 31.12   'Made to measure' treatment: (a) before and (b) after 'mesobotox'.

Injections

- the facial skin is cleansed with an appropriate solution
- injection is done inthe medial dermis with a 32G needle
- a dermal papule will be realized that will allow diffusion in deeper tissue
- dilution:
  - one vial of BOTOX 100 U diluted with 7 ml of physiological saline+0.2 ml xylocaine 2% with adrenaline
  - highly diluted 'mesobotox' for treatment of open pores on the nose and chin, 10 U+1 ml of physiological saline
  - 'mesolift with BOTOX' combination, 10 U BOTOX diluted in a 5-ml syringe (procaine+vitamin C or hyaluronic acid+multivitamins).

The above combination technique consists of mesolift to which we add 10–15 U of BOTOX, for full face and neck. It is not indicated in cases of heavy or lax skin, where it may have devasting consequences including a 'heavy face' sensation, sunken, and a sad, dull, and stiff overall look.

Results

The use of xylocaine 2% with adrenaline allows precise action and the diffusion of 'mesobotox' within marked areas. This made to measure treatment restores the youthful natural beauty of the face, with no tension, and respects the diversity of facial expression (Figure 31.12).

References

1. Lecoz J. Traite de Mésothérapie. Paris: Masson, 2004.
2. Lecoz J. Mesotherapy and Lipolysis. Singapore: Esthetic Medic 2008.
3. Beilin G. Optimisation des résultats en mésolift. J Med Esth Chir Derm 2006; 33: 151–5.
4. Bonnet C. La mesodissolution hypoosmolaire et l'hydrolipodystrophie 'enfin ça marche'. J Med Esth Chir Derm 2006; 33: 11–14.
5. Hertzog B. Le Mesobotox: un concept different de l'injection de la toxine botulique. J Med Esth Chir Derm 2004; 31: 157–62.

32A Injectable collagen

Claude Aharoni and Gérard Flageul

Background

The first clinical research using injectable animal collagen was conducted on burns patients in the 1970s (Stanford).

In 1975, the Collagen Corporation, based in Palo Alto, released Zyderm® I especially designed for cosmetic and esthetic use. Zyderm I (like the later released products Zyderm II and Zyplast®) is a genuine cosmetic medication with controlled manufacture, conservation, and purification processes. Food and Drug Administration (FDA) approval was obtained in 1981. In 1983, Zyderm II was released and in 1985, Zyplast was released.

In France, since 1987, these three products have been legally available (French legal approval for drugs and medical devices). To date, the follow-up with injectable collagen is over 25 years, and several million patients have been treated. More than 280 clinical series have been published in the literature.[1–4]

Product description

This medication is made of natural collagen, harvested, extracted, and highly purified, from bovine dermis (Cheptel Collagen USA). Antigenically inactivated, this material is used as a substitute for altered or lost native collagen.

Biologically assimilable, it is made of 95% type I collagen and 5% type III collagen. This material fits the skin dynamics perfectly, and induces fibroblastic activation with stimulation of neocollagen synthesis. Based on histological studies,[5] Zyderm persistence after injection is 3–4 months. Over this time, protein synthesis of fibrocytes is stimulated, with dermal tissue spread.

Histological Zyplast tissue persistence is longer (18 months).

Nowadays, three complementary presentations are available:

- Zyderm I: 35 mg/ml
- Zyderm II: 65 mg/ml
- Zyplast: reticulated collagen, characterized by interlysine bridges between collagen molecules that enhance fibrillar network cohesion and the stability of the product. This product is available in a 3% lidocaine premixed presentation.

Different dermal tissue depths are targeted, allowing a wide range of indications.

Pre-therapeutic check-up

Operating conditions must be strictly followed.

The usual contraindications are investigated:

- autoimmune disease
- anaphylactic reaction
- acute allergic reaction
- immunosuppressive therapy
- lidocaine hypersensitivity
- acute or chronic skin disease, near to or distant from the area to be treated
- pregnancy or breastfeeding.

An intradermal tolerance double test must be performed prior to any therapeutic procedure.

This test checks for immediate hypersensitivity and delayed hypersensitivity.[6–9] Two 0.1-ml intradermal injections in the forearm separated by a 15-day interval are performed.[10] A wheal lasting a few days is induced. Final results are read 30–45 days after the second injection. The patient is instructed to inform his physician about any abnormal reaction, acute or delayed, local (red spots, pruritus, edema, palpable nodosity) or systemic (fever, arthralgia). These abnormal reactions are absolute contraindications to treatment. During the delay before the results, a filler using hyaluronidate may be proposed.

Series in the literature[6,7,10] report 1.5–3% positive reactions to the tolerance test. These positive reactions are related to bovine collagen allergy. According to the previously cited authors, the double test allows minimization or even eradication of the delayed hypersensitivity risk. In the case of treatment interruption of more than 18 months, a new double test is required.

Antibodies that have been found are targeted toward bovine antigens. No cross-reaction with human collagen has been found. There is no circulating immune complex, and no risk of autoimmune disease induction. It is not necessary to investigate the presence of these antibodies before starting treatment.

Choice of presentation

The choice of presentation depends on the quality and features of the skin to be treated, but also depends on the magnitude and location of wrinkles and skin depressions that are targeted.

Most of the time, all three available presentations are used in combination in the same area:

- Zyplast is used to fill in medium-depth and deep dermis
- Zyderm I and II are used to fill in the superficial dermis.

Injection procedure

The injection procedure is very important, and the final results in terms of quality and duration widely depend on the injection procedure:

- the skin is carefully cleaned using a regular antiseptic
- injection sites are marked
- an appropriate light is required
- small caliber needles are used
- a tracking injection may be performed, or multi-injection in close sites (meaning a 3-mm step between two injection sites)
- when Zyderm I or Zyderm II is used, a whitening of the skin, giving the appropriate subepidermal location of the injection range of effect, is expected
- this whitening is not expected when Zyplast (which is injected in medium-depth and deep dermis) is used
- to ease the injection procedure, the syringe is stabilized with one hand and pressure is applied using thumb and index finger of the other hand
- the skin has to be trapped between the fingers, and tension along the axis of the wrinkle is applied
- overcorrections are not advised; an additional procedure (if needed) is preferable
- within 2 minutes after injection, massage of the treated area is advised in order to homogenize material distribution
- immediate reactions such as edema, red spots, and superficial ecchymosis are minor signs and are expected to vanish within a couple of hours.

Advice to patients

- prior to injection: no alcohol, no aspirin
- after injection:

  - avoid facial mimics for 4 hours
  - avoid sauna and alcohol for 4 days
  - avoid intensive sun exposure for 2–3 weeks.

Injection schedule

Initial treatment is composed of two injection sessions with a delay of 3–4 weeks between.[3] During the first session, Zyplast is injected in the deep dermis. During the second session, Zyderm I or Zyderm II is injected in the superficial dermis.

The results are assessed at 6 months' follow-up. The usual duration of the correction is variable, ranging from 6 to 18 months. This variable duration determines the frequency of maintenance treatment, consisting of Zyderm I or Zyderm II injections. No additional injection of Zyplast in the deep dermis is required.

The more the wrinkle is mechanically stressed, the shorter is the effect.

Overall results

Distribution results of location were:

- nasogenial sulcus: 80%
- glabella (frown lines): 50%
- vertical lip lines: 38%
- jaw: 23%
- lips/vermilion border: 18%
- forehead wrinkles: 15%
- periorbital wrinkles: 15%
- chin: 10%.

Satisfaction distribution results indicated that 80% of patients were satisfied, with:

- very good results: 21%
- good results: 59%
- medium results: 18%
- no result: 2%.

Results duration distribution indicated that:

- 25% of cases underwent a complementary procedure within 6 months
- 60% of cases underwent a complementary procedure within 6–12 months
- 15% of cases underwent a complementary procedure over a year later.

Technical particulars of specific locations

Glabellar wrinkles

This location is a good indication for injectable collagen, in combination with surgical correction of the eyelids. Nevertheless, in spite of repeated injections,

Zyderm II does not allow a total clearing of these wrinkles, because of their depth.

Wrinkles at outer corners of eyes

Zyderm I is effective in this location. This is the first-choice procedure in the treatment of these mild wrinkles situated in thin skin. This procedure may be used in combination with botulinum toxin.

Jaw wrinkles

This location is a good indication for Zyplast plus Zyderm II association, allowing a total filling of these wrinkles, with a long-lasting result. Comparable results may be obtained in the nasogenial sulcus with moderate.

This combination may be used as a complementary procedure to a facelift, in order to treat remaining jaw wrinkles.

Lips

Zyplast injections behind and under the cutaneomucosal junction line of the lips (mainly the upper lip) have a double effect:

- the shape of the lip is restored
- vertical wrinkles are attenuated, and further treatment with Zyderm II is eased (with a significant reduction of the amount of material to be injected).

Paracommissural line (marionette line)

In this location, sufficient effect is not obtained, in spite of massive deep dermis Zyplast injections. Only a surgical procedure may restore these wrinkles caused by ptosis of the buccal commissure.

Incidents and complications

Over two decades of experience with this product, in combination with esthetic surgery (meaning a couple of hundred injections), two cases of intolerance have been observed. The clinical feature was nodosity at the injection site. It resolved within 7 days in the first case, and within a couple of weeks in the second case. These abnormal reactions occurred when only one test was performed prior to therapeutic injection.

The rate of intolerance in our experience is below the 3% reported in the literature. We support the double test that brings the intolerance rate down to 0.25%.

Discussion and conclusion

Injectable collagen is an effective substitute treatment for dermal tissue. It is harmless as long as contraindications are respected. A double test must be performed.

Collagen injections allow a remarkable improvement of most facial and neck wrinkles. This is a non-surgical method which is reliable and harmless. The procedure is performed on ambulatory patients, and may be done in the physician's office. Effectiveness is immediate. Recovery is rapid, and patients may immediately return to a normal social life, leading some to keep the treatment secret.

Two drawbacks have to be mentioned: the treatment is expensive and transient.

Dermal filling is a good procedure in the treatment of facial aging, and may be used as a complementary procedure to surgery. Injectable collegen is flexible, easy to use, rapid, and subtle.

In our experience, patients often ask for reinjection on the occasion of social or family events. It may help the surgeon to choose the more appropriate moment to perform the surgical procedure.

Compared with other injectable materials, collagen is harmless as long as the contraindications are respected, supported by the long-term follow-up of several million patients treated worldwide.

New collagens have appeared, to prevent intolerance. Cosmoderm® and Cosmoplast® have been introduced by Inamed Aesthetics. They are made of highly purified human-based collagen. These new products are claimed to require no pretreatment skin test, after clinical study.

Evolence® achieves its long-lasting effects because it is specifically engineered to enhance stability and mimic the properties of natural collagen found in the skin. The filler is produced via the revolutionary Glymatrix™ technology. The sophisticated production process for Evolence removes the most antigenic part of the collagen molecule – the telopeptides – producing a treatment that is highly immunologically compatible with human collagen.

References

1. Castrow FF 2nd, Krull EA. Injectable collagen implant – update. J Am Acad Dermatol 1983; 9: 889–93.
2. Cooperman LS, Mackinnon V, Bechler G, Pharriss BB. Injectable collagen: a six-year clinical investigation. Aesthetic Plast Surg 1985; 9: 145–51.
3. Flageul G. Le collagène injectable. 20 ans d'expérience. Presented at SOFCPRE, Biarritz, 19–20 May.
4. Inoue K, Nakamoto T, Usui A, Usui T. Evaluation of antibody class in response to endoscopic subureteral collagen injection in patients with vesicoureteral reflux. J Urol 2001; 165: 555–8.
5. Sclafani AP, Romo T 3rd, Parker A et al. Homologous collagen dispersion (dermalogen) as a dermal filler: persistence and histology compared with bovine collagen. Ann Plast Surg 2002; 49: 181–8.

6. Pons-Guiraud A. Réaction d'hypersensibilité retardée aux implants de collagène bovin. Nouv Dermatol 1992; 11: 422–32.

7. Pons-Guiraud A et al (France), Bezzola A (Suisse). Efficacité et tolérance du collagène bovin injectable dans le traitement des rides du visage. Etude multicentrique sur 10 ans et 2800 patients. Officiel Dermatologie, March 1994.

8. Delustro F, Smith ST, Sundsmo J et al. Reaction to injectable collagen: results in animal models and clinical use. Plast Reconstr Surg 1987; 79: 581–94.

9. Schurig V, Konz B, Ring J, Dorn M. Granuloma formation in test and treatment sites caused by intracutaneously administered, injectable collagen. Hautarzt 1986; 37: 42–5.

10. Elson ML. Clinical assessment of Zyplast Implant: a year of experience for soft tissue contour correction. J Am Acad Dermatol 1988; 18: 707–13.

11. Flageul G, Ohana J. Contribution of collagen injectable in the treatment of wrinkles and facial cutaneous depression. Ann Chir Plast Esthet 1988; 33:

32B The different types of injectable collagen

Daniel Cassuto

Background

The first documented clinical use of collagen was in burn patients in the 1970s. In 1975, the Collagen Corporation, based in Palo Alto, California, released Zyderm® I, a bovine-sourced collagen, specifically for cosmetic and esthetic use. Food and Drug Administration (FDA) approval was obtained in 1981 for Zyderm I with Zyderm II and Zyplast® following in 1983 and 1985, respectively.[1,2] These products have been used in France since 1987, with over 20 years' experience and several million patient-exposures.[3] Although bovine collagen is highly effective and well tolerated, its cosmetic use began to decrease with the introduction of human collagen and hyaluronic acid-based dermal fillers. The latter proved to remain in the tissues for a longer period of time, thereby decreasing the number of yearly visits for cosmetic patients. In addition, neither human collagen nor hyaluronic acid fillers required skin pre-testing, making the procedure easier for clinicians and patients. With the introduction of the long-lasting structural Glymatrix™ collagen (Evolence®/Evolence® Breeze™), many clinicians have returned to the use of collagen for the predictable results that are quickly obtainable with minimal patient recovery time following injection.

Product description

Evolence and Evolence Breeze are both porcine-sourced, type I collagen, containing 35 mg/ml of purified xenogenic collagen in a phosphate-buffered saline. The sourced collagen is harvested from controlled livestock herds. Tendons serve as the basis for the purified collagen, and are rendered antigenically inactive through a patented pepsinization and purification process.

Biologically assimilable, Evolence and Evolence Breeze are made of 97% type I collagen and approximately 3% type III collagen. Both products are designed to mimic the collagen that is lost as a person ages. In vivo data have demonstrated a high degree of biocompatibility as evidenced by neovascularization, neocollagenesis, and fibroblastic activity.[4] Clinical studies and post-marketing feedback have consistently demonstrated cosmetic correction and tissue persistence of up to 12 months, regardless of formulation. Evolence, injected with a 27G needle, is reserved for injection into the mid- to deep dermis for the correction of deeper facial wrinkles and folds. Evolence Breeze has different rheological properties from Evolence and a lighter, less fibrous consistency, which enables the product to be injected through a 30G needle into the mid- to upper dermis for finer lines and wrinkles, the vermilion border, and lip body.

Pre-procedure check-up

All patients, regardless of the product chosen for the cosmetic correction procedure, should undergo a thorough assessment of prior existing medical conditions. In addition, every attempt should be made to gather information regarding the patient's cosmetic/esthetic history. Some of the most common precautions include: autoimmune disease; allergy to or anaphylactic reactions to porcine collagen; history of severe multidrug acute allergic reaction; concomitant immunosuppressive therapy; acute or chronic skin disease, near to or distant from the area to be treated; pregnancy or concomitant breast-feeding.

Unlike with Zyderm and Zyplast, an intradermal tolerance skin test is not required prior to the injection of Evolence or Evolence Breeze.

Product selection

The choice of Evolence or Evolence Breeze depends on the experience of the clinician and the location to be injected. Both forms can be injected at the same time into different areas of the face, or sometimes Evolence Breeze is layered over Evolence to increase the degree of cosmetic correction in those hard-to-treat areas.

Injection procedure

The quality of the corrective outcome, patient acceptability, and product durability depend heavily on the skill and technique of the injecting clinician. For maximal patient comfort, a block should be performed. Topical anesthesia may be used for areas such as the nasolabial folds; however, for the lip and vermilion border, a full block is preferred. A combination of topical and injectable blocks can maximize patient comfort and increase the likelihood of a positive experience.

The areas of injection should be carefully cleansed with an antiseptic prior to the injection of Evolence and Evolence Breeze. Antiseptic solutions containing benzalkonium are allowed, unlike hyaluronic acid injections, as this component is prohibited due to the risk of hyaluronate crystal precipitation. Blanching or whitening of the skin should not be evident upon needle placement when using Evolence, since the product should be placed into the mid- to deep dermal area. Slight blanching may be evident upon Evolence Breeze injection due to placement in the mid- to upper dermis. Since Evolence is a fibrous product, occasional needle-clogging may happen with Evolence, but very rarely with Breeze. Pre-injection warming of the syringe in the hand can prevent this. If clogging happens, the syringe should be extracted from the tissue without trying to clear the syringe by using additional pressure. Changing the needle before resuming injection will solve the problem without any untoward effects.

While serial tunneling is the preferred method of placement for both Evolence and Evolence Breeze for beginners, other methods of injection have been employed with great success. These include, but are not limited to, cross-hatching, serial puncturing, and fanning. Regardless of injection technique, the injected areas should receive a gentle, but purposeful massage to ensure a smoothing of the product for maximal corrective acceptance.

Evolence or Evolence Breeze should not be injected to an overcorrected state. While an additional procedure may be preferred in some subjects, data from the US pivotal study demonstrated that touch-up injections did not increase the degree of tissue persistence when compared to those patients who were optimally corrected at visit one.[5]

Important patient considerations

As with any injectable procedure, patients should be instructed to avoid medications and supplements known to affect the body's ability to form clots. This includes the use of common medications such as aspirin, ibuprofen, and naproxen, but also products containing green tea, vitamin e, fish oil and guarana. Patients should discontinue the use of any product known to increase the risk of bleeding at least 5 days prior to the procedure or at the instruction of the treating clinician. In addition, patients should be instructed to limit or refrain from consuming alcoholic beverages within 24 hours before and throughout

the period immediately after placement of the injectable product to minimize the risk of bleeding complications.

Appropriate skin care routines can be resumed quickly following the placement of Evolence or Evolence Breeze. A broad-spectrum sun protectant should be applied prior to exposure to ultraviolet rays.

Injection scheduling

The injection of Evolence and/or Evolence Breeze is often dictated through patient and clinician interaction. Unless directed by the care provider, patients can resume their normal activities quickly following their procedure. The area to be injected should be assessed and the appropriate version of Evolence should be chosen. Both Evolence and Evolence Breeze can be used to restore contour to wrinkles, scars, areas of skin atrophy due to disease and trauma, defects secondary to rhinoplasty, skin graft, or other surgically induced deformities, and other soft tissue defects or deficiencies. Evolence Breeze can also be used for lip enhancement by adding volume to the lip body and/or vermilion border and for finer wrinkles such as those above the lip border (Figures 32B.1 and 32B.2). Caution should be exercised when either product is injected into areas of high vascularity in which blood vessel occlusion may occur.

Clinical information

Data have been collected from at least five clinical trials and over 740 subjects. The early clinical trials were the first to demonstrate the corrective attributes of the new structural Glymatrix collagen and the long-term tissue persistence in patients who underwent corrections in the nasolabial regions of the face.[6,7] Monstrey and colleagues[6] evaluated the use of Glymatrix collagen 30 mg/ml in 12 subjects. Patients received both Zyplast and Evolence[30] in a randomized fashion and were followed for up to 18 months. A touch-up injection could be made at 2 weeks dependent on initial correction. Evolence 30 proved to be superior in corrective durability to Zyplast from 6 months through the 18-month time frame. Rzany and colleagues[7] conducted a similarly designed study with a hyaluronic acid (HA) comparator. This early study supported the long-term durability and safety of Evolence (12–15 months). At the end of the study patients were given a choice to receive further corrections with either product, and 76% of subjects chose to be reinjected with Evolence rather than HA.

For approval in the United States, two clinical trials were conducted. The first study was a single-center, open-label, uncontrolled study in 519 subjects to evaluate the potential of Evolence to elicit allergic reactions in human subjects.[8] Subjects received an intradermal injection of 0.1 ml of Evolence in a forearm and then a subsequent intradermal injection in the contralateral forearm

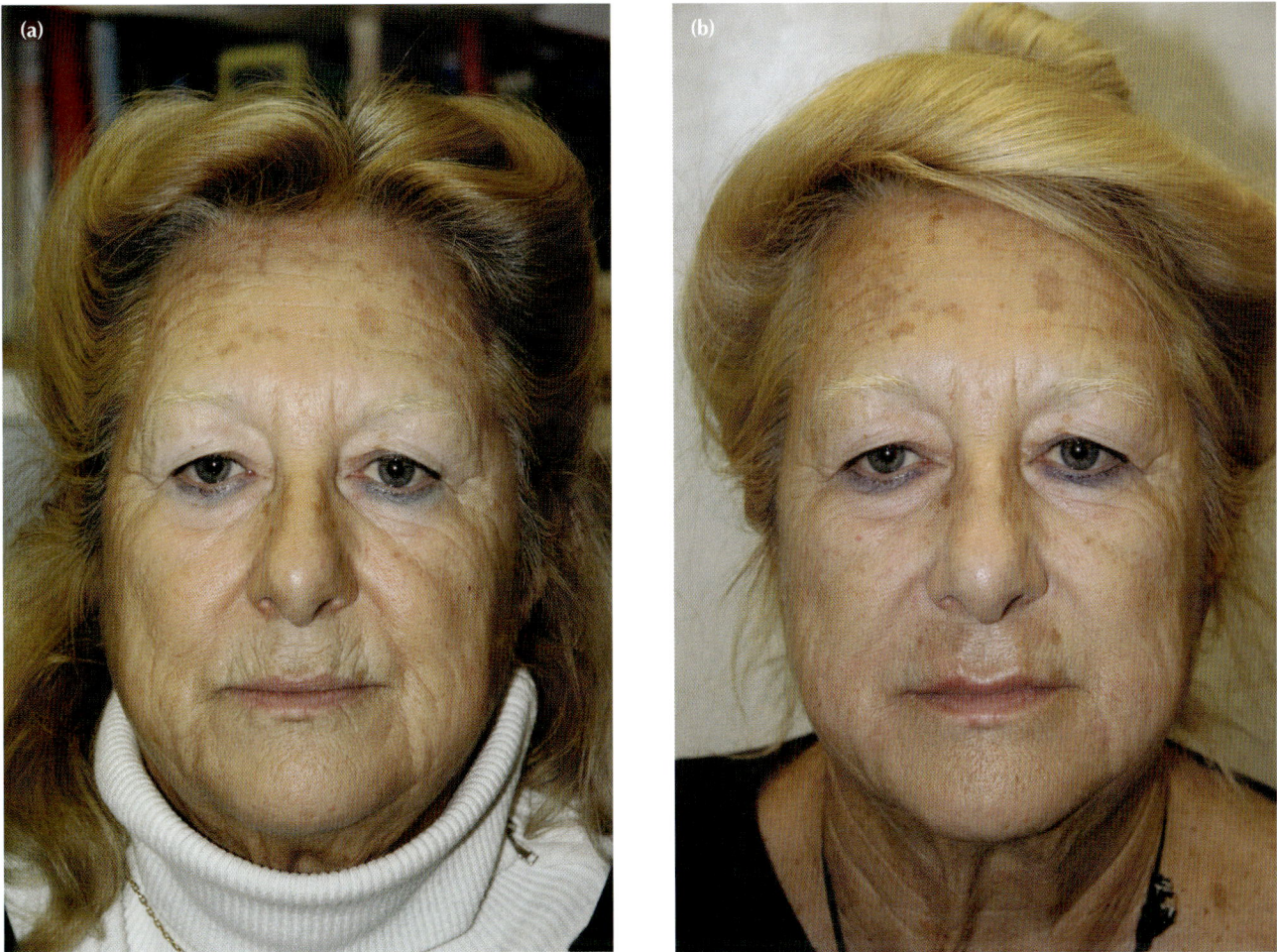

Figure 32B.1   (a) Before and (b) 6 months after volumetric augmentation with Evolence® and superficial wrinkle correction with Evolence® Breeze™.

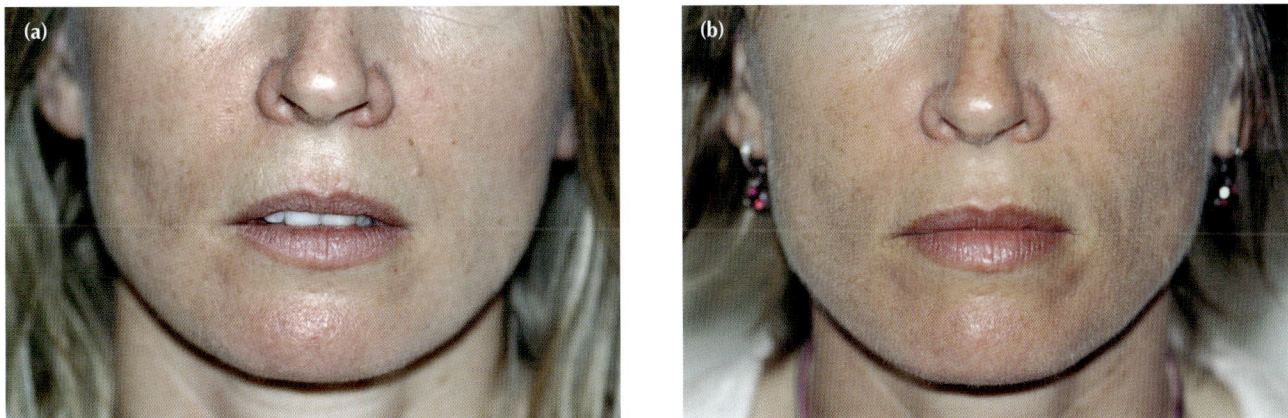

Figure 32B.2   (a) Before and (b) 6 months after lip augmentation and superficial wrinkle correction with Evolence Breeze.

2 weeks later. In addition to skin reactivity, serum samples were obtained from 515 subjects at study entry and again at study completion to assess changes in antibody production (immunoglobulins IgG, IgA, IgM, IgE) using an enzyme-linked immunosorbent assay (ELISA). After the first and second skin tests, there was no evidence of moderate or severe (grade 3 or 4) erythema. Three grade

2 (mild erythema) reactions were noted but were of short duration and did not progress or recur during the evaluation period. There was no evidence of change in antibody status in the majority of subjects as they displayed similar levels of antiporcine type I collagen antibodies at the beginning and end of the study. Although some subjects who received Evolence in this study were found to

possess antibodies against porcine collagen, this was not indicative or predictive of a reaction against Evolence collagen and no evidence of clinical symptoms in those with changed antibody titers was observed during the study. Based on statistical evaluation of the absence of such observations, the upper confidence limit for the possibility of a moderate-to-severe erythematous reaction occurring with Evolence was calculated as 0.58% of subjects. This low level of possible hypersensitivity is comparable to that of other dermal fillers that can be used safely and effectively without a pretreatment skin test, thus providing evidence that Evolence can be safely used without a prior skin test as well.

The effectiveness and non-inferiority of Evolence were demonstrated in a randomized, multicenter, within-subject study of Glymatrix collagen and hyaluronic acid in a large study population in the United States.[9] Subjects were evaluated with the Modified Fitzpatrick Wrinkle Scale, a validated measurement tool used to assess not only the initial depth of wrinkles, but also the improvement following cosmetic correction.[10] In addition, all subjects underwent serum antibody testing (ELISA) before, after, and at the 6-month endpoint. One hundred and forty-nine subjects completed the study. Antibody production proved to be non-predictive of frequency or occurrence of adverse events. Both Evolence and HA were found to be well tolerated and non-inferior to one another at 6 months following the Optimal Cosmetic Result (OCR) for the correction of nasolabial fold (NLF) wrinkles. Adverse effects for both products were typical and expected following the use of a dermal filler for the correction of NLF wrinkles.

Recently, a multicenter evaluation was conducted to support the indication of Evolence Breeze for lip enhancement and augmentation.[11] Patients received treatment for not only lip volume but also vermilion border enhancement. Satisfaction was well over 90% for both subject- and clinician-rated assessments. The incidence of adverse events was very low, and included expected outcomes such as bleeding, bruising, pain on injection, and irregularities.

Complications

Evolence and Evolence Breeze are generally well tolerated following injection. In registration studies, the most common adverse events reported were mild in nature and included pain, erythema, and swelling. In addition, subjects reported being aware of the injected collagen filler immediately following injection when the areas were pressed upon.

Discussion and conclusion

The addition of a long-lasting collagen for esthetic use is welcomed by many clinicians and patients looking for a natural way to correct contour deficiencies. Having a structural collagen such as Evolence or Evolence Breeze with a duration of correction of up to 12 months allows the clinician an opportunity for additional interactions with the patient. In addition, it allows the patient to undergo correction only once a year. Injectable collagen is flexible, easy to use, rapid, and subtle, and the results are predictable. In our experience, patients often ask for reinjection on the occasion of social or family events, and having a long-lasting product with little to no recovery time proves to be an asset.

The author's personal experience privileges the use of Evolence Breeze both for superficial wrinkle correction and for volumetric augmentation. Although the natural 'dermal' color of collagen makes it suitable for superficial injection without the risk of superficial blue shades as with hyaluronic acid, special care must be taken in dark skin types as a lighter shade of color may appear after superficial injection.

Compared with other injectable materials, collagen is harmless as long as contraindications are respected. The esthetic use of collagen is supported by decades of experience, and the safety of these products is well documented. With the introduction of Cosmoderm® and Cosmoplast® the need for skin testing was eliminated, but the corrective duration of action was still far less than optimal and the treatments proved to be expensive. Evolence and Evolence Breeze achieve long-lasting effects because they are specifically engineered to enhance stability and mimic the properties of natural collagen found in the skin. Filler is produced via the revolutionary Glymatrix technology. The sophisticated production process for Evolence removes the most antigenic part of the collagen molecule – the telopeptides – producing a treatment that is highly immunologically compatible with human collagen.

Acknowledgment

The author wishes to thank David A Mays PharmD, MBA, BCPS, for his assistance with aspects of this chapter.

References

1. Castrow FF 2nd, Krull EA. Injectable collagen implant – update. J Am Acad Dermatol 1983; 9: 889–93.
2. Cooperman LS, Mackinnon V, Bechler G, Pharriss BB. Injectable collagen, six years clinical investigation. Aesthetic Plast Surg 1985; 9: 145–51.
3. Flageul G, Ohana J. [Injections of collagen in the treatment of wrinkles and facial cutaneous depressions]. Ann Chir Plast Esthet 1988; 33: 283–7.
4. Nir E, Azachi M, Shoshani D, Goldlust A. Long-term in vivo evaluation of the safety and efficacy of a new porcine collagen dermal filler cross-linked with ribose. Presented at American Academy of Dermatology 66th Annual Meeting, San Antonio, TX, 1–5 February, 2008.
5. Narins RS, Brandt FS, Lorenc ZP, et al. Twelve Months Persistency of the Corrective Response with a Novel, Ribose-

Cross-Linked Collagen Dermal Filler in a Randomized Clinical Trial of Subjects Seeking Correction of Nasolabial Folds. Dermatol Surg, 2008; in press.

6. Monstrey SJ, Pitaru S, Hamdi M et al. A two-stage Phase I trial of Evolence30 collagen for soft-tissue contour correction. Plast Reconstr Surg 2007; 120: 303–9.

7. Rzany B, Monstrey SJ, Hamdi M, Hund M, Shoshani D. High persistency of Glymatrix™ collagen in the correction of facial wrinkles after 15 months. Presented at American Academy of Dermatology 66th Annual Meeting, San Antonio, TX, 1–5 February, 2008.

8. Shoshani D, Markovitz E, Cohen Y, Heremans A, Goldlust A. Skin test hypersensitivity study of a cross-linked, porcine collagen implant for aesthetic surgery. Dermatol Surg 2007; 22; S152–8.

9. Narins RS, Brandt FS, Lorenc ZP et al. A randomized, multi-center study of the safety and efficacy of Dermicol-P35 and non-animal-stabilized hyaluronic acid gel for the correction of nasolabial folds. Dermatol Surg 2007; 33: S213–21.

10. Shoshani D, Markovitz E, Monstrey SJ, Narins D. The Modified Fitzpatrick Winkle Scale: a clinical validated measurement tool for nasolabial wrinkle severity assessment. Dermatol Surg 2008; in press.

11. De Boulle K. Multi-center evaluation of collagen for lip enhancement. Presented at International Master Course on Aging Skin 10th Annual Meeting, Paris, January, 2008.

33 Agarose gel

Daniel Cassuto and Luca Scrimali

Background

Agarose gel is a synthetic polysaccharide. It has been widely used for decades in biomedical research, especially in experimental systems requiring controlled pharmacological releasing systems and in various immunogenicity, mutagenesis, and tissue growth experiments. Its use as a dermal filler began only in 2003. From the preliminary experimental data first presented at the Italian Society of Cosmetic Medicine and Surgery (SIES) in February 2004 until today, the filler based on agarose gel has aroused great curiosity. It is the only resorbable filler, besides collagen and hyaluronic acid, that is authorized in Europe. Its use is relatively easy, safe, and well tolerated, long-lasting, and suitable for a wide range of applications. The idea of using agarose as a filler started from the widely known biocompatibility of this substance in the biological field; during this period, the clinical trials had a large following thanks to the cooperation of a pool of experts, which resulted in a more precise collocation of the filler. The indications for use of this specific implant are similar to those of the other resorbable fillers, but its deployment must be slightly different in order to achieve the best esthetic result.

Product description

Agarose is a purified linear galactan hydrocolloid isolated from agar or agar-bearing marine algae (class Rhodophyceae). (It has nothing to do with agar plates that are used in bacterial culture.) Structurally, agarose is a linear polymer consisting of alternating 3,6-anhydro-L-galactose and D-galactose units rigidly interlocked in a three-dimensional reticulated gel, for slow resorption. The absence of a chemical cross-linking agent is particularly reassuring as it eliminates a possible cause of intolerance. The longer duration can be attributed to the different way it is absorbed. Agarose is not directly degraded by a corresponding enzyme, as for collagen or hyaluronic acid (humans does not produce 'agarase'); it is first digested by macrophages and then degraded by galactosidase that detaches the single chains, 3,6-anhydro-L-galactose and D-galactose, which are finally removed via the pentose cycle. Agarose is considered to be biocompatible[1,2] and non-toxic.[3] It is a non-carcinogenic, transparent, quite homogeneous gel that is stable at room temperature and easily injectable with a 27-, 30-, or 32G needle, depending on the concentration.

Its pH ranges between 5 and 6, due to the physiological serum used for dilution. In the beginning (2002–2003), lactate and other buffers were added to balance the pH and reduce patient discomfort during injection. The buffering salts caused edematous swelling after the injection, and were eliminated in the last formula (2003), which only contains 0.9% NaCl.

There are three available concentrations, packed in 1-ml syringes, under the name of Easy-agarose®: LD – low density at 1%, HD – high density at 1.5%, and VL – volume at 2.5%. A lower concentration (RE) is also available for skin revitalization, often erroneously confused with mesotherapy, which will not be described here, not being a filler.

Easy-agarose LD is used with a 32G needle into the upper dermis for finer lines and wrinkles.

Easy-agarose HD is injected through a 30G needle into the mid- to upper dermis for the correction of deeper facial wrinkles and folds.

Easy-agarose VL is injected with a 27G needle into subcutaneous tissue or the deep dermis; it is also recommended for volume restoration.

Pre-procedure check-up

As recommended before any procedure, all patients, regardless of the product chosen for the cosmetic correction procedure, should undergo a thorough assessment of prior existing medical conditions. In addition, every attempt should be made to gather information regarding the patient's cosmetic/esthetic history. Some of the most common precautions include: acute or chronic skin disease, either near to or distant from the area to be treated; pregnancy or concomitant breastfeeding. No skin test to evaluate tolerance is required prior to the injection of Easy-agarose.

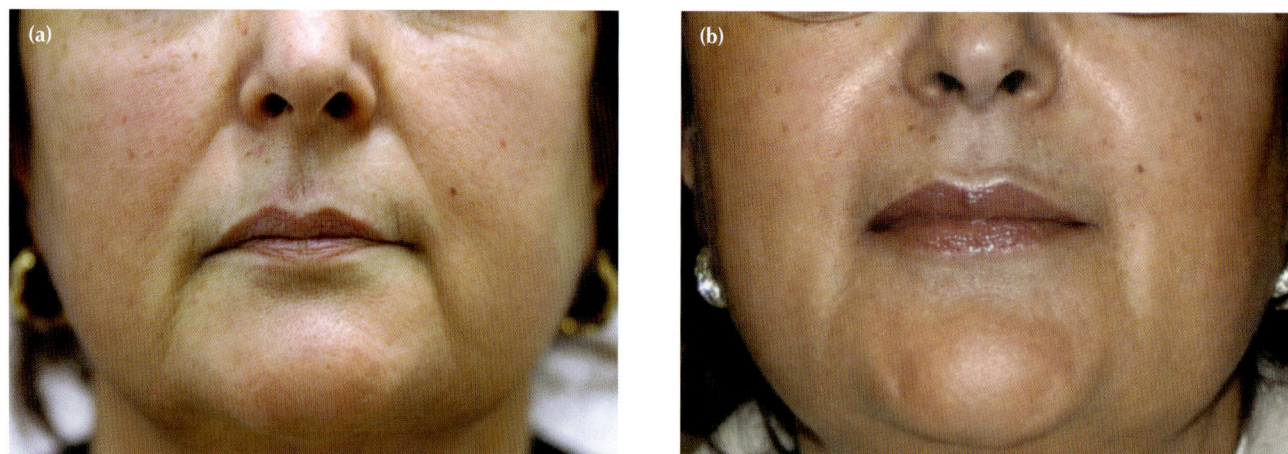

Figure 33.1 A 59-year-old patient (a) before and (b) 6 months after correction of nasolabial folds and marionette lines with Easy-agarose® VL (3 ml). The lips were augmented with 1.5 ml of Easy-agarose HD.

Product selection

The choice of Easy-agarose variety depends on the experience of the clinician and the location to be injected. All forms can be injected at the same time into different areas of the face, or sometimes Easy-agarose LD or HD is layered over Easy-agarose VL to increase the degree of cosmetic correction in those hard-to-treat areas. All concentrations are easily extrudable. The resistance felt by the injector is very low, even lower than with collagen, and much lower than with hyaluronic acid. This is an undoubted advantage in the sensible hands of the busy operator, whose hands are going to be less tired after many procedures.

The author's experience indicates that a skilled user can also inject the more concentrated products (HD, VL) in the superficial layers of the skin to ensure a longer-lasting result. This versatility also allows better exploitation of each syringe. However, this use is not officially recommended by the manufacturer.

Injection procedure

As described for collagen, the quality of the corrective outcome, patient acceptability, and product durability depend heavily on the skill and technique of the injecting clinician. Topical anesthesia should be used for areas such as the nasolabial folds; however, for the lip and vermilion border, a full block is preferred. Subcutaneous use of the VL form can be performed without any anesthesia (Figure 33.1). A combination of topical and injectable blocks can maximize patient comfort and increase the likelihood of a positive experience. The areas of injection should be carefully cleansed with an antiseptic prior to the injection. Antiseptic solutions containing benzalkonium are allowed, unlike when using hyaluronic acid. Blanching of the skin should not be evident upon needle placement when using Easy-agarose

VL, since the product should be placed into the subcutaneous or mid- to deep dermal tissue. Slight blanching with Easy-agarose HD and LD is acceptable, since both products are suitable for superficial use, i.e. in the upper dermis. As with other fillers, beginners are advised to use a serial tunneling technique when injecting Easy-agarose. After gaining experience, other techniques such as cross-hatching, serial puncturing, and fanning can be used. Regardless of injection technique, the injection should be as gentle and uniform as possible in order to ensure maximal corrective acceptance. Particular attention should be given to the exquisite extrudability of the product, which is a cause of great satisfaction in sensitive hands just as in the case of collagen. This feature is extremely interesting when performing deep volume augmentation with Easy-agarose VL. The hypovolemic tear trough and malar, mental, and lower maxillary areas can easily be corrected with the 'key point' technique. The latter consists of positioning a 'lump' of product through a single puncture point. Thanks to the extreme malleability of agarose gel it is possible to manually remodel the lump into the desired form of augmentation (Figure 33.2). The advantage of this technique, especially if compared to thicker hyaluronic acid based deep fillers, is the minimal invasiveness and the small number of injection sites needed to restore facial volumes. Sometimes 6–8 punctures are enough to rejuvenate the face. A further refinement of this technique consists in directing the insertion of the filler by rotating the bevel of the needle while opposing pressure with the fingers of the free hand in order to drive the diffusion in the required direction. Minimizing the diameter of the punctures (27–30G needle) and reducing the trauma caused by multiple punctures is an invaluable means of reducing the risk of edema and bleeding after the injection.

On the other hand, clinicians who usually inject only hyaluronic acid must adjust the pressure exerted on the syringe, or else they might exaggerate and cause

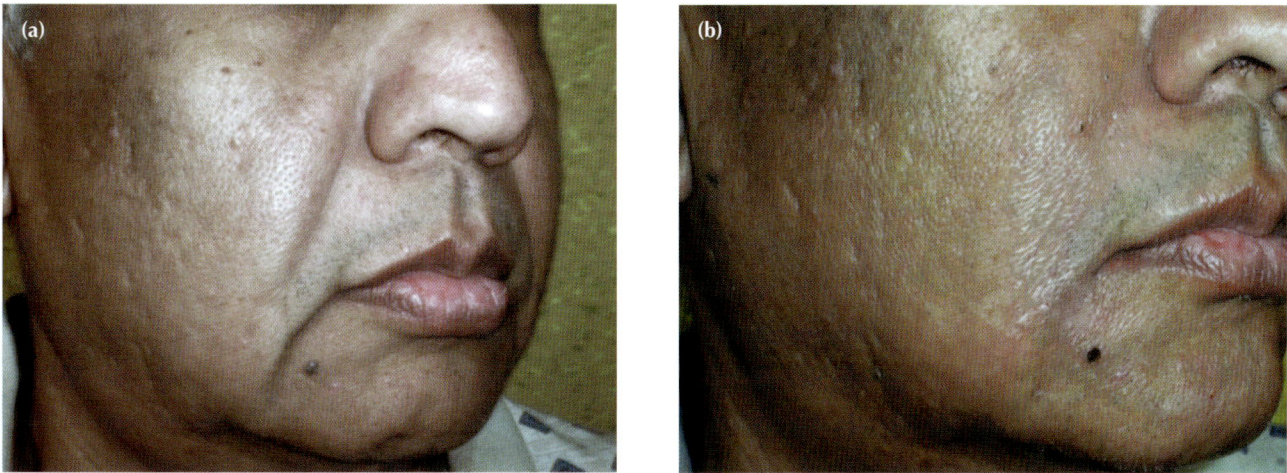

Figure 33.2   A 61-year-old Asian patient (a) before and (b) 7 months after correction of nasolabial folds and marionette lines with 3 ml of Easy-agarose VL.

superficial nodules, which are the only real complication that has been observed during our 5 years' clinical experience. Another frequent error is subcutaneous injection of the lower concentrations, i.e. HD and LD, which almost inevitably leads to diffusion of the substance in the subcutaneous tissue (fat, fascia, or muscle, depending on the area). This diffusion will inevitably cause disappearance of the correction within a few days. When Easy-agarose is **properly** placed, the **minimal** duration of the correction is 6–8 months. None of the products should be injected to an overcorrected state. The European experience shows that initial hypocorrection followed by touch-up injections increases the degree of tissue persistence when compared to those patients who are optimally corrected at visit one.[4]

Important patient considerations

As with any injectable procedure, patients should be instructed to avoid medications and supplements known to interfere with blood coagulation. This includes the use of common medications such as aspirin, ibuprofen, and naproxen, but also products containing green tea, vitamin E, fish oil, and guaranà. Patients should discontinue the use of any product known to increase the risk of bleeding at least 5 days prior to the procedure, or at the instruction of the treating clinician. In addition, patients should be instructed to limit or refrain from consuming alcoholic beverages within 24 hours before and throughout the period immediately after placement of the injectable product, to minimize the risk of bleeding complications. Appropriate skin care routines can be resumed quickly following the placement of Easy-agarose. A broad-spectrum sun protectant should be applied prior to exposure to ultraviolet rays.

Injection scheduling

The injection of Easy-agarose is often decided through patient and clinician interaction. Unless directed by the care provider, patients can resume their normal activities quickly following their procedure. The area to be injected should be assessed, and the appropriate version of Easy-agarose chosen. All forms of Easy-agarose can be used to restore contour to wrinkles, scars, areas of skin atrophy due to disease and trauma, defects secondary to rhinoplasty, skin graft, or other surgically induced deformities, and other soft tissue defects or deficiencies. It is important to place the implant at the appropriate depth for each concentration, as indicated above. Easy-agarose HD can also be used for finer wrinkles such as those above the lip border or at the glabella, or for completing correction by Easy-agarose VL or LD. Caution should be exercised when either product is injected into areas of high vascularity, such as the glabella, in which blood vessel occlusion/spasm may occur.

Clinical information

The biocompatibility of a potential dermal filler is determined by host tissue responses. In vivo experimental analysis of tissue reactions to different substances is a valuable tool for determining the safety and efficacy of a potential tissue filler. First in Italy, Professor Lia Rimondini presented at the 2006 SIES Meeting a comparative evaluation of biomaterials, collagen, hyaluronic acid, and agarose, in the subcutaneous tissue of rats; no significant differences in tissue reaction were observed at 20 weeks with the various materials.[5]

Fernàndez-Cossìo et al, in a recent study, compared tissue responses to agarose gel and collagen in vivo in a rat model. Responses and biocompatibility were assessed by histopathologic and histomorphometric evaluation at 1 week to 8 months after implantation. In this study, agarose gel showed marked bioactivity and biodegradation, although the implants integrated well into tissues: newly formed collagen bands were observed inside the implants and no granulomas were detected. Collagen implants showed low cell infiltration and a significant loss of product over time. No other histological differences were observed between tissues from control and placebo rats either in histopathologic examination or in histomorphometric measurements. The authors concluded that agarose gel is a biocompatible product that can be considered for use as a tissue filler.[6]

Complications

Easy-agarose is generally well tolerated following injection. The most common product-related adverse events are mild in nature and include pain, erythema, and swelling. In addition, subjects have reported being aware of the injected filler immediately following injection when the areas are pressed upon. The reported discomfort is due to the acidic pH, and consists of a burning sensation during injection, as reported for hyaluronic acid. Two main operator-dependent adverse effects have been reported (Ghimas, unpublished data): (1) nodules, and (2) product disappearance after 1–2 weeks:

1. As mentioned above, the extreme extrudability of Easy-agarose is due to its almost watery consistency. In inexperienced hands that are used to applying significant pressure to inject hyaluronic acid, the risk of exaggerated localized injection is significant. This may result in unsightly nodules. The eventual nodules can easily be manually remodeled during the 3–4 weeks following the injections. However, no exogenous degrading substance (such as hyaluronidase for hyaluronic acid) is available for this filler.
2. The physical properties of the lower concentrations, HD and LD, are well maintained if the implants are positioned in the dermis. However, this can be extremely difficult when the dermis overall thickness is similar to the needle gauge, especially in aged skin. If these products are injected below the dermis (fat, fascia, muscle), the watery gel will diffuse and will not maintain the required effect. The inexperienced operator can often erroneously inject too deeply, and blame the product for the lack of result. Deep injection of a superficial-use filler

will shorten the effect of any substance. With Easy-agarose this phenomenon is accentuated.

As with any other implant, infection, though never reported, is possible in perioral injection due to needle contamination from the oral cavity flora. An antiseptic technique is obviously indicated.

Discussion and conclusion

The addition of a long-lasting resorbable filler is valuable for clinicians and patients looking for a natural way to correct contour deficiencies. A structural filler such as Easy-agarose, with a duration of correction of up to 12 months, allows the patient to undergo correction only once a year. Injectable agarose is flexible, easy to use, rapid, and subtle, and the results are predictable. In our experience, patients often ask for reinjection on the occasion of social or family events. A natural appearing long-lasting product with little to no recovery time is indicated in these cases. The author's personal experience favors the use of Easy-agarose VL both for wrinkle correction and for volume augmentation. The watery consistency of agarose gel makes it suitable for superficial injection in fine lines, without the risk of superficial blue shades as with hyaluronic acid, especially in darker skin types, when collagen might show through the epidermis. Compared with other injectable materials, agarose is harmless as long as contraindications are respected. Easy-agarose can achieve long-lasting effects provided it is used in the correct way, since it is specifically engineered to keep its stability while also imitating the behavior of natural skin components, both biomechanically and biologically.

References

1. Margel S, Marcus L. Specific hemoperfusion through agarose microbeads. Appl Biochem Biotechnol 1986; 12: 37–66.
2. Sittinger M, Perka C, Schultz O, Haupl T, Burmester GR. Joint cartilage regeneration by tissue engineering. Z Rheumatol 1999; 58: 130–5.
3. Tashiro H, Iwata H, Warnock GL et al. Characterization and transplantation of agarose microencapsulated canine islets of Langerhans. Ann Transplant 1997; 2: 33–9.
4. Micheels P. Collagène, acide hyaluronique et polylactique: peut-on encore améliorer les résultats? J Med Esthet Chir Dermatol 2004; 31(124).
5. Rimondini L. Comparative evaluation of biomaterials in the subcutaneous tissue of rats. Presented at Congresso SIES, Bologna, 2006.
6. Fernàndez-Cossìo S, Leòn-Mateos A, Sampedro FC, Oreja MT. Biocompatibility of agarose gel as a dermal filler: histologic evaluation of subcutaneous implants. Plast Reconstr Surg 2007; 120: 1161–9.

34 Hyaluronic acids*

Benjamin Ascher, Patrick Bui, and Ahmad Halabi

Introduction

In the early 1990s, after a long period of bovine collagen use, hyaluronic acids (HAs) became the most commonly used biodegradable fillers in Europe in both dermatology and plastic surgery. Currently, HAs are very popular for both soft tissue augmentation and facial volume restoration.

Dermal filler HAs have a high water retention capacity and are both effective tissue volume correctors and well tolerated. Initially, HAs were extracted from rooster combs. Later, techniques were developed to produce HAs by bacterial fermentation. Currently, some of the newer HAs are formed with crosslinking to increase their longevity once injected into human skin.

In addition to the very popular HAs, other European fillers (some of which are not available in the USA) are either non-degradable or slowly degradable. They have now been used for 30 years for the correction of facial volume wasting.

Since some commercially produced HAs and non-degradable fillers can contain residues from the manufacturing process, it is important to understand the latter for each filler. Although two fillers may both be based on HAs, they are not necessarily the same. With the wide availability of so many dermal fillers and the minimal requirements for placing such fillers in the market-place, European physicians must often be concerned about follow-up studies over the short, mid-, and long term.

In Europe, Conformité Européene (CE) marking is obligatory before a manufacturer can market a filler product. However, the presence of a CE mark does not necessarily mean that the product's efficacy and side-effects have been subject to any objective clinical studies. The European approval procedure, which is much less rigorous than that in the USA, is expected to change soon, with the adoption of an approach similar to that used by the US Food and Drug Administration (FDA). It is hoped that soon European approval will be granted only after strict clinical studies critically evaluating both efficacy and safety.

This chapter explores most of the products currently utilized in Europe and in the main locations of the world as of 2008. These fillers are of animal, bacterial, or synthetic origin; they may be reticulated or non-reticulated.

They are used to restore lines, to increase volume, or as filler product vectors.

Before one attempts to use any of the many available products, it is essential to have a thorough understanding of their absolute and relative contraindications, the types of anesthesia required, the differences between the types of wrinkles treated, and the techniques utilized to optimize cosmetic results.

Any injected product may have side-effects, the severity and the outcome of which depend on the nature of the product used. Biodegradable products generally have milder, shorter-lasting side-effects.

In general, allergic reactions are found to occur in 1–3% of patients. With some fillers, a preliminary double allergy test is justified. It is also advisable not to inject biodegradable fillers in a site previously injected with a non-degradable product. Unfortunately, precise statistics, centralized data, results, and side-effects are not available for many currently utilized fillers. This information can only be obtained from double-blinded randomized studies. These data are not only necessary for the safety of patients, but also required to improve physician knowledge and understanding of available products.

Of all the filler agents available in Europe, HAs are the most commonly used. Despite the fact that many questions still remain unanswered, these short-acting fillers do produce very significant results. The other available non-absorbable and/or slowly absorbable fillers, although highly efficient, can be associated with significant (albeit rare) complications. The ultimate goal in Europe is for higher approval standards than the currently used CE mark. Both patients and physicians will be helped when the current filler standards in Europe are brought up to the level of the French Approval for Marketing Medications (AMM) and the US FDA.

Legal aspects of dermal filler use in Europe

HA products in Europe, as in the USA, are classified as medical devices rather than drugs (botulinum toxins, however, are considered to be drugs) (Table 34.1).[1,2] These fillers, like all medical devices in Europe, are

---

*Portions of this chapter were previously published as 'Fillers in Europe' in Goldberg D, *Fillers in Cosmetic Dermatology*, London: Informa Healthcare, 2006.

Table 34.1   Definitions of drugs and medical devices from the French Ministry of Health

Drug definition	Medical device definition
• Any substance or product presented as having curative or preventive properties with regard to human or animal diseases • Any product that can be used in humans or animals in order to establish a medical diagnosis or to restore, change, or modify their organic functions • Any ingested product that contains in its composition a chemical or biologic substance with no food value, but used for medical testing • Products used for disinfecting dental prostheses, and those intended for home use, are not regarded as drugs	• Any instrument, apparatus, equipment, material, product (except products of human origin), or article used alone or in association with accessories and software that is intended by the manufacturer to be used in humans for medical purposes, where the desired principal action is not obtained by pharmacologic, immunologic, or metabolic means, but whose function can be assisted by such means • Medical devices that are designed to be implanted totally or partly in the human body or are placed in natural orifices, and/or which depend for their function on an electrical source of energy or any source of energy other than that generated directly by the human body or gravity, are considered active implanted medical devices

Table 34.2   Definition of risk classes for medical devices from the French Ministry of Health

Class	Class definition
I	Weak potential risk: surgical instruments, non-invasive medical devices, and invasive medical devices for temporary use
IIa	Moderate potential risk: medical devices that are sterile, contact lenses, dental prostheses; invasive medical devices intended for short-term use, invasive surgical devices
IIb	High potential risk: medical devices intended for long-term implantation
III	Critical potential risk: medical intended for long-term implantation in contact with the heart, central circulatory system, or central nervous system, implanted degradable medical devices and/or breast implants

Table 34.3   Rules upon which the risk classification of medical devices is based from the French Ministry of Health. The classification is determined by the characteristics or combination of characteristics in connection with the actual use of the device. The ultimate classification corresponds to the highest rule associated with that device

1. Devices that have no contact with the patient or that come into contact only with intact skin
2. Devices stored for later administration
3. Devices capable of modifying the biologic or chemical composition of blood or other body fluids
4. Devices coming into contact with injured skin
5. Devices that are invasive and introduced through any bodily orifice
6. Devices that are invasive and of a surgical type intended for temporary use
7. Devices that are invasive and of a surgical type intended for short-term use
8. Devices that are invasive and implanted for long-term use
9. Devices that are therapeutic and intended to provide or to exchange energy
10. Devices of diagnostic use
11. Devices that are active and intended to manage or to withdraw drugs or other substances from the body
12. All other active devices
13. Devices containing medical substances
14. Devices used for contraception or for the prevention of sexually transmitted diseases
15. Devices intended specifically to disinfect, clean, or rinse
16. Devices that are inactive and are intended to record images
17. Devices of animal or derivative origin
18. Devices containing blood

classified according to their perceived risk into classes I, IIa, IIb, and III (Table 34.2) on the basis of 18 rules (Table 34.3). Class I devices are considered to be the least dangerous and class III the most dangerous.

Injectable biodegradable fillers are considered to be class III devices, whereas non-biodegradable products are (somewhat paradoxically) considered to be class IIb, i.e. less dangerous devices. If, however, a non-degradable substance is combined with a degradable substance (with the non-degradable substance being considered to be a vector), then the filler device is considered to be of class III.

Table 34.4   The ISO (International Standards Organization) standards

ISO 9000 standard is used as a guide for a group of four standards:

- *ISO 9001:* Quality system, models of guarantee of quality in design, development, production, installation, and associated services
- *ISO 9002:* Quality system, models of guarantee of quality in production, installation, and associated services
- *ISO 9003:* Quality system, models of guarantee of quality for final control
- *ISO 9004:* Management of quality and elements of the quality system

The standard medical NF ISO 13485 related to devices is an adaptation of the general standard ISO 9001. It lays down requirements to be respected by manufacturers of medical devices to satisfy the requirements of international law regarding management of quality and the provision of an effective and secure device

Regulation of filler products, as medical devices, is according to European Directive 93/42/CEE (14 June 1994). This regulation has been incorporated into French law 94–43 of 18 January 1994 as part of the laws of public health and social protection.[3]

Whereas medical drugs in Europe, much as in the USA, are subject to extensive, lengthy, and costly studies, medical devices in Europe can be marketed after CE approval is obtained – a fairly simple, less expensive approach. The CE marking simply attests to 'the conformity of the product to the essential requirements of an obligatory level of health security'. These standards (NF ISO 13485, which are an adaptation of DM standard ISO 90001) (Table 34.4), simply attest to quality assurance regarding the design, development, and production of the product, and to quality assurance regarding the installation and/or the associated services (such as the promotion of the product).

The rules for obtaining a CE marking are uniform throughout the entire European Union (EU). These rules require the following:

1. The manufacturer must classify a device, as described above, according to the 18 rules of European Directive 93/42/CE into one of the four classes I, IIa, IIb, or III. In addition (at least in France), a request must be made to the AFSSAPS (French Agency for Medical Security of Health Products) for the declaration of the product as a medical device (for class IIb and III devices).
2. The manufacturer must maintain a file that tracks the manufacturing quality of a medical device according to NF ISO 13485. Such records document a description of the manufacturing process (including biocompatibility), the results of the validation of the manufacturing process (especially for sterilization), a list of raw materials utilized, a specification of these materials and a list of their components, and a final documentation of the product (labeling and instructions).
3. The manufacturer must establish the conformity of the product with the essential requirements of European Directive 93/42/CE, in particular with regard to biocompatibility (conformity with the international standard ISO 10993–1 and with clinical data).

Indeed, it is the obligation of the device manufacturer to present clinical data on both the efficacy and side-effects of the medical device. However, these data can only be data from the relevant scientific literature. An evaluation of effectiveness and side-effects based on prospective clinical trials must be presented before any group III medical devices (such as HA fillers) can be used.

Ultimately, the situation is that marketing a dermal filler in Europe is constrained more by manufacturing standards than by safety and efficacy standards – which are minimal. The rules are much less stringent than for the development and marketing of a medical drug.[4] Finally, it should be noted that the assignation of a CE marking is only temporary – often for 3 years. This emphasizes the need for more long-term vigilance about these medical materials by the physicians that use them. This policy of vigilance is not a uniform directive throughout Europe.[5] In France, long-term scrutiny of medical devices is assured by AFSSAPS. This agency obliges the manufacturer, users (including expert noting of any complications), or others who have been informed of an incident or a risk of incident that involves either directly or indirectly the death or serious damage to the health of a patient or a user to declare this incident to AFSSAPS. If this rule is violated, the offender risks a 4-year prison sentence and a 75 000 euro fine.[6] However, it is only optional for the manufacturer, users, and others, having been informed of a complication and/or non-desired reaction, to report this problem.[4,7]

In conclusion, marketing of a filler in Europe requires only that a CE mark be obtained – which is a much less stringent requirement than FDA approval. Obtaining a CE mark in no way implies that a particular product was submitted to any clinical trials or any study of its effectiveness and possible short-term or long-term side-effects. The law simply requires (at least in France) that professionals (doctors and manufacturers) declare to AFSSAPS any serious side-effects and 'strongly advises them' to report other less serious side-effects noted after using these products.

Table 34.5   Hyaluronic acid (HA) products

Biorevitalization: non-linked HA	Implants: linked HA	Vectors: slowly linked HA
Animal origin		
AcHyal	Hylaform:	
IAL System	Hylaform Fine Line	
	Hylaform	
	Hylaform Plus	
Bacterial fermentation origin		
Hyaluderm	BeautyGel:	Dermalive (HA + acrylic hydrogel)
Juvélift	BeautyGel	Dermadeep (HA + acrylic hydrogel)
Mac Dermol:	BeautySphere (HA + dextran)	
Mac Dermol Bio	Dethail (HA + dextran):	
Mac Dermol S	Dethail Coilingel	
Restylane Touch Line	Dethail Lastingel	
Revitacare	Esthelis:	
	Esthelis Basic	
	Esthelis Men	
	Esthelis Soft	
	Hyaluderm:	
	Hyaluderm	
	Hydra Fill:	
	Hydra Fill 1	
	Hydra Fill 2	
	Hydra Fill 3	
	Juvéderm:	
	Juvéderm 18	
	Juvéderm 24	
	Juvéderm 30	
	Juvéderm 24HV	
	Juvéderm 30HV	
	Mac Dermol:	
	Mac Dermol R	
	Matridur:	
	Matridur	
	Matridex (HA + dextran)	
	Puragen:	
	Puragen	
	Restylane:	
	Restylane Fine Line	
	Restylane	
	Perlane	
	Restylane Sub-Q	
	Rofilan Gel:	
	Rofilan Hylan Gel	
	Reviderm Intra (HA + dextran)	
	Surgiderm:	
	Surgiderm	
	Voluma:	
	Voluma	

Biodegradable absorbable products available in Europe

A wide range of absorbable products are currently available in Europe (Tables 34.5 and 34.6).[8]

It should be noted that collagen products from the USA (CosmoDerm®/CosmoPlast®; Inamed) as well as the Israeli collagen product Evolence® (Colbar Laboratories) are not described in this chapter.

Linked hyaluronic acids of animal origin

Hylaform®

Hylaform® (Genzyme; distributed by Allergan) received its CE mark in 1995 and FDA approval in 2004. Hylaform is still marketed in some markets. Some sales in Germany, Italy, Benelux and Nordics show the highest sales. Hylaform products are HA extracted from rooster combs. Although the manufacturer at one time suggested that the product is free from any associated proteins, the

Table 34.6 Linked hyaluronic acid (HA) products

Product (CE marking/FDA approval)	Origin	Syringe	Needle
Hylaform (1995/yes, 2004):			
Hylaform Fine Line	Rooster comb	0.55 ml	32G½
Hylaform		0.55 ml	30G½
Hylaform Plus		0.55 ml	27G½
BeautyGel (yes/no):			
BeautyGel	Bacterial fermentation	1 ml	30G½
BeautySphere (HA + dextran)		1 ml	30G
Hyaluderm (yes/no):			
Hyaluderm (weak reticulated HA)	Bacterial fermentation	1 ml	30G
Dethail (2005/no):			
Dethail Coilingel	Bacterial fermentation	1 ml	30G½
Dethail Lastingel		1 ml	27G½
Esthelis (2004/no):			
Esthelis Basic	Bacterial fermentation	0.6 ml	27G½
Esthelis Men		0.6 ml	27G½
Esthelis Soft		0.6 ml	30G½
Hydra Fill (yes/no):			
Hydra Fill 1	Bacterial fermentation	0.6 ml	30G½
Hydra Fill 2		0.6 ml	27G½
Hydra Fill 3		0.8 ml	27G½
Juvéderm (2000, France/no):			
Juvéderm 18	Bacterial fermentation	0.6 ml	30G½
Juvéderm 24		0.6 ml	27G½
Juvéderm 30		0.6 or 0.8 ml	27G½
Juvéderm 24HV		0.8 ml	30G½
Juvéderm 30HV		0.8 ml	30G½
Mac Dermol (yes/no):			
Mac Dermol R	Bacterial fermentation	0.6 ml	30G½
Matridur (yes/no):			
Matridex (HA + dextran)	Bacterial fermentation	1 ml	
Matridur		0.6 ml	
Puragen (2005/no):			
Puragen	Bacterial fermentation		
Restylane (1996, Sweden/yes, 2003):			
Restylane Fine Line	Bacterial fermentation	0.4 ml	31G
Restylane		0.7 or 0.4 ml	30G
Perlane		0.7 ml	27G
Restylane Sub-Q		2 ml	
Rofilan (yes/no):			
Rofilan Hylan Gel	Bacterial fermentation	1 ml	
Reviderm Intra (HA + dextran)			
Surgiderm (2005/no):			
Surgiderm 18	Bacterial fermentation	0.8 ml	30G½
Surgiderm 30		0.8 ml	27G
Surgiderm 24XP		0.8 ml	27G
Surgiderm 30XP		0.8 ml	30G½
Surgilips		0.6 ml	27G
Voluma (2005/no):			
Voluma	Bacterial fermentation	2 ml	21G

medical literature suggests that there may be some traces of potentially antigenic residue.[8] In Europe, the material is currently marketed in three forms:

- Hylaform Fine Line is slightly crosslinked HA, in a 0.55-ml syringe with a 32G, ½-inch needle
- Hylaform is more strongly crosslinked HA, in a 0.55-ml syringe with a 30G, ½-inch needle

- Hylaform Plus is even more strongly crosslinked HA, in a 0.55-ml syringe with a 27G needle.

Linked hyaluronic acids of non-animal origin

These products are manufactured by bacterial fermentation.

BeautyGel®

BeautyGel® (Rofil Medical International, Germany, distributed in France by Philoderm®) has received its CE mark but does not have FDA approval. This material is marketed in two forms:

- BeautyGel is crosslinked HA, in three 1-ml syringes with 30G, ½-inch needles
- BeautySphere® is HA together with dextran.

Dethail®

Dethail® (Phitogen, Italy; distributed in France by Phitogen France) received its CE mark in 2005 but does not have FDA approval. This HA is dextran-associated. The material is marketed in two forms:

- Dethail Coilingel is slightly crosslinked HA, in one 1-ml syringe with two 30G, ½-inch needles
- Dethail Lastingel is more strongly crosslinked HA, in one 1-ml syringe with two 27G, ½-inch needles.

Esthelis®

Esthelis® (Anteis SA; distributed in France by Anteis France) received its CE mark in 2004 but does not have FDA approval. The material is marketed in three forms:

- Esthelis Soft is slightly crosslinked HA, in two 0.6-ml syringes with two 30G, ½-inch needles
- Esthelis Basic is more strongly crosslinked HA, in two 0.6-ml syringes with two 27G, ½-inch needles
- Esthelis Men is the same as Esthelis Basic, but marketed for male patients.

Hyaluderm®

Hyaluderm® (LCA Pharmaceutical) has received its CE mark but does not have FDA approval. It is marketed as:

- Hyaluderm which is slightly crosslinked HA, in one 1-ml syringe with a 30G needle.

Hydra Fill®

Hydra Fill® (Allergan) received its CE mark in 2002 but does not have FDA approval. The product is available, but not marketed/promoted across EAME. It is marketed in five forms:

- Hydra Fill Grade 1 is slightly crosslinked HA in two 0.6-ml syringes with four 30G, ½-inch needles
- Hydra Fill Grade 2 is more strongly crosslinked HA in two 0.6-ml syringes with four 27G, ½-inch needles
- Hydra Fill Grade 3 is even more strongly crosslinked HA in two 0.8-ml syringes with four 27G, ½-inch needles
- Hydra Fill Softline
- Hydra Fill Softline Max.

Hydra Fill grades 1, 2 and 3 have been discontinued and upgraded to Softline and Softline MAX, which are still marketed across EAME.

Juvéderm®

Juvéderm® (Allergan) received its CE mark in 2000 and the US FDA in 2006. It is marketed in five forms:

- Juvéderm 18 is slightly crosslinked HA in a 0.6-ml syringe with a 30G, ½-inch needle
- Juvéderm 24 is more strongly crosslinked HA in a 0.6-ml syringe with a 27G, ½-inch needle
- Juvéderm 30 is even more strongly crosslinked HA in a 0.6-ml or 0.8-ml syringe with a 27G, ½-inch needle
- Juvéderm 24HV is very strongly crosslinked, and highly viscous, in a 0.8-ml syringe with a 30G, ½-inch needle
- Juvéderm 30HV is yet more strongly crosslinked, and highly viscous, in a 0.8-ml syringe with a 30G, ½-inch needle.

The new Juvéderm Ultra® is quite clothed to the surgiderm. See Chapter Surgiderm.

Mac Dermol®

Mac Dermol® (Orgév, France; distributed in France by Centrale des Peelings) has received its CE mark but does not have FDA approval. It is marketed as:

- Mac Dermol, which is slightly crosslinked HA in a 0.6-ml syringe with a 30G, ½-inch needle.

Matridur®

Matridur® (bioPolymer GmbH, Germany; distributed in France by Florelle) has received its CE mark but does not have FDA approval. It is marketed in two forms:

- Matridur is slightly crosslinked HA in a 0.6-ml syringe
- Matridex is HA together with dextran in a 1-ml syringe.

Puragen®

Puragen® (Mentor, USA) received its CE mark in 2005 but does not have FDA approval. It is marketed as:

- Puragen, which is a double crosslinked HA – this may allow better resistance to degradation. The product is dedicated to deep to moderate lines.
- Prevelle® (Mentor, USA) received its CE mark in 2007 but does not have FDA approval. It is marketed as: Prevelle lees croos linked than Pruragen. The product is dedicated to moderate to fine lines.

Restylane®

Restylane® (Q-Med, Sweden; distributed in France by Q-Med) received its CE mark in 1996 and FDA approval in 2003. It is marketed in Europe in three forms (plus Restylane Sub-Q: see below):

- Restylane Fine Line: 200 000 particles/ml in a 0.4-ml syringe with a 31G needle; Restylane Fine line is now replaced by Restylane Touch: 500 000 particles/ml in a 0.4-ml syringe.
- Restylane: 100 000 particles/ml in a 0.4-ml or 0.7-ml syringe with a 30G needle
- Perlane®: 10 000 particles/ml (more viscous than Restylane) in a 0.7-ml syringe with a 27G needle.

Rofilan®

Rofilan® (Rofil Medical International, The Netherlands; distributed in France by Rofil Medical International) has received its CE mark but does not have FDA approval. It is marketed in two forms:

- Reviderm® Intra is HA with associated dextran
- Rofilan Hylan Gel.

Surgiderm®

Surgiderm® (Allergan) received its CE mark in 2005 but does not have FDA approval. It is marketed in the following forms:

- Surgilift plus, non linked HA
- Surgiderm 18 is slightly crosslinked HA in a 0.8-ml syringe with a 30G, ½-inch needle
- Surgiderm 30 is more strongly crosslinked HA in a 0.8-ml syringe with a 27G needle
- Surgiderm 24XP is more strongly crosslinked (similar to Surgiderm 30) plus XP technology
- Surgiderm 30XP is even more strongly crosslinked HA, marketed in a 0.8-ml syringe with a 30G, ½-inch needle
- Surgilips® is marketed specifically for lips, in a 0.6-ml syringe with a 27G needle.

Teosyal®

Teosyal® (Teoxane, Switzerland; distributed in France by Teoxane) received its CE mark in 2004 but does not have FDA approval.

Visagel®

Visagel® (Dermatech, Germany; distributed in France by Dermatech) received its CE mark in 2005 but does not have FDA approval.

Volumetric products (see Chapter 39)

Restylane

Restylane Sub-Q® (Q-Med, Sweden; distributed in France by Q-Med) received its CE mark in 2004 but does not have FDA approval. Its reticulation is chemical. According to the laboratory's documentation, it does not contain any protein residue, and its rate of stabilization should be identical to the other Restylane (NASHA process) products, differing only in the size

and number of the particles. The product is marketed in a 2-ml syringe, injected using an 18- or 21G nozzle.

Voluma®

Voluma® (Cornéal; distributed in France by Cornéal) received its CE mark in 2005 but does not have FDA approval. Its reticulation is chemical, and according to laboratory documentation does not have any protein residue. The product is marketed in a 2-ml syringe injected with a 21G nozzle.

Fortelis® (Anteis SA; distributed in France by Anteis France) received its CE mark in 2007 but does not have FDA approval.

Ultradeep® (Teoxane Switzerland; distributed in France by Teoxane) received its CE mark in 2007 but does not have FDA approval.

Non-linked mesotherapy products

The following HAs are used in mesotherapy rather than generally for true filling.

Hyaluronic acids of animal origin

- AcHyal® (Tetec-Meiji Farma, Japan; distributed in France by Filorga) has received a CE mark but does not have FDA approval. This is a non-linked HA
- IAL System (Phitogen; distributed in France by Phitogen France) received its CE mark in 2005 but does not have FDA approval. This is marketed in 0.6- and 1.0-ml syringes with a 30G needle.

Hyaluronic acids resulting from bacterial fermentation

- Hyaluderm (LCA Pharmaceutical; distributed in France by LCA Pharmaceutical) has received a CE mark but does not have FDA approval
- Juvélift® and Surgilift® (Allergan) received its CE mark in 2004 but does not have FDA approval. This is marketed in a 0.55-ml syringe with a 30G, ½-inch needle
- Mac Dermol (Orgév; distributed in France by Centrale des Peelings) has received a CE mark but does not have FDA approval. This is marketed in two forms:
  - Mac Dermol S is a non-linked HA
  - Mac Dermol Bio is a non-linked HA with associated chondroitin sulfate
- Restylane Touch Line (Q-Med; distributed in France by Q-Med) has received a CE mark but does not have FDA approval. This is marketed in a 0.5-ml syringe with a 30G needle. It is now also available in a new presentation called Vital Restylane, marketed in a 1-ml syringe
- Revitacare® (Revitacare Biorevitalisation, France; distributed in France by Revitacare) received its CE mark in 2004 but does not have FDA approval. This is marketed as 4 ml of HA to be diluted in 10 ml of multivitamins.

Hyaluronic acid with associated vectors

- Dermadeep® (Biocristal France; distributed in France by Derma Tech) received its CE mark in 1999 but does not have FDA approval. This contains an association of 40% acrylic hydrogel (particles of 80–110 μmol) and 60% slightly crosslinked bacterial fermentation-derived HA, marketed in a 1.2-ml syringe with a 26G, ½-inch needle
- Dermalive® (Biocristal France; distributed in France by Derma Tech) received its CE mark in 1998 but does not have FDA approval. This contains an association of 40% acrylic hydrogel (particles of 45–65 μmol) and 60% slightly crosslinked bacterial fermentation-derived HA, marketed in a 0.8-ml syringe with a 27G, ½-inch needle.

Finally, it should be noted that most laboratories manufacturing HAs do not specify the presence of protein-associated residues. Only the manufacturers of Restylane and Hylaform have done this. This is important because the incidence of filler-related reactions may be related to these protein residues. There has been extensive research and considerable clinical experience associated with both products. Currently these two fillers, as well as Juvéderm and Surgiderm, are the most popular HA products in Europe.

Complications of biodegradable absorbable products seen in Europe

The two commonly used biodegradable products are collagen and HAs. Complications can occur from any filler. It is important to recognize potential complications, attempt to avoid them, and finally treat them when possible.

Immediate reactions

During or immediately after injection, the following can appear:

- erythema, which appears to be more common after HA injections than after collagen injections (Figure 34.1a)
- slight bleeding at injection sites – most common at certain locations, such as the peribuccal and oral commissure regions (Figure 34.1b)
- edema
- ecchymosis
- pain, pruritus, or skin hypersensitivity at the injection site.

These immediate reactions generally disappear within 72 hours and are very common. Many measures are available to prevent or to stop the progression of these side-effects. These include homeopathic granules (Apis and Arnica) and creams containing vitamin K (Auriderm XO®, Auriga Laboratory). Some have recommended the

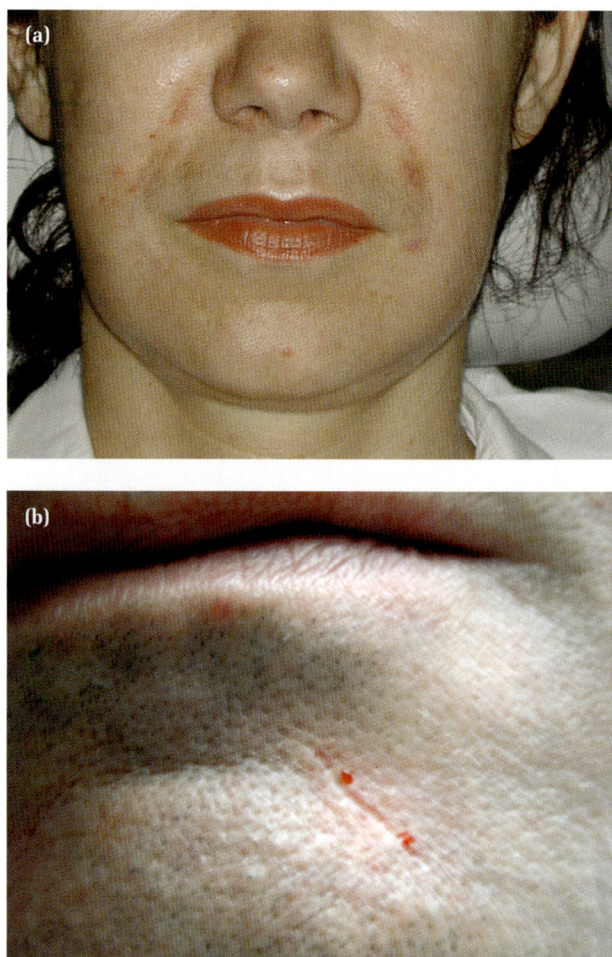

Figure 34.1 Erythema appears to be more frequent with hyaluronic acid products than with collagens: (a) inflammatory general reaction and erythema, disappearing within the following 8 days; (b) bleeding at several points. Courtesy of B Ascher.

immediate application of a steroid-based cream (epithelial HA, Sensibio, Bioderma) and/or the use of cold packs on the injected areas to minimize short-term complications. Finally, some authors[9] suggest that all anticoagulation, including aspirin, be stopped at least 4 days before treatment. This, along with good injection techniques, makes the avoidance of these side-effects more likely.

When dermal fillers are injected into the lips, an inflammatory sensitive edema can appear in less than 12 hours. This may persist from 2 to 7 days. Its disappearance is facilitated by the use of topical steroids.[10]

Longer-lasting problems

Papules or fine white lines, or palpable or visible nodes, at the injection site generally represent poor technique. Either the filler has been injected too superficially or was poorly selected for that location (for example a product that was too concentrated or too crosslinked for the area to be corrected). An immediate and vigorous massage, repeated daily for several days, may help disperse the filler material. However, some papules can persist for months.

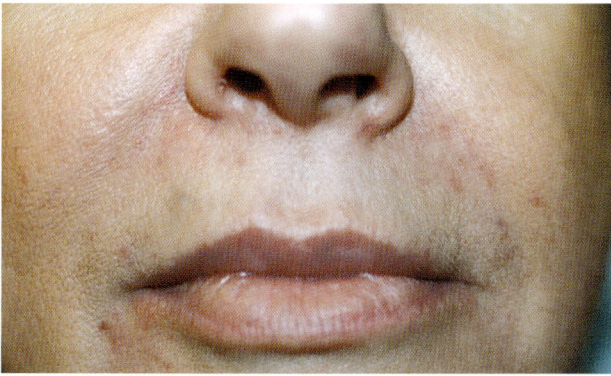

Figure 34.2 Bluish-gray, linear, painless pigmentation has been described after HA injection. This pigmentation usually disappears within 3–6 months, but can last for up to 1 year. It is a contraindication for all new injections before complete disappearance of the pigmentation. The cause of this pigmentation is unknown and there is no known treatment. At best, cover-up products are suggested. Courtesy of Martine Baspeyras.

Bluish-gray, linear, painless pigmentation has been described after HA injection (Figure 34.2). This pigmentation usually disappears within 3–6 months, but can last for up to 1 year. Further injections to the same area are not recommended, as this may lead to permanent pigmentation. The cause of this pigmentation is unknown and there is no known treatment. At best, cover-up products are suggested. In Europe, the principal products to mask these colors are Color Control (Cosmodex), Couvrance (Avene), Dermablend (Vichy), and Unifiance (La Rochel-Posay).

Insufficient correction of the treated side can simply be improved with reinjection of the filler soon after the initial injection.

Overcorrection with frankly visible implant can last for about 1 year. This is best avoided with the correct technique.

More serious semi-delayed complications

These occur in the days following the injection:

- abscesses at the injection site are generally related to poor sterile technique
- hematomas and ecchymoses appear in the hours following the injection, usually localized to the peribuccal region;[11] they can be seen in numerous areas after mesotherapy.

An immediate compression with the added application of cold packs will limit this type of complication, which can last for more than 1 week.

Paresthesia and allergy to local anesthetic are rare complications.

Delayed complications

These generally appear at least a day after the injection. The reactions are quite varied in nature and tend to be localized within the injection site. They have been reported with both bovine collagen and HAs.[12,13] They can take the following forms:[11,14]

- intense and hardened erythema
- non-specific blue–purple granulomas
- hardened folliculitis
- pseudocysts and nodes.

It should be noted that these reactions are more frequent with collagen than with HA. They generally appear 1–4 weeks after injection (even later reactions have been reported with collagen). They can appear at the time of the first injection, but also after any later injection (Figure 34.3).

These complications must be treated as soon as possible. With the appearance of erythema, a local and perhaps even a systemic steroid must be prescribed for 15 days. Fortunately, total disappearance of this type of complication is usual, but they can last some months. Some experts suggest that these lesions be incised or punctured to accelerate cure, but the risk of scarring is always present.[11]

These delayed local complications have been classified into two types: of immunologic and non-immunologic origin.

The immunologic reactions are thought to be delayed hypersensitivity reactions. These are T-lymphocyte-mediated and are induced by antigen present in the injected dermal filler. The specific immune reaction is due to the presence of various proteins (residues, bacteria, and impurities).

Non-immunologic local reactions such as granuloma represent foreign body reactions (Figure 34.3), with the host's phagocytic cells producing inflammatory cytokines at the time of filler injection. These non-specific reactions cause an infiltrate around the implant. Other non-specific inflammatory reactions that have been described after HA injections are thought to be secondary to the presence of postmanufacturing residues of linkage or stabilization. Other contaminants can also be implicated in the formation of such reactions. Only Restylane and Hylaform appear to have produced rare reactions to residues – this may be because they have been on the market for a considerable time, are widely used, and have been the subjects of extensive, published safety studies. Treatment is by injection of a small amount of hyaluronidase, which leads to rapid disappearance of the granuloma.

Rare cases of necrosis have been described, particularly after collagen (Zyplast®) injection into the glabellar area.[15] To date, there are no published studies documenting any case of necrosis after injection of HA.

Patient satisfaction is always an issue with any cosmetic procedure. A basic psychologic profile of patients can occasionally sort out the patient with totally unrealistic expectations.

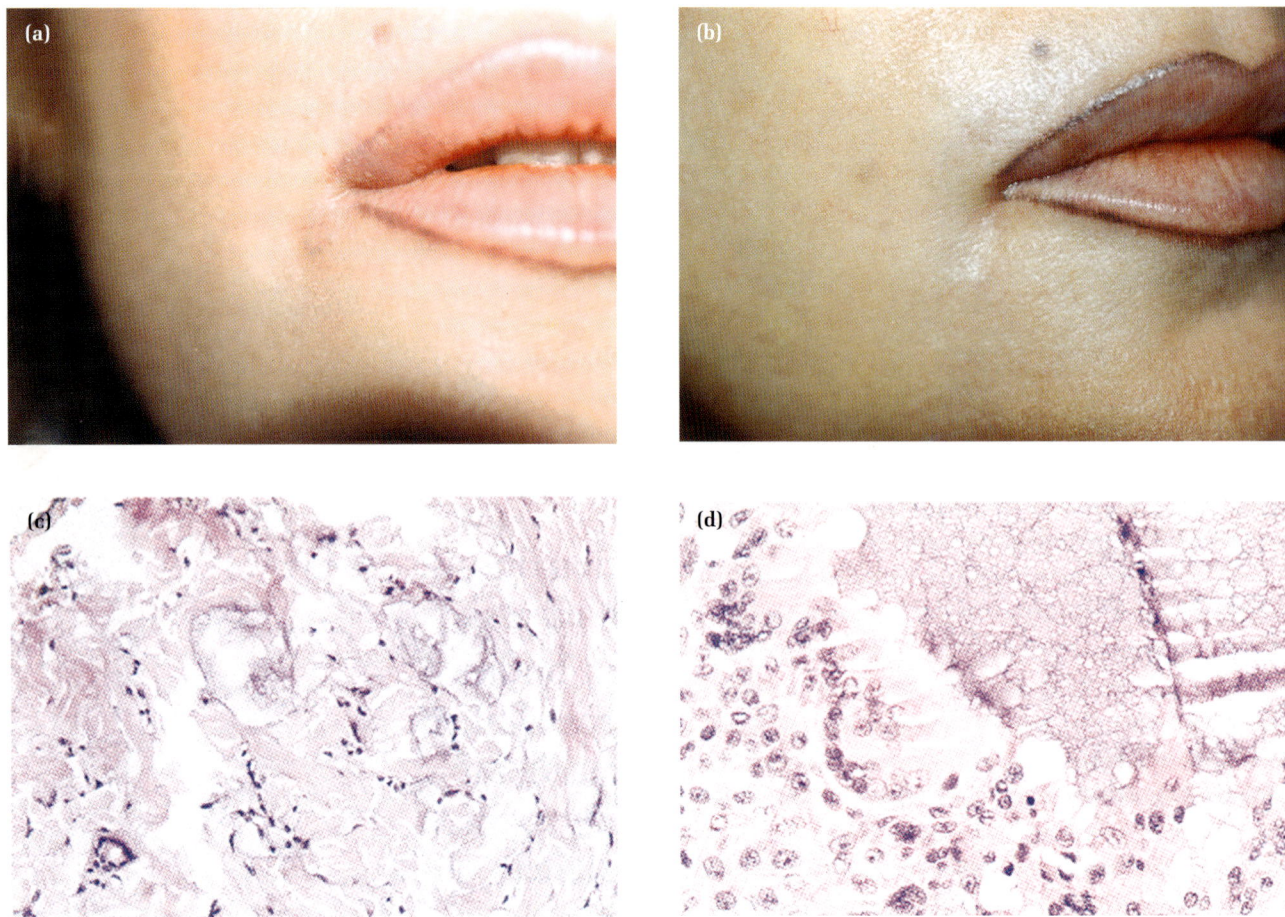

Figure 34.3   (a) Clinical representation of granuloma, representing a foreign body reaction after a hyaluronic acid filler injection. Treatment was with a small quantity of hyaluronidase and a quick resolution was seen in a few days. Such findings rarely occurred with older hyaluronic acid fillers. They are distinctly uncommon with today's purified products. (c, d) Histologic evidence of granuloma formation.

Generally, absorbable products have mild side-effects and are short-lasting – which is why they are generally considered as reliable and safe products. More serious side-effects have been reported with the injection of absorbable products at the same site where non-absorbable products were injected. These side-effects include granulomas, whose treatment is often partial and difficult.[16,17] It is therefore necessary to avoid any injection of a slowly absorbable product in a site already treated with a non-absorbable product. When granulomas appear, they are generally due to the most recent injection at the affected site.

Declaration of the complications in France

As described above, any serious complication that may threaten the life of a patient must be declared to avoid legal repercussions. Other less severe complications should also be reported (even if this is not legally required) so that treating physicians can improve their knowledge base and potentially avoid such complications in the future.

In France, the following declarations should be made:

- at the AFSSAPS website (www.afssaps.sante.fr)
- to liability insurers, to be certain that coverage will be available
- at the VIGIPIL website – a website organized by French dermatologists that provides a registry for complications seen after the performance of esthetic medical procedures (Martine-baspeyras@ wanadoo.fr).

In conclusion, side-effects after HA injection are generally not severe and are usually short-lived. Finally, because complications from non-absorbable products are generally more severe and long-lasting, it is best to avoid HA injections at the site of a previously injected non-degradable product.

Conclusions

The majority of HA fillers, from Europe and the main locations of the world, in current use have been reviewed. New fillers are constantly coming onto the

European market. Thorough understanding of their pharmacology, clinical results, and associated complications is necessary before they should be used widely by cosmetic surgeons.

Acknowledgments

The authors would like to thank Mariane Cerceau MD, Bernard Rossi MD, Annick Pons-Guirard MD, and Roger Kuffer MD for their technical assistance and advice in the preparation of this chapter. We are especially grateful to Martine Baspeyras MD and Patrick Mikeels MD for their help with images and for their editorial assistance.

References

1. Code de la Santé Publique (Partie Législative). Article L5111–1.
2. Code de la Santé Publique (Nouvelle Partie Législative). Article L5111–1.
3. Code de la Santé Publique (www.legifrance.gouv.fr). Code de la Santé Publique livre II: Dispositif médicaux et autres produits et objets réglementés dans l'intérêt de la Santé publique. Titre 1er. Dispositifs médicaux. Articles L5211–1 et suivants.
4. Lemperle G, Morhenn V, Charrier U. Human histology and persistence of various injectable filler substances for soft tissue augmentation. Aesthetic Plast Surg 2003; 27: 354–66.
5. Code de la Santé Publique (Partie Réglementaire – Décrets en Conseil d'Etat). Article R665–48.
6. Code de la Santé Publique (Nouvelle Partie Législative). Article L5461–2.
7. Code de la Santé Publique (Partie Réglementaire – Décrets en Conseil d'Etat). Article L665–50.
8. Manna F, Dentini M, Desideri P et al. Comparative chemical evaluation of two commercially available derivatives of hyaluronic acid (Hylaform® from rooster combs and Restylane® from Streptococcus) used for soft tissue augmentation. J Eur Acad Dermatol Venereol 1999; 13: 183–92.
9. Pons-Guiraud A. Matériaux de comblement: techniques et effets indésirables. EMC Dermatol Cosmét 2004; 1: 59–74.
10. Hoffman C, Schuller-Petrovic S, Soyer HP, Kerl H. Adverse reactions after cosmetic lip augmentation with permanent biologically inert implant materials. J Am Acad Dermatol 1999; 40: 100–23.
11. Pons-Guiraud A. Actualisation des effets secondaires des produits de comblement. Nouv Dermatol 2003; 22: 205–10.
12. Barr R, Stegman SJ. Delayed skin test reaction to injectable collagen implant (Zyderm). The histopathologic comparative study. J Am Acad Dermatol 1984; 10: 652–8.
13. De Lustro F, Fries J, Kang J et al. Immunity to injectable collagen and autoimmune disease; a summary of current understanding. J Dermatol Surg Oncol 1988; 14 (Suppl 1): 57–65.
14. Bergeret-Galley C. Comparison of resorbable soft tissue fillers. Aesthetic Surg J 2004; 24: 33–45.
15. Cucin RL, Barek D. Complications of injectable collagen implant. Plast Reconstr Surg 1983; 71: 731.
16. Bui P, Pons-Guiraud A, Kuffer R. Injectables lentement et non résorbables. Ann Chir Plast Esthet 2004; 49: 486–502.
17. Ascher B, Cerceau M, Baspeyras M, Rossi B. Soft tissue filling with hyaluronic acid. Ann Chir Plast Esthet 2004; 49: 465–85.

35 The injectable products: slowly resorbables and non-resorbables

Patrick Bui, Annick Pons-Guiraud, Roger Kuffer, Françoise Plantier, Pierre J Nicolau, and Gilbert Zakine

Introduction

Research into materials to fill wrinkles has included products that are biodegradable such as collagen or hyaluronic acid as well as non-biodegradable materials such as silicone oil (Table 35.1). The requirement for a biocompatible, efficacious, permanent or long-term filler is increasing continually.

The main characteristic of slowly resorbable and non-resorbable products, besides the durability of their action, is principally the volumetric effect. These products are for injection into deep wrinkles; for superficial wrinkles such products are forbidden.

Implants are unfortunately responsible for more frequent complications, as well as side-effects. The prevention of their complications, their analysis, their identification, and their treatment have been for some years a significant part of their use, and will be particularly itemized in this chapter.

For these products, the holding of CE marking (Conformité Européene), which is minimally obligatory for their marketing and their circulation in Europe, seems to us to be deficient. The marking gives a hygiene and manufacturing guarantee certainly, but assures neither their efficacy nor their tolerance in situ for the short or the long term. Clinical studies are particularly important for this range of products.

Pharmacology

It is necessary to differentiate between products that are slowly resorbable, whose life is estimated at between 12 and 36 months, and those that are permanent. Among the permanent products are those containing various amounts of resorbable material such as collagen or hyaluronic acid, and others are purely non-resorbable products.

In fact, the modes of deterioration are not really known. The manufacturers say that it occurs by hydrolysis, division, and phagocytosis of the fragments.

Table 35.1   The different filler products (at 01/09/2006)

Biodegradables		Non-biodegradables
Medium term (6–18 months)	Long term (18 months–3 years)	
Collagens	*Hyaluronic acid*	*Polymethylmethacrylate (+ collagen)*
Animal origin Zyderm®, Zyplast®, Résoplast®	Non-animal origine Matridex®	*Artefill®*
	Polylactic acid	**Acrylic hydrogel (+ hyaluronic acid)**
Human origin Cosmoderm® Cosmoplast®	New-Fill®	*Dermalive®* *Dermadeep®*
Hyaluronic acid Animal origin Hylaform®	**Polyacrylamide gel** Outline® (*biodegradable?*)	**Polyacrylamide gel** *Evolution®* *Aquamid®*
Hylaform-Plus®, Hylaform FL® Mac Dermol	**Hydroxyapatite** *Radiesse®*	**Alkylimide** *Bio-Alcamid®*
Non-animal origin Restylane®,		**Dimethylsiloxane** *Bioplastique®*
Restylane FL®, Perlane®, Sub Q® Hyaluderm® Juvederm® 18–24HV– 30HV Matridur® Esthelis®		**Silicone oil** *Silikon 1000®* *Adatosil 5000®*
Polyvinylic acid Bioinblue®		

Studies seem necessary to specify the perfect harmlessness of the degradation of these products, notably with regard to the acrylic hydrogels.

Table 35.2   Products on the market

Name	Active agent	Date of CE marking	Duration	Indication
Long-term resorption: life duration 12–18 months				
Reviderm®/ Beautysphere®	Hyaluronic acid + microspheres of dextran	1204/031130 2005/04	12–18 months	Deep dermis Tractate type of injection
Bioinblue®	Reticulated polyvinylic acid	0123, class	12–18 months	Deep dermis Tractate type of injection
Outline® Fine	Acrylic polymeric gel, acrylamide, PAAG	L0042994-01, 09/06/00	Half-life: 12 months	Deep dermis Tractate type of injection
Partial resorption: life duration > 36 months				
New-Fill®	Polylactic acid hydrogel, PLA		36–48 months	Deep dermis, hypodermis Tractate type of injection
Outline® Original	Acrylic polymeric gel, acrylamide, PAAG	L0042994-01, 09/06/00	Half-life: 2 years	Deep dermis, hypodermis Tractate type of injection
Permanent				
Artecoll®	Polymeric acrylic microspheres, methylmethacrylate, PMMA	0344 51490TE01 grade III	Permanent	Deep dermis, hypodermis Tractate type of injection
Radiance/Radiesse®	Hydroxyapatite microspheres	0086, class IIb	Permanent	Hypodermis Tractate type of injection
Dermalive®	Acrylic polymer, hydroxyethyl-methacrylate, HEMA and ethyl-methacrylate, EMA (45–65 μm)	DGM-318, 30/03/1, class IIb	Permanent	Hypodermis Tractate type of injection
Dermadeep®	Acrylic polymer, hydroxyethyl-methacrylate, HEMA and ethyl-methacrylate, EMA (80–110 μm)		Permanent	Hypodermis Tractate type of injection
Outline® Ultra	Acrylic polymeric gel, acrylamide, PAAG	L0042994-01, 09/06/00, and L0042994-02, 19/06/03	Half-life: 5 years	Hypodermis
Aquamid®	Acrylic polymeric gel, acrylamide PAAG	DGM-318, 30/03/01, IIb	Permanent	Deep dermis, hypodermis Bolus injections 3–15 ml
Bio-Alcamid®	Polymeric acrylic gel, alkylimide	0123, 2001	Permanent	Deep dermis, hypodermis Bolus injections 3–15 ml
Evolution®	Microspheres of polyvinyl hydroxide	L0042994-02, 19/06/03	Permanent	Deep dermis, hypodermis Tractate type of injection
Isolagen®	Suspension of autologous fibroblasts	FDA	Permanent	Deep dermis, hypodermis Tractate type of injection

Legislation

This is the same for all injectable products:

- Food and Drug Administration (FDA) approval for the USA, and CE marking for Europe, assure security of manufacture and allow their marketing

- this approval or obligatory marking does not guarantee the existence of clinical study, or prejudge a product's effectiveness or the appearance of side-effects
- practitioners have a legal obligation to declare determined side-effects to AFSSAPS (Agence Française de Sécurité Sanitaire des Produits de Santé) for Europe, and to the laboratory in question.

Different products on the market (Table 35.2)

Aquamid®

PAAG, polyacrylamide 2.5% gel in 97.5% water.
Marking: DGM-318, CE 0543, March 2001.
Not approved by the FDA.
Producer: Ferrosan A/S, Copenhagen, Denmark.
Commercialized by: International Contura SA, Sydmarken 23, DK-2860 Soeborg, Denmark.
Presentation: one syringe of 1 ml, injection with a needle of 27 G.
Must be kept at room temperature and protected from light.
Histology: the acrylamide gel creates a fine fibrocellular capsule which becomes more pronounced between 6 and 9 months, and it presents in the form of millions of microdrops of product. These capsules are enveloped by fibroblasts and macrophages. The half-life of polyacrylamide in the human body is about 20 years for a large quantity, but 0.1 ml of Aquamid is absorbed in 9 months. Practically, the implant remains palpable for 9 months.[1]

Aquamid is authorized in Europe, Australia, South America, and the Middle East, but not in the USA.

Indications: injections in the lips, nasolabial fold, peribuccal wrinkles, glabella, chin, cheekbones, and nose.[2]
Website: http://www.aquamid.com
Australian distributor: http://www.aquamid.info
Clinical studies: http://www.aquamid.info/CSAquamid. pdf

ArteFill®

Microspheres of acrylic polymer, methylmethacrylate, PMMA, 30–50 µm microspheres in a suspension of bovine collagen molecules, in 3.5% and 0.3% lidocaine.
Marking: CE 0344 51490TE01 Grade III, ISO 13485:2003.
Producer: Artes Medical, Inc., San Diego, CA, USA.
Commercialized by: Artes Medical, Inc, San Diego, CA, USA.
Presentation: three syringes of 0.8 ml and two syringes of 0.4 ml, needles of 26G1/2.
Storage: between 2 and 10°C, and let warm up to room temperature before use.
Histology: microspheres of 30–50 µm are polymerized and have a smooth, round surface with the absence of electrical charge that allows them to resist phagocytosis or dislocation. One month after injection we find the microspheres encapsulated by a fine coat of collagen, macrophages, and fibroblasts. Between 3 and 6 months the bovine collagen is absorbed and replaced by human collagen. For 9 months microspheres remain unchanged.[1,3]
Website: http://www.artecoll-usa.com/
Contact information: Artes Medical Corp, 4660 Jolla Village Drive, Suite 825, San Diego, CA 92122, USA.
Preclinical review: http://www.fda.gov/ohrms/dockets/ac/03/briefing/3934b1_02_precl-fda.pdf

Bio-Alcamid®

Polymeric acrylic gel, alkylimide 4% gelled in 96% apyrogenic water.
Marking: CE 0123.
Producer: Polymekon, via Savona 19/A, 20144 Milan, Italy.
Commercialized by: Medi Form, 77/79 rue Marcel Dassault, 92100 Boulogne, France.
Presentation:

- Bio-Alcamid Lips: two syringes of 1 ml with 23G needle
- Bio-Alcamid Face: one syringe of 3 ml with 19G needle
- Bio-Alcamid Body: two syringes of 5 ml with tip catheter.

Website: http://www.bioalcamid.com

Bioinblue®

Reticulated polyvinyl alcohol 8% in 92% apyrogenic water.
Marking: CE 0123.
Producer: Polymekon, via Savona 19/A, 20144 Milan, Italy.
Commercialized by: Medi Form, 77/79 rue Marcel Dassault, 92100 Boulogne, France.
Presentation: two syringes of 0.7 ml.
Website: http://www.polymekonresearch.com

Bioplastique®

Solid, vulcanized methylpolysiloxane microspheres (100–400 µm), suspended in polyvinylpyrolidone.
Producer: Uroplasty BV, The Netherlands.
Bioplastique is not yet approved by the FDA.
Marking: CE

Dermadeep®

Gelled acrylic polymer, hydroxyethylmethacrylate, HEMA, and ethylmethacrylate, EMA (80–110 µm), 40% in 25% water in reticulated hyaluronic acid 60%.
Marking: CE DGM-318, 30/03/01, IIb.
Producer: Dermatech, 10 rue Saint-Claude, 75003 Paris, France.
Commercialized by: Dermatech, 10 rue Saint-Claude, 75003 Paris, France.

Presentation: two syringes of 1.2 ml with 26G1/2 needles.
Website: http://www.dermadeep.com

Dermalive®

Gelled acrylic polymer, hydroxyethylmethacrylate, HEMA, and ethylmethacrylate, EMA (45–65 μm), 40% in 25% water in reticulated hyaluronic acid 60%
Marking: CE DGM-318, 30/03/01, IIb.
Producer: Dermatech, 10 rue Saint-Claude, 75003 Paris, France.
Commercialized by: Dermatech, 10 rue Saint-Claude, 75003 Paris, France.
Presentation: two syringes of 1 ml.
Website: http://www.dermalive.com

Evolution®

Microspheres of polyvinyl suspended in a hydrophilic gel of polyacrylamide, PAAG.
Marking: CE L0042994-02, 19 June, 2003.
Producer: Procytech, 4 rue J. Monod, 33650 Marcillac, France.
Commercialized by:
Presentation:
Not approved by the FDA.
Action: microspheres of polyvinyl 40 μm are positively charged and attract glucosaminoglycans (GAG) which are negatively charged and favor the production of collagen.

Isolagen®

Suspension of autologous fibroblasts obtained from punch culture of a 3-mm retroauricular biopsy which must be sent within 24 h; 1.2 ml is obtaineded in 8 weeks. An additional 1.2 ml can be obtained every 2–3 weeks. Descendent cells are stored indefinitely in liquid nitrogen by the laboratory.
Marking: CE
Producer: Isolagen Europe, Calle Azcona 46n, 28 028 Madrid, Spain.
Commercialized by: Isolagen Europe, Calle Azcona 46n, 28 028 Madrid, Spain.
Presentation: tube of 3.5 ml to transfer in a syringe with a 21G needle.

Outline® Fine

Gelled acrylic polymer, acrylamide, PAAG, 30% in 70% apyrogenic water.
Marking: CE L0042994-01, 09/06/00.
Producer: Procytech, 4 rue J. Monod, 33650 Marcillac, France.

Commercialized by:
Presentation: one syringe of 1 ml or two syringes of 0.5 ml, needle of 27 or 30G.
Action: the hydrophilic polyacrylamide gel, which is positively charged, attracts GAG, which are responsible for the formation of collagen.
Not approved by the FDA.

Outline® Original

Gelled polymer acrylic, acrylamide, PAAG, 30% in 70% apyrogenic water.
Marking: CE L0042994-01, 09/06/00.
Producer: Procytech, 4 rue J. Monod, 33650 Marcillac, France.
Commercialized by:
Presentation: one syringe of 1 ml or two syringes of 0.5 ml, needle of 27 or 30G.

Outline® Ultra

Gelled acrylic polymer, acrylamide, PAAG, 30% in 70% apyrogenic water.
Marking: CE L0042994-01, 09/06/00, and L0042994-02, 19/06/03.
Producer: Procytech, 4 rue J. Monod, 33650 Marcillac, France.
Commercialized by:
Presentation: one syringe of 1 ml or two syringes of 0.5 ml, needle of 27 or 30G.

Radiance/Radiesse®

Microspheres of hydroxyapatite (75–125 μm) in gel of carboxymethyl cellulose, constituted by 30% microspheres in 70% gel.
Marking: CE 0086.
Producer: BioForm Inc, Franksville, WI, USA.
Commercialized by: BioForm Medical Europe BV, Everdenberg 11, 4902 TT Oosterhout, The Netherlands.
Presentation: one syringe of 1.3 ml and 0.3 ml.
Histology: no foreign body reaction.[4] In 3 months the fine capsule is constituted by fibrin, fibroblasts, and macrophages which envelop the microspheres. These become irregular and begin to be resorbed in the 9th month.[5] The electron microscope shows particles of extracellular calcium and microspheres in macrophages.[1]
Website: http://www.bioforminc.com or radiesse.com

Reviderm/Beautysphere®

Hyaluronic acid microspheres of Sephadex®: microparticles of 40–60 μm of dextran, physiological serum.
Marking: CE 1204/031130, April 2005.
Producer: Rofil Medical International, Heusing 16, 4817 ZB Breda, The Netherlands.

Not approved by the FDA.
Website: http://www.rofil.com

Sculptra®

Hydrogel of polylactic acid, PLA, 15% in suspension, in 9% sodium carboxymethylcellulose and apyrogenic mannitol 12%, to be reconstituted with 5 ml of apyrogenic water. It is constituted by a powder of microspheres of polylactic acid, 1–63 μm, combined with the carboxymethylcellulose, mannitol, and sterile water for injection.
Marking: CE 0459.
Approved by the FDA in the USA for the treatment of secondary facial lipodystrophies in human immunodeficiency virus (HIV)-positive patients treated with antiretroviral drugs.
Producer: Sanofi-Aventis Laboratories, 1050 Westlakes Dr., Berwyn, PA 19312, USA.
Commercialized by: Dermik Laboratories, Berwyn, PA, a division of Sanofi-Aventis, Bridgewater, NJ, USA.
Presentation: two bottles to be mixed each with 5 ml of sterile water (wait 2 hours before injection).
Lactic acid was synthesized in 1954, and is often used in suturing materials or implantable orthopedic equipment.
Storage: can be kept for 72 h after reconstitution at room temperature.
Histology: polylactic acid is metabolized in carbondioxide and water. Its persisting effect is due to the production of type I collagen by fibroblasts in the site of injection.[6] After 9 months the polylactic acid is no longer detected.
Website: http://www.sculptra.com

New-Fill®

European name of the version covered by French social security as part of treatment of lipoatrophies of the face of medicinal origin, Sculptra being reserved in Europe for cosmetic treatment.[6]
Hydrogel of polylactic acid, PLA, 15% in suspension, in 9% sodium carboxymethylcellulose and apyrogenic mannitol 12%, to be reconstructed with 5 ml of apyrogenic water.
Marking: CE 0459.
Producer: Sanofi-Aventis Laboratories, 1050 Westlakes Dr., Berwyn, PA 19312, USA.
Commercialized by:
Presentation: two bottles to be mixed each with 5 ml of sterile water.
Website: http://www.new-fill.com

Silicone injections (silicone oil)

Technically, purified, medical polydimethylsiloxane oil, often referred to as liquid injectable silicone.
Not approved for cosmetic use by the FDA in the USA, except in ophthalmology.

No CE marking in Europe.
Origin: http://www.fda.gov/opacom/laws/fdcact/fdcact9.htm
Both Silikon 1000® and Adatosil 5000® (originally approved under the name 'Adatomed Silicone Oil 0P5000') are approved for injection into the vitreous cavity of the eye in the event of retinal detachment and/or hemorrhage. The numbers 1000 and 5000 refer to the viscosity in centistokes (cS) (the viscosity of water is 100 cS).
Storage: between 15 and 32°C.
Producer: Adatosil 5000; Bausch and Lomb Pharmaceuticals, Inc, Rochester, NY, USA. Silikon 1000; Alcon Laboratories, Inc, Fort Worth, TX, USA.

Injection techniques

General contraindications are sought; they are variable according to product origin. Routine cutaneous preparation is accomplished.

Block anesthesia of the infraorbitary and mental nerves is often carried out as these injections are painful. They are always deep, into the dermis or hypodermis. Over correction is not necessary due to the non-resorbable nature of the injections.

Indications include the loss of volume of the face, whatever its origin (aging, traumatic or therapeutic origin (human immunodeficiency virus, HIV), deep grooves, atrophy due to malformation).

Side-effects and complications (Table 35.3)

Secondary reactions after injection of biodegradable products

They differ widely according to the delay between the injection and the clinical reaction.

Immediate and minor reactions (often related to observing recommendations)

Puncture site hematomas can be avoided by the application of vitamin K before and/or immediately after injections. Erythema or light edema along the injection line is frequent and transitional; it disappears in 48–72 hours according to the treatment.

Intermediate reactions

After too superficial injection, a visible white line can be noted, which will disappear only with resorption of the product.

In some cases, and notably after implant of hyaluronic acid (HA) at the level of the lips, 12–24 hours after injection there can appear an inflammatory, sensitive edema, sometimes significant, persisting 2–7 days and justifying the application of a local steroid. It always disappears

Table 35.3 Biodegradable products: side-effects and treatment

Reactions	Side-effects	Duration	Treatment
Immediate reactions From 1 day to 1 week	Hematomas Edema Erythemas	8 days	Not systematic, sometimes vitamin K or local steroids
Semi-delayed reactions 1–3 weeks	Pigmentation (hyaluronic acid) Non-specific inflammation	1–6 months 3 months	Any Eventually topical steroids

Delayed reactions
3–24 months
	Allergies
	  erythema
	
	  granulomas ++
	  abscess
		1 month to
		1 year
			Local and general steroids (1–3 weeks)

	Necrosis (technical error)	Variable	Scar by secondary intention

	Granulomas
	  polylactic acid
	  polyacrylamide
		?	Steroid injection inside the lesion ±
			5-fluorouracil + surgery?
			Laser?

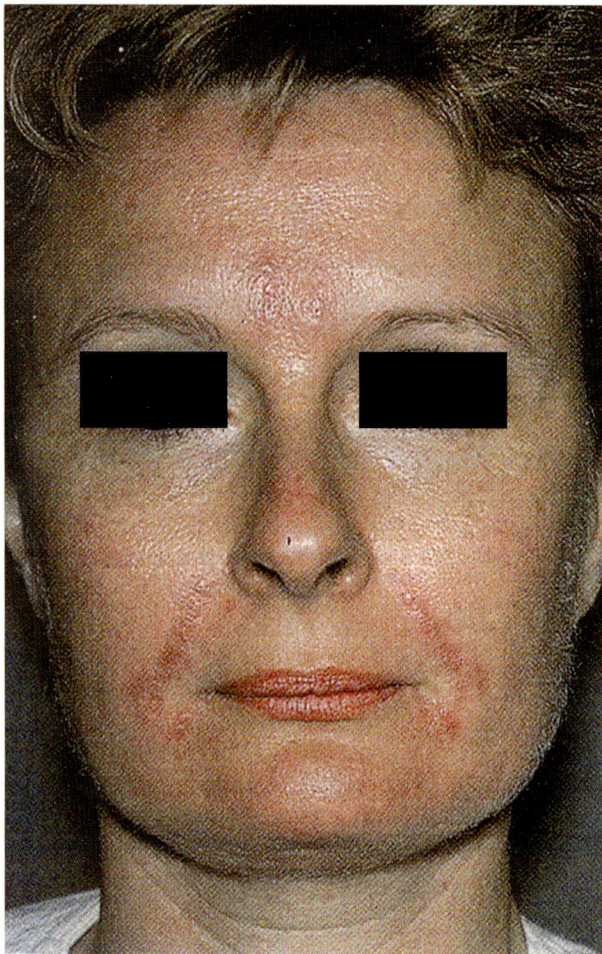

Figure 35.1 Granulomas after collagen injection.

without scarring and should not be confused with an intolerance reaction of retarded hypersensitivity type.

We sometimes note, at the levels of the labiomental region and the nasolabial fold, a variably, intense thin

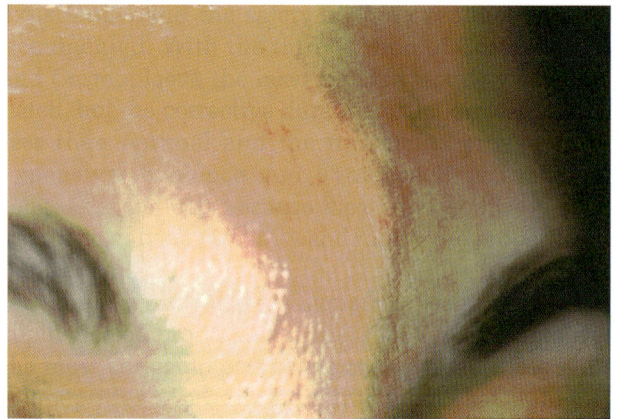

Figure 35.2 Granulomas after injection of hyaluronic acid.

bluish pigmentation; this disappears slowly in 3–6 months, but is a contraindication to any new injection at the same site before completely disappearing.

Concerning the slowly biodegradable products, dextranomer mixed with HA can result in edematous, sometimes significant, inflammatory reactions, for more than 8 days (Matridex®).

Late reactions

Bovine collagen[7–13] and HA[14–16] can sometimes cause, at the injection site level, a variably intense erythema or erythematous, purple, hardened nodule, rarely a pseudocyst, and/or purulent type of abscess. They appear in general 1–4 weeks after injection, sometimes after several months, or even, for the collagen, after several sessions of injection (Figures 35.1 and 35.2).

The treatment of these late granulomatous lesions caused by collagen and HA must be started as quickly as possible. If erythema appears at the level of the

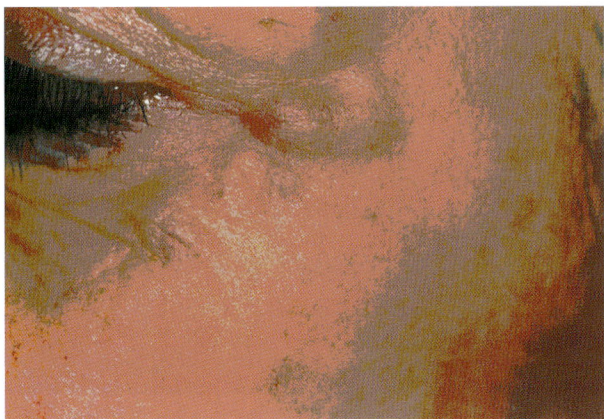

Figure 35.3 Granulomas after injection of polylactic acid.

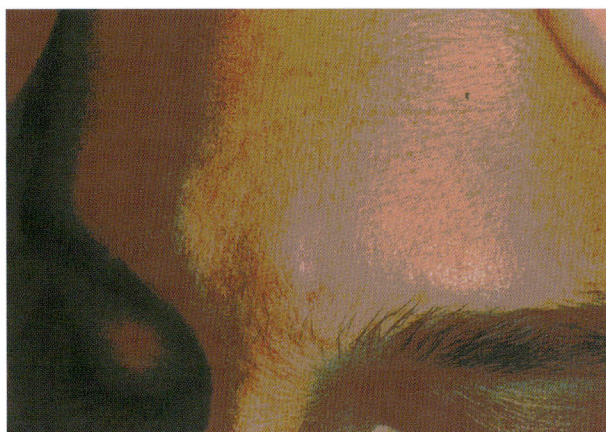

Figure 35.4 Granulomas after injection of polymethylmetacrylate.

injection, even if minimal, it is necessary to prescribe a local steroid, usually oral, for 15 days. As a rule, resorption is rapid at 2–3 weeks, sometimes longer (months), but integral restitution is always complete.

Polylactic acid, probably a slowly biodegradable product, can be the origin of the appearance of late side-effects. Nodules can be granulomatous, purple, very hard, and sometimes very extensive, and can appear between 6 and 24 months after injection, without doubt favored by poor preparation of the product, an elevated concentration, and a too superficial technique of injection, or one not adapted to this type of product. The risk is particularly high in regions where the skin is thin and the injected product superficially has poor resorption. This product is therefore completely contraindicated in certain zones, for example periorbicular and peribuccal; it is even preferable to avoid injections at the level of expression wrinkles where the epidermis is thin and the skin is 'pleated' (Figure 35.3).

Treatment of these granulomas, either local or general, using steroids, does not give sufficient improvement, and treatment by injection of 5-fluorouracil into the lesion does not seem to give the desired resolution. We can also prescribe, at the beginning of treatment, hydroxychloroquine hydrochloride, 2 cps/day for 2 months, which often leads to a reduction of inflammatory reaction (when it exists).

Postponed local reactions in fact concern all the abovementioned filler products and can implicate several immunological mechanisms:

1. Postponed hypersensitivity reactions mediated by T lymphocytes specific to the antigen in the preparation: injectable products have different effects on proteins that can lead to a specific immune reaction (collagen, aviary residue, microbes, impurities). After intradermal injection of the product, antigen-presenting, dendritic cells (Langerhans cells) and/or macrophages predispose the patient to an immune response with specific production of T lymphocytes. These T lymphocytes can then migrate in the skin, proliferate, and thus determine a classical hypersensitivity reaction.[14,17]

2. Local granulomatous reaction to foreign body: an injected product activates phagocytosis, producing inflammatory cytokines that assure recruitment of an infiltrate surrouding the implant, translating to a chronic inflammatory defense reaction with phagocytosis and, with regard to biodegradable products, elimination of the injected product.

3. Non-specific inflammatory reactions: experimental studies have shown that hyaluronic acid fragments can stimulate production by the renal epithelial cells of chemokines, which could lead to induction of a local inflammatory infiltration. It can be assumed that other substances associated with cosmetic filling procedures, therefore, could lead to a non-specific inflammatory reaction.

Secondary reactions after injection of non-biodegradable materials

Non-biodegradable materials are responsible for secondary reactions which can be immediate or very postponed (Figure 35.4).

Immediate reactions

Immediate reactions can be very inflammatory, papulonodulous, and erythematous to purple. They are transitional, and disappear within days to weeks.

Postponed reactions[18,19]

These are in general foreign body granulomas. The diagnosis is made clinically and, if the patient agrees, histologically. Foreign body granulomas after the injection of different semiresorbable or permanent products are probably not rare, but they often remain clinically latent. However, in certain cases the granuloma reaction can be significant, manifested by variably voluminous nodules, palpable or visible, sometimes painful, always unesthetic, which can cause an inflammatory reaction that is difficult to confine.

Polymethylmethacrylate can cause late-appearing granulomas after injection (from 6 months until 2

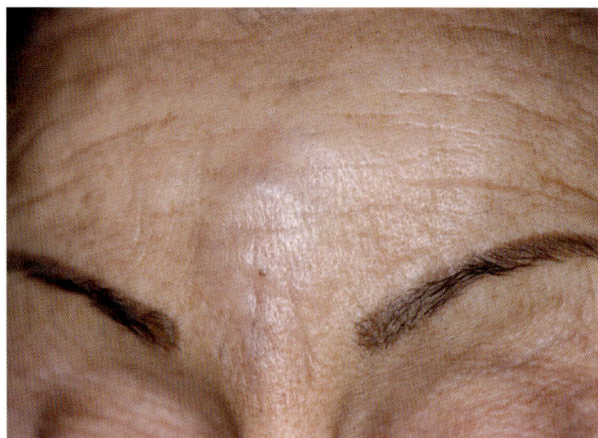

Figure 35.5 Granulomas after acrylic hydrogel injection.

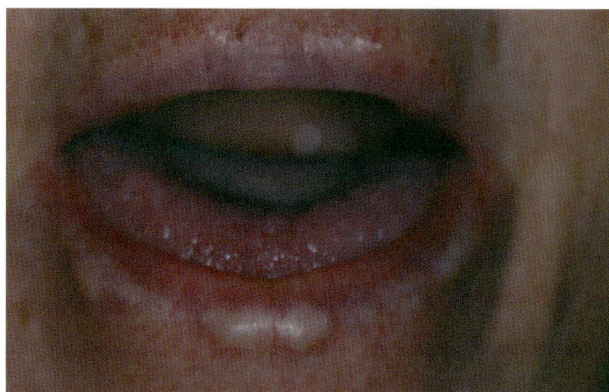

Figure 35.6 Granulomas after acrylic hydrogel injection.

years), erythematous to purple, which might or might not spontaneously diminish. They are improved by intranodular injection of steroids.[20]

Acrylic hydrogel, very widely used in the last 5 years, is the origin of very frequent granulomatous reactions. The nodules, very indurate, of stony consistency, are covered with a normal erythematous tegument. They are often very visible, notably at the level of the lips, and can be isolated between two fingers. Very unesthetic, they can often lead to a marked depressive state of the patient concerned (Figure 35.5 and 35.6).

Due to their non-biodegradability, these nodules do not diminish or improve spontaneously.

Treatments are as follows:

1. Intralesional injections of dermal steroids give only incomplete, minimal improvement, in spite of repetition, which is often short term. The nodules can again increase in volume when corticoids are stopped, and they cannot be used forever.
2. Intranodular injections of a mixture of steroid and 5-fluorouracil (5-FU) or of 5-FU alone give discouraging results. Additionally, 5-FU seems to favor an over- and peri-nodular purple appearance.
3. Due to these observations, patients request surgical removal, which gives immediate and satisfactory results (Figure 35.7), but is sometimes a source of unesthetic, indelible scars. Moreover, after some weeks nodules can reappear at the periphery of the excision. Is this linked to the possible migration of acrylic particles at the time of intervention?

Recently, some physicians have begun to do the excision using CO_2 or long-pulse erbium lasers that seem to give rather satisfactory results, on condition that there is no inflammatory reaction or necrosis after the intervention. We have accomplished the fragmentation of implants using lipostructure, with encouraging results (Figure 35.8).

In certain rare cases, when the nodules are the cause of an inflammatory reaction, with purulent psuedocyst,

the filler product is partially eliminated by spontaneous evacuation.

Polyacrylamide gel can present some weeks after injection a microbeless abscess that can evolve for 3–4 weeks before recovering spontaneously (Figure 35.9).

Alkylimides have recently been commercialized in France. The secondary appearance of granulomas due to these non-resorbable products, if it occurs, must occur in the long term. It is therefore difficult to estimate long-term tolerability. In that case, according to the site, en bloc surgical excision is possible.

Dimethylsiloxane[21–24] has a formula almost identical to fluid silicone, nowadays forbidden in France for use as a wrinkle filler, and which was the cause of some nodular reactions.

Prevention of secondary reactions: practicing intradermal tests prior to treatment

From the perspective of minimizing secondary reactions to these different types of treatment, the aim of which is only esthetic, what is the justification for intradermal testing prior to injection? Such tests cannot discern very postponed reactions. So, are they useful, why, when, how, and for which products?[17,25–27]

Why?

- to detect, before injection of the chosen product, the risk of local reaction which would occur only after the first or second injection; nevertheless, we should not ignore the possibility of sensitization appearing after more than two sessions and therefore not revealed even by double testing prior to injection
- to answer a possible medical action in case of secondary cutaneous reaction to injections of biodegradable filler products
- finally, to study the vigilance of a product before marketing it; nowadays, laboratories do not carry out tests prior to the distribution of a new product, a caution which should, however, be considered.

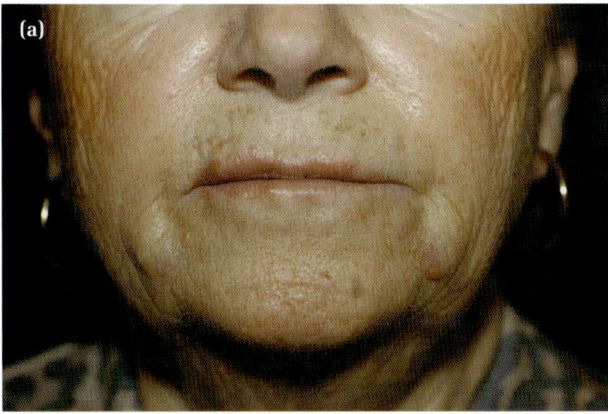

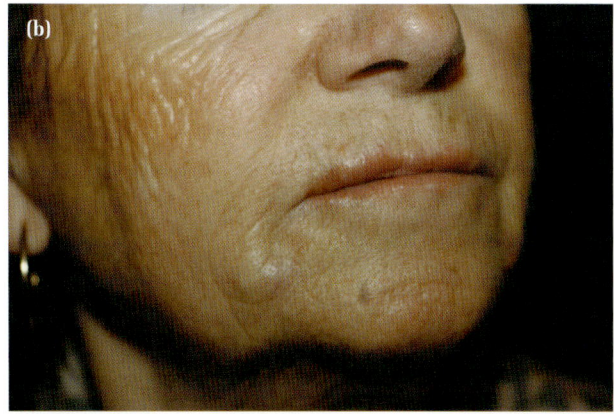

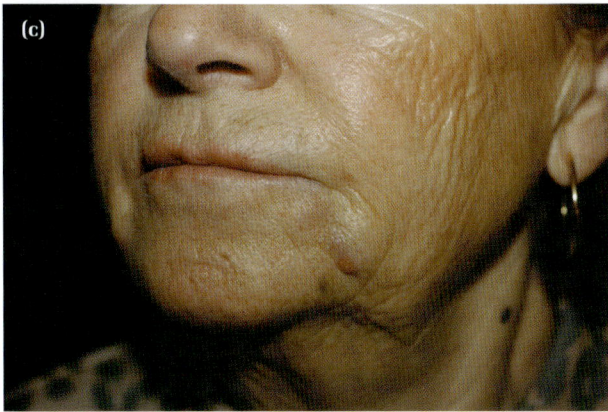

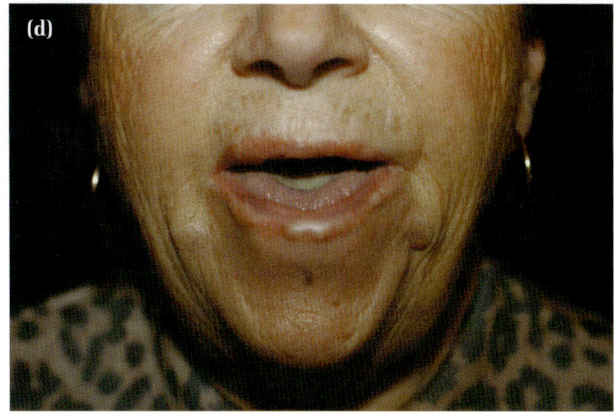

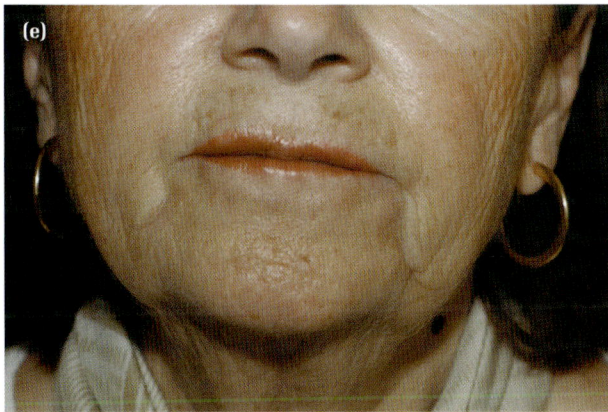

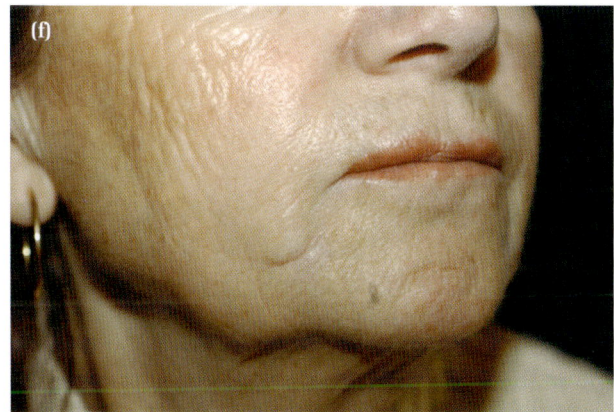

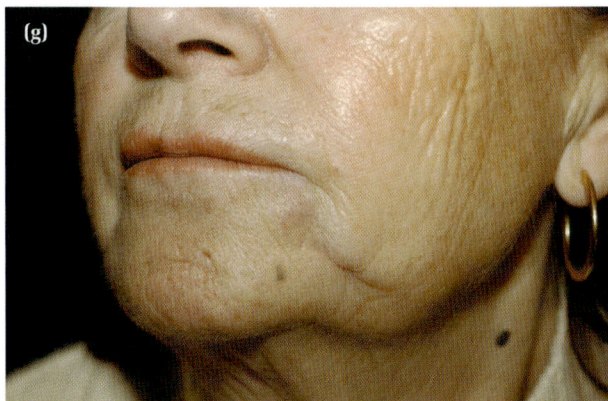

Figure 35.7 (a–d) Granulomas after injection of Dermalive® in lip and paracommissure. (e–g) Results after surgical removal.

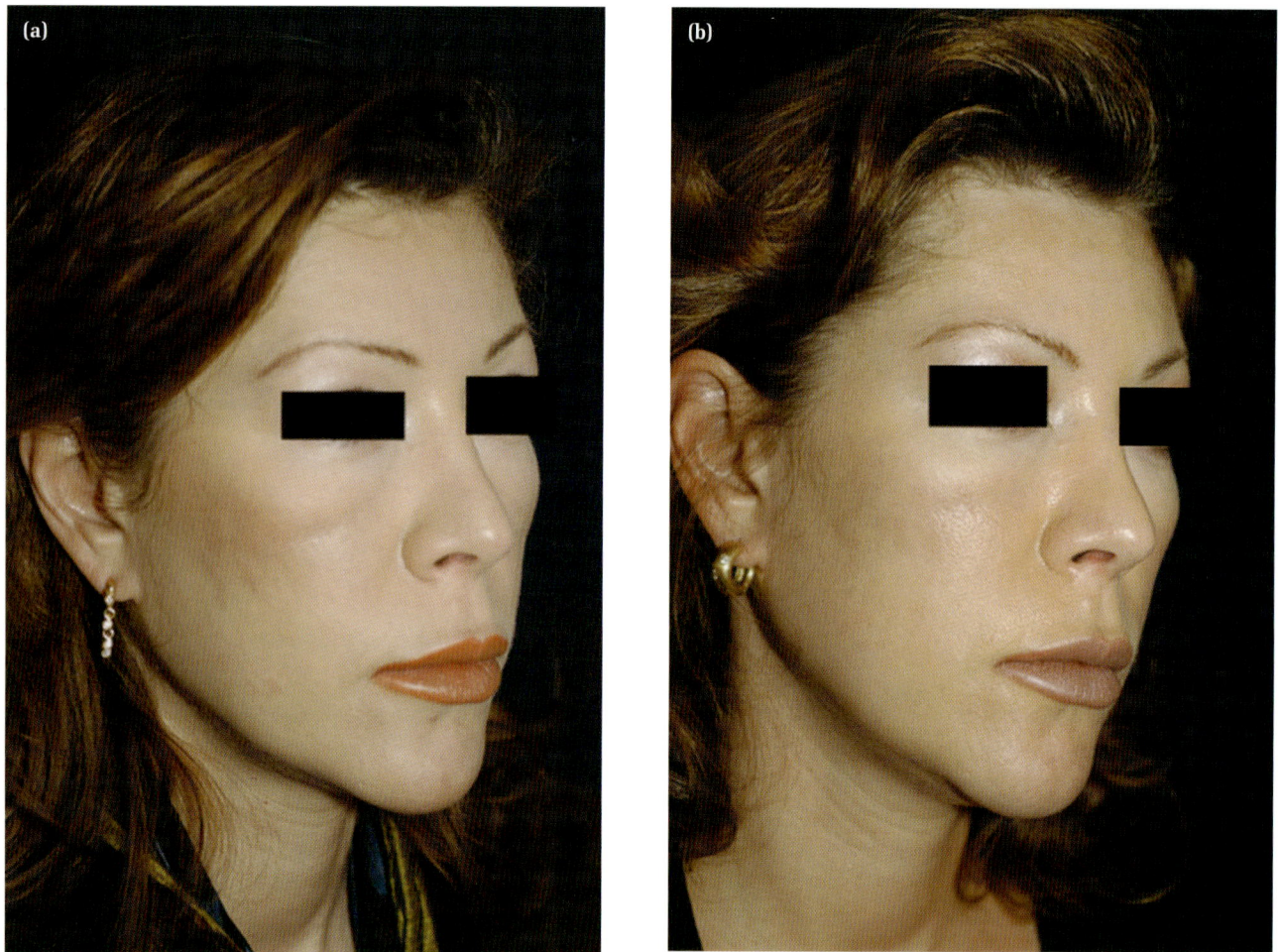

Figure 35.8   (a) Jugal point irregularity after injection of New-Fill® (b) Jugal point filling (right) by means of lipostructure.

When and for which products?

Biodegradable products   The double intradermal test with bovine collagen has been necessary and obligatory since 1991, ensuring both job security and an insignificant number of secondary reactions.

Regarding hyaluronic acid, intradermal testing before injection does not have to be done systematically. Nevertheless, secondary reactions noted after injection of hyaluronic acid, even if not very frequent, encourage the practice of testing in certain cases defined by the examiner.

Hence, we have to take into account:

1. Medical history: autoimmune pathologies and progressive allergic diseases must be taken into consideration (asthma, atopic dermatitis), and perhaps considered to be contraindications, in the same manner as in cases of injections with bovine collagen. In effect, granulomatous reactions secondary to hyaluronic acid injection have been seen principally in patients with autoimmune pathologies (RCH, Crohn's disease, rheumatoid polyarthritis, diabetes, thyroiditis), both unknown at the time of injection and revealed by a later examination, or in cases of atopic illness that are still progressive.

2. Esthetic treatment records: in cases of secondary reactions after injections of one of the biodegradable products (collagen or hyaluronic acid), it is preferable to do intradermal testing when using the other product, even if allergy has not been systematically noted in a concomitant manner in both cases.

3. Psychological history: for certain, particularly anxious, patients, reluctant to have injection of bovine collagen owing to bovine spongiform encephalopathy or simply anxious about the side-effects of any injected product, it is preferable and even recommended to carry out dermal tests before injections.

Preventive measures and indications for testing cannot apply to polylactic acid, which is a slowly biodegradable product. In view of the delay in the appearance of possible secondary reactions (several months), it is useless to do a double test beforehand because it would remain negative and have no predictive significance.

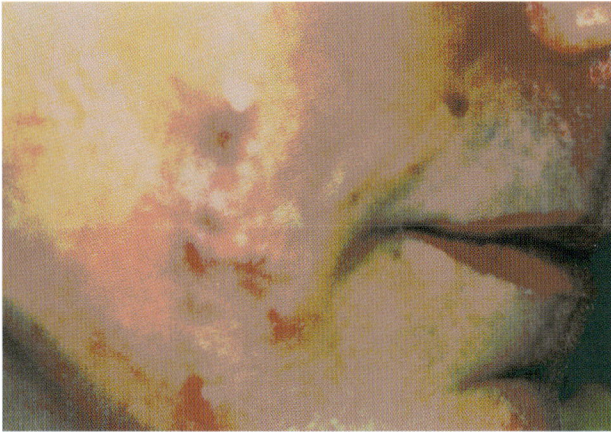

Figure 35.9   Granulomas after injection of polyacrylamide gel.

Non-biodegradable products   In the case of mixed products, i.e. non-biodegradable and biodegradable (PMMA + collagen, acrylic hydrogel + hyaluronic acid), tests have no predictive value regarding a possible postponed reaction to the non-biodegradable fraction of the injected product. Nevertheless, there could be a reaction to the collagen content of Artecoll or to the hyaluronic acid content associated with the acrylic hydrogel in cases of any of the pathologies listed above. That is why it is necessary to perform intradermal testing in these two examples.

If the product is purely biodegradable, the test is useless because reactions (of the foreign body type occur too late (several months or years).

How?

The protocol is always identical: two intradermal tests done, 15 days apart, on the anterior surface of each forearm, with evaluation made by the 'practitioner' 3 days after each injection and about 6 weeks after the first test. Only double-negative tests allow injection at the level of wrinkles.

Moreover, it seems justified, after a period of 2 years (arbitrary duration), to repeat intradermal testing in the case of collagen injection.

Value of testing

Skin   From a retrospective viewpoint, a positive test on the forearm, done after detecting a secondary reaction, confirms the relevance of the injected product to the reaction at the level of the injection site. In terms of predictive value, the interest of testing prior to injection is incontestable. However, the economics is flawed because, in rare cases, reactions to testing appear too late to avoid the first session of injection. Finally, 'sensitization' can appear after several sessions of injection, notably in cases of intermittently occurring pathologies.

Blood   The presence of bovine anticollagen antibody is not predictive of a local reaction after injection. This blood test is simply an indication of a stronger reactivity (× 6). If the skin tests are negative, a positive blood test to bovine collagen is not therefore a contraindication to injection.[3]

Nevertheless, careful surveillance of the slightest indication of a late hypersensitivity reaction is necessary.

With regard to other biodegradable products, research is still too sparse to draw conclusions about anti-hyaluronic acid antibody. However, blood tests carried out in a patient who presented with reactions to Restylane® or Hylaform® showed the presence of antibodies to hyaluronic acid.[16] Supplementary studies, if done systematically after secondary reactions to suspicious implants, will allow us to create a scientific protocol and the minimization of local reactions.

Technique of double testing

The first test is performed on the anterior surface of the left forearm, forming a papule which must be reduced in 24 hours leaving only an insignificant, whitish relief corresponding to degradable products. This first test must be checked by the physician on the third day. The appearance of a modification of the outline of the original injection, such as erythema with or without pruritus, of light edema and/or local hypersensitivity, or rarely an inflammatory nodule or cystic reaction, confirms the diagnosis of a positive reaction to the product and forbids treatment.

If the first test is negative, a second intradermal test is planned 2–3 weeks later, on the anterior surface of the right forearm, and checked 3 days later.

Both tests are checked again, 4–6 weeks after the second. If after this period there is no erythema and no induration, we can start the first injection session.

Points to remember

1. The association of biodegradable and non-biodegradable products, on the same site, can favor the appearance of granulomatous reactions or the 'reactivation' of foreign body granulomas. It is therefore not advisable to inject biodegradable products in a site injected previously with a non-biodegradable or unknown product, even if it was several months or years ago. The risk would be that an inflammatory reaction would appear, the origin of which would be difficult to specify. Moreover, 'unknown products' containing numerous components that are not officially listed also lead to a risk of inflammatory or granulomatous reactions in the case of injection of another product in the same site.

2. For Europe, CE marking guarantees the security of the product at the levels of manufacturing and

materials, but the absence of clinical files does not permit estimation of tolerability in situ in the short and/or the long term. Possibly, an AMM (Autorisation de Mise sur le Marché) should be considered. For the USA, approval by the FDA guarantees reliability and harmlessness of the product.

3. Every side-effect must be declared by the physician to the laboratory of the producer, and AFSSAPS, so that the noxious effects of every type of product are known more definitively, as well as their clinical aspects and their evolution with time. In France, the relevant learned societies centralize side-effects: GEREMI for the French Society of Plastic Surgery and VIGIPIL for the French Society of Dermatology.

4. Actual histological techniques allow definitive identification of the nature of the product, important in the case of a juridicial procedure.

Anatomopathological identification of injected product-provoked facial granulomas

After the injection of various products intended to ameliorate the esthetics of the face, a granuloma, which is a chronic inflammatory defense reaction against the introduced foreign body, can appear. This inflammatory reaction to the product can be minimal or very moderate, but it can cause palpable, variably voluminous or visible nodules, sometimes with pain and inflammatory edema, uncomfortable, and ugly, while the aim was actually to fill a depression. There is currently no explanation as to why certain injections cause granulomas, others latent granulomas, and yet others probably any inflammatory reaction.

Signs appear between 3–6 months and even 10 years after the injection (a visible nodule a week after injection signals a rather latent dispersion of the product). The history of previous injection (or injections) is often forgotten or deliberately skipped. Sites most often affected are the lips, cheeks, nasolabial grooves, and the forehead. Intrabuccal granulomas are noted in cases of deep injection.

The problem of identification of the injected products becomes more complicated due to the fact that patients may have accepted two or three (or more) different products in the same region of the face. They rarely know the product injected; sometimes they remember the most recent, but almost never the previous one, and in general they do not like to speak about it. The physicians who excise the nodules are not usually those who have initially injected the product, and information on previous injections is difficult or even impossible to acquire. Products differ according to the country, and products appear on the market while others disappear.

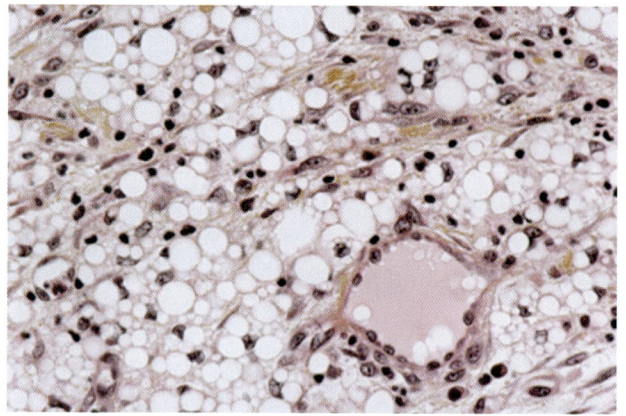

Figure 35.10 Pathology of silicon granuloma of the lower lip: there are vacuoles in the macrophages.

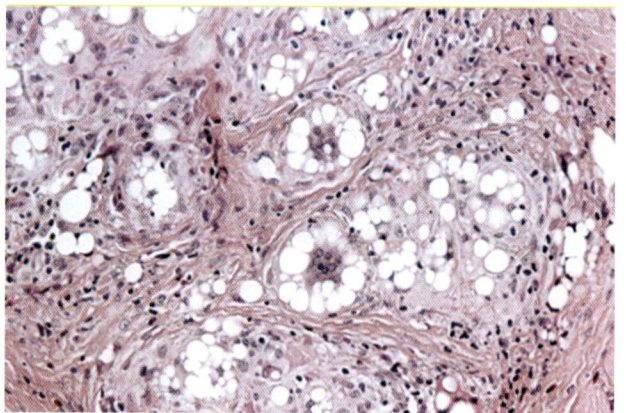

Figure 35.11 Pathology of silicon granuloma of the cheek: giant cell proliferation.

Histological characteristics of granulomas

Histologically, granulomas can be of two different types (but can overlap or juxtapose in cases of numerous esthetic treatments).

Granulomas related to foreign bodies of vacuolar and microcrystalline types are noted after injection of 'permanent' liquid products, in practice, silicone. These are poorly delimited because the product diffuses some distance. They are made up of macrophages that contain clear micro- or macrovacuoles, pushing back the core against the cytoplasmic membrane and causing the macrophages to merge with adipose cells. Large cells are rare, causing peripheral vacuoles that give them an aspect of a 'daisy'. Microcysts are pseudocysts, without a clearly defined epithelial cystic wall, and are constituted by a larger drop of the product. Some lymphocytes can be seen, as well as variably marked collagen fibrosis.

These granulomas can be latent, discovered incidentally during the anatomopathological examination of another lesion.

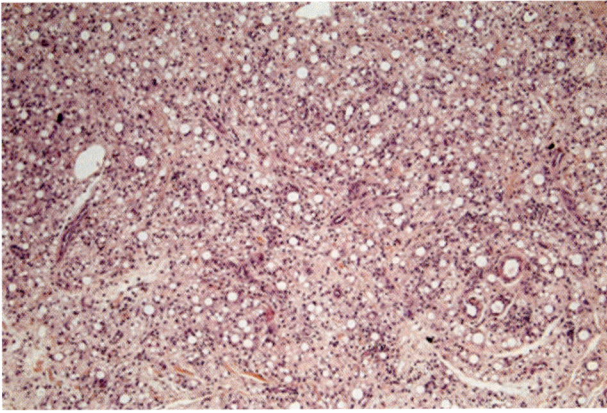

Figure 35.12 Pathology of silicon granuloma of the lower lip: prevalent macrophages.

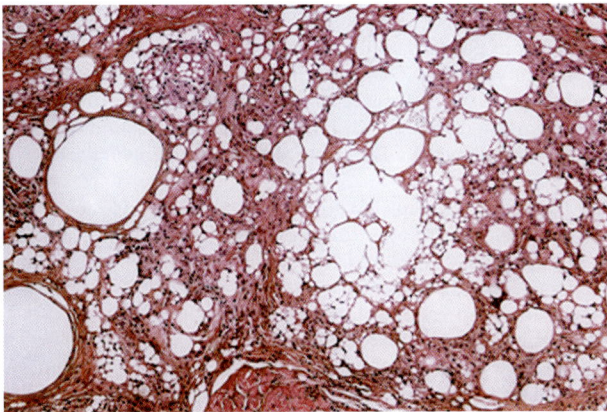

Figure 35.14 (a) Granuloma of the cheek after Arteplast® injection. (b) Granuloma of the upper lip after Artecoll injection.

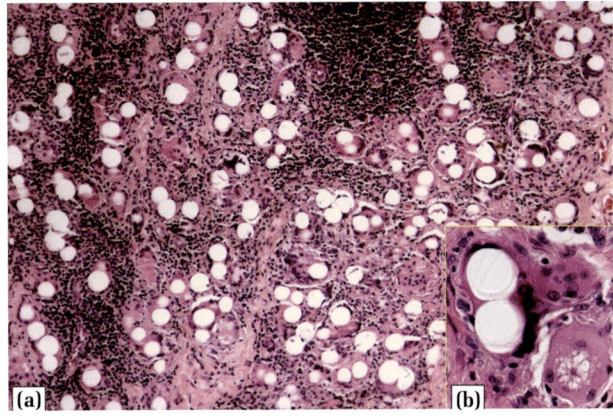

Figure 35.13 Pathology of silicon granuloma of the cheek: microcystic view.

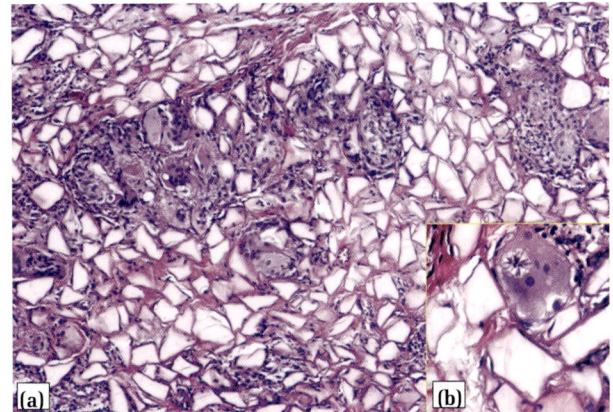

Figure 35.15 (a) Granuloma of the lower lip after Dermalive® injection. (b) Detail.

Silicone is a poorly defined filler product, available as a liquid or a gel, blended with various substances intended to 'fix' it in tissues (Figures 35.10–35.13).

'Classical' foreign body granulomas are noted after injection of products composed of solid particles, either permanent or biodegradable. They constitute well-defined, circumscribed nodules. They are principally made up of histiocytes (macrophages) and giant cells, encircling the foreign body and attempting to phagocytose it with variable success. The giant cells often have an asteroid body in their cytoplasm. Accompanying cells are lymphocytes or plasmocytes. A variable important collagen fibrosis is described.

Products containing the solid particles under discussion can be 'permanent' or 'biodegradable' products. Their identification is made by polarization microscopy.

Permanent products

Polymethylmethacrylate (Artecoll or Arteplast®) This consists of 20% polymethylmethacrylate microspheres with 80% bovine collagen). The foreign bodies are of identical size, round, constituted by a 30–40-μm transparent microsphere and non-birefringence (Figure 35.14).

Acrylic hydrogel (Dermalive or Dermadeep) The foreign bodies are polygonal, irregular particles and of different sizes (20–40 μm), in 'opus incertum', translucent, pale pink, and non-birefringent. They accumulate on a base of pinkish fibrin, necrotic or pseudonecrotic (Figure 35.15).

Silicone elastomer (Bioplastique) The foreign bodies are particles of irregular form. They are transparent and non-birefringent. They are surrounded by giant cells issuing fine projections into microcystic areas in which they are contained.

Biodegradable products

Polylactic acid (New-Fill) The foreign bodies are particles of irregular form, lancelet, with size varying between 10 and 30 μm, transparent but birefringent in polarized light. These characteristics can lead to the diagnosis of silicotic granuloma, i.e. sign of a post-traumatic foreign body (Figure 35.16).

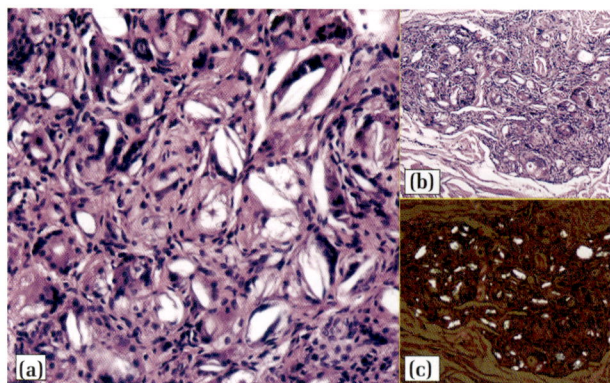

Figure 35.16   (a–b) Granuloma after New-fill® injection in the riasolabial furrow: there are small irregular translucent particles of variable size (10–30 µm) (c) Seen in polarized light.

Foreign body granulomas due to resorbable products (hyaluronic acid, bovine collagen)   These appear to be very rare, but are mentioned in the literature; they can be favored by the presence of another product in the site of injection.

Histological study associated with particular coloration

Tennstedt and Lachapelle[24] have recently perfected histological studies linking six particular colors and examinations using polarized light revealing supplementary information on granulomas and types of injected product.

Summary

The histological analysis of a subsequent cutaneous nodule in injection with an esthetic aim allows identification of the nature of the product having caused the granule, based on coloring and a simple examination in polarized light by Kuffer and Plantier,[28] or using particular coloring by Tennstedt and Lachapelle.[24]

Conclusion

The reconstitution of facial volume is an important component in cosmetic reconstructive and esthetic surgery. Even if fat grafting is the treatment of choice, it is still not always possible or acceptable. Volumetric fillers given by injection offer ease, good performance, and durability. Side-effects are not very numerous, considering the number of patients treated. Biodegradable products can cause secondary, transitional and reversible, reactions, which can be determined by a detailed and selective cross-examination of patients and/or, according to the chosen product, by testing prior to treatment using a well-defined protocol. Biodegradable products can result in the late appearance of long-term or permanent granulomas, and even be the origin of dramatic side-effects. For this reason, in the case of these implants, it would be desirable to consider an AMM, based on clinical and histological studies, as CE marking does not allow an estimation of their tolerability in situ.

References

1. Lemperle G, Morhenn V, Charrier U. Human histology and persistence of various injectable filler substances for soft tissue augmentation. Aesthetic Plas Surg 2003; 27: 354–66; discussion 67.
2. von Buelow S, von Heimburg D, Pallua N. Efficacy and safety of polyacrylamide hydrogel for facial soft-tissue augmentation. Plast Reconstr Surg 2005; 116: 1137–46.
3. Lemperle G, Gauthier-Hazan N, Lemperle M. PMMA-microspheres (Artecoll) for long-lasting correction of wrinkles: refinements and statistical results. Aesthetic Plast Surg 1998; 22: 356–65.
4. Marmur ES, Phelps R, Goldberg DJ. Clinical, histologic and electron microscopic findings after injection of a calcium hydroxylapatite filler. J Cosmet Laser Ther 2004; 6: 223–6.
5. Jacovella PF, Peiretti CB, Cunille DR et al. Long-lasting results with hydroxylapatite (Radiesse) facial filler. Plast Reconstr Surg 2006; 118 (Suppl): 15S–21S.
6. Vleggaar D, Bauer U. Facial enhancement and the European experience with Sculptra (polyl-leactic acid). J Drugs Dermatol 2004; 3: 542–7.
7. Barr R, Stegman SJ. Delayed skin test reaction to injectable collagen implant (Zyderm). The histopathologic comparative study. J Am Acad Dermatol 1984; 10: 652–8.
8. Charriere G, Bejot M, Schnitzler L et al. Reactions to a bovine collagen implant. Clinical and immunologic study in 705 patients. J Am Acad Dermatol 1989; 21: 1203–8.
9. Clark DP, Hanke CW, Swanson NA. Dermal implants: safety of products injected for soft tissue augmentation. J Am Acad Dermatol 1989; 21: 992–8.
10. De Lustro F, Fries J, Kang A et al. Immunity to injectable collagen and auto-immune disease: a summary of current under-standing. J Dermatol Surg Oncol 1988; 14 (Suppl 1): 57–65.
11. Hanke CW, Higley HR, Jolivette DM et al. Abscess formation and local necrosis after treatment with Zyderm or Zyplast collagen implant. J Am Acad Dermatol 1991; 25: 319–26.
12. Pons-Guiraud A. Réactions d'hypersensibilité retardée aux implants de collagène bovin. Etude sur 810 patients. Nouv Dermatol 1992; 11: 422–32.
13. Pons-Guiraud A. Place des tests dans les methodes de comblement des rides. GERDA Prog Dermato-Allergol 2001: 251–61.
14. Larsen NE, Pollak CT, Reiner K, Balazs EA. Hylan gel biomaterial: dermal and immunologic compatibility. J Biomed Mater Res 1993; 27: 1129–34.
15. Lupton JR, Alster TS. Cutaneous hypersensitivity reaction to injectable acid gel. Dermatol Surg 2000; 26: 135–7.
16. Micheels P. Human anti-hyaluronic acid antibodies: is it possible? Dermatol Surg 2001; 27: 185–91.

17. Krasteva M, Kehren J, Nicolas JF. Haptènes et cellules dendritiques. GERDA Prog Dermato-Allergol 1999: 27–42.
18. Requena C, Izquierdo MJ, Navarro M et al. Adverse reactions to injectable aesthetic microimplants. Am J Dermatopathol 2001; 23: 197–202.
19. Rudolph CM, Soyer P, Schuller-Petrovic S et al. Foreign body granulomas due to injectable aesthetic microimplants. Am J Surg Pathol 1999; 23: 113–17.
20. Hoffmann C, Schuller-Petrovic S, Soyer P, Kerl H. Adverse reactions after cosmetic lip augmentation with permanent biologically inert implant materials. J Am Acad Dermatol 1999; 40: 100–2.
21. Faure M. Complication des implants de silicone et autres matériaux dits inertes. Ann Derm Vénéréol 1995; 122: 455–9.
22. Pearl RM, Laub DR, Kaplan EN. Complications following silicone injections for augmentation of the contours of the face. Plast Reconstr Surg 1978; 61: 888–91.
23. Secchi T, Carbonnel E. Correction ambulatoire des lipo-atrophies du visage dans l'infection à VIH par technique de comblement. Nouv Dermatol 2003; 22: 132–3.
24. Tennstedt D, Lachapelle JM. Histopathologie des granulomes tardifs consécutifs aux injections de produits de comblement pour rides (colorations spéciales). A paraître.

36 Side-effects of fillers

Daphne Thioly-Bensoussan

With the slowly increasing demand for wrinkle treatment and lip augmentation beginning in the 1970s, research into collagen production led to a bovine formulation that could be placed in a syringe and injected. For many patients, injectable filling agents gave the promise of facial rejuvenation while offering reduced risks compared to more invasive surgery.

With the increase in products available, it is crucial that both the physician and the patient are fully cognizant of the risks involved in the use of each product.

Reactions can be attributed to the procedure itself, the procedural technique, and the agent injected. Some of these reactions are preventable, whereas others are inevitable.

The temporary nature and the requirement for double testing of collagen implants led to the development and testing of other biodegradable fillers in Europe in the 1990s, such as hyaluronic acid fillers, and because of their few months' duration of effect, permanent fillers were launched on the market. These injectable dermal filler materials consist of either fluid biological fragments or suspensions of particles or microspheres. Particles and microspheres are said to 'migrate', but migration can occur only when they are injected into blood vessels.

The side-effects are immediate, semidelayed, or delayed. The immediate and semidelayed side-effects are minimal and short-lived. They consist of inflammatory reactions, for example hematomas, erythema, or mild edema. When treated promptly, delayed granulomas resolve within a few weeks without leaving any visible marks.

Delayed side-effects may consist of inflammatory and painful edema or pigmentation. Others include erythematous granulomas, which usually develop 1–4 weeks after the injection but may arise even later, or after several injection sessions.

Side-effects associated with biodegradables may be different from those with non-biodegradables by the fact that they resolve with or without treatment; biodegradable implants seem satisfactory in terms of cosmetic results and medical safety.

Legislation

All fillers, except bovine collagen, are classified in Europe as 'medical devices', and rely on the European directive 93/42 CEE of 14 June 1993. Since 15 June 1998, all medical devices must have the CE marking. This means hygiene safety, but does not give any assurance about efficiency or in situ short- or long-term tolerance.

The French Law of 18 January 1994 requires that any incident must be reported to the French National Commission of Materiovigilance.

Information and consent

All patients desiring cosmetic procedures should have a comprehensive medical and social evaluation. Many individuals are well informed because of the media and the internet. When it is determined that fillers are the appropriate therapy, several alternatives should be discussed and a choice made as to the most appropriate.

Outlining normal postoperative sequelae such as bruising, unevenness, and swelling is important, as well as the pretreatment discussion of possible adverse events. If the filler is being used in an off-label manner then this should also be discussed with the patient.

It is important to know the complete medical history, including evolutive allergy (asthma, hay fever, or eczema), psychologic history, and medications.

It is also important to understand the actual expectations of the patient (which may or may not be corrected) and to explain the treatment proposal: filler choice, efficacy, and duration, advantages and risks, and limitations of the technique.

There are very few contraindications to fillers, but a history of previous, long-lasting implant injection might be one.

Choosing the appropriate filler and side-effects

Biodegradable and non-biodegradable implants can be very different if comparing injection sites, quantity needed, in-situ forming implant, type of molecule, and side-effects.

Classification of biodegradable fillers

Collagens

- bovine: Zyderm® I and II, Zyplast®, Resoplast® (Allergan)
- human: Cosmoderm®, Cosmoplast® (Allergan), Fascian® (Fascia Biosystems), Cymetra® (LifeCell Corporation)
- porcine: Evolence® (Colbar Life Science)
- autologous: Isolagen Process™ (Isolagen), synthetic human collagen type III (FibroGen).

Hyaluronic acid (HA)

- animal: Hylaform®, Hylaform Plus (Inamed), Mac Dermol® (Orgev)
- non-animal stabilized HA (bacterial fermentation), NASHA: Restylane®, Restylane Touch®, Perlane®, Restylane SubQ™ (Q-Med); Juvederm™ 18, 24, and 30 (HV24 and 30) (Allergan); Hydrafill® 1, 2, 3, Softline and Softline Max (Allergan); Surgiderm® 18, 24, and 30 (24 and 30HV) (Allergan); Matridur®, Matri®gel, Matridex® (with dextran) (Biopolymer); Esthelis® Soft, Basic, Fortelis Extra (Anteis); Teosyal® (Teoxane); Puragen™, Puragen+, Prevelle™, Prevelle+ with lidocaine (Mentor Corporation–Genzyme Corporation); Hyaluderm® (LCA Pharmaceutical); Rofilan®, Reviderm® (with dextran) (Rofil/Philoderm)
- non-crosslinked or native HA (for mesolift): AcHyal® (Filorga) 1% 1 kDa, Juvelift® (Corneal) 1% 2.5 kDa, IAL System® (Inamed) 1.8% 1 kDa, Hyaluderm® (LCA) 2% 2.4 kDa, Restylane Vital® (Q-Med) 2%, Teosyal® Meso (Teoxane) 1.5% 1 kDa, Surgilift® (Corneal) 1.35% 2.5 kDa, Elastence® (Inamed) 3% 0.9 kDa, Mesolis® 1.4%, Mesolis+ 1.8% (Anteis) 1 kDa, R-fine® (Fame Medical Products) 1% 2 kDa.

Others

- polyvinyl alcohol: Bioinblue™ lips, DeepBlue (Polymekon).

Slowly biodegradable fillers (used in volumetric augmentation of face and folds)

- polylactic acid: New-Fill®/Sculptra® (Sanofi-Aventis), FDA approval August 2004
- hydroxyapatite gel: Radiesse® (Bioform)
- tricalcium phosphate gel: Atlean (ABR Development).

Non-biodegradable implants

- polymethylmethacrylate (+ collagen): Artecoll®, Artefill® (Artes)

- acrylic hydrogel (+ hyaluronic acid): Dermalive®, Dermadeep® (Dermatech)
- silicone: Bioplastique® (Uroplasty), Silikon® 1000 (Alcon), SilSkin® (Richard James) AdatoSil® 5000 (Bausch & Lomb)
- polyacrylamide gel: Outline®, Evolution® (ProCytech), Aquamid® (Contura International), Amazingel (Fuhua High Molecular Matter Company), Beautical® (Rofil/Philoderm)
- alkylimides: Bio-Alcamid® Face, Lips, Body (Polymekon)
- zirconium beads: Embosphere®, Durasphere® (Coloplast Corporation).

Side-effects after biodegradable implant injections

Some products may induce adverse events because of their inherent properties, such as their ability to elicit hypersensitivity reactions. Some reactions occur immediately after treatment, whereas some have a delayed onset.[1,2]

Tissue reactions may occur because of the nature of the filler injected, even if the procedure is correctly done. Sometimes this is due to poor technique. The depth is very important, too: superficial placement of HA or collagen may show visible lines or pale nodules.[3] Other reactions depend on the concentration of the product utilized.

As compared to non-degradable fillers, which cause major side-effects and with which treatment is difficult, biodegradable products seem satisfactory in terms of cosmetic results and medical safety.

Immediate and minor reactions

These side-effects begin after 1–8 days and disappear after 8 days.

They include punctiform hematomas that might be avoided by vitamin K cream application (twice a day, 5 days before and after). Before every injection the patient must stop aspirin and anti-inflammatory drugs, 10 days beforehand (care should be taken with vitamin E and products with ginkgo biloba). Erythemas or mild swelling at the injection site may be easily covered by make-up. Nodule formation (too superficial) must be massaged by the practitioner and the patient.

Swelling and bruising (lips) are especially seen with hyaluronic acid injection. Because of his hygroscopic effect, 2 days' treatment with oral steroids or anti-inflammatory drugs (Celebrex®) may be required.

Deep dermal placement of collagen (Zyplast) may cause a technical spasm or arterial embolism (0.09%). Glabellar necrosis has been observed.[4] This presents as an immediate cutaneous blanch with pain. Immediate vasodilatation with warm compresses and topical nitroglycerin may reduce the spasm.

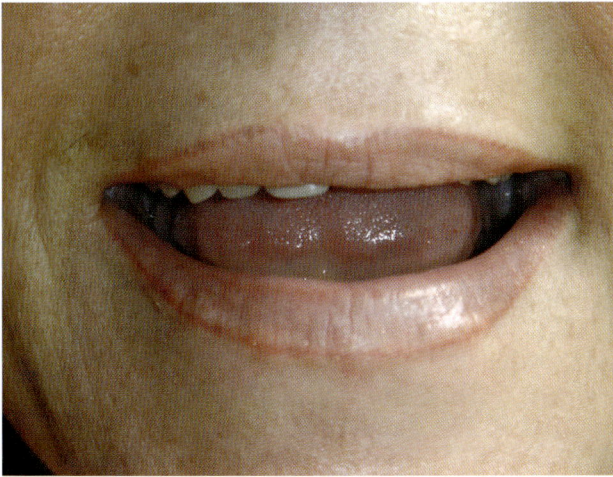

Figure 36.1   Evolence® Breeze: lip nodules appearing 3 days after injection.

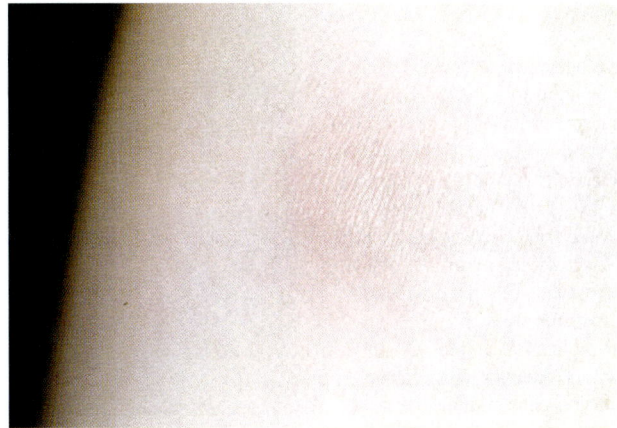

Figure 36.2   Positive hyaluronic acid test.

If tissue necrosis occurs, emotional support and appropriate wound care are essential to expedite a resolution.[5]

Semidelayed reactions

With all injected products, skin discoloration of esthetic significance can occur at the treatment site. After too superficial injection of bovine collagen a white line, visible at the injection site, disappears with product degradation.

A filiform bluish pigmentation (with hyaluronic acid) can be observed in the nasolabial fold, which may disappear slowly (6–8 months); a new injection in the same site is contraindicated. This bluish pigmentation may represent both traces of hemosiderin associated with vascular injury and visual distortion from light refraction to the filler through the skin.[2]

With the slowly degradable implants containing hyaluronic acid and dextran (Matridex), very inflammatory, swelling reactions have been observed, lasting more than 8 days.

We have recently seen nodules after lip injection with Evolence Breeze, and one case of necrosis on the nasolabial fold after Evolence Breeze injection (these effects occurring 1–8 days after treatment) (Figure 36.1).

Delayed side-effects

One to 4 weeks after collagen or hyaluronic acid injection, there may appear bruising, redness, and swelling, red and painful granulomas, papulocystic lesions, or abscesses (1 month to 1 year duration). These granulomas, because of delayed hypersensitivity, are prevented by the double test for bovine collagen and only one test for hyaluronic acid (Figure 36.2).[6]

The double test is essential before injection with bovine collagen. No test is required for porcine collagen (Evolence).

Importance of skin intradermal testing

In this indication the protocol is very precise:

- day 0: first test (right forearm)
- day 3: early analysis of test
- day 15: second test (left forearm)
- day 18: early analysis of second test
- day 45–60: late analysis of two tests
- after 12–18 months without injection a new single test is needed.

Every product containing animal-origin collagen (Artecoll®) needs to have the same tests.

Local reactions to collagen (2–3%) were reduced to 0.25% after double testing.

For hyaluronic acid, the medical history determines testing necessity:

- autoimmune pathology
- evolutive allergic disease (asthma, severe atopy)
- secondary reaction history after resorbable fillers
- anxious patient reassured by testing.

However, even with the double test, there are still a few allergic reactions to bovine collagen (0.04%) and cadaveric human collagen (Cymetra only in the USA, 2.1%).

There are very few cases of delayed hypersensitivity with hyaluronic acid (Figure 36.3).

From 1997 until 2001, in a European survey study[1] the global risk of immediate and delayed hypersensitivity to HA was 0.8%. Since 2000 the amount of protein in the raw product has decreased, and the incidence of hypersensitivity is around 0.6%.

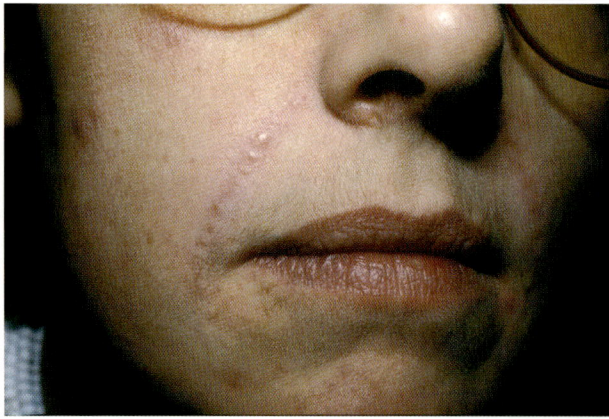

Figure 36.3   Hyaluronic acid hypersensitivity.

With the launch of new HA products (there may be a dozen), we may see reactions (recurrent inflammatory nodules) because of the concentration of crosslinking agent above the regular, which is 0.9–1% BDDE (1,4-butanediol diglycidylether).

The test is necessary if there is a history of food allergy, streptococcal disease, or immunoallergic problems (asthma, atopic dermatitis).

Treatment with topical, intralesional, and oral steroids is effective in 2–3 weeks, sometimes longer, but there is total restitutio ad integrum eventually.

Dissolution of material in erroneous placement and in allergic reactions may be a time saver and a deterrent to patient dissatisfaction: hyaluronidase is an enzyme that dissolves HA in the skin and also assists in the management of granulomatous foreign body reactions to HA (reactions caused by allergy to the material or immunologic response to protein contaminants in the HA preparation). The use of hyaluronidase reduced patient discomfort within 24–48 hours.[7–9]

We also now have collagenase for collagen reactions.

Poly-L-lactic acid (PLLA) (New-Fill or Sculptra in the USA) was used in Europe[10] for correction of human immunodeficiency virus (HIV) facial lipoatrophy and cosmetic rejuvenation of non-HIV patients when launched. It was positioned as a filler, diluted with 1 or 2 ml water. We observed violet then white granulomas 6–12 months after injection, very intense in very thin skin, especially around the lips (Figure 36.4) and the eyes.[11]

Palpable but non-visible and non-bothersome cutaneous micronodules were not uncommon (44%), but by the end of the 96-week study period, spontaneous resolution was observed in 27% of affected patients.[10,12,13]

With 5 ml dilution and very deep dermis injection, subcutaneous nodules were very rare, ≤5%.[14–19]

Such nodules may be transient inflammatory granulomatous reactions, although some have suggested that they are the result of the development of a fibrous reaction as a response to the presence of the implant.

The process of neocollagenesis persists despite the resorption of PLLA particles, and is one putative mechanism by which PLLA adds volume to recontour the face.[10]

The treatment of granulomas with local steroid injection or oral steroids is not always efficient, and neither is that with 5-fluorouracil (5-FU): some need surgery.[15] Lips are very sensitive and should not be injected with PLLA.

Radiesse, another slow degradable implant, is made of bioceramic spheres, ranging 25–125 μm in size, of calcium hydroxyapatite in a gel carrier.[20]

Moderate or important pain can occur during injection, eased by use of an ice pack for 20 minutes. Delayed reactions show persistence of palpable areas in thin skin and nodule formation occurring in about a third of patients.

It is now known that Radiesse cannot be injected in the lips because of numerous problems, as with Sculptra.[21,22]

Only 10% of patients will have nodules that require intralesional steroids, incision, or drainage, especially if injected in the lips.[20,23] Some will need surgery.[24]

Atlean, another slowly degradable implant, made of microspheres of tricalcium phosphate, is used like Radiesse (the first 'ceramics' on the market) for volumetric augmentation and as a tissue stimulant.

The fact that the microspheres disaggregate much more quickly (8 months) than with Radiesse allows the manufacturer to show no granulomas or side-effects after 12 months of study. There is no report of side-effects in the literature.

Non-degradable implants

Products

Polymethylmethacrylate (PMMA)

This consists of microspheres of 30–42 μm diameter suspended in 3.5% bovine collagen (Artecoll/Artefill) associated with 3% lidocaine.

Injection stimulates the tissue fibroblasts to produce patient collagen, which encapsulates the PMMA spheres. It has to be injected in the deep dermis and overcorrection should never be used.

Acrylic hydrogel

Acrylic hydrogel particles, 60 μm, are dispersed in a 60% stabilized hyaluronic acid gel (Dermalive), or the acrylic hydrogel particles can be enhanced in size, 90 μm (Dermadeep).

Injection is in the deep dermis.

Polyacrylamide gel (PAAG)

This consists of crosslinked polyacrylamide gel in a water solution. Aquamid is 2.5% crosslinked hydrophilic PAAG and 97.5% water. Outline uses

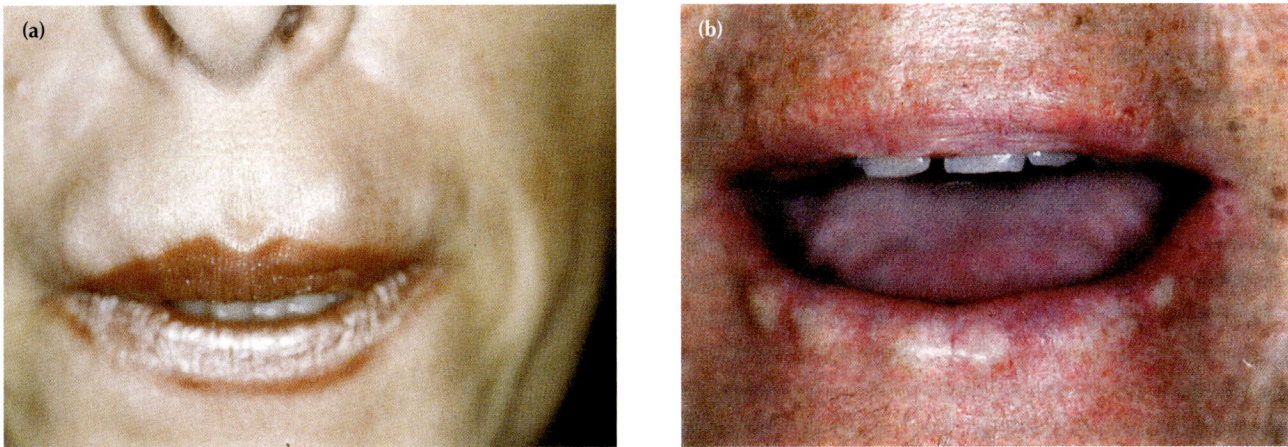

Figure 36.4 (a, b) New-Fill®/Sculptra® lip granulomas. Courtesy of Dr Baspeyras.

absorbable poly(acrylamide-co-DADMA) gel (where DADMA is diallyldimethyl ammonium). Evolution is a mixture of microscopic soft spheres of polyvinyl in a viscoelastic gel of poly(acrylamide-co-DADMA). Beautical 2 and 5 are polyacrylamide gels.

Synthetic alkylimides

Bio-Alcamid consists of 96% water and 4% synthetic reticulate polymer (polyalkylimide). Bio-Alcamid Lips and Face have the same composition, and Bio-Alcamid Body contains more material.

Silicones

Bioplastique contains solid silicone microspheres (100–400 and 600 μm) suspended in a polyvinyl vector. Silikon 1000 is purified, medical grade polydimethylsiloxane oil, 1000 centistokes viscosity. SilSkin and AdatoSil 5000 are polymethylsiloxane oil, 5000 centistokes viscosity.

Side-effects

Non-biodegradable fillers are responsible for immediate and delayed side-effects.

Immediate

Common acute side-effects include redness, swelling, and moderate pain in the first 2 days. One must be aware of infection (staphylococcus or mycobacteria) and therefore the injection must be made in strict asepsy.

Reactions might be very inflammatory, papulous, or nodular, erythematous or violet; they are transitory and disappear in days or weeks (same allergic side-effects as with products made of collagen and HA).

Delayed

Non-erythematous nodules can form immediately after injection as a result of uneven distribution of the product. Such nodules are distinct from the inflammatory response that is to be expected early following injection, whether a reaction to injury (which should disappear within days) or to infection.

Nodules might be single or multiple with inflammatory signs, dermal or subcutaneous, and may be painful.[13] In addition, treatment-associated hypersensitivity can lead to nodules that are usually inflammatory (need to establish a diagnosis of hypersensitivity through skin testing).

In addition to infection, inflammation, maldistribution of the product, hypersensitivity, and the process of neocollagenesis, foreign body reactions can occasionally precipitate the appearance of 'lumps and bumps' by leading to granulomatous inflammation (impossible diagnosis without histology).[2,25] Granulomas are violet, stony nodules, but sometimes of skin color; some of them can be very thick and hard, and evolve with inflammatory periods. They persist for years, and may be visible on the lips, isolated between two fingers.

Sometimes poor technique (too superficial, too much product) is the cause of these side-effects, and sometimes it is due to a foreign body reaction.

Treatment is very often disappointing and unpredictable: restitutio ad integrum is very rare, or with only diminution or persistence of lesions. Intralesional or oral steroids have a temporary effect, which does not prevent local relapse.

Mixtures of 5-FU added to betamethasone and triamcinolone are not very effective. Antimalarial, cyclines, and other treatments have not shown real efficacy. The only possibility is surgery, which leaves scars.

Polymethylmethacrylate (Artecoll) This may give, 6 months to 6 years post-injection, granulomas, violet

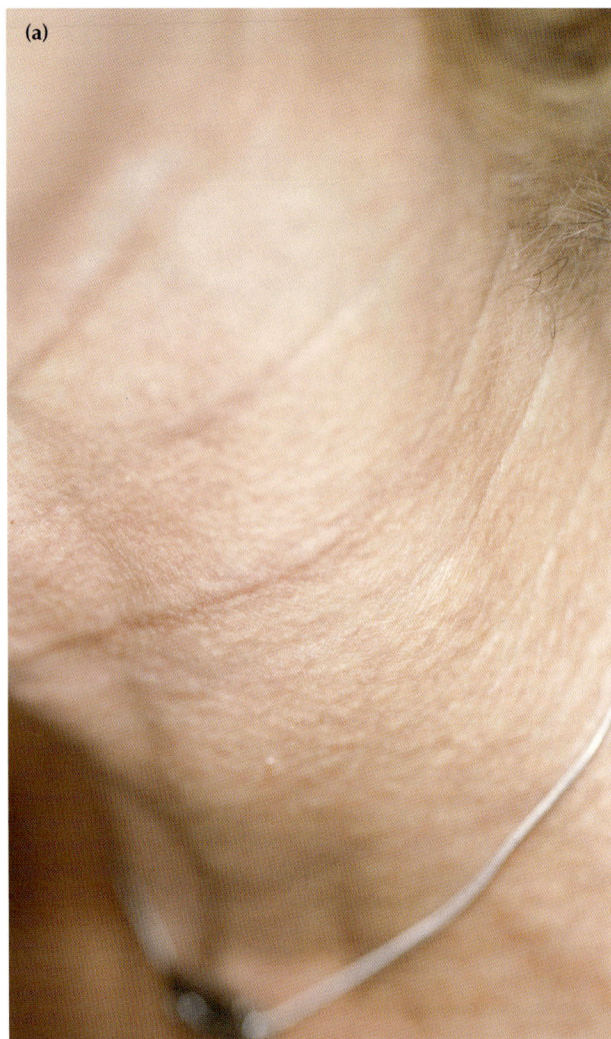

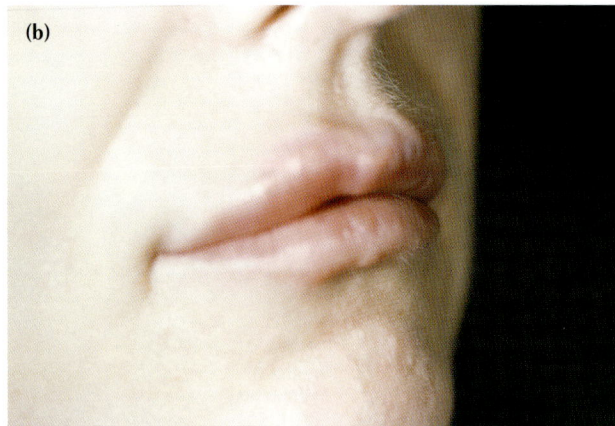

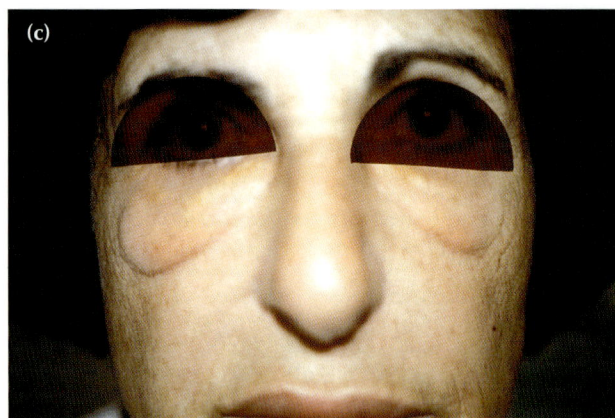

Figure 36.5 (a) Artecoll®/Arteplast® granulomas owing to poor technique. (b) Artecoll granulomas on lips. (c) Artecoll swelling and deep nodules 8 months after injection.

or white; they might be secondary to overcorrection or too superficial injection (Figure 36.5).[25–28]

These granulomas differ histologically from the expected foreign body reaction in that there is a wide distance between the microspheres, filled with macrophages, giant cells, fibroblasts, and a broad band of collagen fibers.

There is one case report of blindness and total ophthalmoplegia after glabella injection.[29]

Treatment includes intralesional steroids, or excision to remove the unwanted nodules.

Acrylic hydrogel (Dermalive, Dermadeep) These products have been widely used since they were launched, and quite often give reactions (Figure 36.6).[28,30,31]

The nodules are very hard, and erythematous or skin colored. They are extremely visible, especially on the lips, and very unattractive, associated with a depressive state.

Their particularity is treatment difficulty and inefficiency. Steroid injection, 5-FU injection, and oral steroids have been tried, as well as surgical excision, but after a few weeks, the nodules reappear around the

scar. Some patients have been treated by CO_2 laser and vascular laser, with unpredictable results.

Polyacrylamide gel (Outline, Aquamid) Foreign body granulomas are always delayed by months (less than 1 year). It's very difficult to give an average percentage of granulomas; the first study showed no real side-effects after 2 years.[32] Inflammatory nodules show an increased foreign body reaction as well as non-microbial abscesses with Aquamid (seem to resolve in 6–8 weeks) and it is better to excise them early.[33–36] One case of Aquamid abscess, after trying different broad-spectrum antibiotics with no success, resolved with intralesional steroid injections.[3]

Very hard granulomas have been described with Outline.

Alkylimides (Bio-Alcamid) This should be viewed as an injectable liquid endoprosthesis. Hence, it is prone to the potential drawbacks of an endoprosthesis such as excessive capsule formation, dislocation or migration, and infection. The onset of complications can be after 1 month to 3 years (Figure 36.7).[8,37]

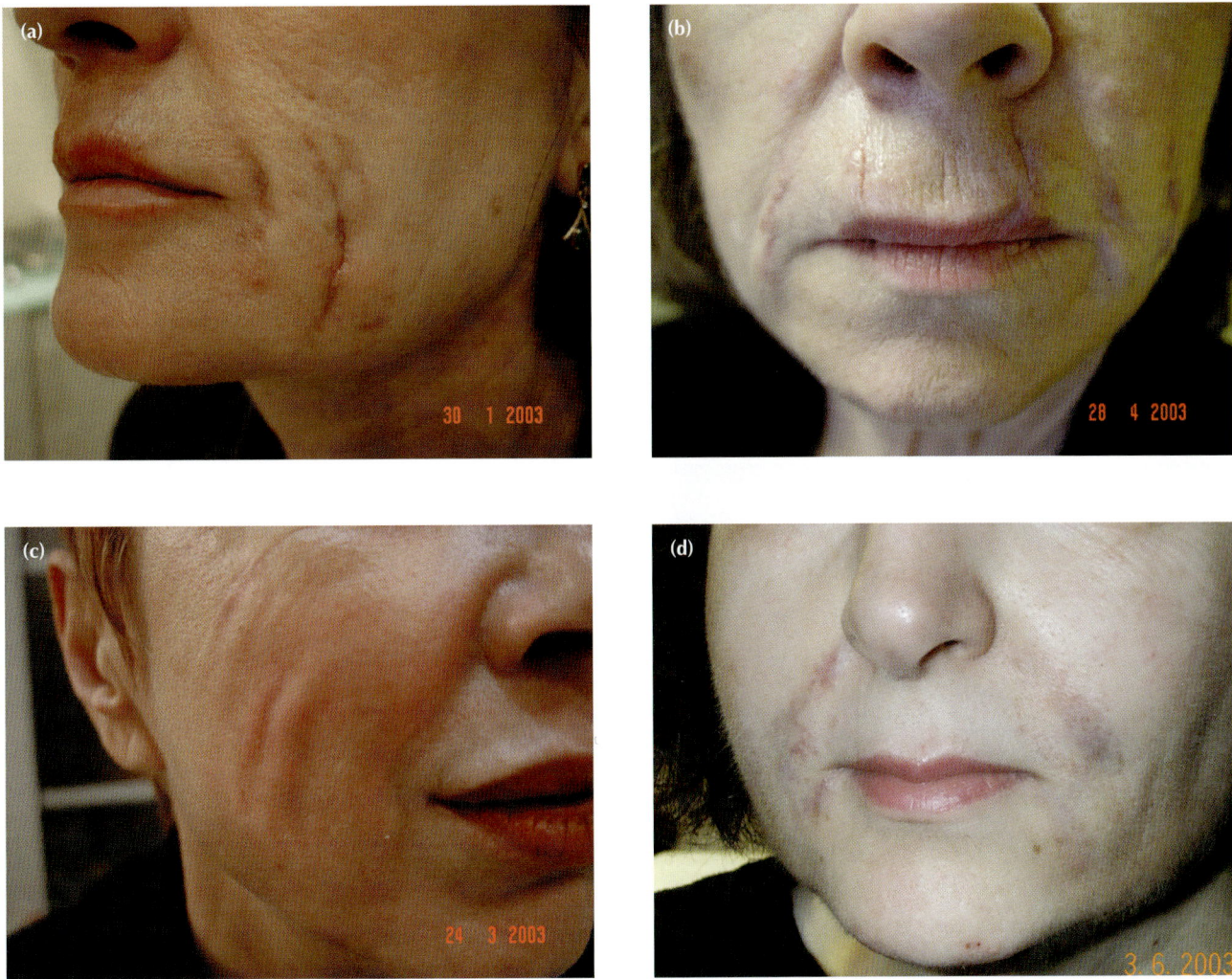

Figure 36.6 (a–c) Dermalive® granulomas, Courtesy of Dr Baspeyras; (d) Dermalive granulomas: reproduced courtesy of Dr de Goursac.

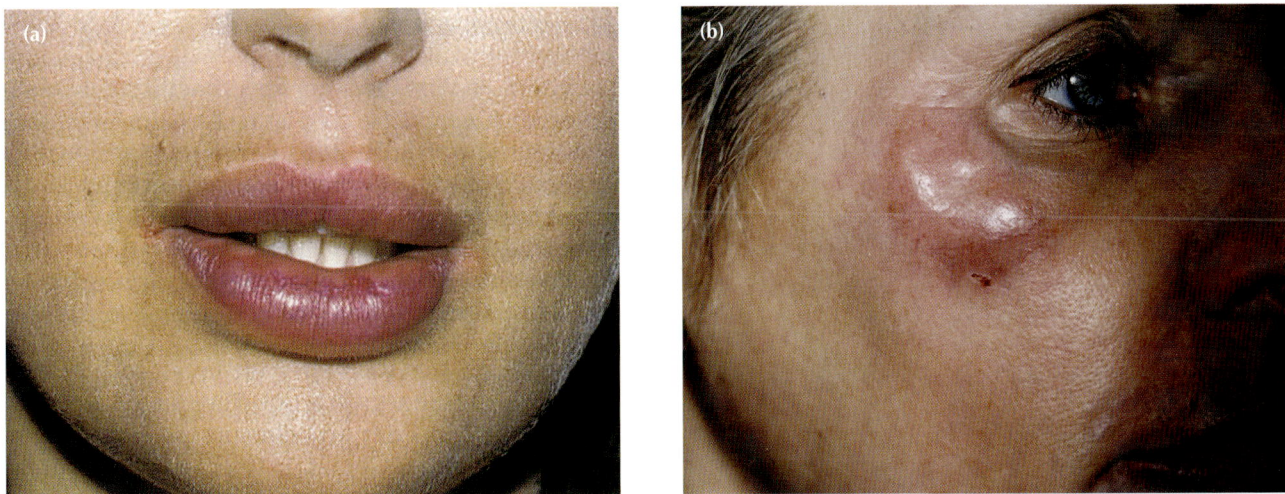

Figure 36.7 (a) Bio-Alcamid® lip granulomas; (b) Bio-Alcamid granulomas.

Injectable polyalkylimide induces fibroblast proliferation and capsule formation, and the severity of capsule formation is unpredictable and varies between patients: this capsular contraction will change the shape of the injection and severely diminish the initial cosmetic effect.

Contrary to manufacturer's claims, puncturing and squeezing cannot easily remove the stony deposit, and

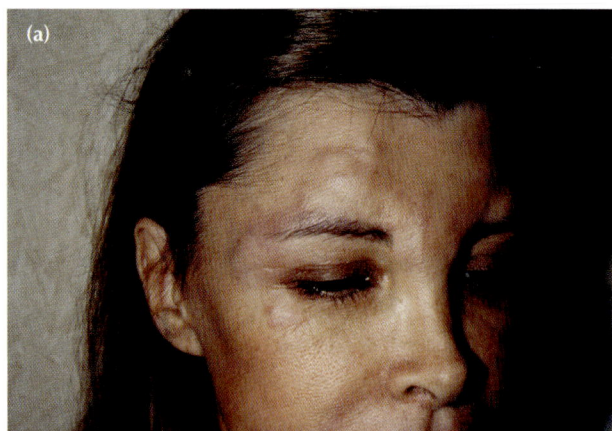

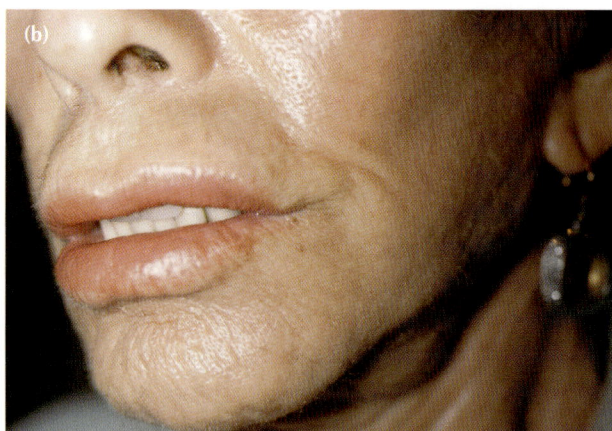

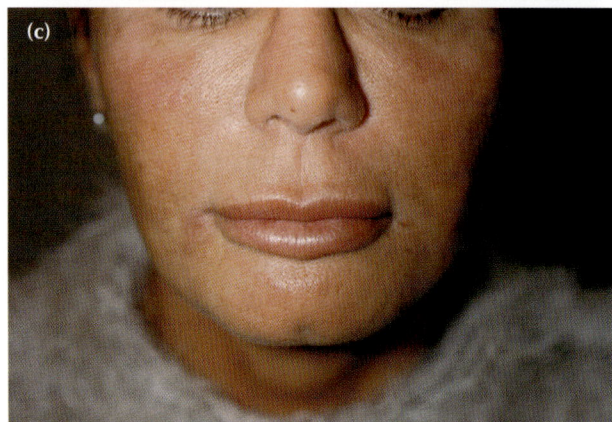

Figure 36.8   (a) Silicone granulomas 6 years after injection. (b, c) Hypertropic lips due to silicone injection.

surgery may be needed to remove all the injected material.

Infection of the injected material gives redness, swelling, and sensitivity, painful to touch. A localized festering mass with no macroscopic remnants of filler material is seen on magnetic resonance imaging (MRI).[8,38]

Systemic or intralesional corticosteroids or antibiotics may temporarily reduce the symptoms of infection, but will not cure it.[38] Sometimes even injections of 5-FU have been tried to treat such inflammation, but this is highly controversial as its therapeutic value in these cases has not been proven, and also it holds the risk of destruction of draining lymph vessels. More often, the foreign material has to be removed surgically to treat the infection adequally.

Moreover, some complications typically occur after additional invasive treatment subsequent to the polyalkylimide injections, and the incidence then may be far higher.

Silicones   Medical grade liquid injectable silicone was used 30 years ago to correct and replace lost volumes of subcutaneous tissue, and as a permanent filler.[39] Patients did not know the type of implant they were receiving all those years ago.

Reactions may happen after 28 years, and granuloma treatment with minocycline[11] or steroids (local and oral) does not always work (Figure 36.8).[2] Nodules and violet lumps can show a cystic and macrophagic type of foreign body granuloma, easy to recognize.[40–42]

Because of cases of burst granulomas after CO_2 laser treatment, it is better not to do the procedure if the nature of implant injected previously is not known.[43]

Retrospective diagnostic histology

With the anatomopathologic study of granulomas, we are able today to understand granuloma structure, immunogenicity, and nature of the filler injected.[2]

Medicolegal assistance may permit identification of the product that causes granulomatous inflammation, which is a histologically distinctive form of chronic inflammation that occurs in particular circumstances in response to foreign material. The function of such reactions is to isolate and prevent the migration of material that cannot immediately be removed by enzymatic breakdown or phagocytosis.

Granulomas can be characterized as aggregates of particular types of chronic inflammatory cells that form nodules containing macrophages, epitheloid cells, and lymphocytes. Macrophages are commonly modified to become multinucleate giant cells.[2,40,41,44]

Histologically, the severity of foreign body granulomas can be classified according to types and numbers of cells present.[45] Duranti et al proposed a classification based on the extent of granulomatous inflammation:[46]

- grade 1: slight inflammatory reaction with few inflammatory cells
- grade 2: clear inflammatory reaction with one or two multinucleate giant cells
- grade 3: more giant cells, presence of lymphocytes and fibrous tissue with inflammatory cells
- grade 4: granulomas with encapsulated implants and a clear foreign body reaction.

If available, histologic examination cannot only confirm the granuloma, it can also potentially point to the type of implant that caused the foreign body reaction. The configuration of the cystic space associated with the granuloma has the potential to differ.[47,48]

Commentary

Because of the possibility of inducing a granuloma reaction at the same injection site associated with a degradable filler injected after a non-degradable filler (even years afterward), it is not advisable to inject a biodegradable product in a location injected previously with an unknown product or a permanent product. An inflammatory reaction may occur, and it would be difficult to assign imputability.

Conclusion

A good pharmacological and chemical knowledge of fillers may help the dermatologist to choose the best implant for each patient.

The side-effects of fillers are not numerous compared to the number of patients injected. Besides, resorbable implants may cause secondary transitory and reversible reactions which may be prevented by medical history inquiry and testing.

When selecting a treatment, patients should be made aware of the potential results and the risks involved in undergoing a procedure.

Non-biodegradable implants may induce very late and long-lasting granulomas, sometimes even permanent because of the treatment difficulty. Given the potentially disfiguring therapy needed to treat these complications, it is important to warn against the use of such fillers for cosmetic indications. For this reason, it is justified to prefer resorbable implants which impart physical security and psychologic satisfaction to the patient.

References

1. Andre P. Evaluation of the safety of a non-animal stabilized hyaluronic acid (NASHA-Q-Med, Sweden) in European countries: a retrospective study from 1997 to 2001. J Eur Acad Dermatol Venereol 2004; 18: 422–5.

2. Lowe NJ, Maxwell CA, Patnaik R. Adverse reactions to dermal fillers: review. Dermatol Surg 2005; 31: 1616–25.

3. Amin SP, Marmur ES, Goldberg DJ. Complications from injectable polyacrylamide gel, a nonbiodegradable soft tissue filler. Dermatol Surg 2004; 30: 1507–9.

4. Hanke CW, Hingley HR, Jolivette DM et al. Abscess formation and local necrosis after treatement with Zyderm or Zyplast collagen implant. J Am Acad Dermatol 1991; 25: 319–26.

5. Ruiz-Esparza J, Bailin M, Bailin PL. Necrobiotic granuloma formation at a collagen implant site. Cleve Clin Q 1983; 50: 163–5.

6. Mullins RJ, Richards C, Walker T. Allergic reactions to oral, surgical, and topical bovine collagen. Anaphylactic risk for surgeons. Aust NZ J Ophthalmol 1996; 24: 257–60.

7. Brody HJ. Use of hyaluronidase in the treatment of granulomatous hyaluronic acid reactions or unwanted hyaluronic acid misplacement. Dermatol Surg 2005; 31: 893–7.

8. Lambros V. The use of hyaluronidase to reverse the effects of hyaluronic acid filler. Plast Reconstr Surg 2004; 114: 277.

9. Soparkar CN, Patrinely JR, Tschen J. Erasing Restilane. Opththal Plast Reconstr Surg 2004; 20: 317–18.

10. Valantin MA, Aubron-Olivier C, Ghosn J et al. Polylactic implants (New-Fill) to correct facial lipoatrophy in HIV-infected patients: results of the open-label study VEGA. AIDS 2003; 17: 2471–7.

11. Stewart DB, Morganroth GS, Mooney MA et al. Management of visible granulomas following periorbital injection of poly-L-lactic Acid. Ophthal Plast Reconstr Surg 2007; 23: 298–301.

12. Broder KW, Cohen SR. An overview of permanent and semi-permanent fillers. Plast Reconstr Surg 2006; 118 (Suppl): 7S–14S.

13. Christensen L, Breiting V, Janssen M, Vuust J, Hogdall E. Adverse reactions to injectable soft tissue permanent fillers. Aesthetic Plast Surg 2005; 29: 34–48.

14. Beljaards RC, de Roos KP, Bruins FG. NewFill for skin augmentation: a new filler or failure? Dermatol Surg 2005; 31: 772–6; discussion 776.

15. Cromheeke M. Survey among 68 plastic surgeons in The Netherlands about side effects of soft tissue fillers. Presented at Spring Meeting of the Dutch Society of Plastic Surgery, Apeldoorn, The Netherlands, 11 June, 2005.

16. Dijkema SJ, van der Lei B, Kibbelaar RE. New-fill injections may induce late-onset foreign body granulomatous reaction. Plast Reconstr Surg 2005; 115: 76e–8e.

17. Douglas RS, Cook T, Snorr N. Lumps and bumps: late surgical inflammatory and infectious lesions. Plast Reconstr Surg 2003; 112: 1923–8.

18. Woerle B, Hanke CW, Sattler G. Poly-L-lactic acid: a temporary filler for soft tissue augmentation. J Drugs Dermatol 2004; 3: 385–9

19. Bauer U, Vleggaar D. Response to 'New-fill injections may induce late-onset foreign body granulomatous reaction'. Plast Reconstr Surg 2006; 118: 265; author reply 265–6.

20. Sklar JA, White SM. Radiance FN: a new soft tissue filler. Dermatol Surg 2004; 30: 764–8.

21. Beer KR. Radiesse nodule of the lips from a distant injection site: report of a case and consideration of etiology and management. J Drugs Dermatol 2007; 6: 846–7.

22. Sankar V, McGuff HS. Foreign body reaction to calcium hydroxylapatite after lip augmentation. J Am Dent Assoc 2007; 138: 1093–6.

23. Tzikas TL. Evaluation of the Radiance FN soft tissue filler for facial soft tissue augmentation. Arch Facial Plast Surg 2004; 6: 234–9.

24. Wolfram D, Tzankov A, Piza-Katzer H. Surgery for foreign body reactions due to injectable fillers. Dermatology 2006; 213: 300–4.

25. Lemperle G, Romano JJ, Busso M. Soft tissue augmentation with Artecoll: 10 years history, indications, techniques and complications. Dermatol Surg 2003; 29: 573–87.

26. Alcalay J, Alkalay R, Gat A, Yorav S. Late onset granulomatous reactions to Artecoll. Dermatol Surg 2003; 29: 859–62.

27. Cohen SR, Holmes RE. Artecoll: a long lasting injectable wrinkle filler material. Report of a controlled, randomised, multicenter clinical trial of 251 subjects. Plast Reconstr Surg 2004; 114: 964–76.

28. Lombardi T, Samson J, Plantier F, Husson C, Kuffer R. Orofacial granulomas after injection of cosmetic fillers. Histopathologic and clinical study of 11 cases. J Oral Pathol Med 2004; 33: 115–20.

29. Silva MT, Curi AL. Blindness and total ophthalmoplegia after aesthetic polymethylmethacrylate injection: case report. Arq Neuropsiquiatr 2004; 62: 873–4.

30. Bergeret-Gallet C, Latouche X, Illouz YG. The value of a new filler material in corrective and cosmetic surgery: Dermalive and DermaDeep. Aesthetic Plast Surg 2001; 25: 249–55.

31. Sidwell RU, Dhillon AP, Butler PE, Rustin MH. Localised granulomatous reaction to a semi permanent hyaluronic acid and an acrylic hydrogel cosmetic filler. Clin Exp Dermatol 2004; 29: 630–2.

32. De Cassia Novaes W, Berg A. Experiences with a non biodegradable hydrogel (Aquamid): a pilot study. Aesthetic Plast Surg 2003; 27: 376–80.

33. Breiting V, Aasted A, Jorgensen A, Opitz P, Rozetsky A. A study on patients treated with polyacrylamide hydrogel injection for facial corrections. Aesthetic Plast Surg 2004; 28: 45–53.

34. Christensen L, Breiting V. Complications induced by polyacrylamide hydrogen injection. Plast Reconstr Surg 2005; 116: 1168–9.

35. Niedzielska I, Pajak J, Drugacz J. Late complications after polyacrylamide hydrogel injection into facial soft tissues. Aesthetic Plast Surg 2006; 30: 377–8.

36. Kawamura JY, Domaneschi C, Migliari DA, Sousa SO. Foreign body reaction due to skin filler: a case report. Oral Surg Oral Med Oral Pathol Oral Radiol Endod 2006; 101: 469–71.

37. Karim RB, Hage JJ, Van Rozelaar L, Lange CAH, Paaijmakers J. Complications of polyalkylimide 4% injections (Bio-Alcamid): a report of 18 cases. J Plast Reconstr Aesthet Surg 2006; 59: 1409–14.

38. Von Eiff C, Jansen B, Kohnen W, Becker K. Infections associated with medical devices: pathogenesis, management and prophylaxis. Drugs 2005; 65: 179–214.

39. Hexsel DM, Hexsel CL, Iyengar V. Liquid injectable silicone: history, mechanism of action, indications, technique, and complications. Semin Cutan Med Surg 2003; 22: 107–14.

40. Morhenn VB, Lemperle G, Gallo RL. Phagocytosis of different particulate dermal filler substances by human macrophages and skin cells. Dermatol Surg 2002; 28: 484–90.

41. Rohrich RJ, Potter JK. Liquid injectable silicone: is there a role as a cosmetic soft tissue filler? Plast Reconstr Surg 2004; 113: 1239–41.

42. Senet P, Backlez H, Ollivaud L. Minocycline for the treatment of cutaneous silicone granulomas. Br J Dermatol 1999; 140: 985–7.

43. Zager W, Huang J, McCue P, Reiter D. Laser resurfacing of silicone injected skin: the 'silicone flash' revisited. Arch Otolaryngol Head Neck Surg 2001; 127: 418–21.

44. Zimmermann US, Clerici TJ. The histological aspects of fillers complications. Semin Cutan Med Surg 2004; 23: 241–50.

46. Duranti F, Salti G, Bovani B, Calandra M, Rosati ML. Injectable hyaluronic gel for soft tissue augmentation. Dermatol Surg 1998; 24: 1317–25.

45. Lemperle G, Morhen V, Charrier U. Human histology and persistence of various injectable filler substances for soft tissue augmentation. Aesthetic Plast Surg 2003; 27: 354–66.

47. Lowe NJ, Maxwell C, Lowe P, Duick M, Shah K. Hyaluronic acid skin fillers: adverse reactions and skin testing. J Am Acad Dermatol 2001; 45: 930–6.

48. Rudolph CM, Soyer HP, Sculler-Petrovic S. Foreign body granulomas due to injectable aesthetic microimplants. Am J Surg Pathol 1999; 23: 113–17.

37 Fillers and granuloma: anatomopathological and clinical analysis and treatments

Nelly Gauthier and Gottfried Lemperle

The increasing use of dermal filler substances in the treatment of wrinkles, as well as the immense variety of new products and introduction of new names without proper disclosure of their chemical contents – at least in some countries – makes any overview difficult.[1] Unfortunately, the general lack of reliable scientific evidence ('a hydrogel') and trustworthy data ('patient satisfaction'), and the general habit of the manufacturers to provide the most positive data ('duration 2–7 years'), meet with a general lack of scientific interest and criticism on the side of the injecting physician. No wonder then, that the sudden occurrence of a complication leads to astonishment, negligence, blame directed at the product, and wrongful treatment of these often troublesome complications. Only proper education of physicians and patients will draw a realistic picture of this new field of injectables, currently filled with enthusiasm and negligence, warnings and hypotheses, and widespread happiness, but some disasters too.

In general, all injectable substances exerting a positive effect may be expected to also cause side-effects. All current dermal fillers, resorbable and non-resorbable, are associated with adverse effects.[2] Biological substances such as collagen or hyaluronic acid may cause allergies, lumps, long-lasting redness, sterile abscesses, and eventually early foreign body granulomas (FBGs) (Figure 37.1); longer-lasting artificial substances such as the many polymers used in medicine may cause lumps, long-lasting redness, and late FBGs (Figure 37.2).

The following opinion on successful treatment of late adverse events is based on a joint experience with various injectable filler substances and their complications, as well as a thorough review of the existing literature. The problem of all here enclosed statistics is obvious: late adverse events after fillers have to be reported neither to the manufacturer nor to the health authorities in most countries, and when they have to be reported they seldom are. This accounts for the low

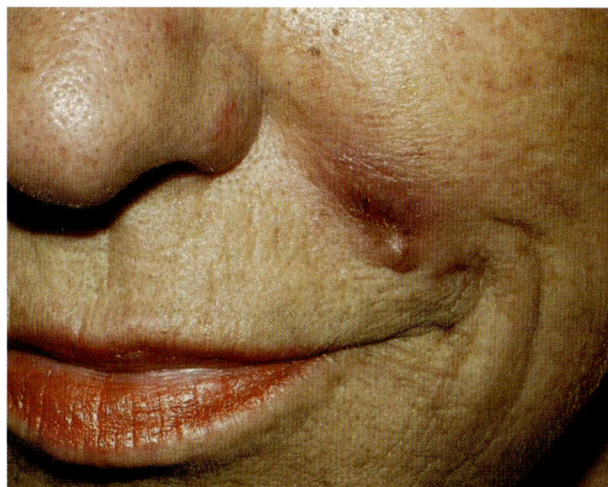

Figure 37.1 Cystic or inflammatory granulomas in both nasolabial folds appearing 3 months after Restylane® injections. The same reaction can appear after collagen injections.

rates that the manufacturers produce. Until official statistics are available, we have to rely on those of single physicians! In order to get reliable and trustworthy numbers, calculations were limited here to reports on case-numbers above 500 patients. It is estimated that the calculated range of occurring genuine FBGs varies between 1 in 100 (1%) and 1 in 5000 (0.02%) patients, depending on the injectable used.

Description of a foreign body granuloma

The word granuloma is a compound of the Latin 'granulum' meaning little grain, and the Greek 'onkos' meaning tumor or nodule. In histopathology it describes a granulomatous tissue reaction to bacteria (tuberculosis, leprosy, dental granuloma), fungi (*Actinomyces*), eggs of

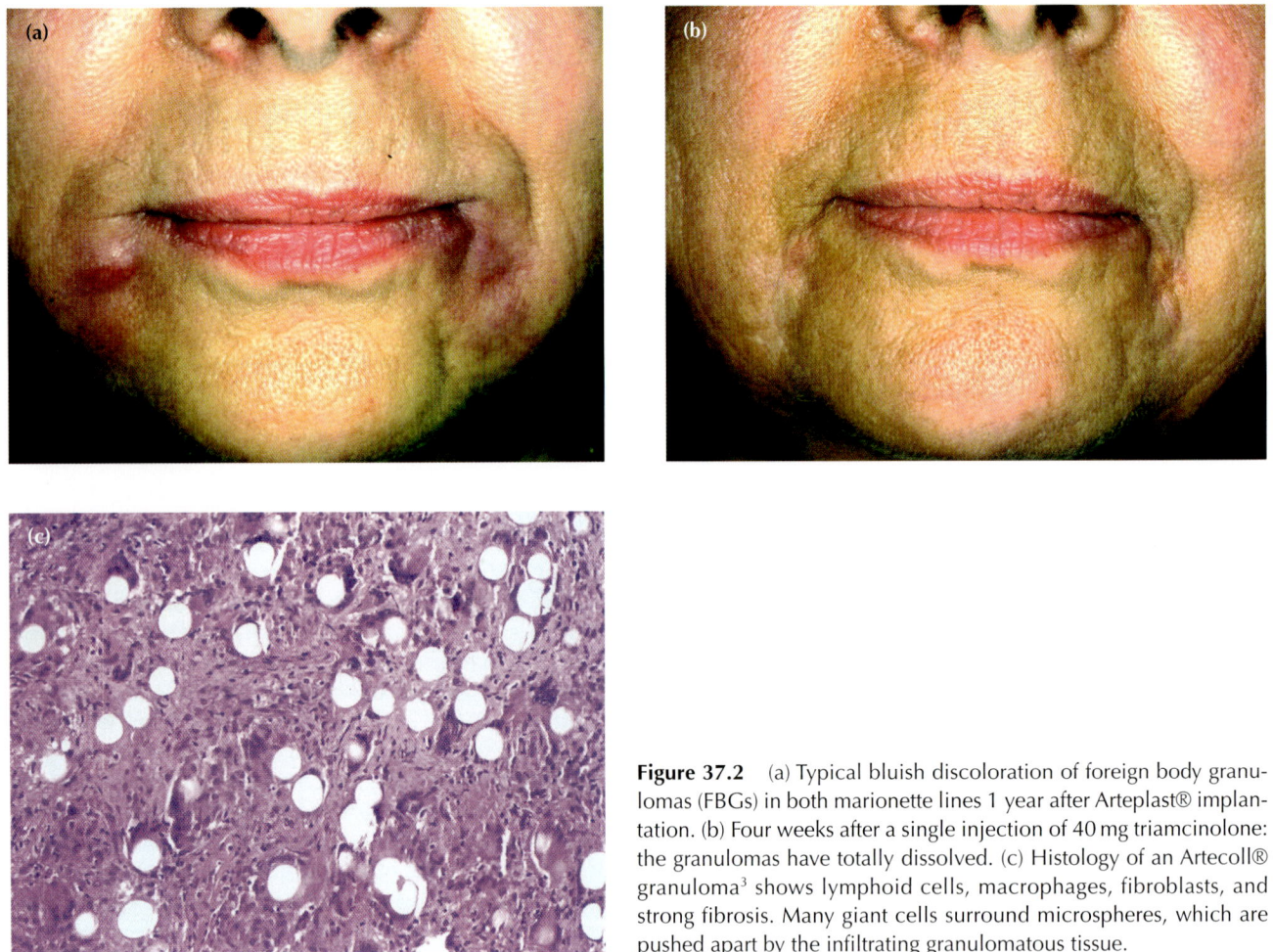

Figure 37.2   (a) Typical bluish discoloration of foreign body granulomas (FBGs) in both marionette lines 1 year after Arteplast® implantation. (b) Four weeks after a single injection of 40 mg triamcinolone: the granulomas have totally dissolved. (c) Histology of an Artecoll® granuloma[3] shows lymphoid cells, macrophages, fibroblasts, and strong fibrosis. Many giant cells surround microspheres, which are pushed apart by the infiltrating granulomatous tissue.

dermal parasites, unknown stimuli (lymphogranulomatosis, erythema nodosum, granuloma annulare, pyogenic and eosinophilic granuloma), or foreign bodies (spines or stings, sutures, fat necrosis, surgical powder, tattoos, injectable filler substances); it is the body's attempt to get rid of the intruded material. Histologically they differ mainly by the amount of epitheloid cells/histiocytes or macrophages/lymphocytes/inflammatory cells and eosinophils/polymorphous exudates, and multinucleated giant cells.

Clinical appearance of foreign body granulomas

Irrespective of its histological picture, a true FBG is and remains a clinical diagnosis! It can develop slowly or rapidly in certain patients after the injection of any existing dermal filler. It occurs significantly less after implantation of microspheres with a smooth surface (Artecoll®, Sculptra®) than with particles of irregular or edged surfaces (Bioplastique®, Dermalive®). Its appearance is usually less dramatic with resorbable implants (collagen, hyaluronic acid) than with longer-lasting implants. The time interval between the

injection and the first appearance of a FBG is usually 6–24 months. However, its appearance has been reported up to 10 years following implantation.[4] Some granulomas develop years after the material has long been absorbed,[5] while others develop only after a second or third injection:

1. After an uneventful and satisfying period of many months or years, one of the implanted areas suddenly increases in size and ends up as an unsightly, painless, plump, non-confined nodule (Figure 37.2a). It may be accompanied locally by uncomfortable tension, persistent or transitory edema, erythema, or purplish pigmentation. It may show periods of 'flare-ups' and temporary regressions.

2. Soon all other implantation sites will develop a similar growth, major differentiation from a nodule due to inadequate implantation. The growths remain in the injected areas and never involve tissues free of material.

3. True FBGs are growing; congested dermal capillaries widen and give the lump an unattractive purplish appearance. If not treated intralesionally with corticosteroids (Figure 37.2b) they may

Table 37.1 A synopsis of data from the literature on the approximate rate of granuloma formation after individual fillers. All fillers have gone through a phase of development and improvement

Product	References	Data collection	Number of granulomas in number of patients	Calculated granuloma rate Individual	Calculated granuloma rate Overall
Collagen gel	Cooperman[10]	1975–1984	15* in 5109	0.3%	
	Charriere[17]	1986–1988	8* in 656	1.2%	=~0.34%
	Castrow[18]	1981–1982	21* in ~7000	0.3%	
	Hanke[19]	*1981–1989*	*?* in ~470 000*	*0.04%*	*=~0.04%*
Hyaluronic acid gel	Lowe[20]	1996–2000	3* in 709	0.4%	
	Andre[21]	1997–2001	18* in 4320	0.4%	=~0.4%
	Friedman[12]	*1999*	*Some in ~ 144 000*	*0.07%*	
	Friedman[12]	*2000*	*Rare in ~ 262 000*	*0.02%*	*=~0.04%*
PMMA microspheres	Lemperle[22] (Arteplast)	1989–1993	15 in 587	2.5%	=~1.51%
	Gauthier (Arteplast)	1993–1994	9 in ~ 1000	0.9%	
	Gauthier (Artecoll)	**1995–1999**	**3 in ~2000**	**0.15%**	
	Lemperle (Artecoll)[13]	**1994–1998**	**7 in ~3500**	**0.24%**	
	Dansereau**	**1998–2005**	**2 in ~ 2000**	**0.10%**	**=~0.16%**
	Canderm Canada**	*1998–2005*	*14 in ~50 000*	*0.03%*	*=~0.02%*
	Hafod China**	*2002–2005*	*2 in ~ 30 000*	*0.01%*	
	TRM Korea**	*1996–2005*	*9 in ~60 000*	*0.01%*	
Ca - hydroxyapatite microspheres	Jansen[23]	2002–2004	> 1 in 609	0.16%	
	BioForm Medical[16]	*2002–2005*	*> 2 in ~ 35 000*		*=~0.005*
PLA microspheres	**Gauthier (3 ml dilut.)**	**1999–2002**	**15 in ~1500**	**1.0%**	**=1.0%**
	Gauthier (5 ml dilut.)	**2002–2005**	**2 in ~1500**	**0.13%**	
	Bauer[24]	**2000–2004**	**5 in 722**	**0.7%**	**=~0.25%**
	Vleggar (personal communication)	**2000–2003**	**3 in 2131**	**0.14%**	
	Aventis Germany**	*1999–2004*	*? in ~150 000*	*0.2%*	*=~0.2%*
HEMA particles	**DeGoursac (personal communication)**	*1998–2000*	**17 in > 800**	**2.1%**	
	Bergeret[15]	**1998–2000**	**9 in 455**	**2.0%**	**=~ 1.25%**
	Harrer (personal communication)	**1998–2004**	**10 in 1630**	**0.6%**	
	Dermatech France	*1998–2005*	*? in ~170 000*	*0.225%*	*=~ 0.22%*
Silicone oil	**Greenberg[25]**	**1980–1990**	**1 in ~1000**	**0.10%**	
	Orentreich[26]	**Since 1985**	**1 in ~5000**	**0.02%**	**=0.12%**
	Fulton[27]	**2002–2005**	**5 in 608**	**0.82 %**	
	Jones[28],**	**2003–2005**	**1 in 500**	**0.20%**	

*Based on our interpretation of granulomas used in this presentation we classified 'sterile abscess' and 'chronic inflammation' as granulomas if they occur at least 2 months after injection at all sites at approximately the same time.

**Answers to enquiries to the manufacturers in 2006 and personal communications 2005 with Prof. Lemperle: data on file.

increase in size to the volume of a pea or bean, and remain unchanged in their clinical appearance until they eventually resolve spontaneously after some years.[6,7]

A prediction or preselection of patients is not yet possible since the reasons for the development of a granuloma in an individual are not yet known. In general, FBGs are of non-allergenic origin: many former granuloma patients, years after successful corticoid treatment, did not react to a later test injection with the same material and did not form granulomas at the test sites. A typical FBG is not a late allergic granulomatous reaction of type IV.[8]

Genuine granulomas occur rarely, but at an incidence rate ranging from 1:100 (1.0%) to 1:5000 (0.02%) patients after injection of any dermal filler substance such as collagen,[5,9,10] hyaluronic acid,[11,12] polymethylmethacrylate (PMMA)/Artecoll,[13] poly-L-lactic acid (PLA)/New-Fill® (Sculptra),[6] liquid silicone,[7] acrylamides,[14] hydroxyethylmethacrylate (HEMA)/Dermalive,[15] and dextran/Reviderm®[16] (Table 37.1).

Differentiation from a nodule due to technical error

All injectables bear the danger of being overinjected, misplaced, remodeled, or dislocated when deposited into or close to facial muscles.

Similar to the muscle of a shell forming a pearl, constant movement may help to form a 'grain' or a nodule from a falsely deposited strand. This may be especially obvious in the corner of the mouth, the crow's feet, and the soft tissues of the lips (Figure 37.3). The formation of these nodules must be blamed on an inadequate implantation technique, and must not be confused with genuine FBGs. Clinically, implant nodules are isolated, single lumps in the implanted area, visually evident and palpable a few weeks postinjection. Often white and much harder than a genuine granuloma, their fibrous capsule confines them well from the surrounding tissue (Table 37.2). They do not grow. If untreated they will remain the same, as long as the product injected will last. Histology reveals the appearance of a dense foreign material and a typical, but deliberate, foreign body 'reaction' with scattered macrophages and giant cells.[8,29] Giant cells per se are not the typical sign of granulomas, but of a foreign material too large to be engulfed by macrophages, which fuse in an attempt to be more powerful; Eppley et al call them 'frustrated macrophages'.[30] Intralesional injections of corticoids are rather difficult to perform due to their hardness and are often non-effective because the substance is in excess, not because of the cellular reaction. In the lips they are best excised from the inside. Nodules occur rather often at the beginning of a new technique or a new implant for a given physician, which outlines the importance of thorough training for all injection techniques.

Another common misdiagnosis occurs when a dermal filler containing microspheres has been implanted

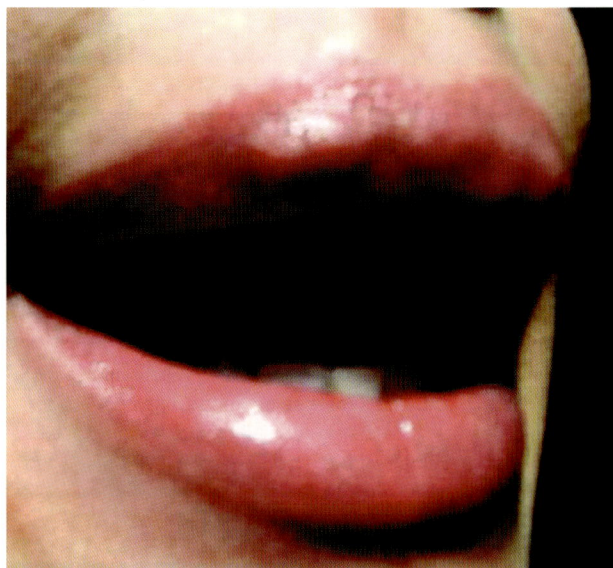

Figure 37.3 Nodules in the lips from compressed Radiesse® strands do not react to triamcinolone and therefore should be excised.

too superficially into the dermis, instead of at the dermal–subdermal junction. In some cases, a hyperreaction of the skin may take place, 2–3 months after implantation, that clinically and histologically resembles a hypertrophic scar or a keloid (Figure 37.4) with the typical coloring of the skin. In such cases the predominant cells present are not macrophages and giant cells as seen in FBGs, but are fibroblasts and broad collagen strands that are pushing the particles apart. Although they respond to intralesional steroids they are usually difficult to treat, which further outlines the need to master the technique of implantation.

Unfortunately, all these pathological misdiagnoses of granulomas, while in reality involve an intended normal foreign body reaction to an inadequately implanted material, add to the confusion of the clinician.

Table 37.2	Differences between granuloma and implant nodule	
	Granulomas	**Nodules**
Appearance	6–36 months after injection, suddenly	1–3 months after injection, after swelling vanishes and reaction settles
Location	All injected sites, at approximatively the same time	Single nodules in some implanted areas, close to facial muscles (++ the lips)
Size	Growing to the size of a bean, skin discoloration and edema	Remain the same size as a lentil or a pea, no edema
Borders	Fingerlike projections into surrounding tissue	Well confined by fibrous capsule
Persistence	If untreated the reaction disappears after 1–5 years	As long as filler remains, until absorption – or permanent
Histology	*Scattered* material in *strong cellular* reaction. Foreign body *granuloma*	*Packed* material in *scarce cellular* reaction. Normal foreign body *reaction*
Treatment	React well to intralesional corticosteroids (or systemic)	Little effect of corticosteroids, waiting for absorption or excision
Cause	*Still unknown*	*Technical error*

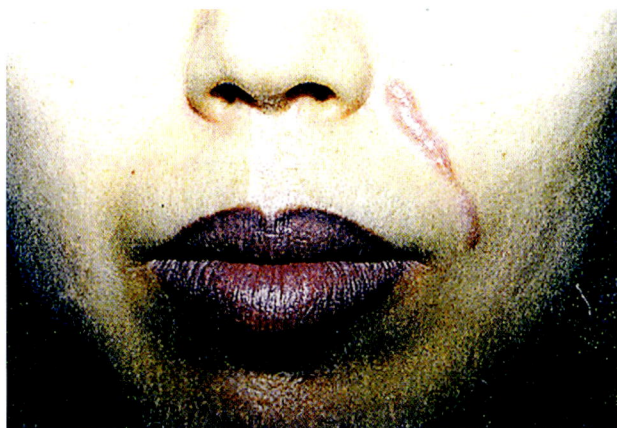

Figure 37.4 Hypertrophic scar in one nasolabial fold only, after mistaken 'intradermal' implantation of Artecoll in an Asian woman.

Histology of a normal implanted material

Since the histology caused by dermal fillers has not yet been introduced into modern textbooks of pathology and is rarely mentioned in the general pathological literature,[8] most histopathologists will diagnose a normal deliberate 'foreign body reaction' to a material containing particles as a 'foreign body granuloma'.[31–33] In fact, the particulate materials are implanted intentionally to stimulate a 'foreign body reaction', i.e. the ingrowth of cells and the encapsulation of each particle (or microsphere) with fibrous tissue in order to ensure a softer and more pliable implant.

All injected substances cause an initial influx of mononuclear cells. Immediately after implantation, macrophages attach to the particles and occasionally fuse in a failed attempt to ingest the same particle,[34] thus converting into giant cells: 5–10 giant cells in a field at ×100 is a normal picture. In general, the particles cause a low turnover reaction: little mitosis and no epitheloid cells. The turnover of macrophages is striking: their half-life is only a few hours, while the half-life of a giant cell is about 1 day.[3] Monocytes differentiate into fibroblasts to produce a collagen network in order to sustain the foreign body 'reaction'. This active phase of fibrosing is probably determined by the length of time the carrier of the particles will take to dissipate. If collagen is the carrier substance (as in Artecoll), after 6–12 months most giant cells have disappeared,[33] and, because PMMA microspheres are permanent and not constantly irritating, the histological picture can remain stable.[13] In cases of faster resorbable carrier substances (Sculptra, Dermalive, Radiesse®), once the carrier is absorbed, the particles are usually packed, with little space for tissue ingrowth. They are then broken down through enzymatic dissolution in the following months and subsequently phagocytosed by macrophages and giant cells,[35] until their complete dissolution.

Histological diagnosis of a true foreign body granuloma

Histologically as well as clinically, three predominant types of FBG can be distinguished after injection of different dermal tissue fillers. Of course, some histological pictures can be a blend of two or three types.

Cystic granuloma

Cystic granuloma (synonyms: inflammatory, necrobiotic, palisading) can develop after intradermal injections of biological gels such as collagen and hyaluronic acid (Figure 37.1). This disturbing adverse event may develop slowly at all injected sites with induration, erythema, and sometimes fluctuation. Intense redness, swelling, and pain are the predominant clinical signs. Small and superficial, they occur 2–12 months after injection and disappear spontaneously within 3–12 months.

Late complications after bovine collagen have been described in the literature as 'palisaded foreign body granuloma'[36] and 'necrobiotic granuloma',[36–39] where the collagen implant, palisaded with macrophages and giant cells, is floating in a sea of neutrophils and lymphoid cells. This form of granuloma is sometimes believed to be a manifestation of cell-mediated delayed hypersensitivity reaction,[19] in which cases patients may have elevated collagen antibody titers[40] and a positive reaction at a second test site.[37,41] In our own experience, none of the patients with cystic FBGs showed positive tests against collagen or hyaluronic acid at the time of onset. The bacterial cultures were uniformly negative.[42,43] Fluctuation may be present, but the term 'sterile abscess'[9,40,44] is incorrect, since the induration and redness will persist for many months after puncture and squeezing of all contained white collagen or hyaluronic acid that lies within a palisaded granuloma. The induration usually absorbs spontaneously in less than a year,[8,19,36,45] but macrophages are known to be 'memory cells', even if they move away after complete degradation,[34] and granuloma-producing agents must persist within cells for a long time.[5]

Edematous granuloma

Edematous granuloma (synonyms: 'lipogranuloma',[36] 'Swiss cheese pattern',[5] 'honeycomb' appearance) may develop suddenly many years after the implantation of permanent artificial fluid, such as silicone and acrylamide gel. Its characteristic is the usually rapid development of the reaction, like an allergic reaction, and the large amount of surrounding inflammation. If it happens in the glabella or the cheeks, the eyelids can be swollen over months (see Figure 37.7). The original implant is usually felt as a rather soft nodule, and erythema of the area implanted is often present.

Histologically, edematous granuloma represents an infiltration of the surrounding tissue mainly by lymphocytes and macrophages, but seldom giant cells.

This type of FBG results from a slow infiltration by the gel of the surrounding tissue, and the subsequent swelling appears to facilitate migration of lymphoid and other mononuclear cells from the capillaries to the implant. For one reason or another, after many years, this can lead to a hypersensitivity reaction,[46] which may remain for several years if left untreated. Local injections into the inflammatory 'capsule', or systemic corticosteroids if the reaction is extended, are the therapy of choice.

Sclerosing granuloma

Sclerosing granuloma (synonyms: sarcoidal, xanthelasmized) may develop after subdermal implantation of all types of particulate material (e.g. Artecoll/Artefill®, New-Fill/Sculptra, Dermalive/Dermadeep®, Radiance®/Radiesse, and Matridex®). Note that 'sarcoid-like' granulomas have also been related to a number of systemic diseases and/or proteins and chemical elements.[34]

They can occur 6–24 months after injection, and will remain for several years if left untreated. Clinically the sclerosing FBG is slowly developing with a very mild inflammation. In all implanted areas nodules eventually become visible, rather hard, and often bluish, with congested dermal capillaries on their surface. Histologically, the foreign particles are characteristically seen as microparticles or as their empty vacuoles and voids left by the preparation of the section (Figure 37.2c). Innumerable giant cells, macrophages, and fibroblasts are present, and occasionally small lymphocytes infiltrate.[47] Typical of the sclerosing granulomas is the production of a large fibrous network of different dimensions,[47] resulting in wide separation between individual microspheres (Figure 37.2c). This wide separation of individual particles and the presence of numerous giant cells are the histological signs of a growing FBG on particulate material (and its histological differentiation from an implant nodule). The granuloma infiltrates the surrounding tissue with finger-like projections; no fibrous capsule is surrounding the FBG, and no confined separation toward the normal surrounding tissue exists. Intralesional injections of high doses of corticosteroid are the best treatment. Identification of the type of injected filler[47] may be further supported by polarized light, which helps differentiate birefringent (PLA) and non-birefringent materials (collagen, hyaluronic acid (HA), silicone, PMMA, HEMA).

Granulomas after different substances

The following concerns the most used fillers with enough history to show a relevant picture. For example, dextran microspheres (Reviderm® Intra and Matridur®) suspended in hyaluronic acid are in clinical trials. Both stimulate a heavy granulomatous tissue[35] but are too recent on the market to get any idea of late complications, although a dextran granuloma has been described to cause urinary obstruction.[16] This section reviews the literature on granulomas secondary to various fillers. Although estimates of granuloma rates are presented in this section and in Tables 37.1 and 37.3, it is difficult to obtain reliable data for several reasons:

1. The number of patients treated was often only an estimate by the manufacturer based on the units of product sold; alternatively, the number of patients was sometimes based on a clinician's recollection of patients treated.
2. Physicians are not required to report late adverse events to manufacturers or health authorities in most countries.
3. The descriptions of adverse events in the literature are often incomplete. Therefore, the estimates given in Tables 37.1 and 37.3 are open to interpretation, and invite commentary on these important data.

For the purposes of this chapter, the following definition of granulomas is used: 'Chronic inflammatory responses, which appear at all injected sites after at least 2 months and/or which last for at least 2 months'.

Silicone fluid

Dow Corning introduced medical grade silicone oil (polydimethylsiloxane) in the late 1950s for soft tissue augmentation.[39,48] Liquid injectable silicone (LIS), with a viscosity of 350 cSt (meaning 3.5 times the viscosity of water), was banned in 1967 by the Food and Drug Administration (FDA) and some countries, but continued to be used in Latin America, Europe, and Asia.[46,49] In the USA, the currently marketed silicone gels have FDA approval for intraocular injections and a viscosity of 1000 cSt: Silikon® 1000 (Alcon Laboratories) and Silskin® (RJ Development Corporation). Through the FDA's modernization act of 1997, they are allowed to be used 'off-label' for other indications such as the treatment of wrinkles and lip augmentation.[28] Even though these 1000-cSt viscous gels remain pliable (they still contain a certain amount of monomers), they should be judged differently.

Public pressure for long-lasting fillers and the introduction of the microdroplet technique have led to a revival of silicone gels and their off-label use in cosmetic surgery, in the USA as well.[50] LIS appears to be safe when applied in small quantities using the microdroplet technique: Orentreich et al[26] reported that none of his patients had yet experienced FBGs after using the puncture technique to administer LIS. In Europe, the wide use of LIS (350 cSt) for lip augmentation in very small quantities seems to have yielded the lowest rate of FBGs in comparison to other permanent fillers.

The amount of published literature on complications after silicone injection is quite remarkable;[4,7,36,39,48,51–54] longer and more wide use of an injectable produces more patient exposure and the potential for a higher number of reported side-effects. Also, because LIS stimulates a very thin-walled fibrous capsule, when large quantities were injected in the past, dislocation by gravity along the fascias and muscle planes was a serious concern (especially in patients with loose connective tissue). It was improperly called 'migration',[26] but 'dead' silicone droplets cannot migrate actively. However, late sclerotic reactions around free silicone oil droplets can develop, as is well known after 'bleeding' occurring from earlier breast implants.[55] Silicone FBGs have developed even at the entry points after acupuncture with siliconized needles.[56]

Histologically, the silicone FBG shows typical vacuolated spaces measuring 1–30 µm in diameter, surrounded by numerous histiocytes (macrophages), lymphocytes, plasma cells, some eosinophils, and scattered giant cells.[57] In 10 volunteers injected with LIS 350 cSt,[17] the histology revealed lymphocytic infiltration and a characteristic reaction of delayed hypersensitivity. In immunohistology, small local deposits of immunoglobulin G (IgG) and IgA were observed around the walls of small vessels. In later biopsies of these volunteers, the inflammation had progressed to a fibroblastic reaction, and, when large doses had been implanted, they appeared to provoke giant cell granulomas.[29]

Clinically, what is impressive is the rather late onset of these FBGs, up to 10–15 years following injection.[46,51] They appear suddenly, like an allergic reaction, with redness, extreme swelling (sometimes of the whole face), and multiple areas of firm, rather soft, fixed nodules. No pain is involved, but submandibular adenopathy is often palpable and disturbing.

Steroid injections into the cellular tissue surrounding the implants or systemic corticotherapy is the best treatment. Spontaneous disappearances of silicone FBGs have been reported after a 3-year follow-up period.[7] Systemic minocycline (100 mg orally twice daily) has resulted in complete remission of silicone FBGs in two patients.[58] 'Liposuction' of larger LIS implants has sometimes been possible, but surgical excisions of true LIS FBGs should be avoided because of their finger-like insertions into the surrounding tissue.

Bovine collagen (Zyderm®/Zyplast®)

Bovine collagen in Zyderm® and its cross-linked form Zyplast® (Inamed Aesthetics, CA) was introduced in 1981 and 1983, respectively. Both have kept their safety standards and are still considered 'the gold standard' of injectable dermal fillers.[19]

Histologically, bovine collagen stains paler and is less fibrillar than native collagen. As early as 7 days after bovine collagen injection, there is a mild perivascular lymphohistiocytic infiltrate which gradually resolves by 3 months.[35] There is little evidence of active cellular degradation or foreign-body reaction, but, consequently, it is not colonized by active fibroblasts.

Even though bovine and human collagen implants are the least toxic and irritating biomaterials known,[44] erythematous dermal nodules can develop at the implantation sites.[5,10,17,19,59,60] The manufacturer reports that they occur at a rate of 1:1000 patients, and often convert into localized tissue necrosis, in approximatively 1:2500 patients.[19] In a study of more then 5000 patients[10] receiving injectable collagen, 67 developed an adverse reaction (1.3%); of these, 14 were clearly late FBGs (0.3%), which resolved under steroid therapy within a year. One patient experienced polyarthralgia over the entire period of effect of the collagen,[41] and another patient developed a histologically similar granuloma annulare at the site of the collagen test injection.[60] Moscona et al[5] described a woman who developed severe FBGs at all injection sites 2.5 years after implanting Zyderm I in the nasolabial folds, glabellar frown lines, and a few areas around the lips. Although high doses of oral prednisolone (up to 60 mg/day) made the swelling reduce, it rapidly recurred as the treatment was stopped. Intralesional triancinolone injections (no doses reported) resulted in almost complete regression, but the FBG recurred 4–6 weeks later. Over the following years, low daily doses of 5–10 mg of Dexacort® resulted in a slight improvement.

Collagen-associated late complications have been described as palisaded foreign body granuloma[36] and as necrobiotic granuloma.[36–39] Intense redness, swelling, and pain of all injected areas are the predominant signs; the palpation reveals induration and sometimes fluctuation. In an early trial in 656 patients of atelocollagen (Koken Ltd, Tokyo), eight patients (1.2%) reacted with an 'abscess' of long persistence.[17] After injection of human collagen (Dermalogen®), the same reaction of an indurated papule was described.[59] It contained macrophages and giant cells, and, although it disappeared in 2 months, a second test injection showed no positive reaction.

Hyaluronic acid (Restylane®)

Restylane® (Q-Med, AZ) was introduced in 1997 and is actually the leading filler worldwide. Numerous similar products from bacterial origin have also reached the market. The human body contains approximatively 15 g of hyaluronic acid (HA) distributed mainly in the connective tissue, and its primary function is to bind water.

Table 37.3   Numbers of treated patients and rates of granulomas, estimated from the literature. All numbers are disputable

Product	Persistence	Patients	Markets	Granuloma rates Authors	Granuloma rates Manufacturers
Collagen (Zyderm®, Zyplast®)	6 months	> 5 million	USA 1982 Worldwide 1983	~1:300	~1:2500*
Hyaluronic acid (Restylane®, Hylaform®)	6 months	> 3 million	Europe 1998 Worldwide 2001 USA 2004	~1:250	~1:2500*
PLA microspheres (Sculptra®/New-Fill®)	> 12 months	> 250 000	Europe 1999 USA 2004	~1:400 (in 5 ml suspended)	~1:500*
Ca-hydroxyapatite microspheres (Radiance®/Radiesse®)	> 12 months	> 150 000	USA 2002 Europe 2004	~1:600	Very few
HEMA particles (Dermalive®)	> 12 months	> 200 000	Europe 1998 Canada 2003	~1:100	~1:500*
PMMA microspheres (Artecoll®)	Permanent	> 400 000	Europe 1994 Worldwide 1998	~1:650	~1:5000*
Silicone gel (3.5 cSt)	Permanent	> 400 000	USA 1953 Banned 1992	~1:1000	No data
Polyacrylamide gel (Aquamid®, Bio-Alcamid®)	Permanent	> 200 000	Russia 1983 China 1998 Europe 2002	No data	~1:5000*

The half-life of an injected molecule is only 1–2 days, so the manufacturers have cross-linked molecules to achieve 3–6 months' duration period with injectable HA (no proof exists that it lasts longer then any of the collagen products). Its absorption has a similar pattern to that with collagen: mainly by hydrolytic enzymes, some macrophages, and scattered giant cells.[35]

Hyaluronic acid (Hylan G-F 20, Synvisc®) is also injected into osteoarthritic knee joints, and several cases have been reported of granulomatous inflammation with palisading granulomas and prominent histiocytic and giant cell cuffing, which required synovectomy.[61] Late complications after dermal injections appear to be similar to those reported with collagen. Early reported complications, such as long-lasting erythema and induration, have been blamed on fermentation residues from *Streptococcus equi*;[2,11,12,62] Bergeret-Galley[63] reports a rate of 12 FBGs in 10 000 patients (0.1%) before further cleaning of Restylane during manufacturing was implemented in 2000, and four cases in 10 000 patients (0.04%) since 2000. But a number of publications between 2000 and 2005[22,29,64–72] describe late adverse events such as localized granulomatous inflammations (Figure 37.2), and, adding up these numbers, one arrives at a granulomatous rate of 0.8%. If one takes into account the low manufacturer's rate reported by Friedman et al,[12] it diminishes to 0.03%. The problem with all the above statistics is clearly exposed: most late adverse events after fillers are not reported to the

manufacturers, so until official statistics are available we should rely on those of single physicians, providing that they report a large number of patients, thus excluding the technical errors of the beginning for a given implant (Tables 37.1 and 37.3).

The histology of HA FBGs is similar to that of collagen FBGs, with palisaded granulomatous tissue, macrophages, and giant cells.[73] This granulomatous tissue often encapsulates the injected HA like a 'sterile abscess', giving the histological picture of a 'cystic granuloma' and preventing absorption of the HA injected. Whether these are 'delayed hypersensitivity reactions' or a special kind of FBG has yet to be proven. In some cases,[20,74,75] a predominantly lymphocytic and plasmatic infiltrate with scattered giant cells has been found. An impressive histological picture is shown by Fernandez-Acenero et al.[74]

Clinically, the granuloma develops 2–11 months after injection, with intense redness and induration, and lasts 2–10 months without treatment. Although some were treated with intralesional triamcinolone,[62,76] most cases resolved without treatment within 1 year. Systemic or local antibiotics were ineffective, but puncture and squeezing out the whitish gel sped up the resolution.[62] Surgical excision of this cellular reaction[77] will certainly be the last solution. Interestingly, Lambros[78] reports the case of a woman who developed lumps in her tear troughs 1 week after injection of a hyaluronic acid filler, which immediately disappeared after intralesional injections of hyaluronidase. This possibility for the treatment of early nodules of hyaluronic acid by depolymerization should be kept in mind.

PMMA microspheres (Arteplast®/Artecoll/Artefill)

Artecoll (Rofil Medical, The Netherlands) and Artefill (Artes Medical, CA) are a 20% suspension of non-resorbable microspheres of PMMA in bovine collagen. PMMA is known to be an inert substance that has been used as bone cement powder for over 50 years in millions of patients. The microspheres are round with smooth surfaces, 30–40 μm in diameter. First the collagen is replaced by a granulation tissue, later by a fibrous tissue. The microspheres act as a stimulus for constant tissue regeneration so that ultimately the Artecoll implant consists of 80% of the patient's own connective tissue.[13]

Artecoll's predecessor, Arteplast®, contained a high number of nanoparticles (less than 20 μm), which was the cause of a high 2.5% rate of FBGs until 1994.[64,65] When the dry sieving process was changed to wet sieving in 1994, the number of nanoparticles in Artecoll was drastically reduced, and the rate of granulomas dropped below 0.1% between 1995 and 2002.[13] True sclerosing FBGs after Artecoll implantation have been reported since 1994,[6,13,35,47,66–69] and, from all cases reported to manufacturers worldwide, the occurrence rate is estimated at 0.02% (Tables 37.1 and 37.3). Since the FDA required even stricter controls on microsphere dimensions for US clinical testing in January 2003, an improvement was made to a third-generation product Artefill (Artes Medical, CA), and the rate of FBGs is expected to further diminish.

The pathologists Requena[47] and Lombardi[6] and their groups gave a detailed description of Artecoll FBGs. The histology reveals round and empty vacuoles (after alcohol dissolution of the PMMA) in wide distances from one another: 2–3 times the diameter of a microsphere, instead of the usual 0.5–1. The tissue between the vacuoles consists of many multinucleated giant cells and macrophages attached to the vacuoles, with many fibroblasts and collagen fibers in between. Occasionally, lymphocytic infiltrates and epitheloid cells are seen (Figure 37.2c).

Clinically, the FBGs develop many months or years following implantation. In a matter of weeks and at approximately the same time, all injected areas show a mild inflammation, with uncomfortable tension but no pain. Nodules become visible, rather hard, and often bluish with congested dermal capillaries on their surface (Figure 37.2a). One of the authors (NG) saw a granuloma develop as late as 10 years after injection, which responded well to high doses of local steroids and a pulsed-light treatment.

Because of the high amount of fibrous network produced in these granulomas, intralesional corticosteroid injections are the best treatment. A few cases of resistance to this treatment have been signaled, but it is our belief that they were due to insufficient initial doses of steroids. If widened capillaries remain, they can be treated by different types of light therapy. Excision should be the very last option (as with all granulomas) because of the FBG insertions into the surrounding tissue.

PLA microspheres (New-Fill/Sculptra)

Sculptra (formerly New-Fill) is a suspension of microspheres composed of resorbable crystalline PLA in methylcellulose, presented as a lyophilisate (Avantis, Europe/Dermik Laboratories, PA). It was introduced to the European market in 1999, with recommendations to dilute it in 3 ml of water for injection and to implant it intradermally as well as subdermally. By 2002 intradermal implantations had been discarded, and physicians reached a consensus to raise the dilution to 5 ml minimum, resulting in a lower rate of granulomas. Renamed Sculptra, it was introduced to the US market in 2004.

In surgery, aliphatic polyesters have been used safely and widely in resorbable suture materials (Vicryl®, Dexon®) and are resorbed within 3–6 months by hydrolytic enzymes and a few macrophages, lymphocytes, and scattered giant cells.[6,70] Large quantities of crystalline PLA microspheres may last up to 2 years.[71,72] PLA is partly dissolved by hydrolysis; the lactate enters the Krebs cycle and is metabolized to CO_2 and water, and partly phagocytosed. Injected PLA microspheres cause a typical foreign body 'reaction' which is the true histological substrate of the filling effect (and not the fibrosis as reported in references 71 and 72): the moment the last PLA bead is absorbed, the induced fibrosis probably recedes as well.[22]

PLA has an excellent biocompatibility profile, but the occurrence of FBGs associated with PLA suture materials is well known to surgeons, usually in the form of extrusions. In orthopedic surgery, PLA in absorbable plates and screws is also known to have produced some delayed hypersensitivity reactions resulting in the development of FBGs. Similar anecdotal cases have been reported after New-Fill injections.[24,73,79–83] The occurrence rate varies from one author to another,[24,84,85] (Vleggaar, personal communication) and overall an estimated rate of 0.4% appears to reflect the reality (Table 37.1). It is expected to further diminish since the dilution of the beads has been raised to 5 ml.

Clinically the granuloma appears 6–24 months after implantation, and involves all injected areas with visible, rather hard nodules, often bluish. If left untreated they remain for 2–5 years, very slowly subsiding. They respond to high doses of steroid injections (Figure 37.5), advantageously combined with intense pulsed-light (IPL) therapy. Here too, resistance to intralesional

Library
College of Physicians & Surgeons of B.C.
400 – 858 Beatty Street
Vancouver BC V6B 1C1

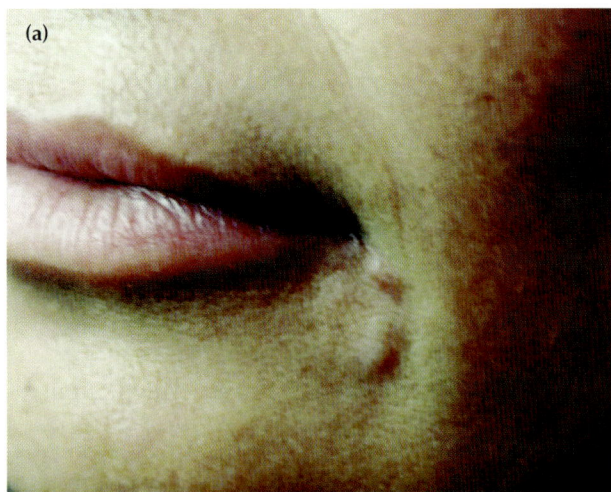

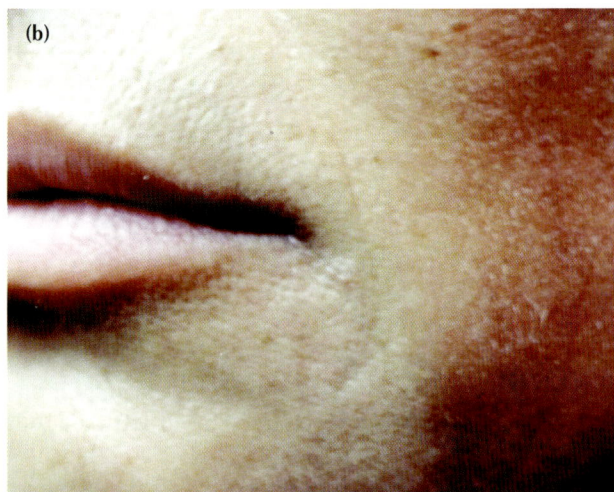

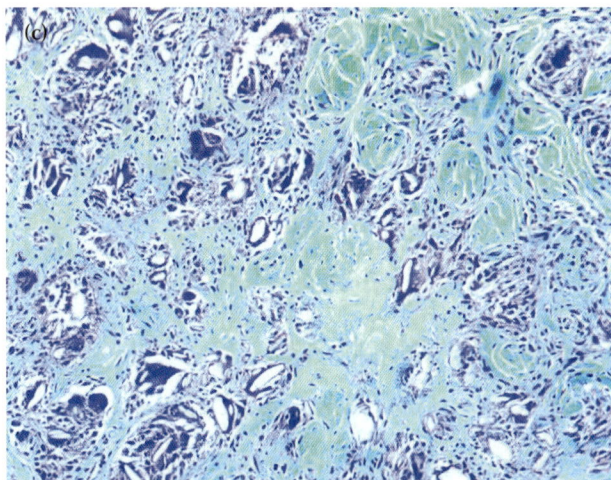

Figure 37.5   (a) Sclerosing granulomas in both marionette lines that developed 18 months after New-Fill® injections. New-Fill granulomas can remain for many years if left untreated. (b) Effective treatment with 2×5 mg betamethasone undiluted intralesionally with a concomitant intense pulsed-light (IPL) treatment (NG). (c) Histology of a New-Fill granuloma shows multiple giant cells surrounding the residues of poly-L-lactic acid (PLA) microspheres.

steroids has been experienced, but the initial doses were probably insufficient and/or the implantation too superficial. Excision should not be an option.

Histologically, it is a typical sclerosing FBG in which the PLA beads have lost their round shape due to the advance of their absorption by hydrolysis; they are seen as numerous translucent particles of irregular shape and size, some of which are very small and spiky. The particles, birefringent in polarized light (Figure 37.5c), are surrounded by macrophages, a few lymphocytes, and many giant cells, some of which contain asteroid bodies.[6]

In one study[71] in 50 human immunodeficiency virus (HIV)+ patients with facial lipodystrophy, large volumes (up to 32 ml in maximum five sessions) of New-Fill diluted at 3 ml were injected into the cheeks. No serious side-effects were observed but 44% of the patients had palpable but non-visible nodules of 3–5 mm in size over the entire period of 96 weeks, with spontaneous resolution in six patients only. It might well be that suspending the microspheres in 5 ml and using the microdroplet technique prevents

this nodule formation, which may be due to clumping of the beads immediately after injection.

HEMA particles (Dermalive/Dermadeep)

Dermalive (Dermatech SA, France) is a 40% solution of resorbable HEMA fragments (10–60 µm) in cross-linked hyaluronic acid of bacteriological origin.[15] It is a by-product of the manufacture of intraocular lenses, and was introduced to the European market in 1998. Because of a rather high incidence of FBGs, it is now mainly used in the form of Dermadeep, with HEMA fragments of 80–110 µm in size, recommended for deep dermal and epiperiosteal implantation. Since hypersensitivity reactions and FBGs occur much less in the subcutaneous tissue and are also less visible, Dermadeep will surely cause fewer side-effects – as did Bioplastique[86] when implanted epiperiosteally compared to subdermally.

The histology of a Dermalive implant looks promising within the first few months since the hydrophilic,

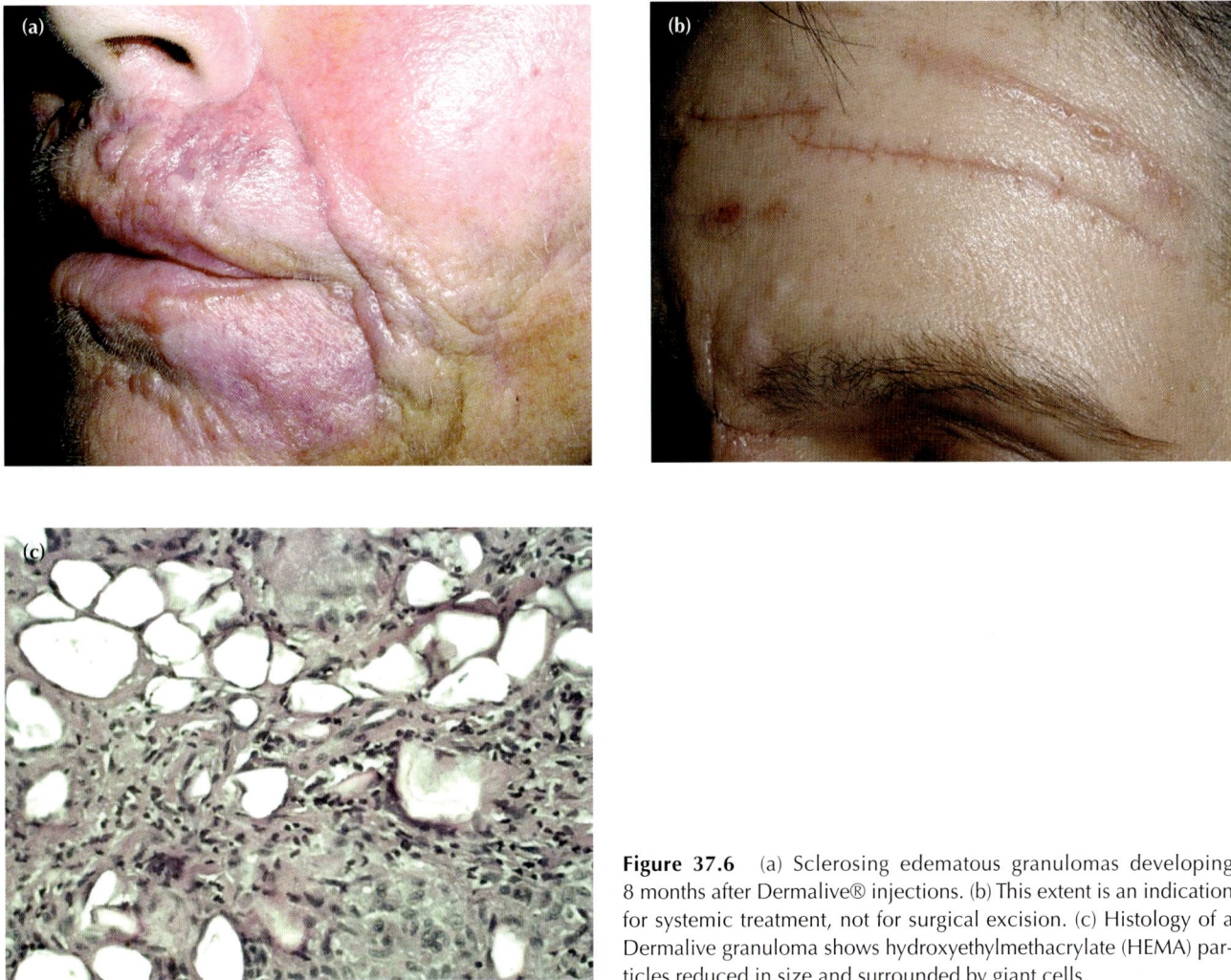

Figure 37.6   (a) Sclerosing edematous granulomas developing 8 months after Dermalive® injections. (b) This extent is an indication for systemic treatment, not for surgical excision. (c) Histology of a Dermalive granuloma shows hydroxyethylmethacrylate (HEMA) particles reduced in size and surrounded by giant cells.

polygonal, translucent, non-birefringent particles swell and round up.[22] At an early stage the HEMA particles are packed closely inside the implant, and the hyaluronic acid carrier is found in separate pools outside the clusters of particles.[22] This is probably due to diminished viscosity of the hyaluronic acid carrier medium (in contrast to the high viscosity and persistence of collagen as a carrier). Tissue ingrowth is non-existent at this stage, and the histology gives the picture of an inert and ideal biocompatible substance. Since little host tissue formation is stimulated, more Dermalive has to be injected compared to other fillers. On the other hand, HEMA has a free OH group, which should stimulate macrophage activity. Endogenous esterases in serum and the liver break down HEMA.

Interestingly, the amount of tissue reaction is no indication of the rate of granuloma formation: Dermalive causes the least foreign body 'reaction', but reports indicate that it causes the highest rate of late FBGs in Europe (Tables 37.1 and 37.3), even though the claim of the manufacturer is that of a 0.225% incidence.

If a granuloma formation occurs (Figure 37.6c), lymphocytic infiltrates increase, the fibrillar network thickens, and giant cells appear suddenly, forming islands in a patchy distribution, some of them containing asteroid bodies.[6,47]

Clinically, granulomas occur 6 months to 3 years after Dermalive implantation.[6,87,88] Some patients react with discoloration and telangiectasia, others with edematous sclerosis in the surrounding dermis (Figure 37.6a). It should be treatable with high doses of intralesional steroid injections (see Figure 37.9), but some cases of resistance to steroids have been experienced. One of our group (MW) saw a 63-year-old patient suddenly develop a generalized granulomatosis of about 1000 red infiltrates (up to 3 cm in diameter), 1 year after perioral Dermalive injections and 6 months after laser resurfacing. They did not react to local steroids and 5-FU injections. Another of our group (ME-K) saw one patient develop a localized sclerosing edema at all injection sites in the face, and who is still under systemic steroids as well as surgical treatment (Figure 37.6).

Calcium hydroxyapatite microspheres (Radiance/Radiesse)

Microspheres of this well-known constituent of bone and teeth suspended in methylcellulose had been developed for the treatment of urinary incontinence,[89] and received FDA approval for injection into a paralyzed vocal cord, as a tissue marker, and as an onlay graft in oral surgery. Since October 2001, Radiance FN, renamed Radiesse, a suspension of round and smooth (25–45 μm) calcium hydroxyapatite microspheres in methylcellulose, has been used off-label in the USA for wrinkle treatment and lip augmentation. While Radiesse is well tolerated beneath wrinkles, it should not be recommended for lip augmentation, where the orbicularis muscle compresses every injected strand to a lump (Figure 37.3). A rather high incidence of nodule formation in the lip,[90,91] where steroid injections are ineffective, has led to caution.

So far, no independent physician has published a study on the long-term effect with Radiesse. True granuloma formation in the above sense has been reported only twice to the main clinical investigators between 2002 and 2004, in approximately 35 000 patients treated in the USA (Graivier, personal communication). This may be due to the little cellular reaction and the few macrophages that Radiesse stimulates,[22] as well as dissolution of the calcium microspheres through predominantly enzymatic activity. One of the cases reported was that of a male acne patient who received 0.55 ml of Radiesse in many depressed scars on both cheeks and who developed nodules, mainly in three areas, far beyond the prior injection sites (3 × 2 × 0.5 cm). Low doses of steroid (up to 15 mg) caused only short-lasting improvement and, as a result, the biggest inflamed area was excised. Histologically, calcium hydroxyapatite triggers little tissue ingrowth and a complete absence of granulomatous tissue. Corticosteroid injections will only be effective if Radiesse microspheres have induced a kind of foreign body reaction.

The only study on long-term effects and adverse events of 609 patients after Radiesse treatment[23] revealed 42 of 338 subjects (12.4%) with lip nodules. However, the histology of one excised nodule (their Figure 5) shows clearly a FBG – and not 'densely packed' microspheres as histology of a normal Radiesse specimen does.[72]

Polyacrylamide gels (Aquamid®/Bio-Alcamid®)

Polyacrylamides are used as flocculants in industrial water clarification and, like dextran beads, in protein electrophoresis. Since its oral application caused stomach tumors in animals, the US Environmental Protection Agency classified monomer acrylamide as a medium-hazard probable human carcinogen.[92]

The use of polyacrylamide as an injectable filler material was initiated in 1983[93] and applied clinically in thousands of patients in Russia as Formacryl® (Interfall Ltd, Ukraine), and in China as Interfall® or 'Amazing Gel' (FuHua Aesthetics Ltd, China). These gels have been injected in large quantities in breast, buttock, and calf augmentation as well as in facial lipodystrophy and congenital malformations.[93] Because of its perfect early biocompatibility, Formacryl was called an 'endoprosthesis'.[94] It is estimated that 30 000 patients[95] received polyacrylamide injections in Kiev. However, during the past 4 years there have been about 20 articles in the Russian and Chinese literature[92,96,97] with figures and descriptions of dislocated, perforated, and hardened 'endoprostheses', which are then difficult to remove. Polyacrylamide clinical and histological behavior is very similar to that of silicone fluid. Its good biocompatibility does not stimulate capsule formation and even less cellular ingrowth,[97] which is the reason for its ease of dislocation when injected in large quantities. In patients with very loose connective tissue, large quantities have 'migrated' – or more accurately dislocated – from the face to the neck, from the breast to the groin, or from the buttock to the hollow of the knee.[97] Recently, polyacrylamides have been banned as injectables in Russia and in Bulgaria – and China is considering a similar step.

Since Interfall's European patent expired in 1995, at least five European companies are marketing polyacrylamides as dermal fillers: Argiform® (which contains antibacterial silver ions), Outline® (absorbable), Evolution® (non-resorbable microspheres in fast absorbing polyacrylamide),[22] Aquamid, and Bio-Alcamid.[98] They may all differ in the amount of free endings; Aquamid[99] has more of them because it is less cross-linked. Aquamid (Contura International SA, Denmark), approved in Europe but not in North America, is a clear 2.5% cross-linked gel from polyacrylamide (PAAG). The manufacturer of a similar product, Bio-Alcamid (Polymekon, Italy), approved in Europe, Israel, and Mexico, reveals its chemical formula as polyalkylimide,[100] probably an acrylamide polymer cross-linked with imide–amide and an additional alkylene group (US patent 20040209997). In an early stage after implantation, it can be withdrawn through a 14G needle if overcorrection or dislocation should occur.

Polyacrylamide FBGs are generally of the 'inflammatory' or 'edematous' type (Figure 37.7). They often begin with a granulomatous stage containing basophilic mononuclear cells and giant cells which corresponds to a tender capsule formation. It is followed by a seromatous stage with fluid accumulation within the capsule and consequent tension, pain, and surrounding edema.[95] Perivascular and focal aggregates of lymphoid cells, and inflammatory walls with macrophages that have phagocytosed PAAG, can lead to a sterile abscess, necrosis, and perforation[96] (Figure 37.8a). Stab incisions have generally led to fistula formation. The involvement of bacteria in the 'biofilm' surrounding PAAG as a cause of FBGs has been suggested;[101] proof for this is insufficient so far.

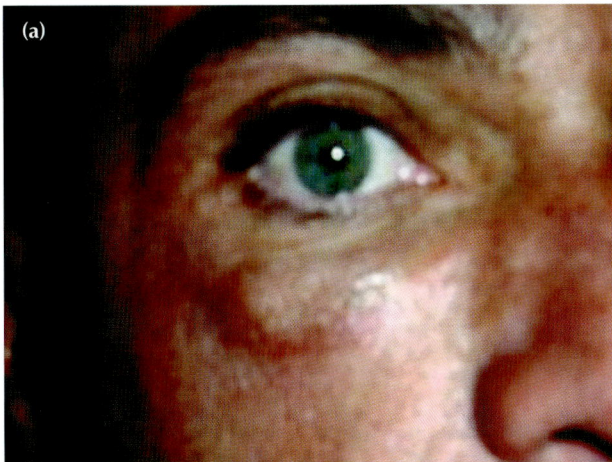

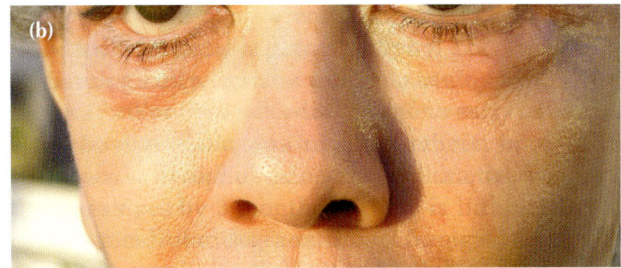

Figure 37.7   (a) Edematous granuloma occurring 12 months after Bio-Alcamid® injection. There was no resolution by puncture or under local or systemic triamcinolone. (b) Edematous granulomas in both cheeks and lower lids, 9 months after Interfall® injections.

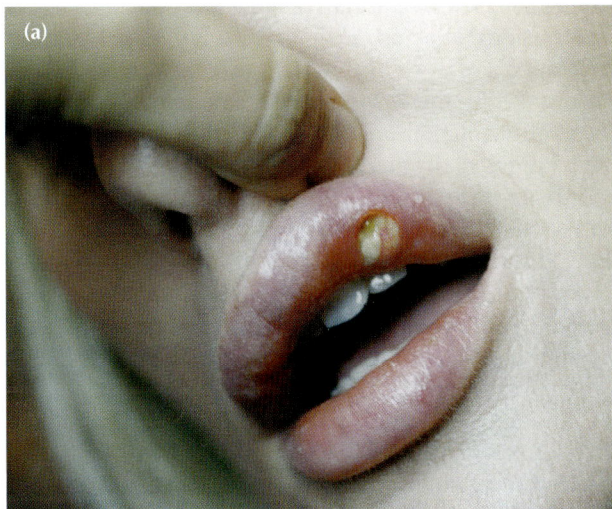

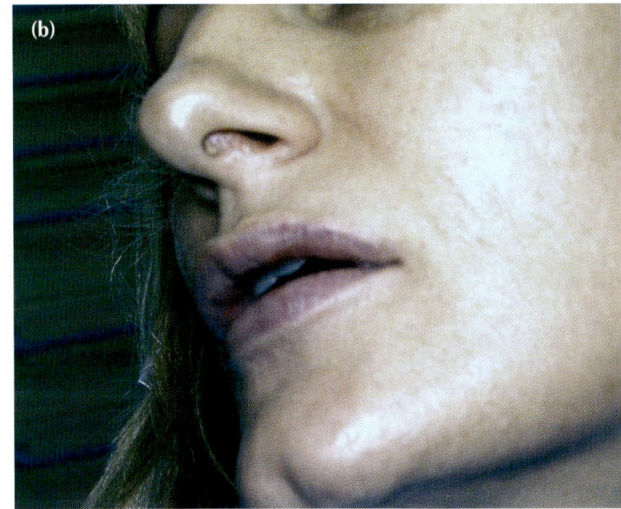

Figure 37.8   (a) Secondarily infected granuloma from acrylamide with consequent ulceration. (b) After surgical removal and closure – and 40 mg methylprednisolone into the residual upper lip granulomas, once (NG).

The Russian articles have described severe side-effects after polyacrylamide injections,[95–97] of which three-quarters of the reported complications were palpable indurations, probably all FBGs. Other complications reported were enlarged and palpable lymph nodes in 12%, migration of gel in 3%, and edema in 2%.[102] The Chinese papers mention an overall complication rate ranging from 1.4 to 18.2%, among which palpable indurations and aseptic inflammations are the most frequent.[103–105] Mazzoleni et al[94] describe four FBGs among 626 patients (0.3%) treated between 1997 and 1999. In our own experience with Aquamid (MW), in 35 patients one developed a FBG after 5 months. Two FBGs on Aquamid have been reported in the USA.[106]

Possible causes of granuloma formation (Table 37.4)

Why do all these injectable dermal fillers cause late and sudden foreign body granulomas in very rare patients after months and years of inconspicuous integration in the skin?

The injected volume of a dermal filler has been blamed to be a cause of granuloma formation.[30,37] In fact, the first messenger cell is the macrophage, of 10–20 μm in diameter, and it cannot recognize the size of the material it is supposed to phagocytose, whether it is 2 mm or 2 cm in diameter. Furthermore, the microdroplet technique, which produces a much larger surface area than a single injection of a bigger volume, should theoretically stimulate many more macrophages and yield more granulomas, which is not the case. The concentration of particles within the implant could play a role in the incidence of FBGs, since it has been observed that PLA diluted at more then 5 ml yields less granuloma than PLA diluted at 3 ml, but this is still lacking scientific proof. Equally, there is no proof today that the additional injection of a different filler into the same location will trigger or activate a FBG of the prior substance.

The concentration of impurities within a filler substance has been blamed convincingly,[13,26,28] since the

Table 37.4   Reported possible connections to infections or trauma that occurred 3–6 months before the onset of foreign body granulomas (FBGs)

Systemic infections[13,26,52,107,108]
Sinusitis[15]
Pharyngitis[15]
Bronchitis[15]
Pneumonia (MW)
Severe flu (MW)
Pleurisy[95]
Enteritis (NG)
Flu-like syndrome[7]
Autoimmune thyreosis (NG)
Hyperthyreosis[109] (MW)
Colitis ulcerosa[101]
Crohn's disease[101]
Pemphigus[101]
Sarcoidosis (NG)
Breast cancer (NG)
Psychological shock[15]
Encephabol®[35]
Facial trauma[35]
Facelift operation[101]

Table 37.5   Reported successful treatment regimens of FBGs

Triamcinolone (Kenalog®, Volon A®) 20–40 mg intralesionally[111,112]
Prednisolone (Depo-Medrol®) 40–80 mg undiluted (NG)
Betamethasone (Diprosone®) 5–7 mg intralesionally[15]
1/3 Diprosone (3.5 mg + 1/3 5-fluorouracil (5-FU) (1.6 ml) + 1/3 lidocaine intralesionally[113]
Kenalog (1 mg/ml) + 5-FU (50 mg/ml) intralesionally[114,115]
Intralesional steroids (high doses) + intense pulsed light (NG)

FBG rate of almost all filler substances has decreased as product improvements have been developed over the years.[13,63] In Arteplast/Artecoll/Artefill,[13] the correlation shown between the drastic decrease of the number of small particles (less than 20 μm) in each product and the significant decrease of FBG formation is an example. Obviously, phagocytosis and therefore the immunological memory of the macrophages are far more stimulated by many small particles than by a few big ones. On the other hand, in some injectable fluids such as silicone and acrylamide, a supposed difference in the amount of impurities between 'industrial grade' and 'medical grade' was incriminated; in reality the composition is the same: a 'medical grade' product has only been subjected to more biological testing (toxicity, pyrogenicity, histology, etc.) and has been submitted in a masterfile to the FDA.[110]

The irregularity of the particle surface appears to be another cause of increased granuloma formation. The best examples are the high incidence of FBGs with Teflon® flakes, Bioplastique clouds,[107] and Dermalive particles with pointed edges and corners. Interestingly, the amount of early foreign body reaction does not relate at all to later formation of FBGs, as seen in the cases of Dermalive, acrylamides, and silicone: these substances show the same lack of cellular ingrowth as Radiesse[24] during the first months after injection.

The only events that have been detected significantly to trigger FBGs are severe systemic infections.[13,26,52,107,108] Patients with permanent injectables should be warned, and cautioned to take antibiotics at the very onset of a severe infection for the next 10 years following implantation. One of the authors (NG) saw FBGs on an Artecoll

implantation, occurring 1 month after an episode of severe bronchitis, another after surgery for sinusitis, and two after acute abdominal infections. In one case the FBG developed 2 years after Artecoll injection and 3 months after the diagnosis of an autoimmune thyroiditis. One patient injected with LIS for lip augmentation developed a silicone FBG 6 years after the procedure and 8 months after the onset of a systemic sarcoidosis. After New-Fill implantation, one patient developed a granuloma immediately after the discovery of advanced breast cancer, another at the onset of a vocal cord tumor, and one at the onset of a new hormone replacement therapy (HRT) treatment. Christensen et al[101] describe a patient who had a facelift 2 months before the onset of a FBG. A patient in one case[109] was diagnosed with hyperthyreosis 2 years after Artecoll injections, and developed FBGs which disappeared with thyreostatic treatment. One of the authors (GL) saw[35] a woman who developed redness and swelling at all Artecoll implantation sites each time she took pyritinol (Encephalbol®). Bergeret-Galley et al[15] report that 12% of their patients who developed FBGs did so during or after infections (bronchitis, pharyngitis, and sinusitis) or a severe psychological shock. Bigata et al[7] describe a patient who developed granulomatous lips 8 months after silicone injections and 1 week after a flu-like syndrome. A case of pleurisy[95] was thought to be the cause of granulomas with scleromyxedema of the skin after hyaluronic acid injections. Another patient acquired severe flu with polynephritis and subsequent inflammatory redness at all injected sites, and because she was in her lactation period she refused antibiotics and steroids. However, the redness and the infiltrations in her face subsided when she finally took the treatment later on.

Obviously, granuloma formation is a single event triggered by a traumatic, infectious, immunologic, or pharmacological stimulus (Table 37.4). If treated early and with sufficient doses of steroids, it does not recur.

The treatment of granulomas and implant nodules (Tables 37.5 and 37.6)

FBGs consist mainly of a cellular multiplication which has, by itself, little therapeutic effect: most particulate

Table 37.6   Anecdotal treatment possibilities of FBGs

Triamcinolone intralesionally + cryotherapy[114]
Bleomycin (1.5 IU/ml) intralesionally[116]
Prednisone (1 mg/kg/day) orally[58]
Prednisone (60 mg/day) orally + ibuprofen (1800 mg/day)
Cortivazol (3.75 mg/1.5 ml) intralesionally
Minocycline (2 × 100 mg/day) orally[58]
Minocycline (2 × 250 mg/day) + prednisolone (4 mg/day)[65]
Cyclosporine (5 mg/kg/day) orally[43]
Allopurinol (200–600 mg/day)[65]
Imiquimod (Aldara®) cream 5%[43,79]
Tacrolimus cream 0.5%[117]
Laser 532 nm and 1064 nm[42]

or artificial materials – even resorbable ones – cannot be broken down faster by a granuloma formation. Granulomas are more a sign of a frustrated reaction, such as the conglomeration of macrophages into giant cells, in no way more effective. The goals in the treatment of FBGs must be to stop the multiplication of cells, as well as the increased secretion of interstitial substances, to restore the normal appearance of the skin, and to leave no scar.

Intralesional injections of steroids

Triamcinolone decreases both cellular proliferation and collagen production by dermal fibroblasts. Alteration of cytokine levels[118] may mediate these effects, for example an increased production of transforming growth factor (TGF)-β1 by the dermal fibroblasts.

In a rat model,[119] dexamethasone drastically interferes with both synthesis and degradation of type I and III collagen and significantly decreases fibril collagen content, which explains why it impairs wound healing and causes occasional skin atrophy. Local steroids suppress all aspects of acute and chronic inflammatory processes. They inhibit[111] fibroblast activity and collagen deposition, macrophage activity, and giant cell formation, and clinically they reduce the swelling, itching, or pain.

Therefore, the attempt of radical surgical removal of FBGs is never indicated in the first place. The treatment of choice is – as soon as possible – the strictly intralesional injection of triamcinolone (Kenalog®, Volon A®)[120] or betamethasone (Diprosone®)[15] or methylprednisolone (Depo-Medrol®, Pharmacia & Upjohn) (Table 37.5). Intralesional triamcinolone has FDA approval for the treatment of keloids, hypertrophic scars, and granuloma annulare but not for FBGs – even though it has been the treatment of choice for FBGs since the early 1960s.[112]

The initial dose has to be sufficiently high (Figure 37.9), making temporary skin depression a risk but thereby avoiding recurrences of the FBG. So far inexplicable is the fact that FBGs treated with sufficiently high initial doses of corticosteroids very seldom recur, contrary to low frequent doses which often result in insufficient treatment and recurrences.

Technique

Because of their high cellular content, granulomas are much easier to inject than nodules. A 1:1 mixture of lidocaine and triamcinolone (Kenalog or Volon) or methylprednisolone (Depo-Medrol) up to 40 mg, or betamethasone (Diprosone) up to 7 mg, can be injected safely through a 1-ml insulin syringe (eventually a Luer Lock) and a 30G needle. Methylprednisolone and betamethasone are often injected undiluted, but this is

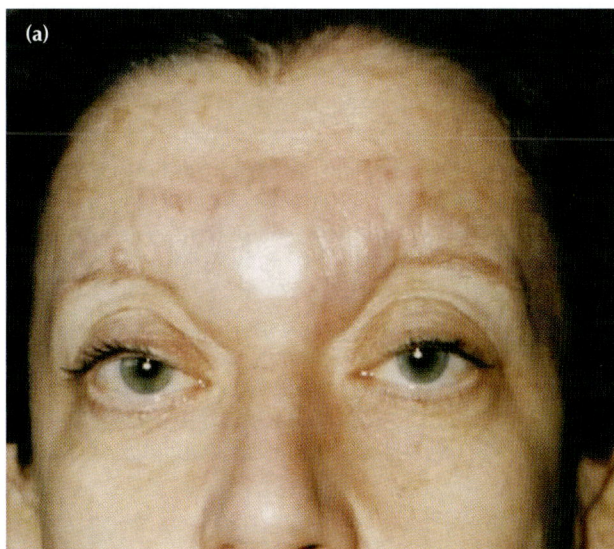

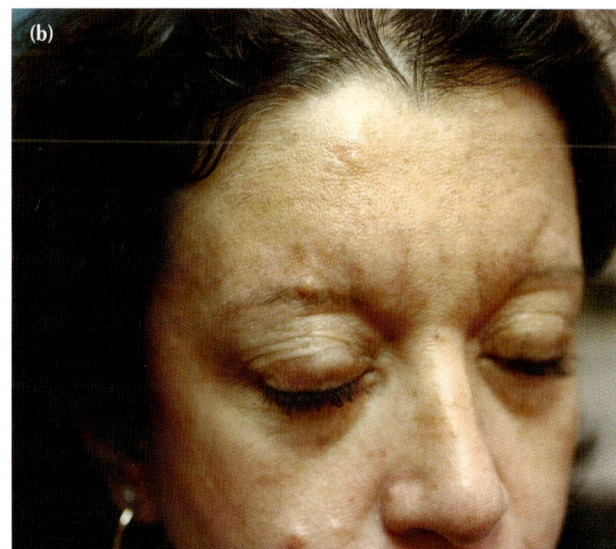

Figure 37.9   (a) Dermalive FBGs 2 years after injection and 3 months after onset. (b) Total resolution after intralesional methylprednisolone 80 mg. However, there was recurrence 9 months later: methylprednisolone 80 mg, then 30 mg 3 months after. Touch-up 1 month later: betamethasone 5 mg and concomitant IPL treatment. There has been no recurrence for 2 years (NG).

not recommended for triamcinolone. The injection must be strictly into each nodule: the nodule is held firmly between two fingers while guiding the needle back and forth into its tight resistance. Since corticosteroids injected into the surrounding tissue may cause temporary skin atrophy, one should stop injecting as soon as the tight resistance to the injection pressure diminishes and start again from a different angle, until it releases the remaining tension in other parts. Two to five sessions at 3-week intervals may be necessary. The combination of triamcinolone injections with cryotherapy has been advocated.[114]

All formations with a high percentage of connective tissue content, such as implant nodules after Artecoll–Artefill/New-Fill–Sculptra/Bioplastique/Reviderm Intra/Matridex, and genuine FBGs of these products, react well to intralesional crystalline corticosteroids. The same volume reduction can be expected if nodules are accidentally dislocated by muscle movement, if too much implant material was injected, or if hypertrophic scarring occurred because of superficial intradermal injection.

There is an inherent reserve against local corticosteroids in many physicians because they can cause skin atrophy in 20–30% of patients, independent of dose. The patient should be fully aware of this side-effect. Since every patient reacts differently to corticosteroids, a way to prevent skin atrophy could be to test the appropriate dose first with a lower one:[68] if there is no improvement after 2–4 weeks, the dose should be doubled. However, in some cases of huge keloids in Asian and African children, up to 160 mg of triamcinolone intralesionally was injected every 4 weeks over a period of 6 months until the keloids remained flat, and we cannot recall any visible systemic effect in these children.

In the case of a skin atrophy,[115] temporary filling with collagen or hyaluronic acid[111] will level the indentation until natural recovery occurs within 3–12 months.[15]

If this therapy is begun early and aggressively, surgical excision will not be an issue. In general, the resolution of granulomas and nodules by corticoids is a matter of dosage, compliance, guidance, and patience on both sides. Some lumps will be reduced satisfactorily after one shot (Figure 37.2b). Some may require 6–10 injections over a period of 3–6 months. Some may recur and need a touch-up treatment with triamcinolone or another steroid. Some react preferably to betamethasone or methylprednisolone, which are supposed to be less damaging for the surrounding tissue than triamcinolone. Some may react to cytostatics alone.

Antimitotic agents

The risk of cortisone skin atrophy might be reduced by the injection of antimitotic agents such as 5-FU mixed with a third Diprosone and a third lidocaine 2% without epinephrine, injected intralesionally every 3 weeks, if necessary.[113] The anti-inflammatory action is astonishing: the painful tension and redness sometimes associated with FBGs subsides immediately, growth stops, and the FBG diminishes within a few weeks.

The pure intralesional mixture of 1.6 ml of 5-FU (50 mg/ml) with 0.4 ml of betamethasone (7 mg/ml) has been shown to decrease cell proliferation and release collagenase activity within the granuloma.[113]

Besides inhibiting tumor growth, cytostatics inhibit collagen synthesis and are effective in the treatment of keloids and hypertrophic scars. From their 9 years' experience in treating hypertrophic scars, Fitzpatrick[121] and Narins[122] and their groups recommend pure 5-FU (50 mg/ml) intralesionally, or mixed with 1 mg/ml Kenalog. Frequent initial injections administered 1–3 times per week were found to be more efficacious than higher single doses.

Bleomycin (1.5 IU/ml) has been injected intralesionally into keloids and hypertrophic scars, and should work successfully in granulomas as well.[116]

Systemic corticoids

Systemic doses of corticosteroids must be much higher than those used for local intralesional injection. A starting dose of 30 mg/day of prednisone[41,46] had to be increased to 60 mg/day because of the recurrence of FBGs, and ibuprofen (1800 mg/day) had to be added in order to achieve a successful treatment in 16 weeks. At 2 years the patient remained asymptomatic.

Alternative drugs

Because many patients have experienced spontaneous improvement of their condition over time, at least five patients should be treated with every new regimen before it can be recommended as an effective therapy for FBGs (Table 37.6).

The following have been reported in the literature:

1. In one report[58] the authors relate the antigranulomatous properties of minocycline's immune-modulating effect in diffuse silicone granulomas developing 8 and 5 years after injection, respectively. Minocycline (2 ×100 mg daily) was the replacement therapy; the prednisolone treatment (1 mg/kg/day) had to be interrupted because of glucose intolerance.
2. Reisberger et al[65] successfully treated a patient with Arteplast granulomas on the forehead with allopurinol (an effective treatment for gout) at 200–600 mg/day administered over a period of 24 weeks.
3. Baumann and Kerdel[43] reported the successful treatment of a silicone FBG of the lips with an immune modulatory cream Aldara® (imiquimod 5%),

known to increase levels of interferon-α. The release of cytokines, interferon, and tumor necrosis factor (TNF) enhances antiproliferative properties and collagenase activity. The swollen lips improved dramatically after 2 weeks of topical treatment twice daily, and the applications could be stopped after 2 months of consecutive treatment. They also successfully treated acute allergy to bovine collagen with cyclosporine (5 mg/kg/day = 175 mg orally twice a day) as it did not respond to oral or intramuscular steroids (40 mg prednisone over 3 days and additional 9 mg celestone intramuscularly): after 2 weeks the reaction subsided.

4. Tacrolimus cream appears to be effective in granuloma annulare, and has solved the local symptoms of collagen allergy as well.[117] Tacrolimus has a similar mechanism of action to cyclosporine: both inhibit T-cell activation, interferon release, and the release of preformed mediators from mast cells and basophils.

5. Whether injections of hyaluronidase[78,123] work in Restylane-associated late FBGs is doubtful – maybe in the early stages in combination with triamcinolone. To our knowledge, the effect of injected collagenase into collagen nodules has not been reported.

The combined treatment of telangiectasia

One combination that has been beneficial with intralesional steroid injections is treatment of the area with a pulsed-light lamp (also called IPL or flashlamp). It is efficient on the blue discoloration of the skin over some sclerosing FBGs. Four or five sessions not only impede the neovascularization but also appear to soften and diminish the volume of the underlying granuloma – probably by reducing its blood supply from above.

Small non-inflammatory granulomas have responded well to long-pulsed 532-nm laser. Larger inflammatory granulomas have shown some favorable responses to 1064-nm long-pulsed laser.[42]

No surgical excisions!

Plastic surgeons tend to excise all lumps where they do not belong, whereas dermatologists in general try corticoid creams first. Both approaches are contraindicated in FBGs.

Surgical excision of genuine granulomas will be incomplete because of their insinuated invasiveness and their non-confined borders with the surrounding tissue. Attempts to excise and extricate injected fluids such as silicone or acrylamide met with dire results, causing fistulas, abscesses, continuous granulation tissue, and marked deformities.[112] In addition, a complete surgical excision will leave long scars on the face or the lips.

On the other hand, normal implant nodules and FBGs which have little capsule formation and little tissue ingrowth will not react to intralesional corticosteroids or antimitotic drugs at all: for example the cystic FBGs after collagen[124] or hyaluronic acid[125,126] and the packed nodules of Radiesse/Dermalive/silicone fluid/polyacrylamide gels. Especially in the lips, surgical removal of these cysts and nodules is probably the method of choice. Also, in a facial fold, if excision of misplaced material becomes necessary, the scar can be well hidden in that fold, especially in elderly patients.

In the soft tissue of the lips, when some hard nodules do not react to steroids and are disturbing to the patient, surgical excision always approached from the inside will be the best solution (Figure 37.8). In general, foreign body nodules can be removed, like a small atheroma, by blunt dissection (due to the presence of the fibrous capsule that develops within 3–6 months). In the vermilion, surgery is absolutely contraindicated because of the implant closeness to the thin dermis of the vermilion border ('white roll') and the possibility of uncontrolled scarring. Similarly, radical excisions of implants or genuine FBGs from enlarged lips should be avoided under all circumstances. We are aware of two cases of radical excision after lip augmentation, one in Frankfurt in 1998 and one in Stockholm in 2004: in both cases the orbicularis muscle had been compressed for years by the implants and could not recover at all (as we know it happens to fat and breast tissue after removal of the implant). Instead, stepwise horizontal volume reduction with the help of a 16G trocar should be tried.

Nevertheless, if surgery has been chosen and indentations or irregularities have occurred, they can be treated with superficial touch-ups of absorbable filler substances such as collagen or hyaluronic acid and/or additional corticoid injections if necessary.

Conclusion

All filler materials have side-effects: they can be diminished but not erased.

One fact is indisputable: the dermis is by far the most sensitive and allergic reacting organ: the deeper the implants are injected, the less is the possibility of FBG formation (see Bioplastique/Macroplastique® or Dermalive/Dermadeep) and the less is the visibility of that reaction if it should occur. Subdermal injections into the dermal–subdermal junction will definitely cause less FBG than intradermal injections.

The use of absorbable or non-absorbable tissue fillers has divided the community. Permanent implants are not followed by a higher rate of FBGs – per se – than temporary implants; however, their clinical appearance is usually more pronounced and their persistence longer if not treated adequately. Autologous fat injections pose a whole different kind of problem, and, even though they do not react with foreign body granulomas, they do not always represent an alternative!

It is estimated that the calculated range of occurring FBGs varies between 1:100 and 1:5000 patients, depending on the injectable used (Table 37.3).

The pathogenesis of FBGs is still not known. The injection of a large volume as a causative factor has been discussed,[28,42] but is still lacking statistical proof. The same is true with the microdroplet technique, which may theoretically prevent lumping and hardening but not FBGs. Chemical and particulate impurities have been blamed convincingly,[13,26,28] since the FBG rate of almost all filler substances has decreased as product improvements have been developed over the years.[13,63]

Dormant allergens with low immunogenicity are able to produce a clinical response during the boost in the immune system that occurs with infections and with HAART (highly active antiretroviral therapy; immune reconstitution syndrome). The memory of the macrophages and the mechanism of a later trigger such as infection or drugs could explain the unpredictability of FBG occurrence, even many years after absorption of the implant.[4] On the other hand, the lack of later proof of antibodies, eosinophilic cells, and positive skin tests does not exclude the possibility that the trigger of certain FBGs may be a late – type IV – cellular allergic reaction.

We, as physicians, should be aware of the rate of adverse events of each injectable filler substance, and we should never rely on the claims of manufacturers but on the reports of a still to be established independent 'Central Registry of Dermal Fillers'.[127] Better knowledge of the basics, and honesty in reporting, will bring improvement and safety – as well as effective treatment of side-effects – into this expanding field.

References

1. Rohrich RJ, Rios JL, Fagien S. Role of new fillers in facial rejuvenation: a cautious outlook. Plast Reconstr Surg 2003; 112: 1899–902.
2. Lowe N. New filler agents: what can we learn from Europe? Pract Dermatol September 2004: 29.
3. Coleman DL, King RN, Andrade JD. The foreign body reaction: a chronic inflammatory response. J Biomed Mater Res 1974; 8: 199–211.
4. Duffy D. Silicone: a critical review. Adv Dermatol 1990; 5: 93–107.
5. Moscona RR, Bergman R, Friedman-Birnbaum R. An unusual late reaction to Zyderm I injections: a challenge for treatment. Plast Reconstr Surg 1993; 92: 331–4.
6. Lombardi T, Samson J, Plantier F et al. Orofacial granuloma after injection of cosmetic fillers. Histopathologic and clinical study of 11 cases. J Oral Pathol Med 2004; 33: 115–20.
7. Bigata X, Ribera M, Bielsa I et al. Adverse granulomatous reaction after cosmetic dermal silicone injection. Dermatol Surg 2001; 27: 198–200.
8. Shapiro PE. Noninfectious granulomas. In: Elder D, Elenitsas R, Jaworsky C, Johnson B, eds. Lever's Histopathology of the Skin, 8th edn. Philadelphia: Lippincott Raven, 1997: 317–40.
9. Hanke, C.W. Adverse reactions to bovine collagen. In: Klein AW, ed. Tissue Augmentation in Clinical Practice: Procedures and Techniques. New York: Marcel Dekker, 1998: 145–54.
10. Cooperman LS, Mackinnon V, Bechler G et al. Injectable collagen: a six-year clinical investigation. Aesthetic Plast Surg 1985; 9: 145–51.
11. Shafir R, Amir A, Gur E. Long-term complications of facial injections with Restylane (injectable hyaluronic acid). Plast Reconstr Surg 2000; 106: 1215–16.
12. Friedman PM, Mafong EA, Kauvar NB et al. Safety data of injectable nonanimal stabilized hyaluronic acid gel for soft tissue augmentation. Dermatol Surg 2002; 28: 491–4.
13. Lemperle G, Romano JJ, Busso M. Soft tissue augmentation with Artecoll: 10-year history, indications, techniques, and complications. Dermatol Surg 2003; 29: 573–87.
14. Niechajev A. Lip enhancement: surgical alternatives and histologic aspects. Plast Reconstr Surg 2000; 105: 1173–83.
15. Bergeret-Galley C, Latouche X, Illouz Y-G. The value of a new filler material in corrective and cosmetic surgery: DermaLive and DermaDeep. Aesthetic Plast Surg 2001; 25: 249–55.
16. Bedir S, Kilciler M, Oezgoek Y, Deveci G, Erduran D. Long-term complication due to dextranomer based implant: granuloma causing urinary obstruction. J Urol 2004; 172: 247–8.
17. Charriere G, Bejot M, Schnitzler L et al. Reactions to a bovine collagen implant. J Am Acad Dermatol 1989; 21: 1203–8.
18. Castrow FF, Krull EA. Injectable collagen implant – update. J Am Acad Dermatol 1983; 9: 889–93.
19. Hanke CW, Higley HR, Jolivette DM et al. Abscess formation and local necrosis after treatment with Zyderm or Zyplast collagen implant. J Am Acad Dermatol 1991; 25: 319–26.
20. Lowe NJ, Maxwell A, Lowe P et al. Hyaluronic acid skin fillers: adverse reactions and skin testing. J Am Acad Dermatol 2001; 45: 930–3.
21. André P. Evaluation of the safety of a non-animal stabilized hyaluronic acid (NASHA, Q-Medical, Sweden) in European countries: a retrospective study from 1997 to 2001. J Eur Acad Dermatol Venereol 2004; 18: 422–5.
22. Lemperle G, Morhenn VB, Charrier U. Human histology and persistence of various injectable filler substances for soft tissue augmentation. Aesthetic Plast Surg 2003; 27: 354–66.
23. Jansen DA, Graivier MH. Evaluation of calcium hydroxylapatite-based implant (Radiesse) for facial soft-tissue augmentation. Plast Reconstr Surg 2006; 118: 22S.
24. Bauer U. Improvement of facial aesthetics at 40 months with injectable poly-L-lactic acid (PLLA). Presented at ISAPS Congress, Houston, TX, August 28–31, 2004: P164.
25. Greenberg JH. Information postal survey of selected physicians in dermatology. Amer Acad Dermatol Meeting, Dallas, TX, USA, December 1991.
26. Orentreich DS. Liquid injectable silicone. Techniques for soft tissue augmentation. Clin Plast Surg 2000; 27: 595–612.
27. Fulton JE Jr, Porumb S, Caruso JC, Shitabata PK. Lip augmentation with liquid silicone. Dermatol Surg 2005; 31: 1577.
28. Jones DH, Carruthers A, Orentreich D et al. Highly purified 1000-cSt silicone oil for treatment of human immunodeficiency virus-associated facial lipoatrophy: an open pilot trial. Dermatol Surg 2004; 30: 1279–86.
29. Naoum C, Dasiou-Plakida D, Pantelidaki K et al. A histological and immunhistochemical study of medical-grade fluid silicone. Dermatol Surg 1998; 24: 867–70.
30. Eppley BL, Summerlin D-J, Prevel CD et al. Effects of positively charged biomaterial for dermal and subcutaneous augmentation. Aesthetic Plast Surg 1994; 18: 413–16.
31. Hubmer MG, Hoffmann C, Popper H et al. Expanded polytetrafluoroethylene threads for lip augmentation induce

foreign body granulomaous reaction. Plast Reconstr Surg 1999; 103: 1277–9.

32. Maas CS, Gnepp DR, Bumpous J. Expanded polytetrafluoroethylene (Gore-Tex Soft Tissue Patch) in facial augmentation. Arch Otolaryngol Head Neck Surg 1993; 119: 1008–14.

33. Rudolph C, Soyer HP, Schuller-Petrovic S et al. Foreign body granulomas due to injectable aesthetic microimplants. Am J Surg Pathol 1999; 23: 113–17.

34. Williams CT, Williams WJ. Granulomatous inflammation – a review. J Clin Pathol 1983; 36: 723–33.

35. Lemperle G, Gauthier-Hazan N, Lemperle M. PMMA – microspheres (Artecoll) for long-lasting correction of wrinkles: refinements and statistical results. Aesthetic Plast Surg 1998; 22: 356–65.

36. Morgan AM. Localized reactions to injected therapeutic materials. J Cutan Pathol 1995; 22: 289–303.

37. Barr RJ, King F, McDonald RM et al. Necrobiotic granulomas associated with bovine collagen test site injections. J Am Acad Dermatol 1982; 6: 867–9.

38. Brooks N. A foreign body granuloma produced by an injectable collagen implant at a test site. J Dermatol Surg Oncol 1982; 8: 111–14.

39. Rapaport MJ, Vinnik C, Zarem H. Injectable silicone: cause of facial nodules, cellulites, ulceration, and migration. Aesthetic Plast Surg 1996; 20: 267–76.

40. Drake LA, Dinehart SM, Farmer ER et al. Guidelines of care for soft tissue augmentation: collagen implants. J Am Acad Dermatol 1996; 34: 698–702.

41. Garcia-Domingo MI, Alijtas-Reig J, Cistero-Bahima A et al. Disseminated and recurrent sarcoid-like granulomatous panniculitis due to bovine collagen injection. J Investig Allergol Clin Immunol 2000; 10: 107–9.

42. Duffy DM. Tissue injectable liquid silicone: new perspectives. In: Klein AW, ed. Tissue Augmentation in Clinical Practice: Procedures and Techniques. New York: Marcel Dekker, 1998: 237–63.

43. Baumann LS, Kerdel F. The treatment of bovine collagen allergy with cyclosporin. Dermatol Surg 1999; 25: 247–9.

44. Stegman SJ, Chu S, Armstrong RA. Adverse reactions to bovine collagen implant: clinical and histologic features. J Dermatol Surg Oncol 1988; 14 (Suppl): 39–48.

45. Heise H, Zimmermann R, Heise P. Temporary granulomatous inflammation following collagen implantation. J Craniomaxillofac Surg 2001; 29: 238–41.

46. Ficarra G, Mosqueda-Taylor A, Carlos R. Silicone granuloma of the facial tissue: a report of seven cases. Oral Surg Oral Med Oral Pathol 2002; 94: 65–73.

47. Requena C, Izquierdo MJ, Navarro M et al. Adverse reactions to injectable aesthetic microimplants. Am J Dermatopathol 2001; 23: 197–202.

48. Hexsel DM, Hexsel CL, Iyengar V. Liquid injectable silicone: history, mechanism of action, indications, technique, and complications. Semin Cutan Med Surg 2003; 22: 107–14.

49. Maas CS, Papel ID, Greene D et al. Complications of injectable synthetic polymers in facial augmentation. Dermatol Surg 1997; 23: 871–7.

50. Rohrich RJ, Potter JK. Liquid injectable silicone: is there a role as cosmetic soft-tissue filler? Plast Reconstr Surg 2004; 113: 1239–41.

51. Salmi R, Boari B, Manfredini R. Siliconoma: an unusual entity for the internist. Am J Med 2004; 116: 67.

52. Achauer BM. A serious complication following medical grade silicone injections of the face. Plast Reconstr Surg 1983; 71: 251–4.

53. Schoeller T, Gschnitzer C, Wechselberger G et al. Chronisch rezidivierende, local destruierende Silikonome nach Brustaugmentation durch fluessiges Silikonoel. Chirurg 2000; 71: 1370–3.

54. Spira M. Failure to remove soft tissue injected with liquid silicone with the use of suction and honesty in scientific medical reports. Plast Reconstr Surg 2000; 105: 1909.

55. Mupparapu M, Mozaffari E. Bilateral calcifications secondary to synthetic soft tissue augmentation of the cheeks: report of a case. Dentomaxillofac Radiol 2002; 31: 388–90.

56. Alani RM, Busam K. Acupuncture granulomas. J Am Acad Dermatol 2001; 45: S225–6.

57. Zimmermann US, Clerici TJ. The histological aspect of fillers complications. Semin Cutan Med Surg 2004; 23: 241–50.

58. Senet P, Bachelez H, Ollivaud L et al. Minocycline for the treatment of cutaneous silicone granulomas. Br J Dermatol 1999; 140: 985–7.

59. Moody BR, Sengelmann RD. Self-limited adverse reaction to human-derived collagen injectable product. Dermatol Surg 2000; 26: 936–8.

60. Rapaport MJ. Granuloma annulare caused by injectable collagen. Arch Dermatol 1984; 120: 837–8.

61. Chen AL, Desai P, Adler EM et al. Granulomatous inflammation after Hylan G-F 20 viscosupplementation of the knee: a report of six cases. J Bone Joint Surg Am 2002; 84-A: 1142–7.

62. Lupton JR, Alster TS. Cutaneous hypersensitivity reaction to injectable hyaluronic acid gel. Dermatol Surg 2000; 26: 135–7.

63. Bergeret-Galley C. Comparison of resorbable soft tissue fillers. Aesthetic Surg J 2004; 24: 33–46.

64. Mang WL, Sawatzki K. Fremdkoerperreaktion nach Implantation von PMMA (Polymethylmethacrylat) zur Weichteilaugmentation. Z Hautkrankheiten, H+G 1998; 73: 42–4.

65. Reisberger E-M, Landthaler M, Wiest L et al. Foreign body granulomas caused by polymethylmethacrylate microspheres. Arch Dermatol 2003; 139: 17–20.

66. Alcalay J, Alkalay R, Gat A et al. Late-onset granulomatous reaction to Artecoll. Dermatol Surg 2003; 29: 859–62.

67. Kim K-J, Lee H-W, Lee M-W et al. Artecoll granuloma: a rare adverse reaction induced by microimplant in the treatment of neck wrinkles. Dermatol Surg 2004; 30: 545–7.

68. Carruthers A, Carruthers J. Polymethylmethacrylate microspheres/collagen as a tissue augmenting agent: personal experience over 5 years. Dermatol Surg 2005; 31: 1561–4.

69. Hoffmann C, Schuller-Petrovic S, Soyer HP et al. Adverse reactions after cosmetic lip augmentation with permanent biologically inert implant materials. Am Acad Dermatol 1999; 40: 100–2.

70. Giordano GG, Chevez-Barrios P, Refojo MF et al. Biodegradation and tissue reaction to intravitreous biodegradable poly(D,L-lactic-co-glycolic) acid microspheres. Curr Eye Res 1995; 14: 761–8.

71. Valantin M-A, Aubron-Olivier C, Ghosn J et al. Polylactic acid implants (New-Fill®) to correct facial lipoatrophy in HIV-infected patients: results of the open-label study VEGA. AIDS 2003; 17: 2471–7.

72. Moyle GJ, Lysakova L, Brown S et al. A randomized open-label study of immediate versus delayed polylactic acid injections for the cosmetic management of facial lipoatrophy in persons with HIV infection. HIV Med 2004; 5: 82–7.

73. Micheels P. Human anti-hyaluronic acid antibodies: is it possible? Dermatol Surg 2001; 27: 185–91.

74. Fernandez-Acenero MJ, Zamora E, Borbujo J. Granulomatous foreign body reaction against hyaluronic acid: report of a case after lip augmentation. Dermatol Surg 2003; 29: 1225–6.

75. Raulin C, Greve B, Hartschuh W et al. Exudative granulomatous reaction to hyaluronic acid (Hylaform). Contact Dermatitis 2000; 43: 178–9.

76. Distante F, Bandierea, Bellini R et al. Studio multricentrico italiano sull'efficacia e la tollerabilita dell'acido

ialuronico di origine non animale (Restylane) nel trattamento degli inestetismi del volto. G Ital Dermatol Venereol 2001; 136: 293–301.

77. Hoenig JF, Brink U, Korabiowska M. Severe granulomatous allergic tissue reaction after hyaluronic acid injection in the treatment of facial lines and its surgical correction. J Craniofac Surg 2003; 14: 197–200.

78. Lambros V. The use of hyaluronidase to reverse the effects of hyaluronic acid filler. Plast Reconstr Surg 2004; 114: 277.

79. Beljaards RC, de Roos K-P, Bruins FG. NewFill for skin augmentation: a new filler or failure? Dermatol Surg 2005; 31: 772–6.

80. Oppel T, Schaller M, Flaig M, Korting HC. Fremdkoerpergranulome nach dermaler Injektion eines auf Polymilchsaeure basierenden Implantates zur Behandlung von Falten. J Dtsch Dematol Ges 2003; 1: 220–2.

81. Dijkema SJ, van der Lei B, Kibbelaar RE. New-Fill injections may induce late-onset foreign body granulomatous reaction. Plast Reconstr Surg 2005; 115: 76e–8e.

82. Pons-Giraud A. Actualisation des effets secondaires des produits de comblemment des rides. Nouv Dermatol 2003; 22: 205.

83. Corbiget-Escalier F, Petrella T, Janin-Magnificat C et al. Episodes d'angio-oedemes de la face avec nodules de granulomes a corps etrangers deux ans après des injections d'un produit de comblement des rides: probable responsibilite du New-Fill. Nouv Dermatol 2003; 22: 136–8.

84. Saylan Z. Facial fillers and their complications. Aesthetic Surg J 2003; 23: 221–4.

85. Burgess CM, Quiroga RM. Assessment of the safety and efficacy of poly-L-lactic aciud for the treatment of HIV-associated facial lipoatrophy. J Am Acad Dermatol 2005; 52: 233–9.

86. Ersek RA. More on Bioplastique. Aesthetic Plast Surg 2000; 24: 461–2.

87. Sidwell RU, Dhillon AP, Butler PEM, Rustin MHA. Localized granulomatous reaction to a semi-permanent hyaluronic acid and acrylic hydrogel cosmetic filler. Clin Exp Dermatol 2004; 29: 630–2.

88. Waris E, Pakkanen M, Lassila K et al. Alloplastic injectable biomaterials for soft tissue augmentation: a report of 2 cases with complications associated with a new material (DermaLive) and a review of the literature. Eur J Plast Surg 2003; 26: 350–5.

89. Jansen DA, Graivier MH. Soft tissue substitutes in perioral augmentation. Semin Plast Surg 2003; 17: 181–98.

90. Zide BM. Radiance: short-term experience. Aesthetic Surg J 2004; 23: 495–9.

91. Sklar JA, White SM. Radiance FN: a new soft tissue filler. Dermatol Surg 2004; 30: 764–8.

92. Ruden C. Acrylamide and cancer risk – expert risk assessments and the public debate. Food ChemToxicol 2004; 42: 335–49.

93. Christensen LH, Breiting VB, Aasted A et al. Long-term effects of polyacrylamide hydrogel on human breast tissue. Plast Reconstr Surg 2003; 111: 1883–90.

94. Mazzoleni F, Dominici C, Lotti T et al. Formacryl® un nuovo biopolimero al servizio della medicina 'piu un endoprotesi che un filler'. Dermatologia 2000; 1: 13.

95. Adamyan AA, Svetukhin AM, Skuba ND et al. Polyacrylamide mammary syndrome: clinical features, diagnosis and treatment. Ann Plast Reconstr Aesthetic Surg (Moscow) 2001; 4: 20.

96. Milanov NO, Donchenko EV, Fisenko EP. Plastic contour correction with polyacrylamide gels. Myth and reality. Ann Plast Reconstr Aesthetic Surg (Moscow) 2000; 4: 63.

97. Evstatiev D. Late complications after injections of hydrogel in the breast. Plast Reconstr Surg 2004; 113: 1878.

98. Pacini S, Ruggiero M, Morucci G et al. Bio-Alcamid: a novelty for reconstructive and cosmetic surgery. Ital J Anat Embryol 2002; 107: 209–14.

99. De Cassia Novaes W, Berg A. Experience with a new nonbiodegradable hydrogel (Aquamid): a pilot study. Aesthetic Plast Surg 2003; 27: 376–80.

100. Casavantes LC, Izabel JM. Estabilidad, tolerancia y seguridad de polialquilimida gel (BioAlcamid™), endoprotesis inyectable para la correction de defectos mayors en tejidos blandos. Dermatologia CMQ 2004; 2: 98–103.

101. Christensen L, Breiting VB, Vuust J et al. Adverse reactions to injectable soft tissue permanent fillers. Aesthetic Plast Surg 2005; 29: 34–48.

102. Breiting V, Aasted A, Jorgensen A, Opitz P, Rosetzky A. A study on patients treated with polyacrylamide hydrogel injection for facial corrections. Aesthetic Plast surg 2004; 28: 45–53.

103. Cheng N-X, Wang Y-L, Zhang X-M et al. Complications of breast augmentation with injected hydrophilic polyacrylamide gel. Aesthetic Plast Surg 2002; 26: 375–82.

104. Xie PB, Shi AP. Application of polyacrylamide hydrogel in augmentation mammoplasty (Chinese). Di Yi Da Xue Bao 2002; 22: 648–9.

105. Xiaoling F, Yi C, Zhang Y et al. Analysis of the complications induced by polyacrylamide hydrogel injection. Plast Reconstr Surg 2004; 114: 261–2.

106. Amin SP, Marmur ES, Goldberg DJ. Complications from injectable polyacrylamide gel, a new nonbiodegradable soft tissue filler. Dermatol Surg 2004; 30: 1507–9.

107. Duffy DM. The silicone corundrum: a battle of anecdotes. Dermatol Surg 2002; 28: 590–4.

108. Rongioletti F, Cattarina G, Sottofattori E et al. Granulomatous reaction after intradermal injections of hyaluronic acid gel. Arch Dermatol 2003; 139: 815–16.

109. Wolters M, Lampe H. Nicht-operative Faltenbehandlung im Gesicht. Plast Chirurgie 2003; 2: 69–82.

110. Winn A. Factors in selecting medical silicones. Med Plast Biomater Mag March 1996.

111. Nuutinen P, Autio P, Hurskainen T et al. Glucocorticoid action on skin collagen: overview on clinical significance and consequences. J Eur Acad Dermatol Venereol 2001; 15: 361–2.

112. Cramer JE. Intra-lesional injection of triamcinolone. Australas J Dermatol 1964; 13: 140.

113. Apikian M, Goodman G. Intralesional 5-fluorouracil in the treatment of keloid scars. Australas J Dermatol 2004; 45: 140–3.

114. Yosipovitch G, Widijanti SM, Goon A et al. A comparison of the combined effect of cryotherapy and corticosteroid injections versus corticosteroids and cryotherapy alone on keloids: a controlled study. J Dermatolog Treat 2001; 12: 87–90.

115. Fisher D. Adverse effects of topical corticosteroid use. West J Med 1995; 162: 123–6.

116. Espana A, Solana T, Quintanilla E. Bleomycin in the treatment of keloids and hypertrophic scars by multiple needle punctures. Dermatol Surg 2001; 27: 23–7.

117. Jain S, Stephens CJM. Successful treatment of disseminated granuloma annulare with topical tacrolimus. Br J Dermatol 2004; 150: 1042–3.

118. Carroll LA, Hanasono MM, Mikulec AA et al. Triamcinolone stimulates bFGF production and inhibits TGF-b1 production by human dermal fibroblasts. Dermatol Surg 2002; 28: 704–9.

119. Oishi Y, Fu ZW, Ohnuki Y et al. Molecular basis of the alteration in skin collagen metabolism in response to in vivo dexamethasone treatment: effects on the synthesis of collagen type I and III, collagenase, and tissue inhibitors of metalloproteinases. Br J Dermatol 2002; 147: 859–68.

120. de Bree R, Middelweerd MJ, van der Waal I. Severe granulomatous inflammatory response induced by injection of polyacrylamide gel into facial tissue. Arch Facial Plast Surg 2004; 6: 204–6.

121. Fitzpatrick RE, Manuskiatti W. Laser, steroid, and 5-FU therapy appear comparable for keloid scars. Arch Dermatol 2002; 138: 1149–55.

122. Narins RS, Brandt F, Leyden J et al. Randomized, double-blind, multicenter comparison of the efficacy and tolerability of Restylane versus Zyplast for the correction of nasolabial folds. Dermatol Surg 2003; 29: 588–95.

123. Soparkar CN, Patrinely JR, Tschen J. Erasing Restylane. Ophthal Plast Reconstr Surg 2004; 20: 317–18.

124. Overholt MA, Tschen JA, Font RL. Granulomatous reaction to collagen implant: light and electron microscopic observations. Cutis 1993; 51: 95–8.

125. Morton AH, Shannon P, Chen AL et al. Increased frequency of acute local reaction to intra-articular Hylan G-F 20 (Synvisc) in patients receiving more than one course of treatment. J Bone Joint Surg Am 2003; 85-A: 2050.

126. Zardawi IM. Granulomatous inflammation after Hylan G-F 20 visco supplementation of the knee. J Bone Joint Surg Am 2003; 85-A: 2484.

127. Woelber L, Zielke H, Wiest L et al. Adverse reactions to injectable filler substances in aesthetic dermatology. – Results of the injectable filler safety-study (IFS-study). J Invest Dermatol 2005; 125: 855.

38 Cell therapy in cosmetic surgery: present and future

Anne Bouloumié

Cell therapy can be defined as replacing diseased or dysfunctional cells with healthy, functioning ones. These new techniques are being applied to a wide range of human diseases, through for example bone marrow transplants in leukemia, grafting of skin cells to burns victims, or growing of corneas for the sight-impaired. In cosmetic surgery, cell therapy represents a promising approach for renewal of the innate aging and photoaging of the dermis.

Fibroblast injection

Autologous cultured fibroblasts, isolated and propagated in culture, are used for face soft tissue augmentation, the approach based on the hypothesis that the injection of collagen-producing cells results in a longer duration of correction of facial wrinkles or dermal and skin contour defects.[1,2] A small tissue sample is taken from the patient, commonly from the retroauricular area. The patient's stroma cells are cultured, cryopreserved, and used for intradermal injection. This approach has been shown to be safe, i.e. no oncogenic properties and no tumor induction in nude mice.[3] However, the efficacy of the treatment is not easily predictable.[4] The culture of fibroblasts on various scaffolds,[5,6] use of a different cell source,[7] or injection combined with filler substances[8] has been suggested to improve the retention time of the implants.

The problems faced with the injection of mature stromal or fibroblastic cells are the limited amount of cellular proliferation, aging of the cells, and the low survival rate probably due to little resistance to ischemic conditions, associated with the risk of fibrosis and calcification. The cells that have shown by far the highest potential for supplying diseased or injured organs with healthy new ones are stem cells.

Stem cells

Stem cells are characterized by three criteria: self-renewal, the ability to differentiate into multiple cell types, and the ability of in vivo reconstitution of a given tissue.[9] Distinct types of stem cells are distinguished depending on their origin and fate. There are totipotent stem cells capable of forming all embryonic layers as well as the extraembryonic trophoblast that supports the growth of the embryo, pluripotent stem cells that give rise to mesoderm, endoderm, and ectoderm, multipotent stem cells that differentiate into multiple cell types, and finally progenitor or precursor cells that are committed cells with limited self-renewal capacity and differentiate into one defined cell type.

The multipotent stem cells, isolated from various adult organs, are considered as reservoirs of reparative cells, ready to mobilize and to differentiate in response to injury or disease. Recent progress in the isolation and characterization of these cells has led to the development and testing of therapeutic strategies in a variety of clinical applications.

Bone marrow-derived stem cells

Stem cells represent a minor fraction of the total nucleated cell population in marrow (0.001–0.01% of total mononuclear cells). The first defined 'adult stem cells' were the hematopoietic stem cells (HSCs), characterized by the expression of several cell surface antigens such as CD34. Mesenchymal stem cells (MSCs) have been shown to reside within the stromal compartment of bone marrow. They have the capacity to differentiate into cells of connective tissue lineages, including bone, fat, cartilage, and muscle, and to provide the stromal support system for the hematopoietic stem cells. They can be expanded 'ex vivo', and were shown to engraft 'in vivo' in multiple tissues.[10] The expression of the Stro-1 and CD105 markers combined with the lack of CD34 is characteristic of MSCs. Multipotent adult progenitor cells are also present in marrow.[11] They can be expanded in culture, and differentiate into endothelial, endodermal, and neural lineages 'in vitro' and 'in vivo'.[12] Finally, endothelial progenitor cells characterized by the coexpression of CD34 and CD133 are also resident in bone marrow. The cells can be expanded for prolonged periods of time in vitro, and have been shown to contribute to neovascularization of ischemic tissues through recruitment at the site of injury.

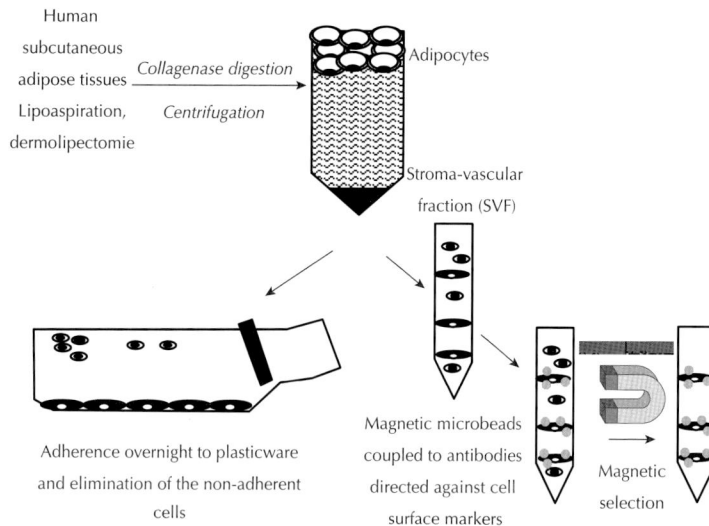

Figure 38.1 Isolation of human adipose tissue-derived stem cells.

Adipose tissue-derived stem cells

In addition to marrow, other sources of multipotent stem cells have been identified, including skin,[13,14] muscle and brain,[15] and adipose tissue.[16] The presence of multipotent stem cells in adult tissues has raised lots of questions and controversies about their origin (are adult tissue-stem cells descendants of circulating bone-marrow stem cells?) as well as about the tissue-specific niche properties, mobilization, and differentiation potential of such populations. Nevertheless, since a large volume of adipose tissue can be harvested without harmful consequences and by a simple, minimally invasive lipoaspiration procedure, the isolation and implantation of adult stem cells derived from the fat mass appears a promising approach for autologous cell therapy.

Cell isolation and in vitro expansion

Human adipose tissue-derived stem cells (hATDSCs) are isolated from several adipose tissue depots such as the infrapatellar fat pad of the knee,[17] the visceral and inguinal fat pad,[18,19] and subcutaneous adipose tissues of the abdomen, hips, and thighs.[16,18,20–22] The stroma-vascular fraction (SVF) obtained after collagenase digestion and differential centrifugation of the fat mass is subjected to adherence to a plasticware surface and subcultured (Figure 38.1). The yield of stem cells is relatively high, and averages approximatively 400 000 cells per ml of lipoaspirate tissue.[23] To overcome contamination with other cell types composing the SVF, such as endothelial cells, lymphocytes, and monocytes, approaches involving immunosorting of cells[18,24] have been developed to generate purified hATDSCs (Figure 38.1). Once isolated, hATDSCs display high proliferative capacity 'in vitro'.[25] For human

applications, standard protocols to isolate and to expand the hATDSCs must be defined to enhance safety. Collagenase as well as fetal bovine serum (FBS), widely used to culture cells in vitro (Table 38.1), may elicit immunogenicity in the host recipient.[32] Several media have recently been developed and proposed to expand hATDSCs.[33,34]

Immunophenotypic features of adipose tissue-derived stem cells

Marked discrepancies in the expression of cell surface markers have been reported by various laboratories, especially concerning CD34, the hematopoietic marker, and Stro-1, the MSC marker (Table 38.1). Such differences led to the hypothesis that hATDSCs are composed of distinct unipotent progenitor cell subsets selected differentially through laboratory-specific isolation procedures and culture conditions. However, recent publications have shown that multilineage differentiation potential was observed at the single cell level by using cloned hATDSCs.[31,35,36] However, to clearly demonstrate hATDSC nature and phenotype, considerable effort has still to be spent on the identification of specific surface markers for selection, detection, and testing of the purity of the hATDSC preparation.

In vitro differentiation

The acquisition of various cell lineage biochemical markers by hATDSCs has been described and characterized by multiple laboratories (Figure 38.2). Adipogenic differentiation of hATDSCs is induced by the addition of an agonist for the peroxisome proliferator-activated receptor γ, such as thiazolidinedione, in the presence

Table 38.1   Immunophenotypic features of human adipose tissue-derived stem cells (hATDSCs)

CD								
13	+	+			+	+		+
14	–	–	–		–			
31	–	–		–	–		–	
34	+	–	–	+	+	+	–	–
44	+	+	+			+	+	+
45	–	–		–			–	
49	+	+				–		+
62	–	–				–		
90		+	+			+		+
105	+	+	+	–		+	+	+
Flk1							+	–
Stro-1	–	+		–				–
Culture	DMEM –F10 10% FBS	DMEM 10% FBS	αMEM 10% FBS		DMEM –F12 10% NCS		DMEM –F12 + MCDB + 2% FBS + suppl	DMEM, low glucose 10% FBS
Freshly harvested cells				Immuno-magnetic selection of CD34+ cells		Immuno-magnetic depletion of CD45+ and CD31+ cells		
Reference	26	20	27	18,28	29	24	30	31

DMEM, Dulbecco's modified Eagle medium; FBS, fetal bovine serum; MEM, minimum essential medium; NCS, newborn calf serum; MCDB, molecular, cellular, and developmental biology; suppl, supplement.

of insulin, tri-iodothyronine (T3), and dexamethasone.[37,38] Osteogenic activation requires the presence of β-glycerol-phosphate, ascorbic acid-2-phosphate, dexamethasone, and vitamin D3.[20,39] Chondrogenic differentiation occurs when hATDSCs are grown in nutrient medium supplemented with transforming growth factor β (TGF-β).[20,40] Induction of myogenesis has been reported after the addition of serum and hydrocortisone.[20] Neurogenesis is induced with β-mercaptoethanol[20] or by media supplementation with butylated hydroxyanisole, valproic acid, forskolin, hydrocortisone, and insulin.[35,41] Acquisition of endothelial cell-specific markers was observed in the presence of vascular endothelial growth factor and insulin-like growth factor[18] or when hATDSCs were cultured in methylcellulose medium[29] or in the absence of serum.[42] Acquisition of cardiomyocyte properties was observed following transient exposure to a rat cardiomyocyte extract.[43] Finally, the expression of epithelial lineage markers has recently been reported in specific media.[44,45]

Fate of implanted human adipose tissue-derived stem cells

The mechanisms that underlie the interactions between implanted hATDSCs and the host recipient are still to be characterized, but several recent works bring interesting observations concerning the host response to stem cell therapy as well as stem cell behavior to distinct local environments.

Host immune response

There is evidence of the non-immunogenic nature of hATDSCs. Indeed, 'in vitro', hATDSCs did not provoke alloreactivity of incompatible lymphocytes[46] and 'in vivo' did not induce accumulation of lymphocytes after implantation in non-immunocompromised mice.[30] This might be related to the low level of cell surface class I and the lack of class II human leukocyte antigen (HLA).[31] Moreover, hATDSCs appear to exhibit immunosuppressive properties at least 'in vitro'.[46] This has broad implications in terms of allogeneic therapy or delivery to a recipient of cells derived from an unmatched donor. To note, the disadvantage of an allogeneic approach is the potential risk of disease transmission from donor to recipient.

Homing mechanisms

hATDSCs, when delivered by intravenous infusion in mice, have been shown to engraft onto various tissues, including brain, thymus, heart, liver, and lung.[47]

In vitro studies   Human adipose tissue-derived stem cells

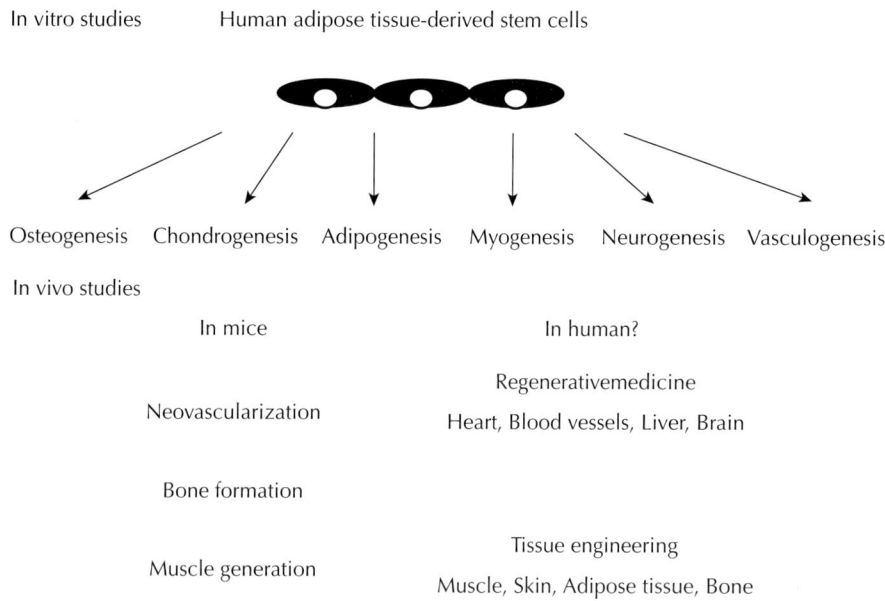

Osteogenesis   Chondrogenesis   Adipogenesis   Myogenesis   Neurogenesis   Vasculogenesis

In vivo studies

In mice   In human?

Regenerativemedicine

Neovascularization   Heart, Blood vessels, Liver, Brain

Bone formation

Tissue engineering

Muscle generation   Muscle, Skin, Adipose tissue, Bone

Figure 38.2   Fate of human tissue-derived stem cells in vitro and in vivo and potential use in regenerative medicine and reconstructive surgery.

Moreover, they exhibited the capacity to migrate to the site of injury. Indeed, partial hepatectomy in mice led to an enhanced engraftment of hATDSCs in the liver.[47] The mechanisms that guide homing of implanted cells are not known, and further research is needed to determine the factors such as chemokines or hypoxia-related signals that are responsible for the attraction of stem cells in injured tissues.

In vivo differentiation

The fundamental principle of stem cell therapy is that undifferentiated cells, following delivery to the injured host and migration to the site of injury, will, under the influence of local signals, differentiate to cells of the appropriate phenotype.

Intravenous injection of hATDSCs has recently been shown to improve neovascularization of an ischemic hindlimb in immunotolerant mice.[18,30,48] However, whether the neoformation of blood vessels is due to 'in situ' differentiation of hATDSCs into endothelial cells[18] and/or to the release of proangiogenic factors by the hATDSCs[48] remains to be clearly determined.

Subcutaneous hATDSC implantation in immunotoler-ant mice has been described to lead to bone forma-tion.[49,50] In an athymic rat with a critically sized femoral defect, implantation of hATDSCs, genetically modified to express an osteoinductive factor (bone morphogenetic protein 2; BMP-2), led to healing of the bone defect.[51]

Finally, transplantation of human multipotent adi-pose-derived stem cells in the tibialis anterior of the mdx mouse, an animal model of Duchenne muscular dystrophy, has been shown to induce dystrophin expression.[31] Once again, the mechanisms underlying muscle generation, i.e. transdifferentiation of the implanted human cells into muscle-specific cells or fusion of the human stem cells with host cells leading to changes in gene expression, remain to be investigated.

In humans, the first report of a phase I clinical trial of cell therapy for the treatment of fistulas in Crohn's disease using autologous stem cells obtained from a lipoaspirate has recently been published. The number of patients included and the uncontrolled nature of the phase I clinical trial did not allow demonstration of the effectiveness of the treatment. However, the results indicated that the protocol was feasible and safe.[52]

Tumor formation

Increasing observations suggest that the neoplastic process involves cancer stem cells.[53] Indeed, cancer stem cells have been identified in several tumor types and have been proposed to derive from normal adult stem cells.[54,55] A recent study points out the risk of transformation of hATDSCs. Indeed, after long-term 'in vitro expansion', the cells have been shown to immortalize and to transform spontaneously leading to tumor formation after injection in immunodeficient mice.[56] Thus, maintaining hATDSCs for a prolonged time in culture may increase the risk that 'mutant stem cells may seed cancer'.[57]

Aging

The decline of tissue regenerative potential is a hall-mark of aging, and may be due to age-related changes in tissue-specific stem cells. Recent studies in mice have shown that the age-related decline of progenitor cell activity can be reverted by exposure to a 'young' systemic environment, and conversely the systemic environment of an old animal either failed to promote or actively inhibited tissue regeneration.[58] Research is now needed to determine the potential effects of aging on adipose tissue-derived stem cells or the consequence of an aged recipient on the implantation and healing capacities of hATDSCs.

Conclusion

hATDSCs may represent, due to the easily available source, a promising cell therapeutic approach for tissue repair and regeneration. They exhibit high proliferative capacity, are able to differentiate into multiple cell types, and have been shown 'in vivo' to contribute to tissue reconstitution (Figure 38.2).

However, several scientific challenges must be overcome. The long-term safety and effectiveness of hATDSC therapy have to be clearly demonstrated in preclinical and clinical approaches using designed and validated standard methods for isolation, characterization, selection, purification, storage, and delivery of the cells. The mechanisms of engraftment and homing must be characterized as well as the relative role of 'in vivo' transdifferentiation, fusion, and release of survival and growth factors in the promotion of local cell regeneration.

References

1. Watson D, Keller GS, Lacombe V et al. Autologous fibroblasts for treatment of facial rhytids and dermal depressions. A pilot study. Arch Facial Plast Surg 1999; 1: 165–70.
2. Boss WK Jr, Usal H, Fodor PB, Chernoff G. Autologous cultured fibroblasts: a protein repair system. Ann Plast Surg 2000; 44: 536–42.
3. Keller G, Sebastian J, Lacombe U et al. Safety of injectable autologous human fibroblasts. Bull Exp Biol Med 2000; 130: 786–9.
4. West TB, Alster TS. Autologous human collagen and dermal fibroblasts for soft tissue augmentation. Dermatol Surg 1998; 24: 510–12.
5. Xiao YL, Riesle J, Van Blitterswijk CA. Static and dynamic fibroblast seeding and cultivation in porous PEO/PBT scaffolds. J Mater Sci Mater Med 1999; 10: 773–7.
6. Kim SS, Gwak SJ, Choi CY, Kim BS. Skin regeneration using keratinocytes and dermal fibroblasts cultured on biodegradable microspherical polymer scaffolds. J Biomed Mater Res B Appl Biomater 2005; 75: 369–77.
7. Wang HJ, Pieper J, Schotel R, Van Blitterswijk CA, Lamme EN. Stimulation of skin repair is dependent on fibroblast source and presence of extracellular matrix. Tissue Eng 2004; 10: 1054–64.
8. Yoon ES, Han SK, Kim WK. Advantages of the presence of living dermal fibroblasts within Restylane for soft tissue augmentation. Ann Plast Surg 2003; 51: 587–92.
9. Lakshmipathy U, Verfaillie C. Stem cell plasticity. Blood Rev 2005; 19: 29–38.
10. Devine SM, Cobbs C, Jennings M, Bartholomew A, Hoffman R. Mesenchymal stem cells distribute to a wide range of tissues following systemic infusion into nonhuman primates. Blood 2003; 101: 2999–3001.
11. Reyes M, Lund T, Lenvik T et al. Purification and ex vivo expansion of postnatal human marrow mesodermal progenitor cells. Blood 2001; 98: 2615–25.
12. Jiang Y, Jahagirdar BN, Reinhardt RL et al. Pluripotency of mesenchymal stem cells derived from adult marrow. Nature 2002; 418: 41–9.
13. Fernandes KJ, McKenzie IA, Mill P et al. A dermal niche for multipotent adult skin-derived precursor cells. Nat Cell Biol 2004; 6: 1082–93.
14. Toma JG, Akhavan M, Fernandes KJ et al. Isolation of multipotent adult stem cells from the dermis of mammalian skin. Nat Cell Biol 2001; 3: 778–84.
15. Jiang Y, Vaessen B, Lenvik T et al. Multipotent progenitor cells can be isolated from postnatal murine bone marrow, muscle, and brain. Exp Hematol 2002; 30: 896–904.
16. Zuk PA, Zhu M, Mizuno H et al. Multilineage cells from human adipose tissue: implications for cell-based therapies. Tissue Eng 2001; 7: 211–28.
17. Wickham MQ, Erickson GR, Gimble JM, Vail TP, Guilak F. Multipotent stromal cells derived from the infrapatellar fat pad of the knee. Clin Orthop Relat Res 2003; 412: 196–212.
18. Miranville A, Heeschen C, Sengenes C et al. Improvement of postnatal neovascularization by human adipose tissue-derived stem cells. Circulation 2004; 110: 349–55.
19. Huang JI, Beanes SR, Zhu M et al. Rat extramedullary adipose tissue as a source of osteochondrogenic progenitor cells. Plast Reconstr Surg 2002; 109: 1033–41.
20. Zuk PA, Zhu M, Ashjian P et al. Human adipose tissue is a source of multipotent stem cells. Mol Biol Cell 2002; 13: 4279–95.
21. Gimble J, Guilak F. Adipose-derived adult stem cells: isolation, characterization, and differentiation potential. Cytotherapy 2003; 5: 362–9.
22. Gimble JM. Adipose tissue-derived therapeutics. Expert Opin Biol Ther 2003; 3: 705–13.
23. Aust L, Devlin B, Foster SJ et al. Yield of human adipose-derived adult stem cells from liposuction aspirates. Cytotherapy 2004; 6: 7–14.
24. Boquest AC, Shahdadfar A, Fronsdal K et al. Isolation and transcription profiling of purified uncultured human stromal stem cells: alteration of gene expression after in vitro cell culture. Mol Biol Cell 2005; 16: 1131–41.
25. Fraser JK, Schreiber RE, Zuk PA, Hedrick MH. Adult stem cell therapy for the heart. Int J Biochem Cell Biol 2004; 36: 658–66.
26. Gronthos S, Franklin DM, Leddy HA et al. Surface protein characterization of human adipose tissue-derived stromal cells. J Cell Physiol 2001; 189: 54–63.
27. Lee RH, Kim B, Choi I et al. Characterization and expression analysis of mesenchymal stem cells from human bone marrow and adipose tissue. Cell Physiol Biochem 2004; 14: 311–24.
28. Sengenes C, Lolmede K, Zakaroff-Girard A, Busse R, Bouloumie A. Preadipocytes in the human subcutaneous adipose tissue display distinct features from the adult mesenchymal and hematopoietic stem cells. J Cell Physiol 2005; 205: 114–22.
29. Planat-Benard V, Silvestre JS, Cousin B et al. Plasticity of human adipose lineage cells toward endothelial cells: physiological and therapeutic perspectives. Circulation 2004; 109: 656–63.
30. Cao Y, Sun Z, Liao L et al. Human adipose tissue-derived stem cells differentiate into endothelial cells in vitro and improve postnatal neovascularization in vivo. Biochem Biophys Res Commun 2005; 332: 370–9.
31. Rodriguez AM, Pisani D, Dechesne CA et al. Transplantation of a multipotent cell population from human adipose tissue induces dystrophin expression in the immunocompetent mdx mouse. J Exp Med 2005; 201: 1397–405.
32. Spees JL, Gregory CA, Singh H et al. Internalized antigens must be removed to prepare hypoimmunogenic mesenchymal stem cells for cell and gene therapy. Mol Ther 2004; 9: 747–56.

33. Kim SJ, Cho HH, Kim YJ et al. Human adipose stromal cells expanded in human serum promote engraftment of human peripheral blood hematopoietic stem cells in NOD/SCID mice. Biochem Biophys Res Commun 2005; 329: 25–31.

34. Lin TM, Tsai JL, Lin SD, Lai CS, Chang CC. Accelerated growth and prolonged lifespan of adipose tissue-derived human mesenchymal stem cells in a medium using reduced calcium and antioxidants. Stem Cells Dev 2005; 14: 92–102.

35. Guilak F, Lott KE, Awad HA et al. Clonal analysis of the differentiation potential of human adipose-derived adult stem cells. J Cell Physiol 2006; 206: 229–37.

36. Rodriguez AM, Elabd C, Amri EZ, Ailhaud G, Dani C. The human adipose tissue is a source of multipotent stem cells. Biochimie 2005; 87: 125–8.

37. Hauner H, Entenmann G, Wabitsch M et al. Promoting effect of glucocorticoids on the differentiation of human adipocyte precursor cells cultured in a chemically defined medium. J Clin Invest 1989; 84: 1663–70.

38. van Harmelen V, Skurk T, Hauner H. Primary culture and differentiation of human adipocyte precursor cells. Methods Mol Med 2005; 107: 125–35.

39. Halvorsen YD, Franklin D, Bond AL et al. Extracellular matrix mineralization and osteoblast gene expression by human adipose tissue-derived stromal cells. Tissue Eng 2001; 7: 729–41.

40. Erickson GR, Gimble JM, Franklin DM et al. Chondrogenic potential of adipose tissue-derived stromal cells in vitro and in vivo. Biochem Biophys Res Commun 2002; 290: 763–9.

41. Safford KM, Rice HE. Stem cell therapy for neurologic disorders: therapeutic potential of adipose-derived stem cells. Curr Drug Targets 2005; 6: 57–62.

42. Martinez-Estrada OM, Munoz-Santos Y, Julve J, Reina M, Vilaro S. Human adipose tissue as a source of Flk-1+ cells: new method of differentiation and expansion. Cardiovasc Res 2005; 65: 328–33.

43. Gaustad KG, Boquest AC, Anderson BE, Gerdes AM, Collas P. Differentiation of human adipose tissue stem cells using extracts of rat cardiomyocytes. Biochem Biophys Res Commun 2004; 314: 420–7.

44. Brzoska M, Geiger H, Gauer S, Baer P. Epithelial differentiation of human adipose tissue-derived adult stem cells. Biochem Biophys Res Commun 2005; 330: 142–50.

45. Seo MJ, Suh SY, Bae YC, Jung JS. Differentiation of human adipose stromal cells into hepatic lineage in vitro and in vivo. Biochem Biophys Res Commun 2005; 328: 258–64.

46. Puissant B, Barreau C, Bourin P et al. Immunomodulatory effect of human adipose tissue-derived adult stem cells: comparison with bone marrow mesenchymal stem cells. Br J Haematol 2005; 129: 118–29.

47. Kim DH, Je CM, Sin JY, Jung JS. Effect of partial hepatectomy on in vivo engraftment after intravenous administration of human adipose tissue stromal cells in mouse. Microsurgery 2003; 23: 424–31.

48. Rehman J, Traktuev D, Li J et al. Secretion of angiogenic and antiapoptotic factors by human adipose stromal cells. Circulation 2004; 109: 1292–8.

49. Hicok KC, Du Laney TV, Zhou YS et al. Human adipose-derived adult stem cells produce osteoid in vivo. Tissue Eng 2006; 10: 371–80.

50. Hattori H, Masuoka K, Sato M et al. Bone formation using human adipose tissue-derived stromal cells and a biodegradable scaffold. J Biomed Mater Res B Appl Biomater 2006; 76: 230–9.

51. Peterson B, Zhang J, Iglesias R et al. Healing of critically sized femoral defects, using genetically modified mesenchymal stem cells from human adipose tissue. Tissue Eng 2005; 11: 120–9.

52. Garcia-Olmo D, Garcia-Arranz M, Herreros D et al. A phase I clinical trial of the treatment of Crohn's fistula by adipose mesenchymal stem cell transplantation. Dis Colon Rectum 2005; 48: 1416–23.

53. Serakinci N, Guldberg P, Burns JS et al. Adult human mesenchymal stem cell as a target for neoplastic transformation. Oncogene 2004; 23: 5095–8.

54. Pardal R, Clarke MF, Morrison SJ. Applying the principles of stem-cell biology to cancer. Nat Rev Cancer 2003; 3: 895–902.

55. Houghton J, Stoicov C, Nomura S et al. Gastric cancer originating from bone marrow-derived cells. Science 2004; 306: 1568–71.

56. Rubio D, Garcia-Castro J, Martin MC et al. Spontaneous human adult stem cell transformation. Cancer Res 2005; 65: 3035–9.

57. Marx J. Cancer research. Mutant stem cells may seed cancer. Science 2003; 301: 1308–10.

58. Conboy IM, Conboy MJ, Wagers AJ et al. Rejuvenation of aged progenitor cells by exposure to a young systemic environment. Nature 2005; 433: 760–4.

39 Developments in management of facial and body lipoatrophy with exogenous volumetric injectables

Benjamin Ascher

What is volumetry?

Volumetry is the science of volume enhancement, and focuses on the analysis of:

- areas where volume loss occurs (above all, the face, but also extrafacial areas such as breast and buttocks)
- causes of volume loss including aging, anti-human immunodeficiency virus (HIV) multitherapy, trauma, cancer, and all causes of substance loss
- therapeutic methods, above all, injectable implants (fatty and exogenous products) and also hard implants (PTFE (polytetrafluoroethylene), Porex®, and silicone), and surgery
- assessment, and measuring methods.[1]

Loss of volume and facial lipoatrophy

Facial lipoatrophy has been observed to occur in a variety of patient populations, with inherited or acquired disease, or even in aging patients as a natural progression of tissue change over time.[1–4] Interest in facial lipoatrophy has recently intensified; this phenomenon is linked to the rise in the number of people adversely affected by the condition, mainly due to aging or a side-effect of highly active antiretroviral treatment for HIV (HAART), combined with the growing number of cosmetic products that claim to be able to correct the appearance of lipoatrophy.[5–16] Loss of volume is caused, to a medium degree, by changes in the skeleton (forehead, zygomatic arches, dental maxillary protrusions) and the dermis, but mostly by the loss of fatty tissue. It is important to understand the anatomy of the different tissues and principally of this fatty tissue. Fat is distributed at three levels: superficial or subcutaneous fat; intermediate fat (on either side of

cutaneous muscles); deep or visceral fat (in contact with temporal and parotid fasciae).

Some regions are more affected than others. Loss of volume first affects the mid-facial area (tear troughs, cheekbones, cheeks, nasogeniae folds, depressed corners of the mouth, and 'marionette lines'), then the mandible and chin, and, more rarely, the neck and the temples. The periorbital and perioral areas, where there is no superficial fat, are less affected, except for the eye sockets and upper orbital rim areas.

Lipoatrophy, the major type of aging, begins at age 20, is noticeable at age 30–40, and is associated with other aging processes. Three types of aging have been identified with a genetic predisposition:

- tissue retraction, which concerns 5% of the population (caused by tissue fibrosis, without hollowing or wrinkles)
- overall sagging, which concerns 55% of the population (caused by posterior and lateral ptosis, wrinkles, excess fat, and loss of anterior fat)
- aging by loss of volume or skeletal deficiencies, which concerns 40% of the population (caused particularly by loss of fat lipoatrophy, but also by loss of muscle and skin, and bone resorption). The resorption comes mainly from demineralization of the upper and lower jawbones, and in general from the upper third of the face versus a degree of bone expansion from the upper orbital rim. As craniofacial support (the 'table') decreases, it leaves less surface area for the outer soft tissue envelope (the 'tablecloth'), causing it to fold or sag.[4]

Techniques useful in measuring lipoatrophy are: X-ray, computed tomography (CT), anthropometric approaches, magnetic resonance imaging (MRI), ultrasound, and the recent advanced three-dimensional photography.[1,2]

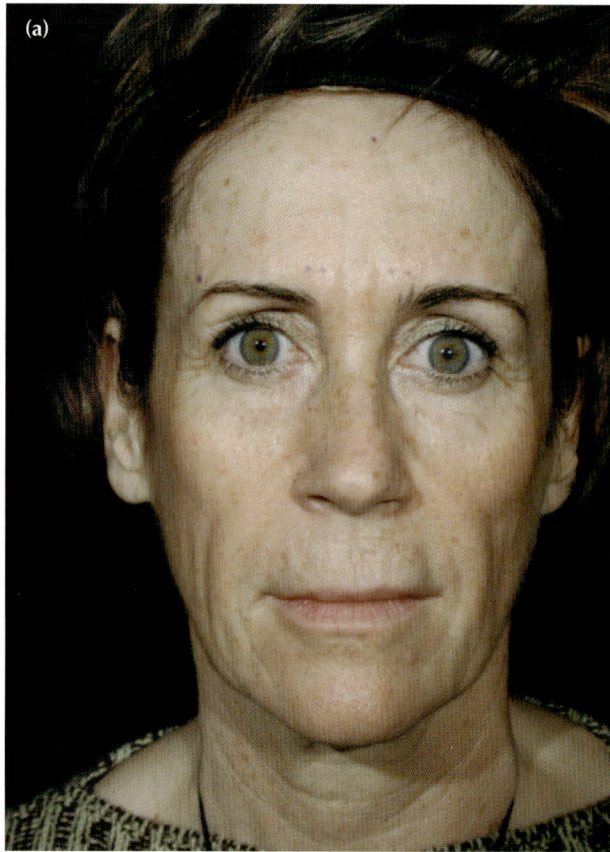

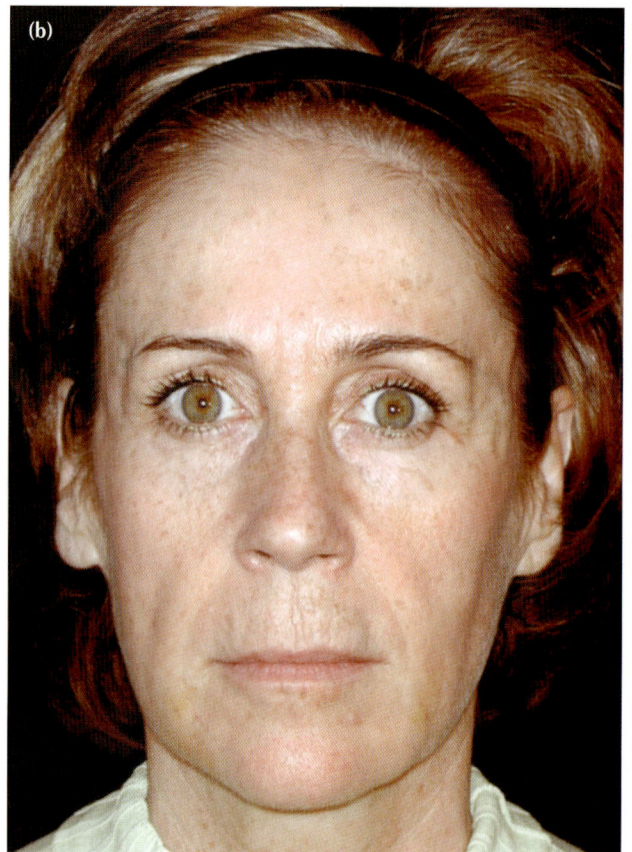

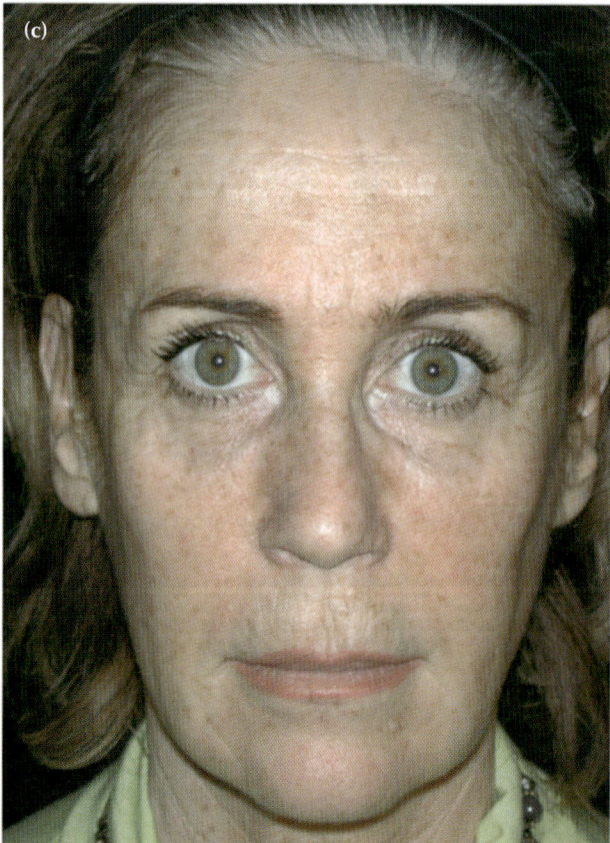

Figure 39.1   (a) Patient presenting lipoatrophy caused by skeletal deficiency on the temples, mid-facial area, and maxillary contour. (b) Results after 12 months, following injection of 2 ml Juvederm Voluma® on both sides, and 0.4 ml Surgiderm® 30 on both sides in the subpalpebral and labial–genial regions. (c) Results at 26 months follow up with a touch up of 1 ml Juvederm Voluma® on both sides, at 18 months.

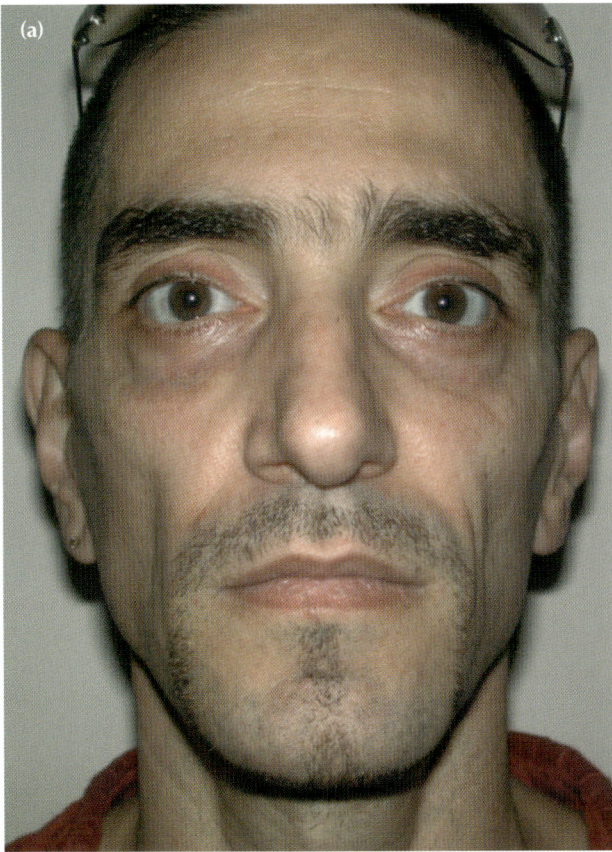

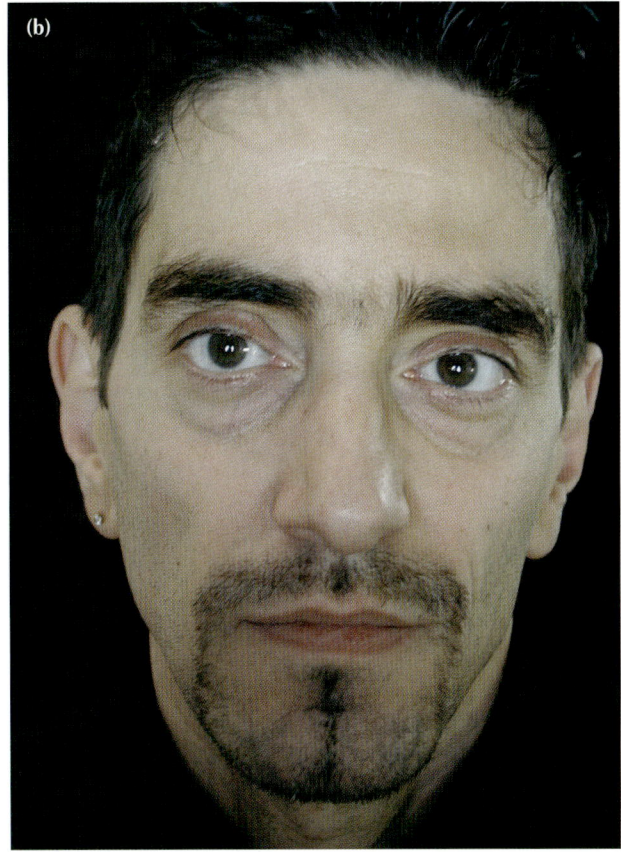

Figure 39.2 (a) Patient presenting congenital lipoatrophy in the mid-facial area. (b) Results after a period of 12 months following bilateral injection of 1 ml Juvederm Voluma.

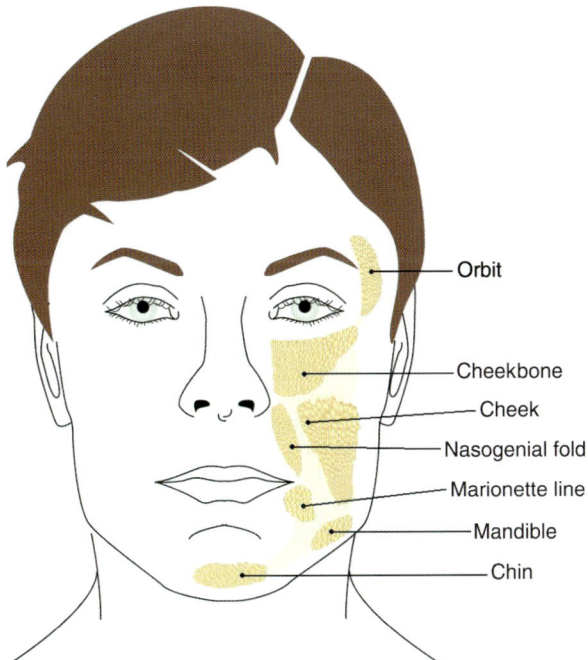

Figure 39.3 Main areas: (1) orbits and tear troughs; (2) cheekbones; (3) cheeks, (4) nasiogenial fold; (5) marionette lines; (6) mandible; (7) chin.

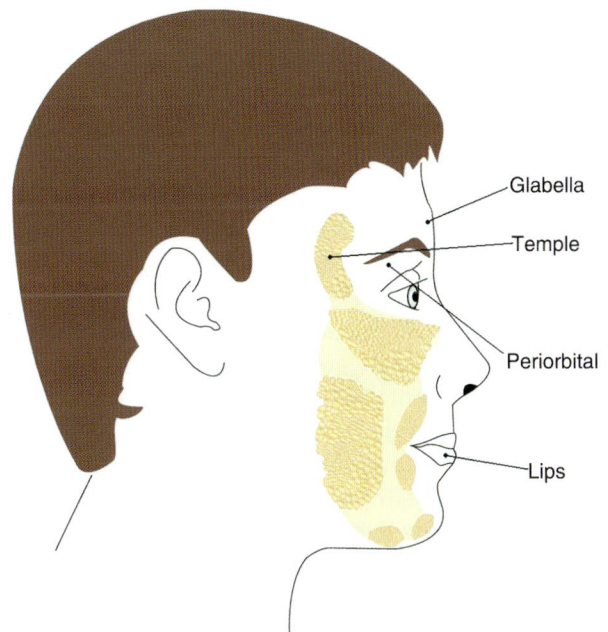

Figure 39.4 Other affected regions: (1) temples; (2) glabella; (3) periorbital; (4) lips.

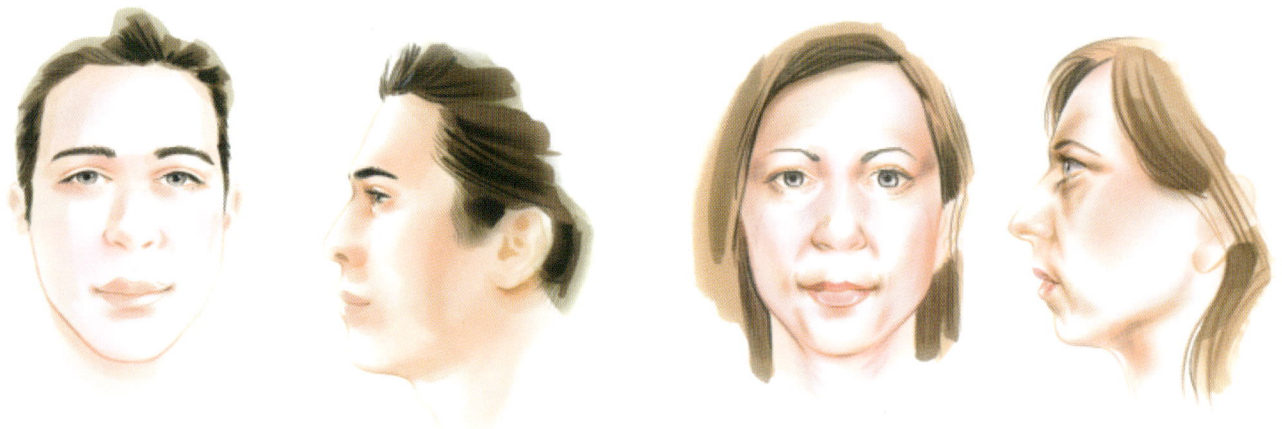

Figure 39.5   Grade 1 facial lipoatrophy (reproduced with permission from reference 2).

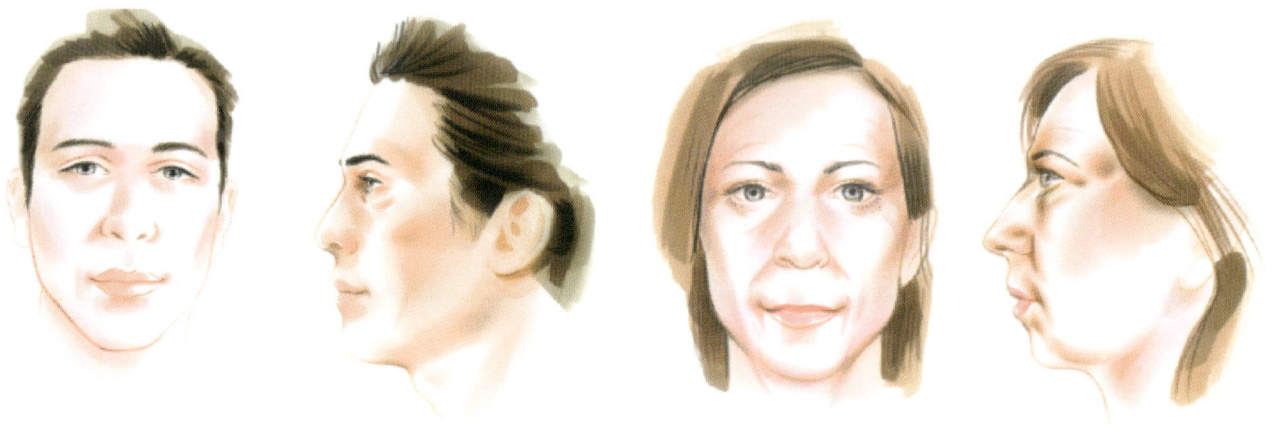

Figure 39.6   Grade 2 facial lipoatrophy (reproduced with permission from reference 2).

The final consensus of our Facial Lipoatrophy Panel encompasses both aging and disease states: 'loss of facial fat due to aging, trauma, or disease, manifested by flattening or indentation of normally convex contours.' The proposed grading scale includes five gradations (grades 1–5, 5 being the most severe), and the face is assessed according to three criteria: contour, bony prominence, and visibility of musculature.[2]

Figures 39.5–39.9 provide a visual guide as to each grade. For each grade, an example of a male and a female, both in profile and straight on, have been given, so all areas of lipoatrophy can be visualized. The use of photography has been avoided because of the inherent difficulty in obtaining sufficiently standardized photographs. Many members of the Panel felt that the ethical issues involved in using actual patient images to exemplify a grade of lipoatrophy could be problematic, particularly because the most severe grades of facial lipoatrophy are typically found in HIV-infected patients.

Grades 1–5 are defined as follows:

- Grade 1 (Figure 39.5): mild flattening or shadowing of one or more facial regions (including the cheek, temple, preauricular, periorbital, and perioral areas); no prominent bony landmarks; no visibility of underlying musculature.
- Grade 2 (Figure 39.6): an intermediate point between grade 1 and grade 3.
- Grade 3 (Figure 39.7): moderate concavity of one or more facial regions (including the cheek, temple, preauricular, perioral, and perioral areas); prominence of bony landmarks; may have visibility of underlying musculature.
- Grade 4 (Figure 39.8): an intermediate point between grade 3 and grade 5.
- Grade 5 (Figure 39.9): severe indentation of one or more facial regions (including the cheek, temple, preauricular, periorbital, and perioral areas); severe prominence of bony landmarks; clear visibility of underlying musculature.

Volumetric facial rejuvenation

This involves restoring lost volume and contours to the face and neck, mainly by filling. Some predispositions

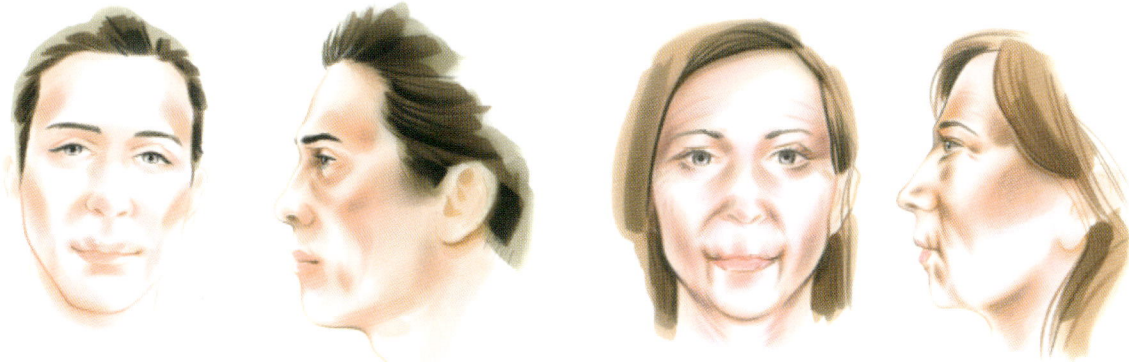

Figure 39.7   Grade 3 facial lipoatrophy (reproduced with permission from reference 2).

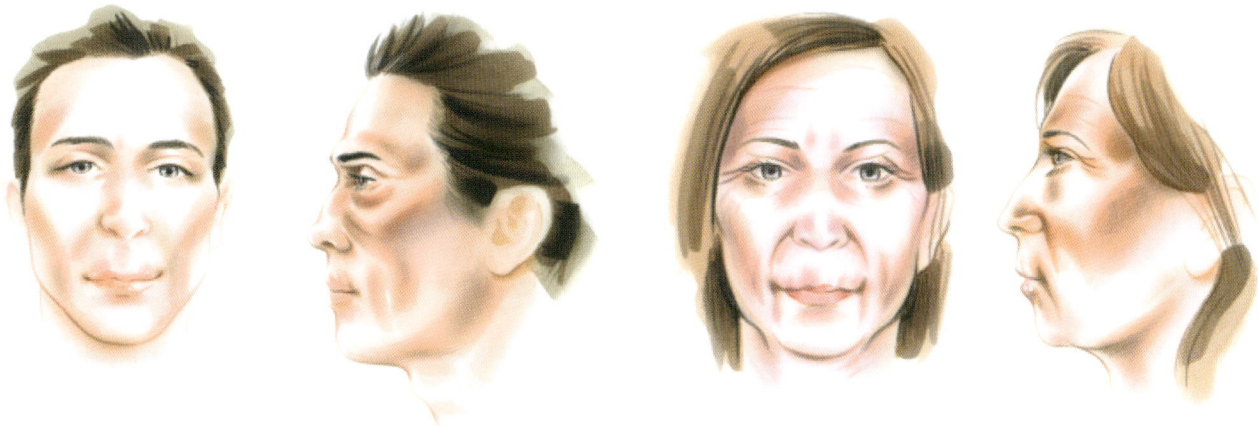

Figure 39.8   Grade 4 facial lipoatrophy (reproduced with permission from reference 2).

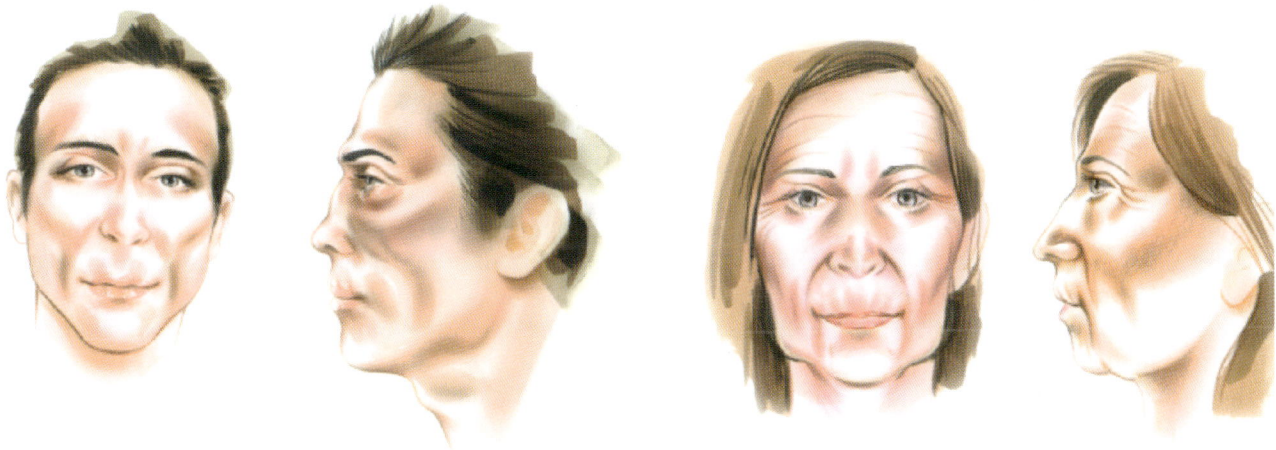

Figure 39.9   Grade 5 facial lipoatrophy (reproduced with permission from reference 2).

derive from face types: long faces can obtain more benefit from filling than short faces.

Rejuvenation from hard implants

These types of implant are being developed in this indication, using porous polyethylene. MedPor® can be fixed against the periosteum,[46] and PTFE can be implanted against the periosteum or inside the deep fatty tissues. Both can be combined with volumetric filler injections at the site of lipoatrophy.[17] Advantages include the permanence of the result, and the possibility of important benefit. Disadvantages include all those associated with the employment of an invasive surgical procedure.

Rejuvenation from resorbable implants

Fat grafts remain one of the best types of implant. Advantages are that a good quantity can be used, and the technique is reliable, with good reproducibility. The average durability is between 12 and 36 months; a touch-up is often required at 12–18 months. A disadvantage is that it is an invasive technique, requiring an operating room, local or neuroleptic anesthesia, and the employment of a 1.5-mm cannula with a 16–18G needle. The side-effects are mainly prolonged edema and ecchymosis.

Exogenous volume-enhancing injectable fillers have many advantages. For instance, they eliminate the need for operating theaters and sampling areas, use local anesthetic, use an 18–27G needle, and do not cause major swelling or ecchymosis. In addition, in the absence of fatty tissue samples, these injectable fillers are the only solution. Disadvantages are that each syringe contains only a low volume, and several injection sessions at between 6 and 18 months are required to obtain durability. Rigorous studies are needed to evaluate the long-term durability and the final cost.

In the past 10 years, there have been many developments in 'slowly resorbable' or 'non-resorbable' volume-enhancing injectable fillers, such as: poly-L-lactic acid (New-Fill–Sculptra®), polyacrylamide gel (PAAG; Aquamid®, Evolution®, Eutrophill®), alkylimide (Bio-Alcamid®), polymethylmethacrylate (PMMA; Artecoll®, Artefill®, Atlean®), acrylic hydrogen (Outline®, Dermadeep®, Dermalive®), hydroxyapatite (Radiesse®, Beautifill®), and dimethylsiloxane. Sculptra and Radiesse attained Food and Drug Administration (FDA) approval for HIV post-treatment patients, and recently Radiesse gained FDA approval for lipoatrophy in the field of esthetic facial indications.[3] The use of poly-L-lactic acid (PLLA) Sculptra, both as a soft tissue volumizer and as an injectable craniofacial implant in a supraperiosteal location, allows both soft tissue volume loss and loss of craniofacial support to be addressed. The most striking result noted was the ability to restore a youthful proportion to the perioral area, which had not been achieved previously with soft tissue treatment alone.[4]

Although improved pharmacology and better injection techniques for these products reduce the risk of side-effects, the delayed appearance of an infection (in rare cases), but above all, of a foreign body granuloma, which is extremely difficult to treat, means that use of these products is appealing but still risky.

Hence, the solution was to develop volume-enhancing resorbable hyaluronic acids (HAs).

These formulas carry few risks, not so much in terms of short-term reactions that occur after any injection (rashes, light bleeding, swelling, punctiform ecchymoses, pain or itching), but rather in terms of papular lesions, bluish pigmentation, or nodules caused by injections made too close to the surface and not accompanied by massage. Granulomas, folliculitis, pseudocysts, and nodules with delayed hypersensitivity, which are rarely described in HA injections, can be avoided by thoroughly questioning the patient to find out about any contraindications to HA and by using corticosteroids if any of these symptoms arise.

In 2004, Restylane SubQ® from Q-Med laboratories was the first volume-enhancing HA to arrive on the market. It was developed according to the NASHA technique (non-animal, stabilized HA), which is based on the concentration and size of particles. Evidence from a preliminary, multicenter, and open-ended preliminary study in 57 patients indicates that Restylane SubQ is safe and effective in creating and maintaining esthetic correction of the cheeks and/or chin for at least 3 months in the great majority of patients. After this one, other published research demonstrated interesting volume-enhancing results and good tolerance, and patients showed a persistence of the benefit up to 64 weeks.[17–23] In the studies with Restylane SubQ® in HIV patients there is an improvement in the Global Aesthetic Improvement Scale for 90% of patients at 52 weeks.[42,43] Some studies show an improvement in contouring with Restylane®, the classic Q-Med filler, in at least 80% of the patients after 12 months.[44,45]

In 2005, Juvederm Voluma®, from Allergan laboratories, was developed, according to the 'three-dimensional hyaluronic acid matrix' technique, which is not based on the size or concentration of particles, but on the optimum use of bridges between cross-linking agents. Our clinical preliminary study from September 2005 to November 2006 in 36 patients with one treatment found no side-effects apart from the usual few short-term reactions which disappear within 72 hours, and visible and lasting volume enhancement, between 12 and 15 months, in 69% of the patients. Multicenter, long-term studies will enable more accurate assessment of the product's results, durability, and tolerance.

In 2007, Fortelis Extra® from Anteis laboratories and Ultradeep® from Teoxane laboratories began to be developed. Fortelis is manufactured according to cohesive polydensified matrix technology with a high level of cross-linking. The first trials are expected to assess the immediate results, duration, and safety. Our first evaluation of this product between October 2007 and June 2008 found visible and lasting volume enhancement during these first 9 months in 65%, with very few side-effects that usually occur after any injection and disappear in 2–8 days (rashes, swelling, ecchymosis), but no papular lesions, bluish pigmentation, or nodules. The employment of a 25- or 26G needle decreases the risk of swelling and ecchymosis.

Injection technique

Before the injection

A cost estimate is provided, informed consent given, and photos taken. Preoperative marking of the lipoatrophy, and pictures of the injection areas and points with the patient at rest, in half-sitting position, and with the head bent forward are essential.

No preliminary medication or tests are required, and any relative contraindications will give rise to a second test carried out 1 month later. To avoid ecchymosis during the injection, cooling with an ice pack for 10 minutes is suitable. Local anesthetic is often administered using 1% xylocaine with adrenaline at the entry point. Nerve block anesthesia is sometimes required, particularly in the infraorbital facial nerve (V2).

The injection

Following thorough disinfection, the injection is administered with the patient in the lying or half-lying/half-sitting position.

For Restylane SubQ (Q-Med), an 18G smooth cannula is used, so we recommend that a pre-slit is made using a 16G needle. For Juvederm Voluma (Allergan) a 21G needle is required, and a 25G needle (20 mm length) for Fortelis Extra (Anteis). The needle or the cannula is inserted perpendicular to the deep planes – in the deep fascia in the temple region, elsewhere in the deep subcutaneous tissue, and more rarely in the subperiosteal tissue. The injection is made using the linear-threading technique, without using the nappage technique or moving the cannula back and forth. The non-injecting hand is essential. It constantly palpates the end of the cannula and assesses the quantity of product being injected. Rigorous massage of the injected areas is required. All three products are quite easy to inject, but Voluma and Fortelis are a little more readily employed in terms of syringability. The 18G cannula due to its length of 60 mm, as well as the 21G cannula measuring 40 mm, is more appropriate for this injection. Research into the development of longer 21G and 25G soft-tipped needles is currently under way. In the event of overcorrection, pressure can be applied to the injected area to immediately remove the product. In the event, to prevent any extrusion to the superficial layers of the dermis, it is suitable to inject 1 ml of saline from the needle before taking it out.

Do not overcorrect. The injection volume required generally varies between 1 and 3 ml on each side, and 2 ml per side is injected for average volume loss. Combination with a regular linked HA filler supplement, usually from the same laboratory range, may be a good solution. For instance, deep dermis injection in the cheeks, upper part of the nasolabial fold (NLF), and maxillary region could be balanced with mid-dermis injections of regular fillers in the same area as well as complementary injections in tear troughs (subperiosteal), marionette lines, and inferior part of the NLF.

After the injection

Immediately after the injection, the patient is systematically checked in the upright position with the head bent forward. An anti-bruise cream and a cold pack are often advisable. Other regulatory procedures include putting the label in the patient's file, correctly disposing of the used solution, and writing a prescription.

During the check-up, which takes place 21–45 days later, retouching with the volumetric HA or with another linked HA supplement from the same laboratory range may be suggested. One year to 18 months after the initial injection, it may be necessary to touch up the area with the same volumetric product and/or a linked filler usually from the same laboratory.

Mammary and body hyaluronic acid volumetric implants

Fat grafts remain one of the best types of implant for these corrections. Fat transfer can provide substantial volume to deficient areas, but the surgery can be complex. A further criticism of fat transfer is its unpredictable efficacy. Non-resorbable materials can accumulate permanently in the body, and may cause granuloma formation or chronic foreign body reactions. Complication and reoperation rates as high as 50% have been reported with silicone implants during the first 3 years following surgery,[25] as well as with alkylimide (Bio-Alcamid).

A new gel HA implant designed for volume restoration and contouring of both the mammary and the body surface has had CE (Conformité Européene) approval since September 2007: Macrolane® from Q-Med laboratories. It is manufactured according to the NASHA technique. The available volumes are 10 and 20 ml, with a maximum recommended per sequence of 100 ml per site and 20 ml as touch-up; a 16G needle is necessary to perform the injection. The injection is mostly done in the deep dermis, and subcutaneous and/or supraperiosteal layers. Good indications are the following: minor body atrophy due to trauma scars, scarring and asymmetry after liposuction, concave body deformities, and enlargement of body areas such as breasts and buttocks. Other indications such as hands, penile enlargement, and vaginal volume reduction, as well as the upper arms, calves, and décolleté are being developed. A touch-up is probably required: 50% of the initial injection at 12–18 months and 25% at 36 months.

Use in female breast hypotrophy has recently gained CE approval. Clinical pilot studies started in 2002, and the results are shortly to be published in *Aesthetic Surgery Journal*. In a first pilot study of NASHA gel for breast enhancement (19 participants), mammography and MRI were performed in five patients following treatment. Injected NASHA gel had increased radiolucency compared with silicone or saline implants, allowing visualization of tissue behind the gel. In addition, MRI results showed persistence of implanted NASHA gel up to 12 months post-injection, albeit with a degree of biodegradation. The second study from Per Heden's group in 20 patients, with an average injection of 97.8 ml per breast, showed on MRI scan 1–5 days after treatment that 80% of the implant was present in the correct location between the muscle and the mammary gland. Breast appearance improvement was 100% in all patients, and 75% at 6 months. The most commonly reported adverse event was injection site pain: eight cases, resolved in 8 days. The second most common was an implant site reaction: six cases, with capsular contracture. The time to recovery was 133 days, with 4–6 encapsulations treated with closed capsulotomy.[25,26]

Legal and practical considerations

In Europe and USA

In Europe, CE marking is a prerequisite for marketing injectable products. However, a CE marking does not necessarily imply that the product's efficacy and side-effects have been assessed objectively in clinical studies. Nevertheless, this marking is expected to fall into line with the US legislation, where the marketing of any medicinal product is subject to FDA approval, based on comprehensive animal and clinical studies and on more systematic and better centralized side-effect reporting.

Different products

We have examined most of the slowly resorbable, non-resorbable, and resorbable products available in 2008, used mainly to increase volume. Before injecting these products, it is essential to have a thorough understanding of their absolute and relative contraindications and anesthetic requirements, differences between types of areas to fill and indicated techniques, differences between concerned regions or tissues, and the impact of associated cosmetic treatments.

Side-effects

The slowly and non-resorbable products are highly efficient, but unfortunately sometimes responsible for complications or even undesirable after-effects. In order to avoid these the following are necessary: clinical and histological analysis of facial granulomas, and a proposal for guidelines for their use which would predict in situ tolerance.[27]

All injections

Thorough questioning is required to find out about the patient's previous history and absolute, relative, or psychological contraindications to these products.

In-depth knowledge of the anatomy of fat, facial lipoatrophy areas, and reshaping techniques is necessary, and a product must never be injected in a contraindicated area (such as the eyelids or lips for most).

Conclusion

It is desirable to avoid, especially at the same site, a mixture of biodegradable and non-biodegradable products, but it is possible to use two different biodegradable ranges. Meticulous investigations of the antecedents and former treatments are of primary importance. Similar to a the health booklet, it would be appropriate to have a booklet of 'health-beauty' in which all esthetic procedures are mentioned in detail. It would be necessary for both the patient and the practitioner to have a copy of the health-beauty booklet containing the dates and labels of the products used.

The reconstitution of volumes of the face is a fundamental chapter in both dermatology and cosmetic and esthetic surgery. Although fat grafting represents the procedure of choice, it is not always available or acceptable; volumetric fillers then offer ease of use, performance, and durability. Volumetric implants have mostly been slowly and non-biodegradable fillers. Their reported side-effects are very few considering the number of treated patients, but can sometimes be the origin of dramatic consequences when the product is permanent. The recent employment of hyaluronic acids as volumetric implants shows that still many factors are unknown; initial results are clearly significant, and those for HAs are indisputable.[25–45]

However, all these volumetric injectables have an undeniable increasingly important place in the search for the ideal implant, being immunologicaly inert and rather slowly biodegradable, and acting optimally by filling and increasing in volume.

References

1. Ascher B, Katz P. Facial lipoatrophy and the place of ultrasound. Dermatol Surg 2006; 32: 702–12.
2. Ascher B, Coleman S, Alster T et al. Full scope of effect of facial lipoatrophy: a framework of disease understanding. Dermatol Surg 2006; 32: 1058–69.

3. Ascher B, Bui P, Halabi A. Fillers in Europe. In: Goldberg D, ed. Fillers in Cosmetic Dermatology. London: Informa Healthcare, 2006: 127–50.

4. Vleggaar D, Fitzgerald R. Dermatological implication of skeletal aging: a focus on supraperiosteal volumization for perioral rejuvenation. J Drugs Dermatol 2008; 7: 209–20.

5. Lichtenstein KA, Ward DJ, Moorman AC et al. Clinical assessment of HIV-associated lipodystrophy in an ambulatory population. AIDS 2001; 15: 1389–98.

6. Carr A, Law M. An objective lipodystrophy severity grading scale derived from the lipodystrophy case definition score. J Acquir Immune Defic Syndr 2003; 33: 571–6.

7. James J, Carruthers A, Carruthers J. HIV-associated facial lipoatrophy. Dermatol Surg 2002; 28: 979–86.

8. Garg A. Acquired and inherited lipodystrophies. N Engl J Med 2004; 350: 1220–34.

9. Valantin MA, Aubron-Olivier C, Ghosn J et al. Polylactic acid implants (New-Fill) (R) to correct facial lipoatrophy in HIV-infected patients: results of the open-label study VEGA. AIDS 2003; 17: 2471–7.

10. Amard P, Saint-Marc T, Katz P. The effects of polylactic acid (PLA) as therapy for lipoatrophy of the face. Antivir Ther 2000; 5 (Suppl): 79.

11. Carr A, Miller J, Law M, Cooper DA. A syndrome of lipoatrophy, lactic acidaemia and liver dysfunction associated with HIV nucleoside analogue therapy: contribution to protease inhibitor-related lipodystrophy syndrome. AIDS 2000; 14: F25–32.

12. Palella FJ Jr, Delaney KM, Moorman AC et al. Declining morbidity and mortality among patients with advanced human immunodeficiency virus infection. HIV Outpatient Study Investigators. N Engl J Med 1998; 338: 853–60.

13. Collins E, Wagner C, Walmsley S. Psychosocial impact of the lipodystrophy syndrome in HIV infection. AIDS Read 2000; 10: 546–50.

14. Dukers NH, Stolte IG, Albrecht N et al. The impact of experiencing lipodystrophy on the sexual behaviour and wellbeing among HIV-infected homosexual men. AIDS 2001; 15: 812–13.

15. Duran S, Saves M, Spire B et al. Failure to maintain longterm adherence to highly active antiretroviral therapy: the role of lipodystrophy. AIDS 2001; 15: 2441–4.

16. Ammassari A, Antinori A, Cozzi-Lepri A et al. Relationship between HAART adherence and adipose tissue alterations. J Acquir Immune Defic Syndr 2002; 31(Suppl 3): S140–4.

17. Mole B. Long term treatment for lipoatrophy associated or not with HIV infections using ePTFE implants and polyacrylamide gel. Aesthetic Surg J 2005; 25: 561–70.

18. Lowe N, Grower R. Injectable hyaluronic acid implant for malar and mental enhancement. Dermatol Surg 2006; 32: 881–5.

19. DeLorenzi C, Weinberg M, Solish N, Swift A. Multicenter study of efficacy and safety of subcutaneous non-animal-stabilized hyaluronic acid in aesthetic facial contouring: interim report. Dermatol Surg 2006; 32: 205–11.

20. Verpaele A, Strand A. Restylane SubQ, a non-animal stabilized hyaluronic acid gel for soft tissue augmentation of the mid- and lower face. Aesthetic Surg J 2006; 26 (Suppl): S10–17.

21. Grover R. Optimizing treatment outcome with Restylane SubQ: the role of patient selection and counseling. Aesthetic Surg J 2006; 26 (Suppl): S18–21.

22. Sito G. Transoral injection of Restylane SubQ for aesthetic contouring of the cheeks. Aesthetic Surg J 2006; 26 (Suppl): S18–21.

23. Belmontesi M, Grover R, Verpaele A. Transdermal injection of Restylane SubQ for aesthetic contouring of the cheeks, chin and mandible. Aesthetic Surg J 2006; 26 (Suppl): S28–34.

24. Strand A, Wolters M. HIV-related lipodystrophy and facial lipoatrophy: the role of Restylane SubQ in reversing facial wasting. Aesthetic Surg J 2006; 26 (Suppl): S35–40.

25. Hedén P, Olenius M. Stabilized hyaluronic acid-based gel of non-animal origin, a promising new development for breast enhancement. Poster presented at AAWC, Paris, 10–12 April, 2008.

26. Hedén P et al. Review article on body contouring including data from first pilot study on breast and concave deformities. Aesthetic Plast Surg 2008;

27. Cucin RL, Barek D. Complications of injectable collagen implant. Plast Reconstr Surg 1983; 71: 731.

28. Lemperle G, Morhenn V, Charrier U. Human histology and persistence of various injectable filler substances for soft tissue augmentation. Aesthetic Plast Surg 2003; 27: 354–66.

29. Code de la Santé Publique (Partie Réglementaire – Décrets en Conseil d'Etat). Art. R665–48. www.legifrance.gouv.fr.

30. Manna F, Dentini M, Desideri P et al. Comparative chemical evaluation of two commercially available derivatives of hyaluronic acid (Hylaform® from rooster combs and Restylane® from Streptococcus) used for soft tissue augmentation. J Eur Acad Dermatol Venereol 1999; 13: 183–92.

31. Pons-Guiraud A. Matériaux de comblement: techniques et effets indésirables. In: EMC, vol, Cosmétologie et Dermatologie esthétique. Paris: Elsevier Masson, 2004: 59–74.

32. Hoffman C, Schuller-Petrovic S, Soyer HP, Kerl H. Adverse reactions after cosmetic lip augmentation with permanent biologically inert implant materials. J Am Acad Dermatol 1999; 40: 100–23.

33. Pons-Guiraud A. Actualisation des effets secondaires des produits de comblement. Nouv Dermatol 2003; 22: 205–10.

34. Barr R, Stegman SJ. Delayed skin test reaction to injectable collagen implant (Zyderm). The histopathologic comparative study. J Am Acad Dermatol 1984; 10: 652–8.

35. De Lustro F, Fries J, Kang J et al. Immunity to injectable collagen and autoimmune disease; a summary of current understanding. J Dermatol Surg Oncol 1988; 14 (Suppl 1): 57–65.

36. Bergeret-Galley C. Comparison of resorbable soft tissue fillers. J Aesthet Surg 2004; 24: 33–45.

37. Ascher B. CPM HA volumetric injectable for facial lipoatrophy: preliminary evaluation. Abstract presented at IMCAS Asia, Singapore, 13 July, 2008.

38. Bui P, Pons-Guiraud A, Kuffer R. Injectables lentement et non résorbables. Ann Chir Plast Esthet 2004; 49: 486–502.

39. Ascher B, Cerceau M, Baspeyras M, Rossi B. Soft tissue filling with hyaluronic acid. Ann Chir Plast Esthet 2004; 49: 465–85.

40. Requena C, Izquierdo MJ, Navarro M et al. Adverse reactions to injectable aesthetic microimplants. Am J Dermatopathol 2001; 23: 197–202.

41. Rudolph CM, Soyer HP, Schuller-Petrovic S, Kerl H. Foreign body granulomas due to injectable aesthetic microimplants. Am J Surg Pathol 1999; 23: 113–17.

42. Secchi T, Carbonnel E. Correction ambulatoire des lipoatrophies du visage dans l'infection à VIH par technique de comblement. Nouv Dermatol 2003; 22: 132–3.

43. Tennstedt D, Lachapelle JM. Histopathologie des granulomes tardifs consécutifs aux injections de produits de comblement pour rides (colorations spéciales). 2008; in press.

44. Pearl RM, Laub DR, Kaplan EN. Complications following silicone injections for augmentation of the contours of the face. Plast Reconstr Surg 1978; 61: 888–91.

45. Faure M. Complication des implants de silicone et autres matériaux dits inertes. Ann Dermatol Venereol 1995; 122: 455–9.

46. Claude O, Domergue Than Trong E, Blanc R et al. Treatment of HIV facial lipoatrophy with a submalar porous polyethilene implant (Medpor®). Annales de chirurgie plastique esthétique (2008), In Press. doi: 10.1016/j.anplas.2008.05.009

40 Adipose tissue, physiology and regenerative medicine

Béatrice Cousin, Valérie Planat, Guillaume Charrière, Patrick Laharrague,
Audrey Carrière, Luc Pénicaud, and Louis Casteilla

Body fat, or adipose tissue, was long considered merely a filler tissue. It has been studied for its involvement in metabolic diseases such as diabetes and obesity. In the course of the past decade, it has evolved in status from being regarded as a simple energy reservoir to being considered as an endocrine and secretory tissue, and it is these characteristics that make it appear likely to play a role in many of the body's physiological responses, including the inflammatory response.

The use of adipose tissue transfer in plastic and reconstructive surgery is not new and has been the subject of numerous studies, especially after the development of lipostructure by Coleman who introduced a procedure based on strict methodology and the use of specific material. Initially aimed for the treatment of facial aging, this technique has been extended to the various fields of plastic surgery such as hand rejuvenation or correction of the deformities of lower members and hips.[1-3] Discovery of the developmental capacities of the great number of lineages from adipose-derived cells and their in vitro culture has opened new research perspectives and clinical applications. Now, the view of adipose tissue is moving to a potentially suitable and huge source of regenerative cells from various perspectives for cell therapy.

Adipose tissue: general presentation

There are several types of adipose tissue. In fact, three types can be distinguished from each other on the basis of their physical, morphological, and functional characteristics: white adipose tissue (WAT), brown adipose tissue (BAT), and medullary adipose tissue, or yellow marrow (Figure 40.1). We will discuss here only the white adipose tissue, which is the most abundant and the only one easy to use in regenerative medicine.

White adipose tissue is the most well known of the three types of adipose tissue. It is found in two forms: a diffuse form made up of more or less isolated cells (for example intramuscular fat), and a form made up of depots situated at various anatomical locations. The largest depots are subcutaneous or deep depots (intra-abdominal or visceral). These WAT depots are the body's main locations for storing energy in the form of lipids. These lipids give the tissue its white color. Distribution of the fat mass is variable according to sex, and is under the control of the sex hormones. This distribution has considerable pathological consequences because the excessive development of abdominal adipose tissue is associated with a higher cardiovascular risk.

WAT develops mainly after birth. It plays a considerable role in the maintenance of energy balance because it can store and release energy according to the organism's needs. It mainly consists of white adipocytes that are specialized tissue cells; they are large cells with a large unilocular lipid droplet and very little cytoplasm. The tissue also contains blood capillaries, nerve endings, connective tissue, fibroblast cells, and macrophages.

WAT mass in the body may vary considerably depending on the body's energy needs, and in pathological situations such as obesity and cachexia. Increases in WAT mass are due to increases in the size and/or number of adipocytes.[4]

White adipose tissue development

There exist very few data on early adipose tissue development. Indeed, no study of the adipose lineage comparable to studies conducted on other tissues has been performed to date. The main data available come from histological studies. WAT was long considered to be a simple filler tissue and classified as connective tissue. Beginning in the 1960s, adipose tissue went from being considered a filler tissue to gaining the status of an adipose organ. WAT is not present in rodents before birth. On the other hand, in larger mammals (humans, for example), it is detectable late in the gestation period.[5,6] In 1964, Wassermann was the first to compare WAT development to the development of other organs.[7] Through an in-depth histological analysis, he observed that adipose depots, then called 'adipose organs', develop from primitive organs. These primitive structures are reticuloendothelial in nature. It is in these primitive organs that the first adipocytes appear in

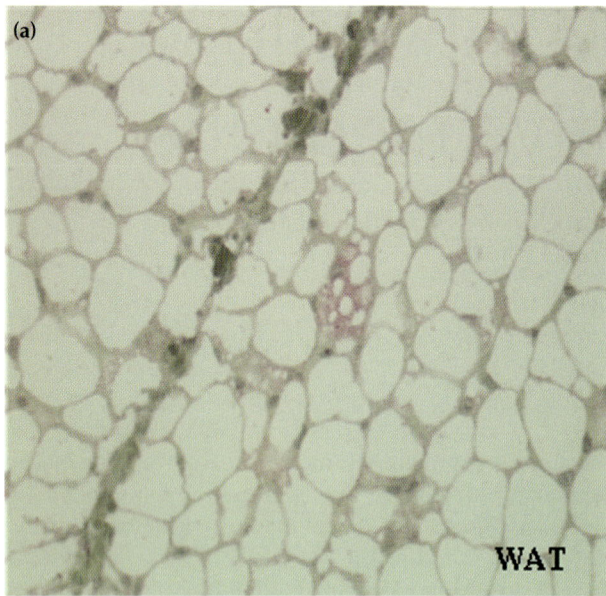

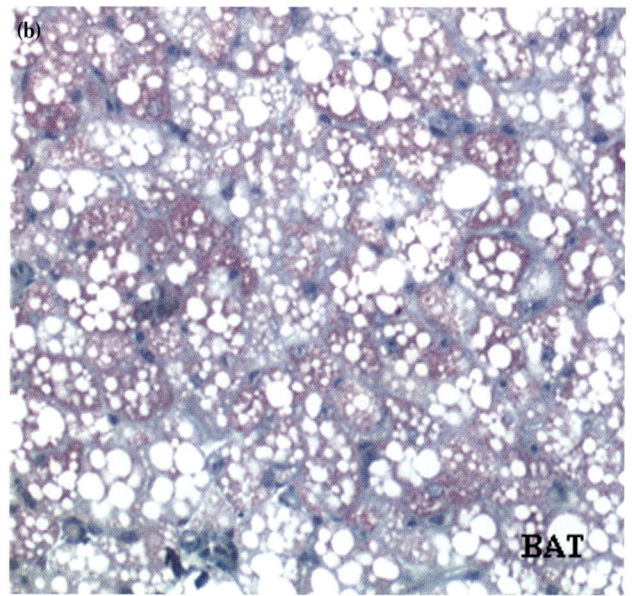

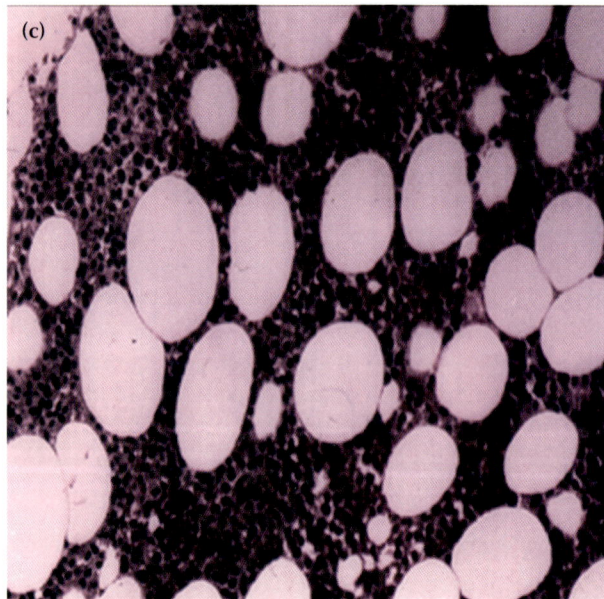

Figure 40.1 Histomorphological aspect and main physiological functions of the three types of adipose tissue. (a) WAT: white adipose tissue. Extramedullary (energy metabolism): energy storage (10–50% of adult body weight), reversible enlargement, endocrine function. (b) BAT: brown adipose tissue. Extramedullary: thermogenesis. (c) Bone marrow adipose tissue: hematopoiesis.

clusters adjacent to blood capillaries. The structures containing the first adipocytes and many blood capillaries are at this stage referred to as adipose tissue lobules. Within these lobules, the adipocyte clusters stem from a mass of mesenchymal cells which are associated with the vascular network development. Mesenchymal cells, stemming from nascent capillaries, begin to accumulate lipids. The most advanced cells in the differentiation are the cells which are farthest from the capillaries. Vascularization plays a key role in the development of adipose tissue: the density of adipocytes correlates to the density of blood capillaries. Angiogenesis and adipose tissue development appear to be related in time and space.[8] Recently, the use of angiogenesis-regulating factors showed the existence of a direct relationship between adipose mass

development and angiogenesis.[9] Furthermore, recent work conducted in our own laboratory found that adipose lineage cells have the ability to give rise to endothelial cells in vivo and in vitro.[10] Therefore, there appears to be a lineage relationship between adipose cells and endothelial cells.

Metabolic and secretory roles of white adipose tissue

Metabolic role

The first roles attributed to WAT were organ cushioning and thermal insulation. It is now widely accepted that adipose tissue is essential to maintaining

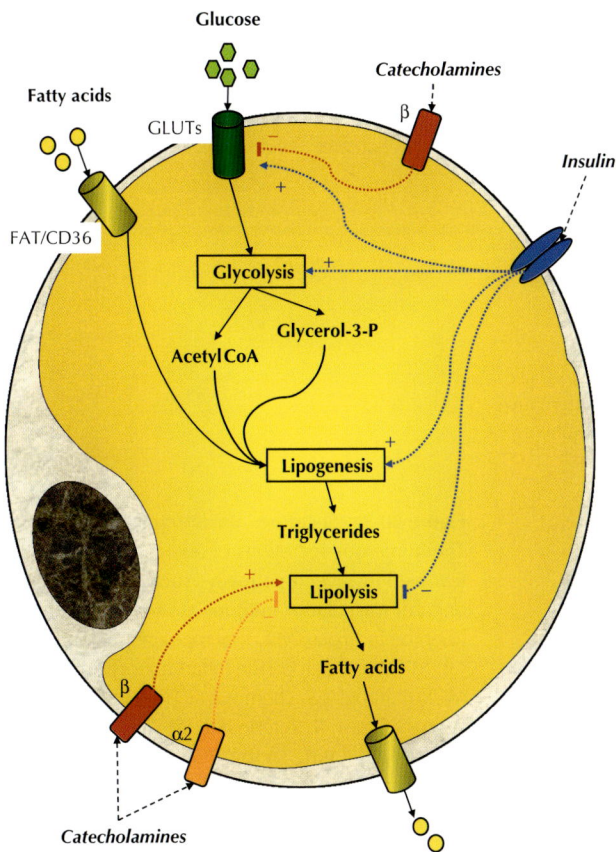

Figure 40.2 Adipocyte metabolism. Adipocytes are able to accumulate triglycerides via lipogenesis that is positively controlled by insulin, or by direct capitation of fatty acids via FAT/CD36. Lipogenesis is dependent on glucose transport and glucose metabolism. Catecholamines inhibit glucose transport. Under some circumstances, triglycerides may be hydrolyzed to give rise to fatty acids via a lipolytic pathway that is inhibited by insulin and α2 receptors of catecholamines. By contrast, catecholamines may also have a positive effect on lipolysis via their β2 receptors. FAT/CD36, fatty acid transporter; GLUTs, glucose transporters; CoA, coenzyme A; P, phosphate.

energy homeostasis. Energy homeostasis is the body's process of maintaining a fine balance between energy intake and expenditure. The most important role of WAT is in energy storage, thereby taking part in energy homeostasis in spite of irregular food intake.

The storage of energy in adipocytes is regulated by hormonal signals and nervous stimuli which depend on the body's energy needs (Figure 40.2). Adipocytes are capable of storing vast quantities of fatty acids in the form of triglycerides. The storage pathways represent a large difference between rodent and human species. Indeed, while lipogenesis (synthesis of triglycerides from glucose) takes place mainly in rodent mature adipocytes, a similar pathway occurs mainly in the human liver, and lipid storage in mature adipocytes is more related to lipid uptake from

lipoproteins. Triglyceride storage within adipocytes is heavily dependent upon insulin. In physiological situations where energy needs are high, the breakdown of triglycerides (lipolysis) is highly stimulated, enabling the release of fatty acids into the bloodstream. This stimulation of lipolysis is generally due to the concomitant action of an insulin decrease and a catecholamine increase.

More recently, it has come to light that adipocytes have a large capacity for cholesterol storage. Indeed, cholesterol is picked up from high density lipoproteins (HDLs). Adipocytes are able to bind to HDLs via the scavenger receptor SR-B1. Cholesterol is then stored within the adipocytes' characteristic intracytoplasmic lipid droplets. Depending on metabolic variations, adipocytes can release stored cholesterol via the ABCA1 transporter.[11]

Endocrine and secretory functions

During the past 20 years, many studies have demonstrated the important secretory abilities of adipocytes. A large number of products secreted by adipocytes are peptidic in nature, and are grouped together under the term adipokines (Figure 40.3). Through its secretory properties, WAT participates actively in the body's energy homeostasis, but it is also involved in other functions such as cardiovascular function and innate immunity.[12] We are not going to list in detail all the different products secreted by adipocytes. The only products to be dealt with here are those which will help illustrate the concept of WAT as a secretory organ and its involvement in the regulation of energy metabolism, the cardiovascular system, and innate immunity.

Secretions and energy metabolism

The 1994 discovery of leptin promoted WAT to the status of endocrine organ. Leptin is a hormone which is mainly secreted by WAT and which plays a major role in energy homeostasis. Leptin secretion is proportionate to body fat mass. Leptin acts within the hypothalamus and reduces appetite by inhibiting the action of neuropeptide Y.[13] Since the discovery of leptin, many studies have shown that it has pleiotropic effects, in particular on reproduction, leukocyte activity, hematopoiesis, angiogenesis, and bone and brain development, as well as on healing.[14,15] It is interesting to note that other cytokines are also secreted by adipocytes and influence energy metabolism. For example, tumor necrosis factor α (TNF-α) is secreted by adipocytes and appears to play an important role in the development of insulin resistance during type II diabetes and during obesity.[16,17] Since the discovery of leptin, other adipocyte-secreted proteins have been found which have significant effects on energy metabolism. This is the case with adiponectin and resistin.[18]

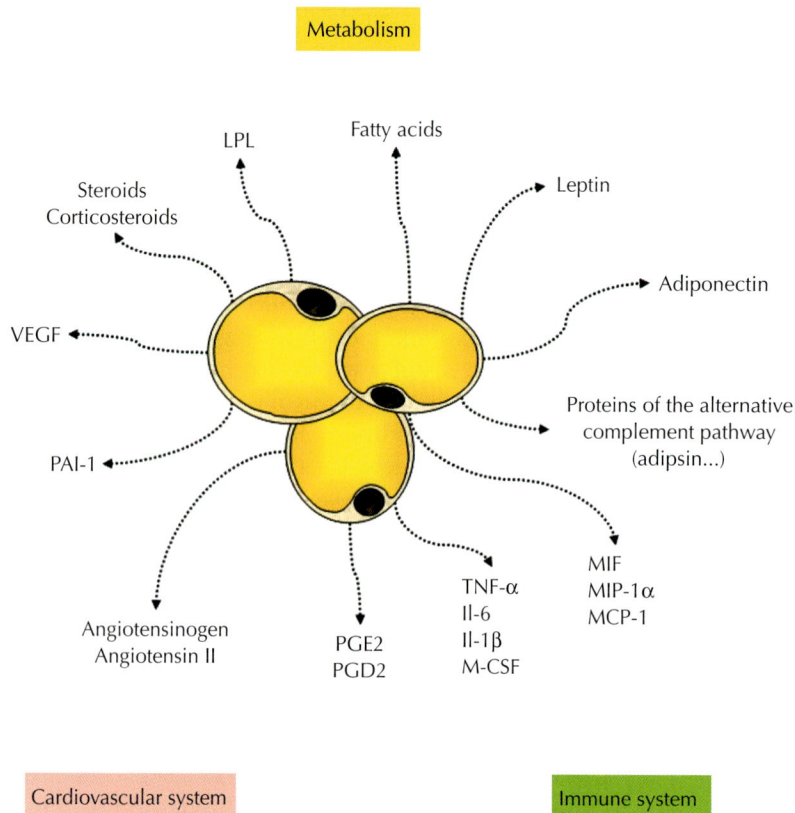

Figure 40.3   Secretory functions of adipose tissue. The numerous secretions of adipose tissue may be involved in several pathways such as metabolism, or cardiovascular or immune system function. LPL, lipoprotein lipase; MIF, macrophage inhibitory factor; MIP-1α, macrophage inflammatory protein 1α; MCP, macrophage chemotactic protein; TNF, tumor necrosis factor; IL, interleukin; M-CSF, macrophage colony stimulating factor; PG, prostaglandin; PAI, plasminogen activator inhibitor; VEGF, vascular endothelial growth factor.

Secretions and the immune system

Adipose tissue is a significant source of complement proteins, inflammatory cytokines, chemokines, and prostaglandins. Among the complement proteins secreted by adipose tissue are the alternative pathway factors: B, C3, factor D, also known as adipsin, and acylation-stimulating protein (ASP).[19,20] Adipsin was the first factor found to be secreted by adipocytes. Another secreted factor which is similar to complement factor C1q, called Acrp30, or adiponectin, was recently identified.[21] The total adipose tissue mass represents almost 15% of a healthy individual's body weight. Therefore, adipose tissue is the main source of the body's complement factors.

As we have already seen, adipocytes secrete TNF-α. They also secrete other inflammatory cytokines such as interleukin 6, interleukin 1β, and chemokines such as macrophage inhibitory factor (MIF), macrophage colony stimulating factor (M-CSF), macrophage inflammatory protein 1α (MIP-1α), and monocyte chemotactic protein 1 (MCP-1). All of these products are protein in nature, and are known to be involved in the inflammatory reaction and to regulate leukocyte functions.[22–24] Other non-protein products secreted by adipocytes such as prostaglandins PGE2 and PGD2 may

regulate immune responses by playing on leukocyte activity.[25]

Secretions and the cardiovascular system

Among the products secreted by adipose tissues, some act on cardiovascular functions. WAT contains the principal components of the renin–angiotensin system, namely angiotensinogen, the angiotensin conversion factor, angiotensin II, and angiotensin receptors. Angiotensinogen appears to play a role in tissue blood flow regulation and therefore in fatty acid flux.[26] Moreover, angiotensin II, angiotensinogen breakdown product, appears to stimulate prostacyclin (PGI2) secretion by adipocytes, and thus promotes autocrine/paracrine regulation which promotes the differentiation of adipocyte precursors.[27–29]

Adipose tissue also secretes plasminogen activator inhibitor 1 (PAI-1). This factor is implicated in cardiovascular pathologies since its levels are increased during situations of myocardial infarction and venous thrombosis. It has also been argued that PAI-1 secretion levels correlate to adipose tissue mass.[30–32] As a consequence, PAI-1 may play an important role in the development of cardiovascular pathologies associated with obesity. Adipose tissue also secretes angiogenic factors such as vascular endothelial growth factor (VEGF) and monobutyrin.[33] VEGF is largely known for its significant role in angiogenesis stimulation. Leptin's angiogenic effects have also been described. Thus, because adipocytes are a major source of angiogenic factors, they are thought to promote the vascularization of adipose tissue itself and therefore its growth.[34]

Preadipocyte and adipocyte differentiation

Highlighting

The increase in mass of adipose depots during the developmental process is due to increases in the number and size of adipose cells. Increases in the number of adipocytes depend on the differentiation of adipocyte progenitors or preadipocytes. They are found within adipose tissue. Preadipocytes can be isolated in the samples of adipose tissue from many species, and they can be induced to differentiate in vitro. The dissociation of adipose tissue cells is carried out by shearing and digestion with collagenase. The cells are then separated based on the difference in density between adipocytes and other types of cells. Since adipocytes are full of lipids, they have a lower density than water and therefore float to the surface, unlike the other types of cells which sink (preadipocytes, endothelial cells, macrophages, and fibroblasts). This fraction of cells is called the stromavascular fraction (SVF). From the cells of the SVF, a fibroblastic population of cells adheres in culture and, from these cells, preadipocytes gradually accumulate lipids and acquire the characteristics of mature adipocytes.

This is observed irrespective of an individual's age. Adipocyte differentiation may be observed even in adipose tissue from particularly old mice.[35] The generation of new adipocytes depends upon the body's energy balance. The number of adipocytes increases in rats subjected to a high-carbohydrate or high-fat diet.[36,37] In cases of severe obesity in humans, an increase in the number of adipocytes is also observed. As we will see, there are currently different models for studying adipocyte differentiation which allow us to understand the characteristics of preadipocytes. However, and although we know a fair amount about the process of adipocyte differentiation, the preadipocyte is not yet a fully understood cell type. There are currently no antigenic markers specific to this cell type; the majority of markers used are in fact markers of more or less early adipocyte differentiation. Consequently, these markers do not allow the identification of cells already engaged in the process of adipocyte differentiation. The only precise definition of the preadipocyte is probably the following: it is a cell which is capable of differentiation into an adipocyte.

The stages of differentiation

Determination

Studies conducted using adipocyte differentiation in vitro have made it possible to identify the major stages in the differentiation process (Figure 40.4). Unlike the myocyte lineage, no master gene controlling the commitment of multipotent cells in the adipocyte lineage has been clearly identified. Recently, only early genes capable of inhibiting the commitment of cells in adipocyte differentiation have been identified. Among these early genes are the transcription factors GATA-2 and -3,[38] the DeltaFosB factor which promotes osteogenesis to the detriment of adipogenesis,[23] and Wnt family factors which promote the commitment of cells to myogenesis to the detriment of adipogenesis[39] (Figure 40.5). In addition, PPAR-γ (peroxisome proliferator activated receptor γ) and C/EBP-α (CAAT enhancer binding protein α) are major players in the control of adipose differentiation. Indeed, the expression of these two transcription factors in myoblasts induces their differentiation into adipocytes.[40] PPAR-γ is expressed early during the process of adipogenesis and controls the expression of numerous genes involved in adipocytic metabolism or differentiation.[41]

Cellular contact

Contact between cells appears necessary to the adipogenic process. When adipocyte precursors/progenitors reach the confluence, intercellular contact is significant, and the cells stop in phase G0/G1 of the cellular cycle. After the arrest of their cellular cycle, adipoblasts express early markers of adipocyte differentiation such as liporotein lipase (LPL)[42] and A2Col6 (an equivalent of the α2 chain of type IV collagen in humans)[43] (Figure 40.4). This expression of early markers of adipogenesis is probably subordinate to the paracrine/autocrine signals unleashed by cellular contact. At this stage adipoblasts go on to become preadipocytes and lose the expression of the surface protein preadipose factor 1 (Pref-1) which has an inhibiting effect on adipocyte differentiation.[44] Pref-1 is a surface protein that contains repetitions of epidermal growth factor (EGF)-like domains. A soluble form of Pref-1 is produced by division, and it is this form which has an inhibiting effect on adipocyte differentiation.

Clonal expansion

A clonal-expansion phase is necessary to the progression of preadipocytes in adipocyte differentiation.[45,46] This phase corresponds to post-confluent mitoses (Figure 40.4). In the course of these mitoses, DNA replication may participate in the modification of the chromatin state and thus uncover the sites which then become

Steps of differentiation

Cell types

Protein expression

Multipotent cell

Wnt
DeltaFosB
GATA-2/3

Determination towards
adipocytic lineage

Adipoblast

Pref-1

Proliferation

Confluence

A2Col6
LPL

PPAR-δ
C/EBP-β/δ

Preadipocyte

Clonal expansion

PPAR-γ
C/EBP-α
ADD1/SREBP1c

Arrest of
proliferation

GLUT-4
aP2
HSL

Young adipocyte

PEPCK
Leptin
Adipsin

Terminal
differentiation

Mature adipocyte

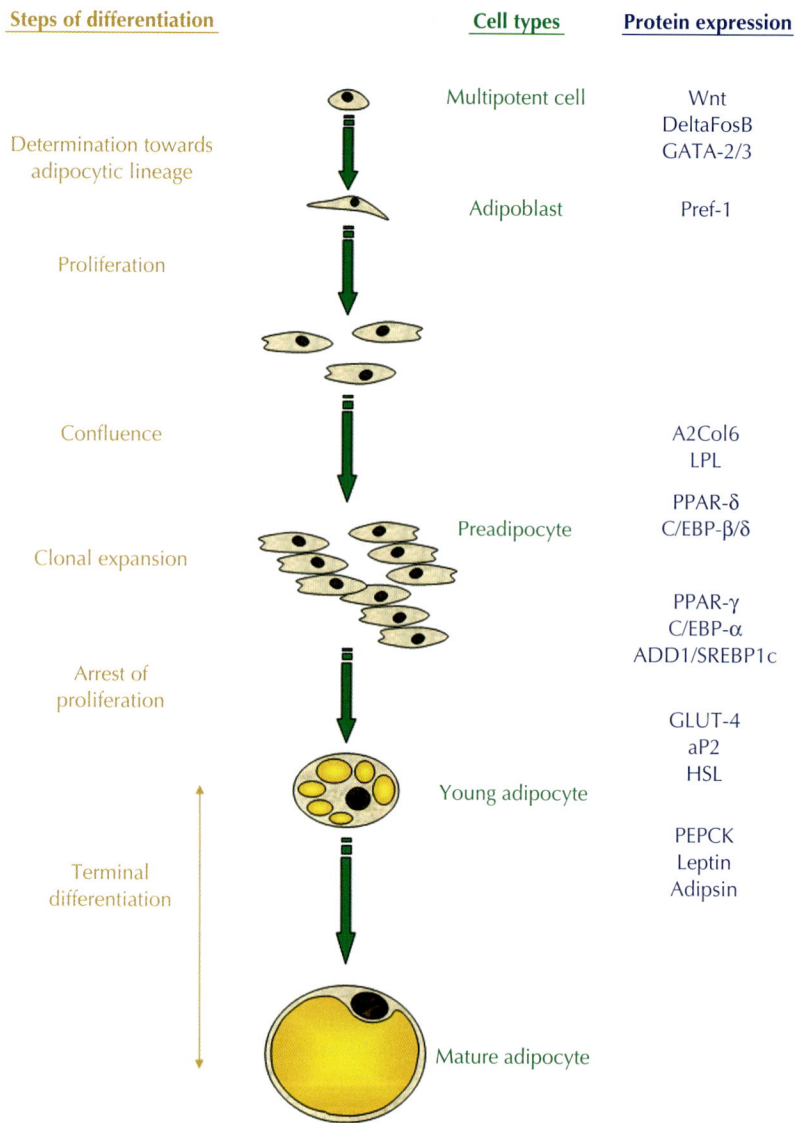

Figure 40.4 Adipose differentiation. To acquire adipocyte phenotype, the immature multipotent cell has to go through numerous steps identified by the expression of several proteins. A2Col6, A2 chain of collagen 6; LPL, lipoprotein lipase; PPAR, peroxisome proliferator activated receptor; C/EBP, CAAT enhancer binding protein; GLUT, glucose transporter; HSL, hormone sensitive lipase; GPDH, glycerol-3-phosphate dehydrogenase; PEPCK, phosphoenolpyruvate carboxykinase.

accessible to adipogenic transcription factors. The existence of mitoses in the preadipocyte stage was demonstrated in vivo by means of pulse-chase experiments.[47] Only the cells whose DNA has been replicated express glycerol-3-phosphate dehydrogenase (GPDH) in vivo, GPDH being a late marker of adipocyte differentiation.[48]

Terminal differentiation

After the clonal expansion phase, the adipocytes stop proliferating and begin to express adipocyte differentiation markers (Figure 40.4). Among these markers are aP2 (ALBP, adipocyte lipid binding protein), a lipid transporter, as well as the glucose transporter GLUT-4, the hormone-sensitive lipase, and GPDH. Most of these markers are involved in adipocyte energy metabolism and, consequently, lipid droplets appear in the cytoplasm of preadipocytes. This accumulation of lipids brings about morphological changes within the cells; they lose their fibroblastic appearance and grow round with the increase in size of the intracytoplasmic lipid droplets.

Throughout this process, the nascent adipocytes express late-differentiation markers such as adipsine, phosphoenolpyruvate carboxykinase (PEPCK), and leptin.[4]

Preadipocytes and immune cells

Analysis of the literature revealed that adipocyte and monocyte/macrophage lineages have many features in common (Figure 40.6). In particular, proteins or functions considered as specific to one lineage have been characterized in the other. For instance, mature adipose cells express a membrane-bound nicotinamide adenine dinucleotide phosphate (NADPH)-oxidase similar to that present in specialized phagocytes.[49] Preadipocytes and adipocytes secrete numerous inflammatory cytokines such as TNF-α, and are sensitive to lipopolysaccharide (LPS) activation. Conversely, aP2, a fatty-acid transporter, or PPAR-γ, long described as specific to adipocyte lineage, have been detected in macrophages.[50,51]

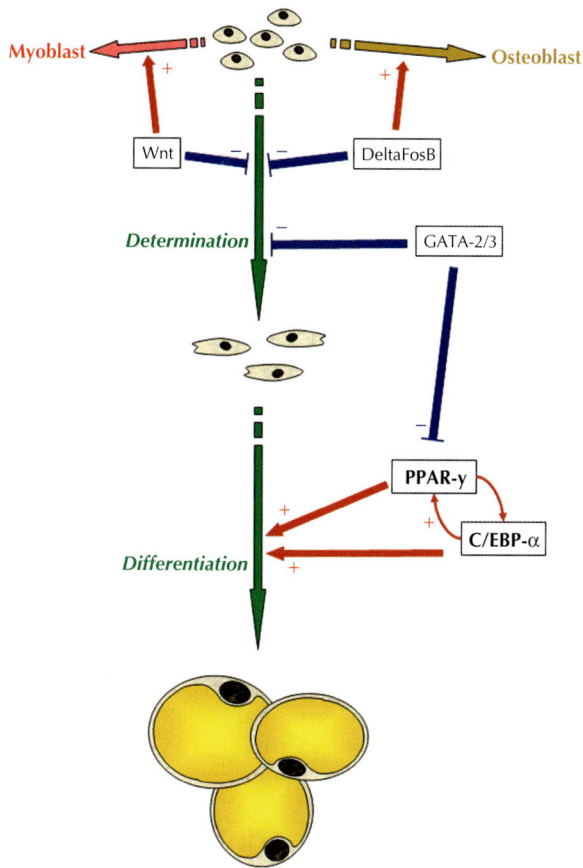

Figure 40.5 Transcriptional control of adipocyte differentiation. The engagement of multipotent cells towards adipocytic lineage is under control of Wnt, DeltaFosB, and GATA-2 and -3. Once the cell is determined, PPAR-γ and C/EBP-α become the major regulators of this process.

In our laboratory, studies have found that preadipocytes have a certain ability to phagocytose and an ability to kill phagocytosed microbes (microbicidal activity).[52] This phagocytic ability is less than that of professional phagocytes, but greater than that of C2C12 myoblasts, and differs according to the fat pad localization.[53] During inflammation, the phagocytic activity of preadipocytes is increased. Surprisingly, the same type of phenomenon is observed in genetically obese mice (ob/ob).[54] The phagocytic activity of preadipocytes is therefore regulated in various body physiopathological situations.

These macrophage functions of preadipocytes are also present in humans. The phagocytic activity of human preadipocytes is significantly higher than that of skin fibroblasts.[55] Furthermore, preadipocytes are able to phagocytose zymosan particles, as well as yeasts and apoptotic bodies. These data support the hypothesis that macrophage-like functions of preadipocytes could be involved in inflammation and tissue remodeling.

A gene profiling analysis between adipocyte and macrophage lineages emphasized similarities between these cell phenotypes. Indeed, preadipocyte gene profiles are systematically associated with macrophage gene profiles.[56]

Finally, preadipocytes can very rapidly convert into macrophage-like cells when they are injected into the peritoneal cavity, considered as a prone environment to support macrophage phenotype.[56] The rapid kinetics of change suggests a trans-differentiation process or/and a stronger lineage relationship between adipocyte progenitors and macrophages than expected.

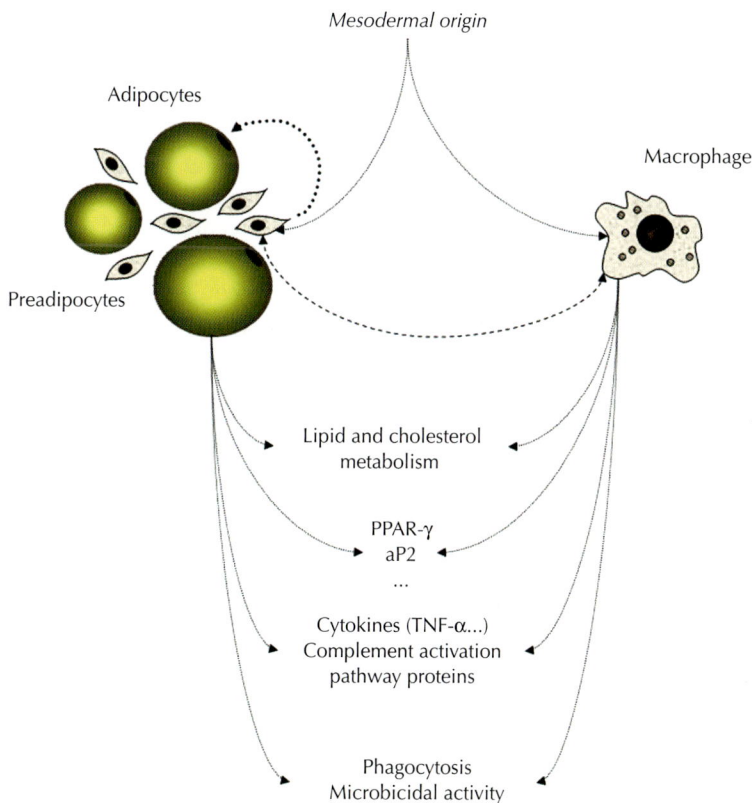

Figure 40.6 Similarities between adipocyte and monocyte/macrophage lineages. Adipose cells and macrophages share numerous similarities, in terms of lipid and cholesterol metabolism, or expression of specific proteins. In addition, both cell types present functional similarities, since they secrete cytokines and are able to phagocytose micro-organisms.

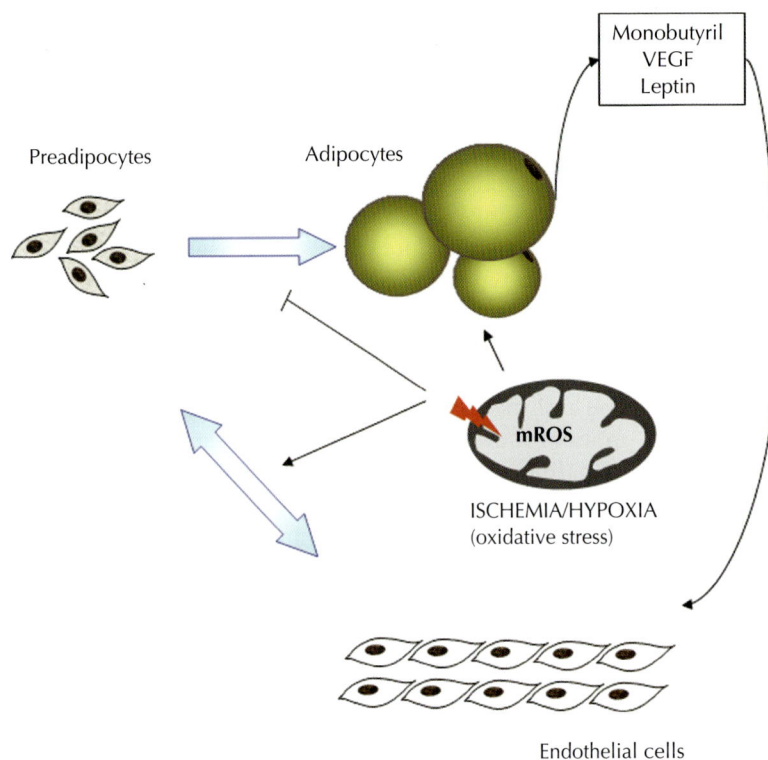

Figure 40.7 Plasticity of adipose-derived cells towards endothelial lineage and its control by mitochondria. Adipocyte precursors have the ability to differentiate into adipocytes and to acquire a functional endothelial phenotype. These two differentiation processes are, at least in part, under the control of reactive oxygen species. mROS, mitochondrial reactive oxygen species.

In fact, it becomes currently very difficult to distinguish without any doubt these two cell types involved in two types of nutritional metabolic diseases, obesity and atherosclerosis. The common point which connects these two pathologies could be the inflammation and the cells which are involved there. These functional analogies between preadipocytes and macrophages suggest that preadipocytes can be involved directly, as well as macrophages, in inflammatory or immune processes of the organism, as well as in adipose tissue remodeling. In support of this hypothesis, two recent studies using the most modern techniques led to the concept that obesity can be regarded as a chronic inflammatory state, as well as atherosclerosis.[57,58]

In addition to its specific relationship with macrophages, adipose tissue contains a specific population of lymphocytes, either gathered in lymph nodes or disseminated among the tissue.[59,60] Cytofluorometric analysis reveals the presence of significant levels of lymphocytes in the stroma-vascular fraction of white adipose tissue. In epididymal fat, lymphocytes display an 'ancestral' immune system phenotype (up to 70% of natural killer (NK), γδ+ T, and NKT cells among all lymphocytes) whereas the inguinal (subcutaneous) immune system presents more adaptive characteristics (high levels of αβ+ T and B cells). The percentage of NK cells in epididymal fat was decreased in obese mice fed with a high-fat diet, whereas γδ positive cells were significantly increased in inguinal fat. These data support the notion that adipose tissue may elaborate immunological mechanisms to regulate its functions which might be altered in obesity.[59]

Preadipocytes and endothelial cells: a common precursor?

During embryonic development, the formation of capillary convolutions is a decisive and specific phase for the development of fat lobules.[7] Later, adipose tissue remodeling and its optimal functioning as a metabolic and endocrine tissue require development of the capillary network. This is consistent with recent data describing that antiangiogenic agents promote adipose tissue loss, thus underlining the functional interaction between adipogenesis and blood vessel formation.[9,61] This close relationship is underlined by the potent proangiogenic factors released by adipose lineage cells (monobutyril, VEGF, and leptin).[62,63] The expression of the marker CD34 by cultured SVF, previously referred to as preadipocytes, led us to postulate that these cells could have an angiogenic potential.[10] Indeed, cultured SVF cells are able to spontaneously differentiate into von Willebrand positive cells in a semi-solid medium. Moreover, in vivo injected adipose-derived cells enhance the neovascularization process in ischemic tissues with direct participation in vascular structure formation and the secretion of angiogenic and antiapoptotic factors. Finally, human mature adipocytes that can dedifferentiate have the potential to differentiate again into mature adipocytes, in vivo and in vitro, to rapidly acquire endothelial phenotype (expression of CD31 and von Willebrand factor (vWF) antigens) and functions. Therefore, it is reasonable to postulate that SVF cells are bipotent cells and can be considered both as preadipocyte and endothelial progenitors[10,64] (Figure 40.7). Identification of the pathways that regulate these plastic processes could lead to the development of new therapeutic strategies for the control of adipose tissue development. The ability of adipocyte lineage cells to differentiate into vascular cells is very consistent with histological observations and with recent reports, which suggest that adipose tissue vessels are in a relatively immature state compared to other organs with a lower plasticity. This could be interpreted as a noncommitted status for adipocyte progenitors or dedifferentiated adipocytes, which can be favored by the culture conditions.

The conjunction in the same cell of macrophagic and angiogenic properties underlies the abundant literature on the nature of endothelial progenitor cells, or EPCs. It is noteworthy that the 'angiogenic' efficiency of adipose-derived cells is as important as that of mononuclear cells of the bone marrow, which are tested in protocols of clinical research.

A perspective in this field would be to determine the different stimuli able to control such plasticity. Among these, hypoxia and mitochondria are prominent. Recently, we provided strong evidence that mitochondrial reactive oxygen species (ROS) negatively control adipocyte differentiation via CHOP-10/GADD153 expression, and could be considered as antiadipogenic signaling molecules.[65] We also suggest that mitochondrial ROS and CHOP-10/GADD153 belong to the intracellular O_2 sensing mechanism of adipose cells. This signaling pathway could be involved in limiting growth of adipose tissue, as described in other tissues.[66] Moreover, ROS generation by mitochondrial dysfunction could be directly involved in adipose tissue alterations associated with the metabolic disorder.[67] It is noteworthy that the same signal promotes both angiogenesis and the secretion of angiogenic factor by mature adipocytes.[68,69] We now propose that the development of adipose tissue is associated to/with local hypoxia situations (Figure 40.7). A similar mechanism could participate in adipogenesis occurring in degenerative processes observed after denervation or during aging.

Other progenitor cells in adipose tissue

Hematopoietic progenitor/stem cells

In 2003, we showed that intraperitoneal injection of SVF cells in lethally irradiated mice prevents mortality and supports the reconstitution of lymphoid and myeloid lineage, suggesting that adipose tissue could be an unexpected source of hematopoietic stem cells.[70] After sex mismatch engraftment, detection of the *sry* gene, identifying the Y chromosome, in the main hematopoietic organs clearly argues that some fat-derived cells have the potential to migrate and possibly undergo hematopoietic site-specific differentiation. Moreover, the presence of hematopoietic stem cells (HSCs) in adipose tissue is clearly reinforced by

the identification of hematopoietic precursors (CD34+, CD45+) in SVF cells. These cells could be among the ones responsible for this striking hematopoietic activity. According to developmental issues, it is not so surprising to find such cells in adipose tissue. Indeed, the large arteries of the embryo are the sites from which HSCs first emerge and where early adipose tissue development takes place.[71] An indirect benefit of fat-derived cell transplantation could be the stimulation of endogenous hematopoiesis. Indeed, the formation of a new stroma could provide a suitable microenvironment for endogenous HSCs via paracrine and/or endocrine processes. This process has been largely documented for stromal cells of the bone marrow,[72] and is also described for stromal cells isolated from adipose tissue (unpublished results).

Spontaneous emergence of cardiac progenitors from adipose-derived cells

An unexpected observation of our group was the spontaneous emergence of functional cardiomyocytes when adipose-derived cells were cultured in a semi-solid medium.[73] These cells express the cardiac specific transcription factors Nkx2.5, GATA-4, and MEF2C (myocyte enhancer factor 2C), the structural cardiac protein β-MHC (myosin heavy chain), and late stage cardiac specification proteins MLC-2v, MLC-2a (myosin light chain), and ANP (atrial natriuretic peptide) as well as functional properties (i.e. calcium transient flux and pharmacological modulation of beating rate). Furthermore, at the early stage of differentiation, they displayed electrophysiological properties (i.e. pacemaker-like activity), characteristic of intermediate stage cardiomyocytes as previously defined in embryonic stem cell-derived cardiomyocytes. In contrast to medullar mesenchymal stem cells,[74,75] this cardiomyocyte differentiation was achieved without 5-azacytidine, as for cardiomyocyte differentiation from embryonic stem cells (ESCs). The concept that potential cardiogenic progenitors reside in the fat tissue ready to express their potential in some specific conditions is remarkable and difficult to understand. This suggests the presence of very immature cells with striking properties in adipose tissue.

Other potentials of differentiation

As long ago as the 1970s, several observations suggested that a relationship exists between marrow adipocytes and bone formation. This relationship was then extended to peripheral adipocytes, and it was shown that adipose-derived cells are able to differentiate in vitro into osteoblasts and to form osteoid in immunodeficient mice.[76]

In 2002, several groups showed that it was possible to obtain, in vitro, myoblasts, osteoblasts, or chondrocytes

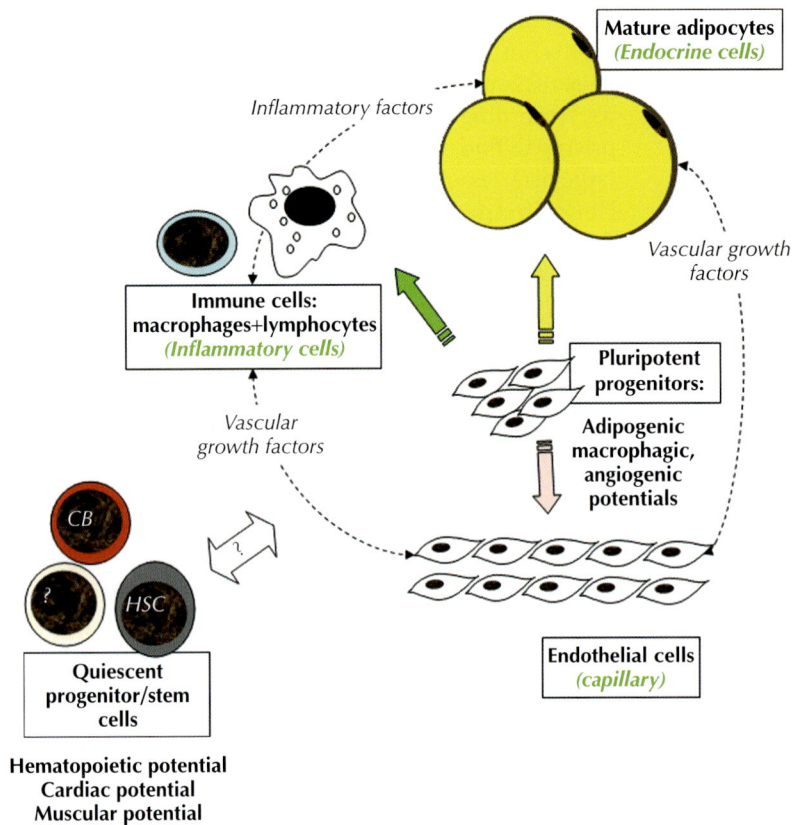

Figure 40.8 Schematic representation of the complexity of adipose tissue.

from human adipose tissue obtained by liposuction.[77,78] Other more recent studies show that it is possible to obtain cells having neuronal characteristics starting from the same samples,[79,80] or to differentiate adipose stromal cells into a hepatic lineage.[81]

Another group has isolated from the adipose tissue of young donors a population of cells that could be extensively expanded ex vivo and that could undergo differentiation into various cell types. These cells injected into mdx mice gave rise to higher levels of dystrophin positive myofibers than primary myoblasts or muscle stem cells isolated from wild type mice.[82] This confirms that adipose-derived cells may participate in damage reparation in skeletal muscles in vivo.[83]

Conclusion: is adipose tissue a suitable source of stem cells for cell therapy?

Altogether, numerous reports have described numerous differentiation potentials for cells derived from adipose tissue. This is consistent with the great plasticity of adipose tissue and leads to the concept that adipose tissue is a subtle and complex cell ecosystem in which different cell populations coexist (Figure 40.8): a large pool of adipocyte precursor cells with a status which needs to be reconsidered and smaller pools of progenitor/stem cells from which hematopoietic, cardiac, or

other cell types can be derived. The isolation and culture procedures of adipose-derived cells seem to be crucial, and are not always similar between reports. This complicates the analysis of data, and further efforts are needed to homogenize procedures and vocabulary. For instance, the delineation between progenitor and stem cell needs to define the self-renewal activity of each subset. Similarly, a complete analysis of adipose-derived cells and medullary mesenchymal stem cells has to be undertaken to clearly establish the mesenchymal status of adipose-derived cells.

Whatever the answers, these recent insights into adipose-derived cell biology already open tremendous perspectives for adipose tissue biology and cell therapy. Although the physiological relevance of these observations needs further investigation, it seems that adipose tissue and the cells derived from it ensure more diverse functions than previously assumed, according to their locations and the physiological and pathophysiological contexts. Moreover, the emergence of adipose cells in non-adipose tissues, such as muscle during degeneration or aging, can be easily understood. In addition, the high degree of plasticity of adipose-derived cells highlights the potential of such cells for cell therapy.

For cell therapy, adipose tissues present several advantages. First, adipose-derived cells are adult cells and avoid ethical issues. Second, their surgical access is very simple, with only a small/minor discomfort for patients, and as their amount is almost non-restrictive, they are convenient for applications in the treatment of a number of disorders. Third, they can be obtained from the patient themselves, avoiding risk of rejection and the need for immune-suppressive drugs.

In ischemia situations, the scarcity of endothelial progenitors, combined with their putative functional impairment, constitutes a major limitation of an endothelial progenitor-based strategy.[84] Thus, the identification of suitable sources of angiogenic cells represents a challenge. Such a challenge seems promising because of the positive effect of bone marrow mononuclear cell-based therapy in the chronic ischemia hindlimb. For adipose-derived cells, the first positive point is that several teams describe the angiogenic properties of such cells, but two crucial steps have to be overcome: (1) the set-up of and the scale-up of adipose cells in GMP (Good Manufacturing Practice) conditions, and (2) the demonstration that adipose-derived cells from patients maintain their angiogenic properties in pathological situations (diabetes, atherosclerosis, inflammation).

The regenerative potential of adult cardiac tissue is limited and not sufficient to prevent tissular degeneration after myocardial infarction. Thus, cell transplantation seems to be an alternative.[85] Different cell types, i.e. embryonic, fetal, and adult cells have been investigated and tested. Among them, mesenchymal stem cells (MSCs) isolated from bone marrow are accepted to give rise to connective tissue cell types. Their differentiation to cardiomyocytes was obtained in vitro and in vivo. However, immortalization of MSCs and their treatment with the DNA demethylation agent 5-azacytidine were necessary to reveal their cardiogenic potential in vitro and cannot be used for medical purposes.[86] For cells derived from human adipose tissues, cardiogenic potential and the benefit of their engraftment on heart function have been demonstrated. Thus, a better understanding of cardiomyocyte differentiation from adipose-derived cells is required to foresee the use of adipose stroma-derived cardiomyocytes in cell based therapy of heart failure.

In conclusion, data demonstrate the existence in adipose tissue of unexpected, particularly promising cells. Knowledge of these may bring new perspectives on the comprehension of adipose tissue development for cell therapy. Because of this new potential, the handicap that fat deposits can represent a large amount of undesirable tissue in some conditions could become its nobility.

Acknowledgments

This work was supported by the European Community (Genostem and Feder-Interreg), Conseil Regional Midi-Pyrénées, and Association Française contre les Myopathies/Inserm.

References

1. Coleman SR. Facial recontouring with lipostructure. Clin Plast Surg 1997; 24: 347–67.
2. Coleman SR. Structural fat grafts: the ideal filler? Clin Plast Surg 2001; 28: 111–19.
3. Coleman SR. Hand rejuvenation with structural fat grafting. Plast Reconstr Surg 2002; 110: 1731–44; discussion 1745–7.
4. Ailhaud G, Grimaldi P, Negrel R. Cellular and molecular aspects of adipose tissue development. Annu Rev Nutr 1992; 12: 207–33.
5. Burdi A. Adipose tissue growth patterns during human gestation: a histometric comparison of buccal and gluteal fat depots. Int J Obes Relat Metab Disord 1985; 9: 247–56.
6. Hausman GJ. Identification of adipose tissue primordia in perirenal tissues of pig fetuses: utility of phosphatase histochemistry. Acta Anat 1987; 128: 236–42.
7. Wasserman F. The concept of the 'fat organ'. In Roddahl K, Issekutz B, eds. Fat as a Tissue. New York: McGraw-Hill, 1964: 22–40.
8. Hahn P, Novak M. Development of brown and white adipose tissue. J Lipid Res 1975; 16: 79–91.
9. Rupnick M, Panigrahy D, Zhang C et al. Adipose tissue mass can be regulated through the vasculature. Proc Natl Acad Sci USA 2002; 99: 10730–5.
10. Planat-Benard V, Silvestre J, Cousin BS et al. Plasticity of human adipose lineage cells toward endothelial cells. Physiological and therapeutic perspectives. Circulation 2004; 109: 656–63.
11. Dagher G, Donne N, Klein C et al. HDL-mediated cholesterol uptake and targeting to lipid droplets in adipocytes. J Lipid Res 2003; 44: 1811–20.
12. Fantuzzi G. Adipose tissue, adipokines, and inflammation. J Allergy Clin Immunol 2005; 115: 911–19.
13. Zhang Y, Proenca R, Maffei M et al. Positional cloning of the mouse obese gene and its human homologue. Nature 1994; 372: 425–32.
14. Ahima RS, Flier JS. Leptin. Annu Rev Physiol 2000; 62: 413–37.
15. Huang L, Li C. Leptin: a multifunctional hormone. Cell Res 2000; 10: 81–92.
16. Hotamisligil GS, Shargill NS, Spiegelman BM. Adipose expression of tumor necrosis factor-alpha: direct role in obesity-linked insulin resistance. Science 1993; 259: 87–91.
17. Ranganathan S, Davidson MB. Effect of tumor necrosis factor-alpha on basal and insulin-stimulated glucose transport in cultured muscle and fat cells. Metabolism 1996; 45: 1089–94.
18. Steppan CM, Bailey ST, Bhat S et al. The hormone resistin links obesity to diabetes. Nature 2001; 409: 307–12.
19. Choy LN, Rosen BS, Spiegelman BM. Adipsin and an endogenous pathway of complement from adipose cells. J Biol Chem 1992; 267: 12736–41.
20. Cook KS, Min HY, Johnson D et al. Adipsin: a circulating serine protease homolog secreted by adipose tissue and sciatic nerve. Science 1987; 237: 402–4.
21. Hu E, Liang P, Spiegelman B. AdipoQ is a novel adipose-specific gene dysregulated in obesity. J Biol Chem 1996; 271: 10697–703.
22. Prins J. Adipose tissue as an endocrine organ. Best Pract Res Clin Endocrinol Metab 2002; 16: 639–51.
23. Mohamed-Ali V, Pinkney JH, Coppack SW. Adipose tissue as an endocrine and paracrine organ. Int J Obes Relat Metab Disord 1998; 22: 1145–58.
24. Gerhardt CC, Romero IA, Cancello R et al. Chemokines control fat accumulation and leptin secretion by cultured human adipocytes. Mol Cell Endocrinol 2001; 175: 81–92.
25. Harris S. Prostaglandins as modulators of immunity. Trends Immunol 2002; 23: 144–50.

26. Frederich RC Jr, Kahn BB, Peach MJ, Flier JS. Tissue-specific nutritional regulation of angiotensinogen in adipose tissue. Hypertension 1992; 19: 339–44.

27. Ailhaud G, Fukamizu A, Massiera F et al. Angiotensinogen, angiotensin II and adipose tissue development. Int J Obes Relat Metab Disord 2000; 24: S33–5.

28. Aubert J, Darimont C, Safonova I et al. Regulation by glucocorticoids of angiotensinogen gene expression and secretion in adipose cells. Biochem J 1997; 328: 701–6.

29. Safonova I, Aubert J, Negrel R, Ailhaud G. Regulation by fatty acids of angiotensinogen gene expression in preadipose cells. Biochem J 1997; 322: 235–9.

30. Alessi MC, Peiretti F, Morange P et al. Production of plasminogen activator inhibitor 1 by human adipose tissue: possible link between visceral fat accumulation and vascular disease. Diabetes 1997; 46: 860–7.

31. Lundgren CH, Brown SL, Nordt TK et al. Elaboration of type-1 plasminogen activator inhibitor from adipocytes. A potential pathogenetic link between obesity and cardiovascular disease. Circulation 1996; 93: 106–10.

32. Shimomura I, Funahashi T, Takahashi M et al. Enhanced expression of PAI-1 in visceral fat: possible contributor to vascular disease in obesity. Nat Med 1996; 2: 800–3.

33. Dobson DE, Kambe A, Block E et al. 1-Butyryl-glycerol: a novel angiogenesis factor secreted by differentiating adipocytes. Cell 1990; 61: 223–30.

34. Bouloumie A, Drexler HC, Lafontan M, Busse R. Leptin, the product of Ob gene, promotes angiogenesis. Circ Res 1998; 83: 1059–66.

35. Kirkland JL, Hollenberg CH, Gillon WS. Age, anatomic site, and the replication and differentiation of adipose precursors. Am J Physiol 1990; 258: C206–10.

36. Faust IM, Johnson PR, Stern JS, Hirsch J. Diet-induced adipocyte number increase in adult rats: a new model of obesity. Am J Physiol 1978; 235: E279–86.

37. Miller WH Jr, Faust IM, Hirsch J. Demonstration of de novo production of adipocytes in adult rats by biochemical and radioautographic techniques. J Lipid Res 1984; 25: 336–47.

38. Tong Q, Dalgin G, Xu H et al. Function of GATA transcription factors in preadipocyte-adipocyte transition. Science 2000; 290: 134–8.

39. Ross SE, Hemati N, Longo KA et al. Inhibition of adipogenesis by Wnt signaling. Science 2000; 289: 950–3.

40. Hu E, Tontonoz P, Spiegelman B. Transdifferentiation of myoblasts by the adipogenic transcription factors PPAR gamma and C/EBP alpha. Proc Natl Acad Sci USA 1995; 92: 9856–60.

41. Lazar MA. PPAR gamma, 10 years later. Biochimie 2005; 87: 9–13.

42. Cornelius P, McDougald OA, Lane MD. Regulation of adipocyte development. Annu Rev Nutr 1994; 14: 99–129.

43. Ibrahimi A, Bertrand B, Bardon S et al. Cloning of a2 chain of type VI collagen and expression during mouse development. Biochem J 1993; 289: 141–7.

44. Smas C, Sul H. Pref-1, a protein containing EGF-like repeats, inhibits adipocyte differentiation. Cell 1993; 73: 725–34.

45. Amri EZ, Dani C, Doglio A et al. Coupling of growth arrest and expression of early markers during adipose conversion of preadipocyte cell lines. Biochem Biophys Res Commun 1986; 137: 903–10.

46. Kuri-Harcuch W, Marsch-Moreno M. DNA synthesis and cell division related to adipose differentiation of 3T3 cells. J Cell Physiol 1983; 114: 39–44.

47. Pilgrim C. DNA synthesis and differentiation in developing white adipose tissue. Dev Biol 1971; 26: 69–76.

48. Cook JR, Kozak LP. sn-Glycerol-3-phosphate dehydrogenase gene expression during mouse adipocyte development in vivo. Dev Biol 1982; 92: 440–8.

49. Krieger-Brauer H, Kather H. Human fat cells possess a plasma membrane-bound H2O2-generating system that is activated by insulin via mechanism bypassing the receptor kinase. J Clin Invest 1992; 89: 1006–13.

50. Pelton PD, Zhou L, Demarest KT, Burris TP. PPARgamma activation induces the expression of the adipocyte fatty acid binding protein gene in human monocytes. Biochem Biophys Res Commun 1999; 261: 456–8.

51. Ricote M, Li AC, Willson TM et al. The peroxisome proliferator-activated receptor-γ is a negative regulator of macrophage activation. Nature 1998; 391: 79–82.

52. Cousin B, Munoz O, André M et al. A role for preadipocytes as macrophage-like cells. FASEB J 1999; 13: 305–12.

53. Villena J, Cousin B, André M et al. Adipose tissues display differential phagocytic and microbicidal activities depending on their localization. Int J Obes Relat Metab Disord 2001; 25: 1275–80.

54. Cousin B, André M, Casteilla L, Pénicaud L. Altered macrophage-like functions of preadipocytes in inflammation and genetic obesity. J Cell Physiol 2001; 186: 380–6.

55. Saillan-Barreau C, Cousin B, Andre M et al. Human adipose cells as candidates in defense and tissue remodeling phenomena. Biochem Biophys Res Commun 2003; 309: 502–5.

56. Charriere G, Cousin B, Arnaud E et al. Preadipocyte conversion to macrophage. Evidence of plasticity. J Biol Chem 2003; 278: 9850–5.

57. Weisberg S, McCann D, Desai M et al. Obesity is associated with macrophage accumulation in adipose tissue. J Clin Invest 2003; 112: 1796–808.

58. Xu H, Barnes G, Yang Q et al. Chronic inflammation in fat plays a crucial role in the development of obesity-related insulin resistance. J Clin Invest 2003; 112: 1821–30.

59. Caspar-Bauguil S, Cousin B, Galinier A et al. Adipose tissues as an ancestral immune organ: site-specific change in obesity. FEBS Lett 2005; 579: 3487–92.

60. Pond C. Interactions between adipose tissue and the immune system. Proc Nutr Soc 1996; 55: 111–26.

61. Hausman GJ, Richardson RL. Adipose tissue angiogenesis. J Anim Sci 2004; 82: 925–34.

62. Bouloumie A, Lolmede K, Sengenes C et al. Angiogenesis in adipose tissue. Ann Endocrinol (Paris) 2002; 63: 91–5.

63. Claffey KP, Wilkison WO, Spiegelman BM. Vascular endothelial growth factor. Regulation by cell differentiation and activated second messenger pathways. J Biol Chem 1992; 267: 16317–22.

64. Miranville A, Heeschen C, Sengenes C et al. Improvement of postnatal neovascularization by human adipose tissue-derived stem cells. Circulation 2004; 110: 349–55.

65. Carriere A, Carmona MC, Fernandez Y et al. Mitochondrial reactive oxygen species control the transcription factor CHOP-10/GADD153 and adipocyte differentiation: a mechanism for hypoxia-dependent effect. J Biol Chem 2004; 279: 40462–9.

66. Yun Z, Maecker HL, Johnson RS, Giaccia AJ. Inhibition of PPAR gamma 2 gene expression by the HIF-1-regulated gene DEC1/Stra13: a mechanism for regulation of adipogenesis by hypoxia. Dev Cell 2002; 2: 331–41.

67. Deveaud C, Beauvoit B, Hagry S et al. Site specific alterations of adipose tissue mitochondria in 3'-azido-3'-deoxythymidine (AZT)-treated rats: an early stage in lipodystrophy? Biochem Pharmacol 2005; 70: 90–101.

68. Lolmede K, Durand de Saint Front V, Galitzky J et al. Effects of hypoxia on the expression of proangiogenic factors in differentiated 3T3-F442A adipocytes. Int J Obes Relat Metab Disord 2003; 27: 1187–95.

69. Rehman J, Traktuev D, Li J et al. Secretion of angiogenic and antiapoptotic factors by human adipose stromal cells. Circulation 2004; 109: 1292–8.

70. Cousin B, Andre M, Arnaud E et al. Reconstitution of lethally irradiated mice by cells isolated from adipose tissue. Biochem Biophys Res Commun 2003; 301: 1016–22.

71. Dieterlen-Lievre F, Pardanaud L, Bollerot K, Jaffredo T. Hemangioblasts and hemopoietic stem cells during ontogeny. C R Biol 2002; 325: 1013–20.

72. Devine SM, Hoffman R. Role of mesenchymal stem cells in hematopoietic stem cell transplantation. Curr Opin Hematol 2000; 7: 358–63.

73. Planat-Bénard V, Ménard C, André M et al. Spontaneous cardiomyocyte differentiation from adipose tissue stroma cells. Circulation Res 2004; 94: 223–9.

74. Liu Y, Song J, Liu W et al. Growth and differentiation of rat bone marrow stromal cells: does 5-azacytidine trigger their cardiomyogenic differentiation? Cardiovasc Res 2003; 58: 460–8.

75. Rangappa S, Fen C, Lee EH et al. Transformation of adult mesenchymal stem cells isolated from the fatty tissue into cardiomyocytes. Ann Thorac Surg 2003; 75: 775–9.

76. Gimble JM, Nuttall ME. Bone and fat: old questions, new insights. Endocrine 2004; 23: 183–8.

77. Erickson G, Gimble J, Franklin D et al. Chondrogenic potential of adipose tissue-derived stromal cells in vitro and in vivo. Biochem Biophys Res Commun 2002; 290: 763–9.

78. Zuk P, Zhu M, Ashjian P et al. Human adipose tissue is a source of multipotent stem cells. Mol Biol Cell 2002; 13: 4279–95.

79. Safford KM, Safford SD, Gimble JM et al. Characterization of neuronal/glial differentiation of murine adipose-derived adult stromal cells. Exp Neurol 2004; 187: 319–28.

80. Fujimura J, Ogawa R, Mizuno H et al. Neural differentiation of adipose-derived stem cells isolated from GFP transgenic mice. Biochem Biophys Res Commun 2005; 333: 116–21.

81. Seo MJ, Suh SY, Bae YC, Jung JS. Differentiation of human adipose stromal cells into hepatic lineage in vitro and in vivo. Biochem Biophys Res Commun 2005; 328: 258–64.

82. Rodriguez AM, Pisani D, Dechesne CA et al. Transplantation of a multipotent cell population from human adipose tissue induces dystrophin expression in the immunocompetent mdx mouse. J Exp Med 2005; 201: 1397–405.

83. Bacou F, el Andalousi RB, Daussin PA et al. Transplantation of adipose tissue-derived stromal cells increases mass and functional capacity of damaged skeletal muscle. Cell Transplant 2004; 13: 103–11.

84. Silvestre JS, Levy BI. Angiogenesis therapy in ischemic disease. Arch Mal Coeur Vaiss 2002; 95: 189–96.

85. Vilquin JT, Marolleau JP, Hagege A et al. Cell transplantation for post-ischemic heart failure. Arch Mal Coeur Vaiss 2002; 95: 1219–25.

86. Makino S, Fukuda K, Miyoshi S et al. Cardiomyocytes can be generated from marrow stromal cells in vitro. J Clin Invest 1999; 103: 697–705.

41 History of fat grafting in cosmetic surgery

Ali Mojallal and Jean Louis Foyatier

From the end of the 19th century, with the aim of producing biomaterials for soft tissue augmentation, fat transfer using autografts or homografts was introduced.

To mark evolution and specify important events, we have classified the history into three distinct periods:

- 1889–1977: the period before lipoaspiration
- 1977–1994: the period of liposuction and reinjection of uncleaned fat
- from 1994: the period of lipoaspiration, purification and atraumatic reinjection
- from 1999: the period of tissue regeneration and fat tissue derived stem cells.

1889–1977: before lipoaspiration

This period corresponded to the introduction of transplants of adipose tissue. It was the period of experimental trial and error, the discovery of techniques and indications.

The first use of fat was in 1889, when van der Meulen[1] accomplished a hepatodiaphragmatic interposition by the large omentum to treat a diaphragmatic hernia.

Use of fat at the level of the face

The first autograft of adipose tissue was accomplished by Neuber in 1893.[2] He took a sample from the forearm as a graft to fill a secondary facial scar in a tuberous ostitis. He introduced, for the first time, the notion of samples of small size, considering that a graft larger in size than an almond does not give good results.

In 1910, Lexer[3] was the first to report the use of fat in plastic surgery by offering a procedure to increase the malar and nasolabial regions, as well as filling of wrinkles and grooves to combat the effects of aging. He transplanted a fat graft of size 12×3 cm taken from the abdominal wall. Brunning[4] reported in 1911 an original method for the correction for the rhinoplasties. Small fragments of fat were reinjected under the skin with the aid of a syringe. The results, which were satisfactory at first, became obscured with resorption of the fat.

In 1925, Lexer[5] reported the survival of adipose tissue grafts for more than 3 years, and concluded that fat tissue must not be damaged either during sampling or during reimplantation. He also reported a case of restoration of the facial outline to a patient suffering from Romberg's syndrome.

Salvat,[6] during the Second World War, accomplished the disguise of allied spies by injecting them with some fat. He used autologous fat for a permanent result and homologous fat for a temporary result.

It was then necessary to wait until 1950 for the research of Peer[7,8] before the next important study on the grafting of adipose tissue. This showed that fragments of grafted adipose tissue lose about 50% of their size and their volume at the end of the first year. Peer was the first to discuss the theory of cell survival (adipocytes), which is in opposition to the theory of replacement by foreign cells.

Use of fat in other locations

Indications progressively increased, and adipose tissue grafting became of interest for almost all parts of the body. The first case of mammary reconstruction using autologous fat was reported by Czerny in 1895.[9] He used a lipoma taken from the hip to repair a mammary tumorectomy.

Lexer, in 1931,[10] introduced mammary reconstruction, after mastectomy for cystic mastopathy, using the fat of the axillary region. The strong rate of resorption which followed was explained by the weak vascularization of this type of fat.

In 1941, a case of bilateral mammary reconstruction was introduced using only adipose tissue on the one side and grafting of fat and the fascia of other side with the idea that the fascia allowed better preservation of fat.[11]

Related to mammary hypoplasia, Bames[12] in 1953 published several cases of mammary augmentation by dermofat grafting, and Schrocher[13] in 1957 reported eight cases of mammary augmentation by fat grafting. About the same time, Peer treated a case of Poland's syndrome by dermofat grafting.[7]

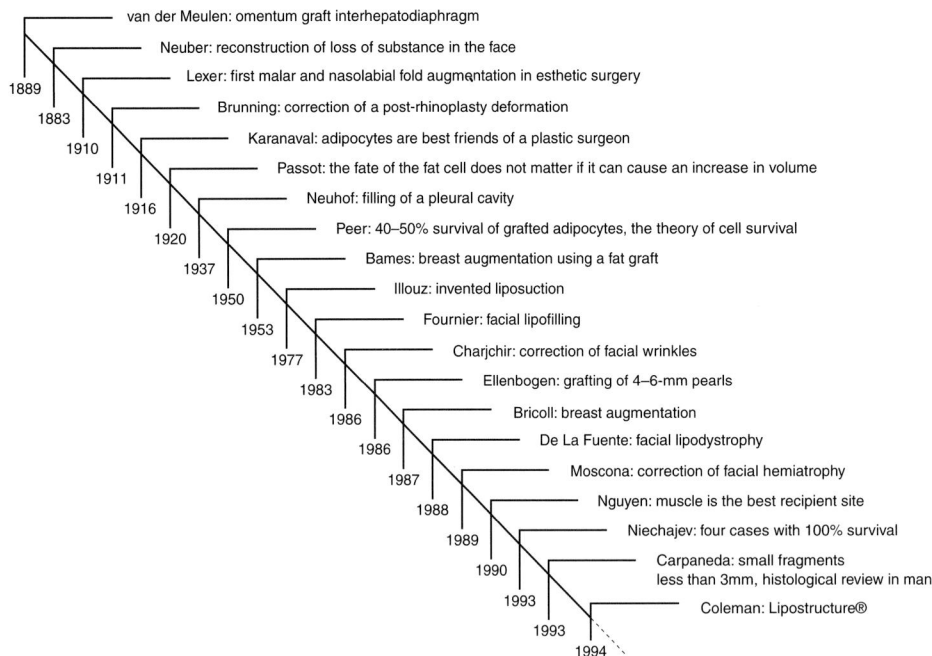

Figure 41.1 Review of the use of adipose tissue.

1977–1994: lipoaspiration and uncleaned fat reinjection

This was the age of reflection.

A bridge had been crossed: adipose tissue could be obtained by a means other than by surgical incision.

Illouz[14] invented the technology of liposuction by cannulation. He was also one of the first to use the raw material of liposuction as filler product.[15,16] His method of taking fat by aspiration opened new horizons on the grafting of adipocytes. In effect, a certain number of fat cells taken by this method remained undamaged, and it was suggested that their reimplantation was possible with a reasonable rate of survival.

Then, Fournier in 1989[17,18] proposed a technology of injection of uncleaned fat which he named liposculpture or lipofilling. The inherent hypercorrection and unreliability of the results did not allow widespread use of this technology.

In 1987, Bircoll and Novack[19,20] introduced several cases of correction of hypoplasia or mammary asymmetry after cancer by injecting small quantities over several sessions. This practice provoked vehement reaction in the scientific community.[21,22] This opposition of the scientific community of cancer research was based on non-justifiable arguments, reasons for which actually did not exist because the techniques of adipose tissue transfer had changed.

Hang-Fu[23] reported a series of breast implants filled with autologous fat to avoid all disadvantages linked to injection into breast tissues. Other authors discussed fat homografts in the breast.[24,25]

Ellenbogen[26] in 1986 described the technique of fat pearls, opening the way to a new series of publications. This procedure injects fragments from 4 to 6 mm in diameter to treat facial wrinkles, palpebral depressions, or acne scars.

From 1994: lipoaspiration, purification and atraumatic reinjection

This is the age of perfection.

The new era of the grafting of adipocytes started following the research of Coleman. From 1986, he reported methods and results using adipocyte precursors and initiated a protocol of fundamental principles based on the atraumatic character of the manipulation of adipose tissue. He published the technique in 1997,[27] which he later named structural fat grafting or Lipostructure®. It encodes distinct stages of technique: sampling, purification by centrifugation, and transfer (reinjection). Any act traumatizing the fat must be avoided. Fat must not be pressed, or constricted, or filtered, or washed, or aspirated at high vacuum, or injected using high pressure, or manipulated in contact with air, or frozen, or blended with different blood factors. Intended initially for the treatment of facial aging, this technique encompassed the different domains of plastic surgery.[28]

Since then, interest in this technique has not stopped increasing, and various research has shown the applicability of this technique and good acquired results.

Toledo,[29] Ellenbogen,[30] Guerrerosantos,[31,32] Teimourian,[33] and other authors have all accomplished grafting of adipose tissue but by using different techniques.

From 1999: tissue regeneration and adipose derived stem cells

Due to better knowledge of the development of adipocytes, research into tissue engineering is evolving. This represents the future of tissular reproduction in vitro.[34] The only adipose cells able to multiply and differentiate are the preadipocytes. In addition, they have capacities of development and resistance to ischemia superior to those of mature adipocytes. These cells are isolated, multiplied, and differentiated in vitro, then they are implanted into humans by means of a biocompatible matrix. Adipose tissue represents a source of 'mother cells'. Mesenchymal stem cells extracted from adipose tissue can be developed into adipocytes, osteoblasts, chondrocytes, myocytes, and neuron-like cells.

Adipose tissue is more than a permanent filter:[35] it has the power to regenerate tissue. It has been used in the treatment of ischaemic lesions and radiodystrophics.[36,37] It also been shown in a histological study that the transplanted adipose tissue improves the quality of tissue in the recipient.[38] The future lies in this form of autologous reconstruction.

References

1. van der Meulen. Considérations générales sur les greffes graisseuses et séro-graisseuses épiploïques et leurs principales applications. Thèse Médecine, Paris, 1919.
2. Neuber GA. Fett Transplantation. Verl Dtsch Ges Chir 1893; 22: 66.
3. Lexer E. Freie Fett Transplantation. Dtsch Med Wochenschr 1910; 36: 640.
4. Brunning P. Contribution à l'étude des greffes adipeuses. Bull Mem Acad R Med Belg 1919; 28: 440.
5. Lexer E. Zwanzig Jahre Transplantatiosforshung in der Chirurgie. Arch Klein Chir 1925; 138: 294.
6. Mojallal A, Foyatier JL. Historical review of the use of adipose tissue transfer in plastic and reconstructive surgery. Ann Chir Plast Esthet 2004; 49: 419–25.
7. Peer LA. Loss of weight and volume in human fat graft, with postulation of a 'cell survival theory'. Plast Reconstr Surg 1950; 5: 217.
8. Peer LA. The neglected free fat graft. Plast Reconstr Surg 1956; 18: 233.
9. Czerny V. Plasticher Ersatz der Brustdrüse durch ein Lipom. Zentralb Chir 1895; 27: 72.
10. Lexer E. Die gesamte Wiederherstellungschirurgie. Leipzig: JB Barth, 1931.
11. Billings E Jr, May JW Jr. Historical review and present status of free fat graft autotransplantation in plastic and reconstructive surgery. Plast Reconstr Surg 1989; 83: 368–81.
12. Bames HO. Augmentation mammaplasty by lipo-transplant. Plast Reconstr Surg 1953; 11: 404.
13. Scrocher F. Fettgewebsverpflanzung bei zu kleiner Brust. Munchen Med Wochenschr 1957; 99: 489.
14. Illouz YG. Adipoaspiration and 'filling' in the face. Facial Plast Surg 1992; 8: 59–71.
15. Illouz YG. Present results of fat injection. Aesthetic Plast Surg 1988; 12: 175–81.
16. Illouz YG. The fat cell 'graft': a new technique to fill depressions. Plast Reconstr Surg 1986; 78: 122–3.
17. Fournier PF. Microlipoextraction et microlipoinjection. Rev Chir Esthet Lang Fr 1985; 10: 40.
18. Fournier P. Facial recontouring with fat grafting. Dermatol Clin 1989; 8: 523.
19. Bircoll M, Novack BH. Autologous fat transplantation employing liposuction techniques. Ann Plast Surg 1987; 18: 327–9.
20. Bircoll M. Cosmetic breast augmentation utilizing autologous fat and liposuction techniques. Plast Reconstr Surg 1987; 79: 267–71.
21. Hartrampf CR, Bennett GK. Autologous fat from liposuction for breast augmentation (correspondence). Plast Reconstr Surg 1987; 80: 646.
22. Gradinger GP. Breast augmentation by autologous fat injection. Plast Reconstr Surg 1987; 80: 868–9.
23. Hang-Fu L, Marmolya G, Feiglin DH. Liposuction fat-fillant implant for breast augmentation and reconstruction. Aesthetic Plast Surg 1995; 19: 427–37.
24. Rosen PB, Hugo NE. Augmentation mammaplasty by cadaver fat allografts. Plast Reconstr Surg 1988; 82: 525–6.
25. Haik J, Talisman R, Tamir J et al. Breast augmentation with fresh-frozen homologous fat grafts. Aesthetic Plast Surg 2001; 25: 292–4.
26. Ellenbogen R. Free autogenous pearl fat grafts in the face—a preliminary report of a rediscovered technique. Ann Plast Surg 1986; 16: 179–94.
27. Coleman SR. Structural fat grafts: the ideal filler? Clin Plast Surg 2001; 28: 111–19.
28. Mojallal A, Breton P, Delay E, Foyatier JL. La greffe d'adipocytes. Applications en chirurgie plastique et esthétique. In: Encyclopédie Médico-Chirurgicale, Traité de Techniques Chirurgicales 45-125. Paris: Elsevier Masson, 2007: IV.
29. Toledo LS. Syringe liposculpture: a two-year experience. Aesthetic Plast Surg 1991; 15: 321–6.
30. Ellenbogen R. Fat transfer: current use in practice. Clin Plast Surg 2000; 27: 545–56.
31. Guerrerosantos J. Simultaneous rhytidoplasty and lipoinjection: a comprehensive aesthetic surgical strategy. Plast Reconstr Surg 1998; 102: 191–9.
32. Guerrerosantos J. Autologous fat grafting for body contouring. Clin Plast Surg 1996; 23: 619–31.
33. Teimourian B. Repair of soft-tissue contour deficit by means of semiliquid fat graft. Plast Reconstr Surg 1986; 78: 123–4.
34. Katz AJ, Llull R, Hedrick MH, Futrell JW. Emerging approaches to the tissue engineering of fat. Clin Plast Surg 1999; 26: 587–603, viii.
35. Coleman SR, Structural fat grafting: more than a permanent filler. Plant Reconstr Surg 2006; 118: 108S–120S.
36. Nakagami H, Maeda K, Morishita R et al. Novel autologous cell therapy in ischemic limb disease through growth factor secretion by cultured adipose tissue-derived stromal cells. Arterioscler Thromb Vasc Biol 2005; 25: 2542–7.
37. Rigotti G, Marchi A, Galie M., et al. Clinical treatment of radiotherapy tissue damage by lipoaspirate transplant: a healing process mediated by adipose-derived adult stem cells. Plant Reconstr Surg 2007; 119: 1409–22; discussion 1423–4.
38. Mojallal A, Lequeux C, Brayer F, et al. Improvement of skin quality: animal studies and clinical cases. In: Coleman SR and Mazzola G (eds), Fat injection: from filling to regeneration. Quality Medical Publishing, 2009.

42 The effect of different factors on the survival of transplanted adipose tissue

Ali Mojallal and Jean Louis Foyatier

Theories of adipose tissue transplantation

Two theories have been proposed.

Adipocyte survival

This theory was proposed by Peer[1,2] in 1950 and revived by Coleman and others.[3,4] According to this theory, transplanted adipocytes survive and continue their cycle of development at the level of the recipient site. On the first day the transplanted adipocytes undergo an ischemic phase, and there is an influx of macrophages, histiocytes, and polynuclear cells to mop up the debris. By the fourth day, revascularization of the transplant by means of neoangiogenesis in the host has commenced. This revascularization starts from the periphery and moves toward the center. The central fat cell therefore undergoes prolonged ischemia and only revascularizes if the fragments are small.

Cellular replacement by the host

According to this theory, transplantation of the cells causes an influx of the host's histiocytes, which are attracted to lipids released by the adipocytes and mop up the cellular debris. There is a fibrous reaction with an influx of fibroblasts.[5,6] The histiocytes take on characteristics of the adipocytes and replace them entirely. In other words, the transplanted adipocytes generate a local tissue increase.

Certain studies found in the literature conclude that the transplanted adipocytes disappear within several months.[7,8] However, it should be noted that the majority of these studies date back several years. It is difficult to compare the results of this procedure between studies, since the techniques used by different authors are not the same and the older procedure differs from that practiced today. One can thus find faults in a technique, but that should not call into question the actual transplantation of the adipocytes. In addition, one should remember that when one speaks about a 50% loss, there is also a 50% survival. The most recent studies all tend in the same direction, toward the survival of adipocytes. In fact, not only does adipose tissue survive and continue its natural cycle of developments; it also induces a change in the local tissue.[9–11] We call this the theory of tissue interactivity: the recipient tissue permits the survival of the adipose tissue, and the latter reacts to the recipient site. Various experimental, clinical, and radiological studies have made it possible to demonstrate this, and a review of the literature on the factors influencing the outcome of transplantation of adipocytes, at each stage of the operational procedure, is presented below.

Factors influencing the survival of adipocytes

Adipose tissue is fragile. The transfer of this tissue requires delicate handling. Each procedural stage of this intervention has been the subject of study to identify factors influencing the viability and the survival of the adipocytes.[12] They are presented in chronological order of the surgical procedure.

Type of anesthesia and infiltration

The type of anesthesia is relevant – particularly the effect of the injected product on the adipose tissue. If the procedure is under local anesthesia it is primarily the effects of Lidocaine and epinephrine that are important. Moore et al[13] compared two collections carried out by aspiration using a syringe of 10 ml with a nozzle of 3 mm, the first after infiltration with Lidocaine® and the second after infiltration with Lidocaine and epinephrine. There was no significant difference in the metabolic activity of the adipocytes and glucose transport between these two samples. On the other hand, when the adipocytes came into contact with Lidocaine, compared to a reference group there was a suppression of glucose transport, lipolysis, and their growth in culture. These effects disappeared once the adipocytes were removed from contact with Lidocaine, for example after washing. There thus exists an effect caused by Lidocaine but not by adrenaline. The injection of vaso-constrictors and/or a large quantity of physiological saline solution at the level of the donor or recipient site decreased the viability of adipocytes.[13] The anesthesia used for the recipient site should preferably be general or locoregional. Local anesthesia, by the modification of volume that it generates, can disrupt accurate visual-ization of the procedure.

We carry out all procedures under general anesthesia, except when only a small quantity of fat tissue is required. Under general anesthesia the donor site is not infiltrated, except in thin patients, by normal saline.[14] The relevance of prior infiltration is to limit any trauma caused during tissue collection.

The donor site

There has been research into the longevity of adipocytes according to the various donor sites. It is known that adipocytes differ in size and lipogenic activity according to their topography.[15] Given these differences, the harvesting must be made in a zone where the adipose tissue resists moderate variations in weight.[16] Such zones are the trochanteric region, the inner sides of the thighs and the knees, and the periumbilical area. Fat tissue harvesting should be from the deeper layer, which is different genetically and metabolically from the subcutaneous layer because of the higher number of α_2 receptors. Hudson et al[15] published a study in 1990 which tended to show a morphological and biochemical difference between adipose tissues taken from various sites. Adipocytes from the trochanteric area were larger and had increased lipoprotein lipase activity, followed by the abdominal region and facial cells.

In our series of 100 cases,[14] collection was carried out at the level of the abdomen 59 times, at the hip 27 times, and at the inner sides of the knees eight times, the remaining six cases combining several sites. We sought to highlight whether the relation of the quantity of adipose tissue centrifuged to the quantity of tissue removed made it possible to deem any site to be superior. This relation was approximately 75%, and there were no significant differences between the various donor sites. However, this related only to the concentration of adipose tissue without taking into account the morphological and meta-bolic differences that can exist between these various zones. Rohrich et al. demonstrate that all donor sites analysed (thigh, knee, flank and abdomen) provide statis-tically equivalent viable cells.[17]

Method of adipose tissue harvesting

Is there a difference between surgical collection, mechanical aspiration, and manual aspiration? Do the

negative pressure exerted for aspiration and the type of cannula have an influence? Studies have compared surgical collection with traditional aspiration and showed the superiority of the surgical technique. Marques et al[18] compared transplantation of adipose tissue carried out in the rat after use of a cannula with lateral aspiration, then a cannula with distal aspiration, and finally after surgical excision. The results obtained after analysis of the graft at the 12th month showed a higher percentage of survival in the surgical group at 45%, compared with 14% and 35% survival for lateral and distal aspiration, respectively. However, Har-Shai et al[19] showed that there were more triglycerides with pump aspiration (1 atm of negative pressure) than with manual aspiration (0.2 atm of negative pressure), which would favor manual harvesting. It is known that har-vesting by machine causes deterioration of the cells because of vaporization in the tube, which dehydrates them, and because of the excessive negative pressure exerted on them.[20] We conducted a study comparing manual fat harvesting using a 10-ml syringe versus a lipoaspiration device with and without assistance at −350 mmHg and 700 mmHg. The cannula sampling was a 3mm cannula regardless of the negative pressure exerted. Our results show a greater number of mature cells and stem cells in the sample than in −350 mmHg assisted liposuction.[21] In the same way, ultrasound aspiration causes deterioration of adipocytes as an effect of mechanical trauma, cavitation, or thermal changes.[22] Niechajev and Sevcuk[23] observed that the negative pressure imposed at the time of aspiration is a factor which influences the viability of adipocytes. With a negative pressure of 0.95 atm there is 66% more cellular damage than at 0.5 atm. Moore et al[13] compared the histologies of adipose cells obtained by atraumatic surgical collection and by aspiration at low pressure using a 3 mm cannula assembled on a 10-ml syringe. There was no significant difference in functional or metabolic terms or in growth between these two groups. Lalikos et al,[24] using an enzymatic technique and a dosage of glyceraldehyde-3-phosphate dehydro-genase (G3PDH), found no difference in deterioration between harvesting by lipoaspiration and by surgical excision. When aspiration was carried out manually and with low pressure, the results matched those of the surgical technique.[19] Moreover, it was not necessary, as was the case after surgical excision, to divide and thus traumatize the sample. Various studies show the direct relationship between the diameter of the needle used to harvest and/or reinject, and the capacity of survival of adipocytes. The morphological aspect of adipocytes was studied under the microscope and displayed a deterioration of the core and the lipid vacuole. In the same way, the capacity of adipocytes to maintain their metabolic activity and lipogenesis was measured via glycolysis according to the size of the needle.[25] The smallest size of needle or cannula was 14G. There was no difference between harvesting/reinjection using a needle or a cannula of 14G. Any harvesting using high negative pressure causes cellular damage and should be avoided. Syringes of 60 ml usually used for aspiration by means of forced operation of the piston exert an excessive negative pressure and cause deterioration of the cells. Only a 10-ml syringe whereby aspiration is manually regulated allows withdrawal at weak pressure. Operation of the piston of the syringe is accomplished gradually to avoid excessive aspiration of adipocytes. When aspiration is carried out with a 10-ml syringe at low pressure, there is no deterioration and no cellular necrosis.[26]

Purification of adipose tissue

The tissue obtained by lipoaspiration, whether manually or mechanically, is a heterogeneous material comprising healthy adipocytes but also a mixture of destroyed adipocytes, collagenous fibers, and blood remnants. The inflammatory reaction that takes place for the recovery of the recipient site by cleaning away this debris is inevitably more intense than just removal of what is harmful for survival of the adipocytes.[27] In order to decrease the inflammatory reaction after reinjection, it is necessary to purify the adipose tissue as much as possible.[11] Moreover, reinjection of all these products would give a false impression of the volume correction; they would be reabsorbed within a few hours[12] because the presence of blood in the transplanted tissue quickly involves it in digestion by proteases. Various methods of purification have been proposed, such as washing of adipose tissue, filtration, decanting, and centrifugation. In all cases the adipose tissue must be in the least possible contact with air. Histological study showed 50% lysis of adipocytes after exposure to air.[29]

Washing

In order to eliminate the debris and to dilute the anesthetic product used, certain authors have proposed washing of the adipose tissue, either with physiological saline solution, or in Ringer's lactate.[30,31] However, some studies have shown that washing in Ringer's lactate does not increase the survival of adipocytes[18] and the results obtained are less good than those of the control group.[32] Washing creates additional mechanical trauma and osmosis that is preferable to avoid. We do not carry out any washing of adipose tissue.

Filtration

As this is carried out with a metal flail[33] or using a filter incorporated in the pipe of the aspirator,[34] it is something that causes too much trauma and consequently should be avoided. New harvesting techniques and filtration by a syringe filter have been described, but have not established their superiority.

Centrifugation

Centrifugation decreases operational time compared to decantation. It allows the separation and elimination of blood debris and triglycerides obtained by bursting of the adipocytes.[14,35] It has been shown that centrifugation does not create any deterioration of the adipocytes.[26] Boschert et al[36] compared centrifugations with variable force and duration. They showed that there were 13% fewer adipocytes in the centrifuged bottle than in the bottle left to form a sediment, but the eliminated adipocytes were those that had been damaged and the remaining cells were healthy. Centrifugation is the only permitted external manipulation; any other handling causes trauma and is to be avoided.[37] Centrifugation has no consequence on the cellular structure; there is no significant difference in the cellular structure of samples with or without centrifugation. It increases the density of the adipose tissue to be reinjected, by eliminating red blood cells and cellular debris.

Anabolic factors

The theory of adipose tissue survival shows that adipocytes undergo an initial period of ischemia. Improvement of the conditions for survival of adipocytes by hormonal or other factors would thus be one way to increase the rate of survival. Comparison of the action of various factors such as insulin (I), IGF-I (insulin-like growth factor I), bFGF (basic fibroblast growth factor), and mixtures of these factors (I+IGF-I, I+IGF-I+bFGF) shows a significant increase in the rate of survival in all cases.[38] This is especially the case for adipocytes with insulin and IGF-I and stromal fraction cells with bFGF. This increase in the rate of survival is explained by the existence of preadipocyte cells in the tissue, on which these growth factors act. The association of several growth factors does not increase survival in any correlated fashion.[38] The addition of a medium enriched in nutritive elements with amino acids, vitamins, glucose, trace elements, growth factors, insulin, and thyroxine makes it possible to increase the survival of adipocytes from 31% to 44% survival at 4 months.[39] Smith[40] measured the concentration of proteins in reinjected material. An association with hyperbaric oxygen treatment (2 atm) for 90 minutes per day after transfer was tested at 5, 10, and 15 days. There was no significant growth in weight or volume of the transplanted adipocytes.

We are thus departing from the principle that transplantation of adipose tissue, realized under good conditions, does not require any additional factor.

The recipient site

It is certain that the quality of the recipient site is a major factor. A zone free of any trauma and pathology (as is the case in cosmetic surgery) is much more favorable to accepting transplanted adipocytes because of its vitality and flexibility. Reinjection into scar tissue is difficult, and one feels resistance during the injection. This mechanical resistance, by the overpressure which it creates, causes deterioration of the adipocytes, and longevity thereby decreases. Certain authors have proposed a preliminary preparation for the recipient site: they placed silicone implants in the rat 3 weeks before transplantation of adipocytes in order to form a prosthetic capsule, to increase the neovascularization.[41] They found that the rate of survival of adipocytes was higher when compared to the control group, but the inflammatory reaction toward a foreign body is certainly more intense than that toward transplanted adipocytes. Probably, due to the effects of an increase in vascularization and type of recipient site, an increased number of sessions of reinjection would increase the rate of survival of adipocytes. Some authors realize multiple subcutaneous tunnels using a cannula of larger diameter and then deposit the adipocytes with a smaller cannula.[19] The purpose of this is to decrease the resistance pressure against the injection of adipose tissue. Other authors[7,24] report that the best recipient site seems to be muscle, and that intramuscular injection of adipocytes increases the rate of survival by its large vascular contribution.[24] In addition, however, injection into muscle is likely to cause a hematoma, which can work against the transplant. The transplantation of adipocytes to bone, tendon, fascia, or nerve is doomed to failure.[24] The head and neck is richly vascularized and represents the recipient site of choice for transplanted adipocytes. The preparation of the recipient site by vasodilators in the hope of increasing vascularization at the time of transplantation did not show any change in longevity of the results.[12] However, adipocytes survive poorly in areas where they do not usually exist;[42] this is why authors use factors to increase the nutritional contribution.[26] Mojallal[14] reported four cases of adipocytes transplanted onto an irradiated region. The results reported after three sessions showed clear clinical improvement. The noted results were particularly good with an improvement of cutaneous nutrition.[14] Rigotti also shows tissue regeneration after fat tissue transfer.[11]

Mojallal[14] tried to show a difference according to the condition of the recipient site – the transfer of adipose tissue in cosmetic surgery (healthy site) as compared to reconstructive surgery (pathological site). The results obtained in each series did not differ statistically except in median number of sessions, which tended toward a difference in the rate of survival by session, even if a similar result was obtained at the end of treatment. Comparison of the results obtained in the two series of surgeries, reconstructive and cosmetic, showed a tendency in favor of better results for cosmetic surgery, but this difference was not statistically significant. However, results are different for the esthetic subunits of the face: the malar and cheek areas produce the best results.

Reinjection

Various points are important.

Pressure with which adipocytes are deposited

This depends on the instrument used (gun or syringe), on its diameter, and on the volume and diameter of the cannula.

Trauma to the recipient site

This depends on the size, shape, and diameter of the cannula or needle used for reinjection. To deposit a minor amount with each transfer, we recommend the use of a 1-ml syringe, with 6–8 tunnels. The cannula must have a non-traumatic tip so as not to damage the tissue or the adipocytes already injected. The cannula should have a side opening, and one must start by introducing the entire cannula and begin reinjection by pulling out. These two elements avoid any intravascular injection of adipocytes. A cannula with a sharp V-shaped tip makes it possible to separate out the fibrous zones and the adherent bridges during its passage. It is important that each deposit must have a diameter of less than 1.5 mm. The injection must produce a three-dimensional lattice resembling 'peas in a pod', which increases surface contact between the adipocytes and the recipient site. The reinjection must be done with the cannula horizontal in order to avoid any damage to the branches of the facial nerve, the channel of Stenson's duct, and the facial artery.

When it is associated with another procedure, we think that adipocye transplantation should be carried out last, because its purpose is to restore volume following associated surgery. Moreover, performing adipocyte transplantation last avoids any additional trauma to the transplanted material. The injection must start deep and involve all levels.

Number of sessions of reinjection in the same site

The rate of survival estimated by researchers is variable. It is seldom 100%, which implies that an overcorrection or a series of sessions – even, sometimes, both – must be considered and explained to the patient. The volume of adipocytes transplanted decreases in two phases: at the beginning there is a reduction in the number of cells, then secondarily there is a reduction in volume by resorption of the lipid vacuoles of the dead cells.[36] The transplanted adipocytes must be small so that rapid neovascularization can take place. This seems applicable for small repairs, but for large defects transplantation over the course of several sessions helps survival. Excess pressure during deposition is a factor that reduces the rate of survival and favors migration of the transplanted material toward a region of lower pressure. This is why it is preferable to envisage several sessions from the start, and to limit the quantity reinjected at each procedure. Under these conditions, it is not necessary to overcorrect. Moreover, the local infiltration of anesthetic if it takes place, the immediate edema, and the possible hematoma created by the injection all make it difficult to predict the exact volume necessary. It is important to explain to patients during the preoperative consultation that the limit of the technique is the quantity of adipose tissue transplanted at each session, and to preempt from the start the need for repeated interventions.

Freezing

In order to facilitate repeated transplant sessions, some authors keep the aspirated material refrigerated or frozen. Coleman[43] preserved excess adipose tissue by freezing, and recommended the procedure after 1, 3, and sometimes 6 months under local anesthesia. This enabled him to decrease the quantity used in each session and thus to achieve a better result and also to shorten the duration of the patient's perioperative social exclusion. Schuller-Petrovic[44] froze the tissue at −20°C for a new session after 2 months. Donofrio systematically anticipated freezing tissue at −30°C for later sessions.[45] Bertossi et al[46] proposed freezing adipocytes at −30°C in order to increase the number of reinjection sessions without having to harvest again further adipose tissue. They reported good clinical results, and histological study at 20 days and 8 months showed adipose tissue survival. These results support the theory of cellular replacement by the host. The fat tissue is extremely fragile. We believe that freezing destroys adipocytes.[47] However, we are currently working on freezing stem cells extracted from fat tissue that could be secondarily differentiated in mature adipocytes.

We do not carry out any storage by freezing the adipose tissue. Patients are told of the possibility of repeated interventions. A minimum period of 3–6 months is necessary between two sessions.

The transplanted adipose tissue is incorporated into the local texture, and is not palpable and identifiable as a foreign body. This is why some patients think that the adipose tissue has been completely reabsorbed, whereas comparison of photographs from before and after the intervention reveals an increase in volume.

Results obtained after the second and then the third session seem to be better. This is probably related to the fact that the subcutaneous structure has been modified and improved by the secretory qualities of the transplanted adipose tissue, which will exert its influence on the local regulation of blood flow, on angiogenesis, on modification of the extracellular matrix, and on the whole of the cicatricial process.[9–11]

Postoperative treatments

Most authors prescribe treatment by antibiotics and non-steroidal anti-inflammatory drugs (NSAIDs) for 1 week. Others add therapy with vitamin E. We institute a double treatment with both antibiotics for 5 days and NSAIDs for 3 days.

Conclusion

The great disparity between various techniques and details reported by researchers is at the heart of difficulties in comparison, because the number of variables among techniques is significant. This diversity also demonstrates that further improvements should be researched and introduced to this procedure.

References

1. Peer LA. Loss of weight and volume in human fat graft, with postulation of a 'cell survival theory' Plast Reconstr Surg 1950; 5: 217.
2. Peer LA. The neglected free fat graft. Plast Reconstr Surg 1956; 18: 233.
3. Coleman SR. Facial recontouring with lipostructure. Clin Plast Surg 1997; 24: 347–67.
4. Rieck B, Schlaak S. Measurement in vivo of the survival rate in autologous adipocyte transplantation. Plast Reconstr Surg 2003; 111: 2315–23.
5. Sadick NS, Hudgins LC. Fatty acid analysis of transplanted adipose tissue. Arch Dermatol 2001; 137: 723–7.
6. Neuhof H. Free transplantation of fat for closure of bronchopulmonary cavities (lattice lung). J Thorac Surg 1937; 7: 23.
7. Nguyen A, Pasyk KA, Bouvier TN, Hassett CA, Argenta LC. Comparative study of survival of autologous adipose tissue taken and transplanted by different techniques. Plast Reconstr Surg 1990; 85: 378–86; discussion 387–9.
8. Eremia S, Newman N. Long-term follow-up after autologous fat grafting: analysis of results from 116 patients followed at least 12 months after receiving the last of a minimum of two treatments. Dermatol Surg 2000; 26: 1150–8.
9. Mojallal A, Lequeux, Damour O et al. Improvement of skin quality. Animal studies and clinical cases of facial reconstructive surgery. In Coleman SR Mazzola RF, eds, Fat injection: from filling to regeneration. QMP, 2009.
10. Coleman SR, Structural fat grafting: more than a permanent filler. Plast Reconstr Surg 2006; 118: 108S–120S.
11. Rigotti G, Marchi A, Galie M et al. Clinical treatment of radiotherapy tissue damage by lipoaspirate transplant: a healing process mediated by adipose-derived adult stem cells. Plast Reconstr Surg 2007; 119: 1409–22; discussion 1423–4.
12. Mojallal A, Foyatier JL. The effect of different factors on the survival of transplanted adipocytes. Ann Chir Plast Esthet 2004; 49: 426–36.
13. Moore JH Jr, Kolaczynski JW, Morales LM et al. Viability of fat obtained by syringe suction lipectomy: effects of local anesthesia with lidocaine. Aesthetic Plast Surg 1995; 19: 335–9.
14. Mojallal A. Greffe d'adipocytes. Intérêt dans la restauration des volumes de la face. A propos de 100 cas. Thèse de Doctorat d'Etat en Médecine, Lyon, 2003.
15. Hudson DA, Lambert EV, Bloch CE. Site selection for fat autotransplantation: some observation. Aesthetic Plast Surg 1990; 14: 195–7.

16. Fournier PF. Réflexion sur la lipoplastie. Rev Chir Esthét. 1985; 10: 41.

17. Rohrich RJ, Sorokin ES, Brown SA. In search of improved fat transfer viability: a quantitative analysis of the role of centrifugation and harvest site. Plast Reconstr Surg 2004; 113(1): 391–5; discussion 396–7.

18. Marques A, Brenda E, Saldiva PH, Amarante MT, Ferreire MC. Autologous fat grafts. A quantitative and morphometric study in rats. Scand J Plast Reconstr Surg Hand Surg 1994; 28: 241–7.

19. Har-Shai Y, Lindenbaum ES, Gamliel-Lazarovich A, Beach D, Hirshowitz B. An integrated approach for increasing the survival of autologous fat grafts in the treatment of contour defects. Plast Reconstr Surg 1999; 104: 945–54.

20. Katz AJ, Llull R, Hedrick MH, Futrell JW. Emerging approaches to the tissue engineering of fat. Clin Plast Surg 1999; 26: 587–603, viii.

21. Mojallal A, Lequeux C, Auxenfans C, Braye B, Damour O. Influence of negative pressure when harvesting adipose tissue on all yield of stromal vascular fraction. Biomed Mater Eng. In press.

22. Rohrich RJ, Morales DE, Krueger JE et al. Comparative lipoplasty analysis of in vivo-treated adipose tissue. Plast Reconstr Surg 2000; 105: 2152–8; discussion 2159–60.

23. Niechajev I, Sevcuk O. Long-term results of fat transplantation: clinical and histologic studies. Plast Reconstr Surg 1994; 94: 496–506.

24. Lalikos JF, Li YQ, Roth TP et al. Biochemical assessment of cellular damage after adipocyte harvest. J Surg Res 1997; 70: 95–100.

25. Campbell GLM, Laudenslager N, Newman J. The effect of mechanical stress on adipocyte morphology and metabolism. Am J Cosmet Surg 1987; 4: 89–94.

26. Jauffret JL, Champsaur P, Robaglia-Schlupp A, Andrac-Meyer L, Magalon G. Arguments in favor of adipocyte grafts with the S.R. Coleman technique. Ann Chir Plast Esthet 2001; 46: 31–8.

27. Goodpasture JC, Bunkis J. Quantitative analysis of blood and fat in suction lipectomy aspirates. Plast Reconstr Surg 1986; 78: 765–72.

28. Carpaneda CA. Study of aspirated adipose tissue. Aesthetic Plast Surg 1996; 20: 399–402.

29. Aboudib Junior JH, de Castro CC, Gradel J. Hand rejuvenescence by fat filling. Ann Plast Surg 1992; 28: 559–64.

30. Fulton JE, Parastouk N. Fat grafting. Dermatol Clin 2001; 19: 523–30, ix.

31. Ersek RA, Chang P, Salisbury MA. Lipo layering of autologous fat: an improved technique with promising results. Plast Reconstr Surg 1998; 101: 820–6.

32. Smith P, Adams WP Jr, Lipschitz AH et al. Autologous human fat grafting: effect of harvesting and preparation techniques on adipocyte graft survival. Plast Reconstr Surg 2006; 117: 1836–44.

33. Cortese A, Savastano G, Felicetta L. Free fat transplantation for facial tissue augmentation. J Oral Maxillofac Surg 2000; 58: 164–9; discussion 169–70.

34. Horl HW, Feller AM, Biemer E. Technique for liposuction fat reimplantation and long-term volume evaluation by magnetic resonance imaging. Ann Plast Surg 1991; 26: 248–58.

35. Toledo LS. Syringe liposculpture: a two-year experience. Aesthetic Plast Surg 1991; 15: 321–6.

36. Boschert MT, Beckert BW, Puckett CL, Concannon MJ. Analysis of lipocyte viability after liposuction. Plast Reconstr Surg 2002; 109: 761–5; discussion 766–7.

37. Coleman SR. Structural fat grafts: the ideal filler? Clin Plast Surg 2001; 28: 111–19.

38. Yuksel E, Weinfeld AB, Cleek R et al. Increased free fat-graft survival with the long-term, local delivery of insulin, insulin-like growth factor-I, and basic fibroblast growth factor by PLGA/PEG microspheres. Plast Reconstr Surg 2000; 105: 1712–20.

39. Ullmann Y, Hyams M, Ramon Y et al. Enhancing the survival of aspirated human fat injected into nude mice. Plast Reconstr Surg 1998; 101: 1940–4.

40. Smith J, Kaminski MV Jr, Wolosewick J. Use of human serum albumin to improve retention of autologous fat transplant. Plast Reconstr Surg 2002; 109: 814–16.

41. Baran CN, Celebioglu S, Sensoz O et al. The behavior of fat grafts in recipient areas with enhanced vascularity. Plast Reconstr Surg 2002; 109: 1646–51; 1652.

42. Van RL, Roncari DA. Complete differentiation in vivo of implanted cultured adipocyte precursors from adult rats. Cell Tissue Res 1982; 225: 557–66.

43. Coleman WP 3rd. Fat transplantation. Dermatol Clin 1999; 17: 891–8, viii.

44. Schuller-Petrovic S. Improving the aesthetic aspect of soft tissue defects on the face using autologous fat transplantation. Facial Plast Surg 1997; 13: 119–24.

45. Donofrio LM. Structural autologous lipoaugmentation: a pan-facial technique. Dermatol Surg 2000; 26: 1129–34.

46. Bertossi D, Kharouf S, d'Agostino A et al. Facial localized cosmetic filling by multiple injections of fat stored at -30 degrees C. Techniques, clinical follow-up of 99 patients and histological examination of 10 patients. Ann Chir Plast Esthet 2000; 45: 548–55; discussion 555–6.

47. Lidagoster MI, Cinelli PB, Levee EM, Sian CS. Comparison of autologous fat transfer in fresh, refrigerated, and frozen specimens: an animal model. Ann Plast Surg 2000; 44: 512.

43 Global approach and techniques of fat grafting

Ali Mojallal and Jean Louis Foyatier

Adipose tissue

It is useful to define the three kinds of adipose tissue, which differ radically in their function within the organism.

White adipose tissue is in fact yellow in man because of the liposoluble carotene pigment content. It contains mainly triglycerides, and its principal function is the storage of energy. Histologically, it comprises mainly adipocytes, but also cells which do not contain lipids such as fibroblasts, macrophages, blood cells, and endothelial cells. These cells compose the fraction known as the 'stromal–vascular' fraction, which also contains preadipocytes, able to form new adipocytes according to the state of the energy balance and the nutritional and hormonal conditions.[1,2]

Brown adipose tissue is particularly important in hibernating rodents or mammals. It does not seem to be active in man, except for the perinatal period, during which it is found in relatively large quantities, in particular around the great vessels.

Medullary adipose tissue is an adaptable tissue, important for metabolic and secretory activities, which is involved in the regulation of hematopoiesis and its environment.[3,4]

The development of adipose tissue

The adipocytes become differentiated from multipotent mesodermal cells, which can be the origin of different and distinct cellular types: adipocytes, myocytes, chondrocytes, hepatocytes, cardiomyocytes, endothelial cells, epithelial cells, and neuron-like cells. It has been shown that adipose tissue is the largest source of readily collectable stem cells. It was thought for a long time that the number of adipocytes increased only at certain periods of life and that, according to Cameron and Senevirante,[5] mature adipose tissue did not have the capacity to proliferate, and the primitive material constituted the principal source of mature adipose tissue. However, it is now known that, even though the rate slows down with age, adipocytes continue to proliferate throughout life. This process starts with the cell precursors, the preadipocytes from stem cells.

In the process of differentiation of the preadipocyte to the adipocyte, one can distinguish proliferation as an early stage and differentiation as a later stage (Figure 43.1).

Metabolism of adipocytes

In addition to its role as heat and mechanical insulator, the principal function of adipose tissue is as a reserve for energy.[6] The stored fatty acids can come from the circulating lipids conveyed in the plasma by lipoproteins, or be synthesized in situ from glucose via lipogenesis.

Regulation of storage

Two types of hormones – insulin and the catecholamines – control in an extremely precise way the activity of lipid storage in adipose tissue. Insulin exerts a positive influence on storage, whereas catecholamines, via the β-adrenergic system, have a negative effect.[6]

Over the last 10 years, a new property of adipose tissue has been discovered – to be able to produce and secrete signals for paracrine or endocrine action. The discovery of this property now makes it possible to consider adipocytes as an endocrine gland, producing hormones (Figure 43.2).

This role was revealed in a particularly striking way by the discovery of leptin.[6] This is a major factor in the autoregulation of adipose tissue, secreted by only adipocytes and not preadipocytes.[7,8] Leptin plays a role in food intake, puberty, fertility,[9] and angiogenesis.[8] This last property is an important component since, parallel with adipocyte hypertrophy, leptin produced by hypertrophic adipocytes could stimulate endothelial cells, leading to an increase in microvascularization of adipose tissue and contributing to the development of vascularization of the fat mass.[8]

Variation in distribution of adipose tissue

Subcutaneous adipose tissue is found around the entire organism, except in the scrotum, penis, and eyelids.[10] In general, one can distinguish two main types of adipose location – subcutaneous (suprafacial) or deep (subfascial) – which differ significantly in their metabolic capacities. This variation is

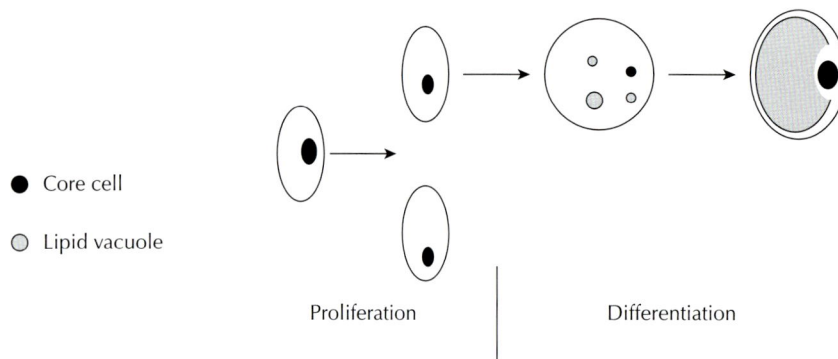

Figure 43.1   Proliferation and differentiation of preadipocytes into adipocytes.

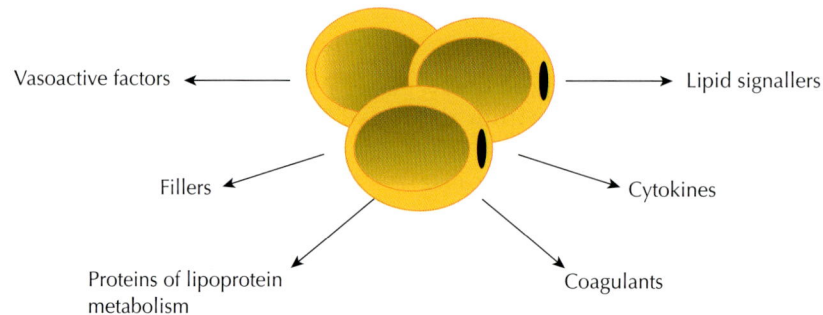

Figure 43.2   Principal adipocyte secretions according to Dugail and Ferre.[6]

related to biochemical and metabolic differences. The relationship between the two receptors, β_1 and α_2, dictates whether adipose tissue is more or less sensitive to lipolysis; thus, α_2 receptors slow down lipolysis in the area of the buttocks, and it can be observed that a woman can lose weight from her entire body apart from in this region.

Theories of adipocyte transplanation

Two theories have been proposed.

According to the theory of adipocyte survival, the transplanted adipocytes survive and continue their development cycle at the recipient site. On the first day, the transplanted adipocytes undergo a phase of ischemia. There is an influx of macrophages, histiocytes, and polynuclear cells to mop up the debris. By the fourth day, revascularization of the transplanted adipose tissue occurs by neoangiogenesis of the host site. This revascularization starts at the periphery and moves toward the center. The central adipose tissue thus undergoes more prolonged ischemia, and revascularizes only if the transplanted material is small.

According to the theory of cellular replacement by the host, the transplanted adipose tissue causes an influx of histiocytes from the host, which come to eliminate the lipids released by the adipocytes and to clear the cellular debris. There is a fibrous reaction with an influx of

fibroblasts.[11,12] The histiocytes take on characteristics of the adipocytes and replace them entirely. In other words, the transplanted adipose tissue generates by induction a local tissue increase.

All authors are in agreement with the theory of cell survival. However, today we know that transplanted fat tissue acts as a dynamic filler: it causes a change in the local physiology of the donor site and induces neosynthesis of collagen fibers and increases neoangiogenesis.[13–15] This combination of two phenomena has been termed the theory of tissue interactivity.

Evidence of adipocyte survival

Various experimental, clinical, and radiological studies have made it possible to demonstrate the survival of adipocytes.

Histological evidence

Niechajev and Sevcuk[16] carried out biopsies at the 7th, 14th, 25th, and 36th postoperative months in patients who had had a transfer of adipose tissue. Histological analysis showed adipocytes of small size (10–70 μm), mature, with lobular organization and fibrous septa. The survival of the adipocytes was thus confirmed histologically.

Peer found a normal aspect to the adipocytes in a biopsy of transplanted material dating back 13 years.[17,18] Ellenbogen[19] carried out a biopsy more than 1 year after a transplantation in the palpebral area, and found adipose tissue of normal morphology.

Carpaneda and Riberiro[20] in 1993 presented the results of a study carried out in humans. Five patients waiting for an abdominoplasty had a transplantation of adipose tissue 60, 30, 21, 15, 8, 5, and 2 days before the operation. At the time of the abdominoplasty, these transplanted zones were analyzed histologically. The study demonstrated approximately 40% survival of adipocytes, in spite of a technique that caused trauma, and also concluded that the most important element is the size of the transplanted adipose fragment. Only 1.5 ± 0.5 mm of the periphery of the transplanted adipose tissue was revascularized and therefore survived.

All these studies show the survival of adipocytes and agree that the material transplanted must be of small size, and transferred to a richly vascularized zone.[12,21]

Biochemical evidence

The amont of a marker of the cellular membrane of adipocytes (PKH26), before and after transplantation of adipose tissue, demonstated a survival of 30.4% of transplanted adipocytes in the mouse model.[22] According to this study, the transplanted adipocytes release their lipid vacuoles and decrease their oxygen uptake throughout ischemia before reconstituting these vacuoles from the third month, which demonstrates survival of the adipocytes.

Clinical evidence

It is difficult to provide clinical and morphological evidence. The best way to evaluate the results, before the standardization of three-dimensional imaging, is the use of pre- and postoperative comparative photographs. We used 3D CT of the surface to calculate the gain in volume by subtracting the preoperative image from the postoperative one. This involves heavy irradiation of the patient and does not have clinical significance. Currently we are working on the use of 3D digital imaging.

Radiological evidence

Magnetic resonance imaging (MRI) is the reference technique for the study of adipose tissue, but it does not provide any additional information for patient follow-up. Some authors carried out follow-up by ultrasound,[23] but this examination supplied little of interest. Postoperative MRI shows on average a loss of 49% at 3 months and 55% at 6 months; then the tissue is stable and there is no change at 9 or 12 months. This proves that, in spite of the traumatizing technique used, approximately 50% of transplanted adipose tissue survives and that the transplanted material is stable from about the 6th month.[24]

It is difficult, for economic reasons, because of availability, and for ethical concerns, to carry out MRI examination before and after each intervention and in all patients. The place of MRI in current practice is therefore as a preoperative examination in complex cases with multitissue involvement.

Technique of adipocyte transplanation

The technique of adipocyte transplantation used and presented here is that described by Coleman, called 'structural fat graft'.[25] Some details vary from its initial description, but the concept remains identical. This technique is rigorous and uses specific material.

The technique comprises three stages: harvesting, centrifugation, and reinjection (Figure 43.3). Anesthesia is usually general, except in the case of a localized procedure requiring small quantities of tissue.

Harvesting

The harvesting must be carried out on the deep subfascial fat tissue, often in the abdominal and flank area, the area of the trochanter, or the inner side of the knees. The harvesting is carried out using a specific aspiration cannula of 3 mm diameter, 15 cm length, with a non-traumatic end and with double lateral openings broad enough to allow passage of the adipocytes. This cannula is mounted on a fixed syringe (Luer Lock) of 10 ml. The vacuum in the syringe is created manually and gradually, in order to avoid too great a negative pressure being imposed on the adipocytes. Multiple tunnels are used in the withdrawal to diminish trauma and hemorrhage (Figure 43.3a,b).

Centrifugation

The 10-ml syringes are sealed using stoppers, the piston is withdrawn, and the syringes are stored in a sterile rack before being introduced into the centrifuge (Figure 43.3c). Centrifugation is conducted for 3 minutes at a speed of 3000 revolutions per minute. Finally, the contents of the syringe are separated into three phases (Figure 43.3d):

- the material floating on top: this is oily, composed of triglycerides from the damaged adipocytes, and constitutes the least dense part; this part is eliminated by plugging (Figure 43.3e)
- the lower part of the syringe contains primarily blood products and debris of hematic origin with remnants of the products of infiltration; this part is also eliminated
- the intermediate portion: this part contains the adipocytes to be transplanted.

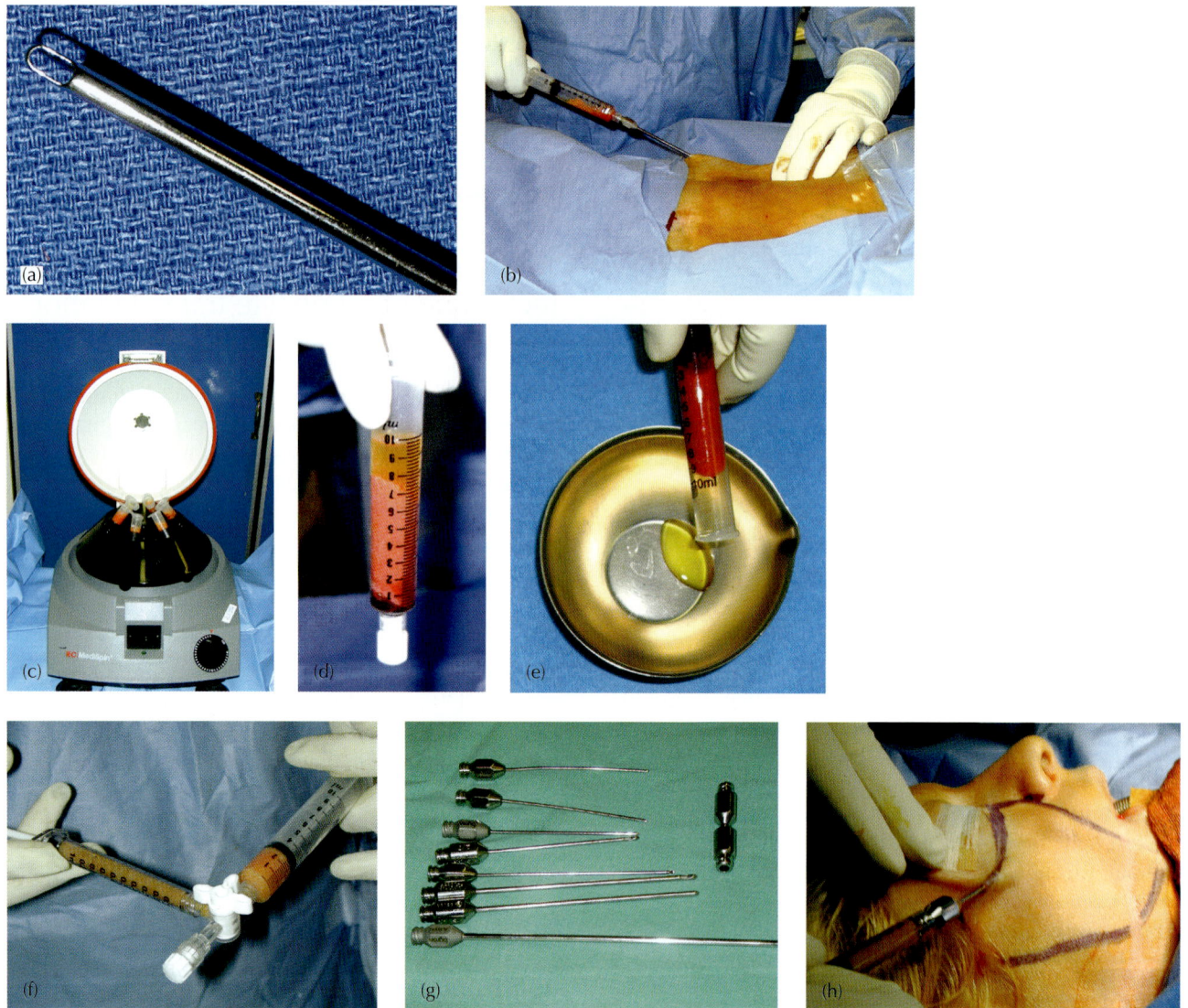

Figure 43.3 Materials used in the transplantation of adipose tissue. (a, b) Harvesting; (c–e) purification; (f–h) injection.

Transfer of adipocytes (reinjection)

The goal is to deposit the smallest possible quantities with each injection. To achieve this, it is necessary to realize a three-dimensional lattice in the tissue to be transplanted. For use in the face and small areas, the purified tissue obtained is transferred from 10-ml syringes to 1-ml syringes using a double or triple tap. This procedure should be done without atmospheric contamination, delicately, and without any pressure exerted on the syringes (Figure 43.3f). The cannulas used for reinjection are 17–18G with variable form and length (Figure 43.3g). In all cases, the end of the cannula is blunt to avoid any additional trauma and to avoid generating a hematoma at the recipient site. The cannula should have a side opening in order to avoid inopportune intravascular injection. The size of the cannula and the opening should be sufficiently large to let the adipocytes pass without damage. The cannula is introduced to its full extent via an incision, and injection is made by withdrawing the cannula (Figure 43.3h). The 1-ml

syringe should permit transplantation of material in 6–8 tunnels. It is important to achieve a multitude of tunnels that criss-cross in order to deposit the tissue in the form of a three-dimensional lattice. All levels are grafted, beginning with the deepest. Incisions are closed using 6/0 surgical thread.

The technique is organized according to 10 principles:

1. The fat tissue harvest must preferably be of fat cells from the abdomen, hips, or inner faces of the knees. The deep tissue must be collected. Only in very thin patients should the harvest involve all adipose tissue zones.
2. Collection of adipose tissue must be the least traumatic possible, by manual aspiration with low pressure, using a 10-ml syringe and a cannula with blunt tip.
3. Any unnecessary handling and exposure to the air must be avoided.

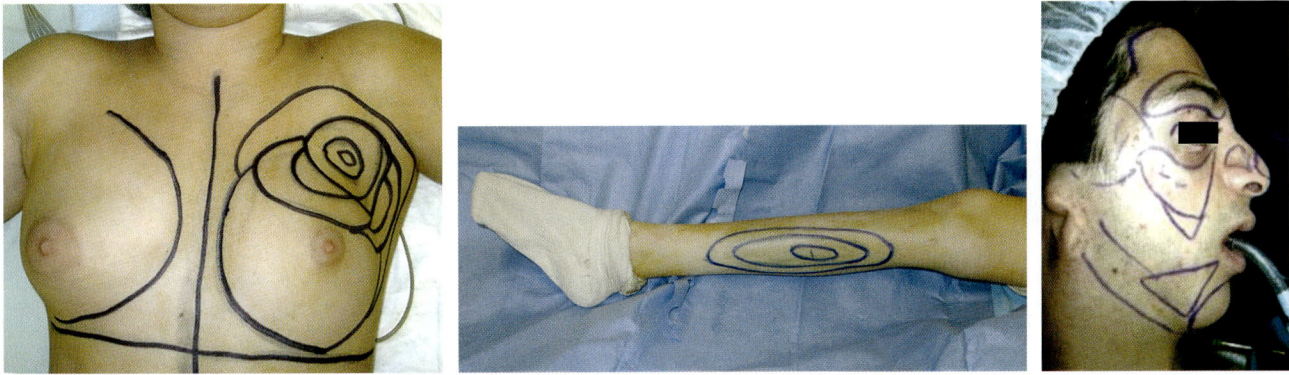

Figure 43.4 Preoperative planning and marking of zones for treatment of breasts, lower extremity, and face.

4. It is necessary to isolate and purify the adipose tissue by centrifugation.
5. The oily material floating on top and the blood debris are carefully eliminated.
6. Reinjection is performed using a fine cannula of 18G, with a non-traumatic end and side openings, fixed on a 1-ml syringe (except for the centre where the tissue is transferred directly using 10-ml syringes).
7. To reinject, it is necessary to introduce the cannula completely and to deposit the material during the removal of the cannula. It is necessary to multiply to the maximum the tunnels for injection in order to insert the fat in very small quantities. There should be a three-dimensional lattice of transplanted adipose tissue, called structural fat grafting.
8. At the end of the intervention, careful and delicate remodeling with the fingers can perfect the result.
9. After closing the incision points, it is recommended that the head should be slightly elevated, and a cooling application of cold compresses made to the face.
10. It is necessary to envisage – and to warn the patient of the possibility of – later sessions.

Combining fat tissue transplantation with other procedures

When fat tissue transplantation is carried out in conjunction with another surgical procedure, two principles should to be respected:

1. Fat tissue transplantation must always be performed last, because it involves an adjustment of volumes after their redistribution. Moreover, a final position for transplantation avoids any additional trauma to the transplanted tissue at the time of the associated intervention.
2. If the associated procedure relates to the same zone, the reinjection of material must be carried out using the exposure from the operative exposure and not performed percutaneously.

Application of fat tissue transplantation to reconstructive and cosmetic surgery procedures

As with all filling products, the purpose of the transplanted tissue is to restore a lack of volume. With mastery of this technique and in view of the good results obtainable, the application of fat tissue transplantation can be extended to other fields for the cosmetic surgeon. Its use can even be advocated in the case of multitissue defects, and the adipose tissue will then substitute for the absence of bone, muscle, or other tissue. However, when there is a functional defect, in particular in facial malformations or of the limbs, this must be treated first. The volumetric restoration will then be done at the end of treatment.

Clinical examination of the patient under good lighting makes it possible to see lack of volume. For the face, it is necessary first of all to look at the zones of projection: the zygomatic arch and the malar projection, the upper orbital rim and the position of the eyebrows, and the mandibular edge and the chin, including the zone where it joins the melolabial sulcus and the so-called 'marionette folds'. Then should come an analysis of the remainder: in the face this would be the periorbital area, upper lip and lower lip, nasoglabellar lines, cheek, nasolabial folds, nose, and temporal area. For the breasts (in reconstructive surgery), the position of the inframammory fold, the median axis, the position of the areolae, and the volume and projection of the various quadrants of the breasts must be compared with those on the opposite side. The superior medial quadrant is the most difficult to correct by traditional techniques, and the most visible in a low neckline. For the limbs, it is necessary to measure the circumference in several levels: each patient should be photographed full face, in profile, at three-quarters, and axially.

Accurate and detailed information should be reported to the patient, enumerating the disadvantages and complications of this technique, but especially the possibility and sometimes the need for repeat sessions to obtain a satisfactory and final result, because the results are inconsistent and variable according to the site. It is necessary to carry out a three-dimensional strategy of treatment. The various subunits and zones to be treated should be marked before beginning the procedure (Figure 43.4), because the instantaneous edema that results can mask the regions of depression.

Advantages

Advantages of adipose tissue

Of all the existing implants, autologous adipose tissue represents the ideal.[25] It has the advantage of being:

- biocompatible, and therefore reliable, not toxic or endangering the health of patients, and resistant to infection, after an initial period of integration
- natural, not felt as a separate entity but forming an integral part of the texture of the tissue
- stable, often after several sessions, while avoiding the deposition of too great a quantity per session
- simple and comfortable for the patient, without major inconveniences
- general-purpose, since the material substitutes for all missing tissue with the same morphological aim
- regenerative effect of adipose tissue with stem cells and growth factors.

Advantages of adipocyte tissue transplantation technique

Compared to other techniques in restorative or cosmetic surgery, this has the advantage of being:

- technically simple
- reproducible
- effective, for small zones as well as for large tissue replacement
- adjustable, allowing correction of the most difficult zones requested
- percutaneous, and non-invasive
- realizable under local anesthesia and in an ambulatory setting, according to the volume of tissue necessary
- the cause of low morbidity for the donor site.

Disadvantages

Contraindications for adipose transplantation are rare. They concern mainly cases of very thin patients, who do not have enough fat tissue to use.

Complications

Edema

This is the most frequent complication. It is related to local trauma generated by the many tunnels created during reinjection. In certain cases it can persist for several weeks. Non-steroidal anti-inflammatory drugs (NSAIDs), the Trendelenburg position, and cooling with ice are all used to decrease the edema.

Ecchymoses

Bruising arises especially when the passage of the cannula was too superficial or if too large a quantity of adipose tissue was transplanted when compared to the elastic capacity of the local tissue. An application of petroleum jelly or glycerol on the recipient site avoids any damage to the skin.

Hematomas

Hematomas are rare. They occur if a vein is injured at the time of local anesthesia or reinjection of tissue. If this occurs, it is necessary to warn the patient of the possibility of resorption of the transplanted adipose tissue.

Undercorrection

This is the most frequent complication. It is due to underestimating the volume necessary, or to a lack of tissue that can be harvested in some very thin people. It can also occur after resorption of part of the transplanted tissue. The treatment is repetition of the procedure.

Overcorrection

This is less frequent than the above but the treatment is also less simple. The transplanted adipose tissue retains its initial characteristics and can be the origin of secondary hypertrophy at the time of an increase in weight.[26]

Pseudocyst and fat necrosis

This occurs when the volume injected is too large compared to the recipient site and its capacity for revascularization. The center of a large fragment is the site of ischemic necrosis, and consequently of a cyst or pseudocyst.[27,28] Such pseudocysts occur 6–12 months after the intervention and contain lipids, triglycerides, fatty acids, and cholesterol.

Migration

Migration can take place when too great a quantity of adipose tissue is deposited in a zone that is under tension when the neighboring zone is flexible. Adipose tissue moves naturally from a zone of high pressure toward one of lower pressure. Therefore, correction in several sessions is necessary when a great volume of adipose tissue has to be transplanted.

Irregularities

These occur when tissue is deposited too superficially in a zone where the cutaneous cover is fine. Large fragments are sites of spontaneous lysis, but often small fragments form 'knots'. The eyelid is often the location for irregularities.

Tattooing

This occurs by dermal penetration in the region of the incisions of the blue ink that was used to mark the various zones, or sometimes by hemosiderin deposit from the degraded blood cells.

Infection

The oral mucous membrane is the principal source of infection in the facial area if a breach is created during injection of the cheek or the lips. A case of erysipelas of a lower extremity has been reported.[29]

Lesion of the underlying elements

The purpose of use of a cannula with a smooth end is to avoid this. Lesions encountered have included parotitis, infraorbital injection by perforation of the orbital septum, and lesion of branches of the facial artery, vein, or nerve. This complication is exceptional.

Intravascular injection

This can occur especially in the periorbital area, with fat embolism leading to thrombosis of the central artery of the retina or a cerebrovascular ischaemic accident.[30,31] These preconditions are necessary to cause a fat embolism:[32] bloody adipose tissue whose injection is carried out under strong pressure, injection into vascular pathways, and introduction of the end of the needle into the vascular lumen.

Conclusion

The transplantation of adipose tissue according to this technique is a delicate operation on fragile tissues, requiring non-traumatizing procedures. It uses a specific material and very strict methodology. Comparative histological studies do not show deterioration of tissue transplanted by this technique. The theory of the survival of transplanted tissue has been demonstrated by various histological, biochemical, radiological, and clinical studies. This is a simple, effective, and reproducible technique, making it possible to obtain good results and a high rate of patient satisfaction. In our opinion, fat tissue transplantation constitutes the best means to adjust volume. The application of this technique to the various fields of cosmetic surgery is a therapeutic tool that is essential not to neglect. Research has contributed to a better understanding of adipose tissue which could, thanks to tissue engineering, be a source of 'stem cells', used to repair or regenerate various connective tissues.

References

1. Dugail I, Ferre P. Développement du tissu adipeux. In: Encyclopédie Médico-Chirurgical. Traité d'Endocrinologie-Nutrition. Paris: Elsevier, 2002: 10-506-A-10.
2. Poznanski WJ, Waheed I, Van R. Human fat cell precursors. Morphologic and metabolic differentiation in culture. Lab Invest 1973; 29: 570–6.
3. Laharrague P, Corberand JX, Cousin B, Pénicaud L, Casteilla L. Adipocytes médullaires et hématopoïèse. Hématologie 1999; 5: 255.
4. Smahel J. Adipose tissue in plastic surgery. Ann Plast Surg 1986; 16: 444–53.
5. Cameron GR, Senevirante RD. Growth and repair in adipose tissue. J Pathol Bacteriol 1947; 59: 665.
6. Dugail I, Ferre P. Métabolisme du tissu adipeux blanc. Encyclopédie Médico-Chirurgical. Traité d'Endocrinologie-Nutrition. Paris: Elsevier, 2002: 10-506-B-10.
7. Markman B. Anatomy and physiology of adipose tissue. Clin Plast Surg 1989; 16: 235–44.
8. Lafontan M, Bouloumie A. Angiogenèse: une implication physiologique de plus pour la leptine. Med Sci (Paris) 1999; 15: 382.
9. Montague CT, Farooqi IS, Whitehead JP et al. Congenital leptin deficiency is associated with severe early-onset obesity in humans. Nature 1997; 387: 903–8.
10. Ryan TJ, Curri SB. The structure of fat. Clin Dermatol 1989; 7: 37–47.
11. Neuhof H. Free transplantation of fat for closure of bronchopulmonary cavities (lattice lung). J Thorac Surg 1937; 7: 23.
12. Sadick NS, Hudgins LC. Fatty acid analysis of transplanted adipose tissue. Arch Dermatol 2001; 137: 723–7.
13. Mojallal A, Lequeux C, Damour O, Foyatier JL, Braye F. Improvement of skin quality. Animal studies and clinical cases of facial reconstructive surgery. In Coleman SR, Mazzola RF, eds, Fat injection: from filling to regeneration. QMP editions, 2009.
14. Coleman SR. Structural fat grafting: more than a permanent filler. Plant Reconstr Surg 2006; 118: 108S–120S.
15. Rigotti G, Marchi A, Galie M et al. Clinical treatments of radiotherapy tissue damage by lipoaspirate transplant: a healing process mediated by adipose-derived adult stem cells. Plant Reconstr Surg 2007; 119: 1409–22; discussion 1423–4.
16. Niechajev I, Sevcuk O. Long-term results of fat transplantation: clinical and histologic studies. Plast Reconstr Surg 1994; 94: 496–506.
17. Peer LA. Loss of weight and volume in human fat graft, with postulation of a 'cell survival theory'. Plast Reconstr Surg 1950; 5: 217.
18. Von Heimburg D, Pallua N. Two-year histological outcome of facial lipofilling. Ann Plast Surg 2001; 46: 644–6.
19. Ellenbogen R. Free autogenous pearl fat grafts in the face – a preliminary report of a rediscovered technique. Ann Plast Surg 1986; 16: 179–94.
20. Carpaneda CA, Ribeiro MT. Study of the histologic alterations and viability of the adipose graft in humans. Aesthetic Plast Surg 1993; 17: 43–7.
21. Guerrerosantos J, Gonzalez-Mendoza A, Masmela Y et al. Long-term survival of free fat grafts in muscle: an experimental study in rats. Aesthetic Plast Surg 1996; 20: 403–8.

22. Rieck B, Schlaak S. Measurement in vivo of the survival rate in autologous adipocyte transplantation. Plast Reconstr Surg 2003; 111: 2315–23.

23. Glogau RG. Microlipoinjection: autologous fat grafting. Arch Dermatol 1988; 124: 1340–3.

24. Horl HW, Feller AM, Biemer E. Technique for liposuction fat reimplantation and long-term volume evaluation by magnetic resonance imaging. Ann Plast Surg 1991; 26: 248–58.

25. Coleman SR. Structural fat grafts: the ideal filler? Clin Plast Surg 2001; 28: 111–19.

26. Latoni JD, Marshall DM, Wolfe SA. Overgrowth of fat autotransplanted for correction of localized steroid-induced atrophy. Plast Reconstr Surg 2000; 106: 1566–9.

27. Mandrekas AD, Zambacos GJ, Kittas C. Cyst formation after fat injection. Plast Reconstr Surg 1998; 102: 1708–9.

28. Maillard GF. Liponecrotic cysts after augmentation mammaplasty with fat injections. Aesthetic Plast Surg 1994; 18: 405–6.

29. de Pedroza LV. Fat transplantation to the buttocks and legs for aesthetic enhancement or correction of deformities: long-term results of large volumes of fat transplant. Dermatol Surg 2000; 26: 1145–9.

30. Dreizen NG, Framm L. Sudden unilateral visual loss after autologous fat injection into the glabellar area. Am J Ophthalmol 1989; 107: 85–7.

31. Teimourian B. Blindness following fat injections. Plast Reconstr Surg 1988; 82: 361.

32. Feinendegen DL, Baumgartner RW, Schroth G, Mattle HP, Tschopp H. Middle cerebral artery occlusion AND ocular fat embolism after autologous fat injection in the face. J Neurol 1998; 245: 53–4.

44 Facial rejuvenation: lipostructure and other techniques

Patrick Bui and Gilbert Zakine

Introduction

Facial aging involves superficial structures such as the skin but also deeper structures such as fat, muscle, and skeleton.[1–5]

During the first 10 years of life, the large quantity of fat in the face and particularly at the level of the cheeks is the origin of 'jowls', which tend to accentuate the nasolabial grooves and labiomental region giving a 'cherub' appearance.

In the young adult fat is abundant, but, unlike in the face of a newborn baby, it is distributed in a regular and diffuse manner, creating a fatty continuum within every esthetic unit of the face and between each of them, their distribution appearing balanced and homogeneous. Fat is at the origin of the 'convex' aspect of the face, where zones of shade are rare. In profile, the arch of the forehead and that of the mid-facial region reflect light. In contrast, the aging face is characterized by a loss of forward projection of the forehead, eyebrows, and mid-facial region. This reduction in projection favors cutaneous excess and ptosis.[3,4]

The aging of the fatty masses at the facial level is especially marked by a decline.[6] The reduction in fat is notable around the orbit, the temporal region, and the submalar region. Some zones can present an excess of fat, particularly in overweight persons, which creates, along with the areas of fat atrophy, an irregular aspect to the facial relief. Storage of facial fat occurs especially at the levels of the medial one-third and the inferior one-third (under chin region, jowls).

The adipose support of the premalar region shows a progressive reduction, with descent of the malar region into the canine fossa, and an overhang of the nasolabial groove. Fat atrophy involves especially the upper part of the face, but can affect the whole face in thin persons.

The injection of fat, allowing its redistribution in zones that have become atrophic with age, seems therefore logical to make the aging face appear younger in a natural manner. Microlipoaspiration of a region where fat is redundant can be combined with the lipofilling of atrophic zones allowing a true balance. Moreover, increasingly numerous authors recommend the injection of autologous fat associated with a cervicofacial facelift to treat tissue prolapse and fat ptosis simultaneously.[7,8]

History

Neuber accomplished the first grafting of adipose tissue in 1893,[9] taking graft samples of small size from the forearm to fill a secondary facial scar in tubercular osteitis. The first to offer the use of fat with esthetic aim was Lexer[10] in 1910, with augmentation of the malar and nasolabial region and the filling of wrinkles and grooves being reported. In 1911, Brunning[11] reinjected at the subcutaneous level small fragments of fat to correct rhinoplasties, but the results become indistinct with time. Peer[12] in 1950 showed that the grafted fragments of fat lost about 50% of their volume in 1 year. Good results were reported using dermofat grafting by Eitner[13] in 1931, Peer[12] in 1950, Boering and Huffstadt[14] in 1967, and Sawhney et al[15] in 1969. The last authors showed resorption of 33% of the graft, and the possibility of replacing adipose tissue with conjunctival tissue in pigs.

The first case of mammary reconstruction using autologous fat was presented by Czerny[16] in 1895. He took a sample from a large lipoma of the back to fill a defect after a tumorectomy. A case of mammary reconstruction after mastectomy was introduced in 1931 by Lexer.[17] Then, in 1941, a bilateral mammary reconstruction using a fat graft on one side and a fasciofat graft on the other side was reported by May.[18] Several cases of mammary augmentation for hypotrophy using dermofat grafting were published by Bames[19] in 1953. Dermofat grafting was used by Schroder[20] in 1957 to treat hypotrophy and by Peer to treat a case of Poland syndrome. At the same time, in ophthalmology,[21] in general surgery,[22] in gynecology,[23] in neurosurgery,[24] and in maxillofacial surgery,[25,26] fat was progressively being offered to fill losses of material.

After the discovery of lipoaspiration by cannula by Illouz,[27] adipose tissue could be obtained other than by surgical removal. Fournier[28,29] in 1989 presented a technology of injection of non-purified fat which was called lipofilling or liposculpture. Bircoll[30,31] in 1988 introduced cases of mammary augmentation and symmetrization after cancer by injecting small quantities over several sessions.

Ellenbogen,[32] in 1986, injected fat fragments of 4–6 mm in diameter to treat facial wrinkles, palpebral depressions, or acne scars.

Cycles of enthusiasm and skepticism accompanied these techniques of fat injection, the quality of results of which was marked by frequent resorption and unpredictability.

In 1995, Coleman[6,33–35] published a defined protocol of fat injection that he described as atraumatic. It encodes in a definite manner the different stages of this technology using centrifugation and redeposition. This leads to the concept of adipocyte grafting, very different from fat injection. This method allows stable and reproducible results to be acquired. Interest in this technique is increasing continuously, and numerous research studies are regularly published. The stable and reproducible character of volumetric reconstruction confirms the combined improvement of texture and skin atrophy. We note also an action on wrinkles, pores, and skin pigmentation as well as the aspect of scarring or after radiotherapy.

Recently, the use of autologous fat has become more widespread in other domains. It has been used for rejuvenation of the hands,[34,36] to treat anal incontinence,[37] to correct limb or trunk atrophy,[38–41] to ameliorate defects in mammary reconstruction after mastectomy and grooves after mammary prosthesis, or to accomplish mammary augmentation without prosthesis. In fact, any zone presenting fat atrophy can benefit from adipocyte grafting and indications are practically unlimited.

Lipostructrure: operating technique

Indications, evaluation, and preoperative search

Morphological and volumetric criteria of the different regions of the face allow the choice of lipostructure. Some cases of excess facial fat can benefit from lipoaspiration at the same time. Indications in esthetic surgery are the restoration of form and volume of the face at the beginning of aging, or in association with a cervicofacial facelift or else secondarily after a facelift to ameliorate particularly the curve of the medial one-third of the face. Indications in reconstructive surgery are tissue filling post-trauma, the correction of secondary irregularity after esthetic lipoaspiration, or the correction of facial lipoatrophy of iatrogenic origin in a human immunodeficiency virus (HIV) patient treated by tri- or quadritherapy (associated particularly with anti-prostheses).

Clinical examination is done with the patient in a sitting or standing position with good illumination to see the zones of depression. Photographs of facial contours including three-quarter and axial views are taken, and comparison made with more youthful photographs. Definitive and detailed information listing disadvantages and complications, and especially the possibility or necessity of supplementary intervention after 6 months, must be given. As for any surgical operation, the anesthetist must be seen in consultation at the latest 48 hours beforehand, and any medication based on aspirin must be avoided for at least 10 days before the intervention. The intervention is performed under general anesthesia or neuroleptic analgesia; this surgery can be accomplished as an ambulatory procedure.

Surgical technology

The injection sites are marked on the conscious and sitting patient; the harvest regions are chosen and explained.

Materials

Instruments include a smooth cannula for fat harvesting, 10-ml Luer-Lock syringes for collection, a special-purpose 3400-rev/minute centrifuge, single-use corks to occlude syringes, one or more 1-ml Luer-Lock syringes for precise injection, and cannulas of 17–18G with smooth ends, 7 and/or 9 cm long, especially manufactured for the reinjection of fat.

Harvesting

This is performed in an atraumatic manner by small incisions using a fine cannula and with a Luer-Lock syringe of 10 ml – the plunger allowing no more than 2 ml aspiration of fat. The zones most often used as donor sites for the face are the medial aspect of the knee and the thigh (depot area), and then the abdomen. It is important to reinject fat of the same origin at the same level, for example, knee fat for cheeks and thigh fat for temples, and not knee fat for one cheek and thigh fat for the other. This symmetry of sampling and injection harmonizes results.

Purification of fat

Coleman recommends centrifugation of 3 minutes at 3400 rev/minute with an appropriate centrifuge. This allows separation of the adipocytes from the blood products. Adipocytes are harvested and grafted in the living state, which assures theoretically the permanence of results. Numerous authors propose washing or decantation, with identical results. It is important to attain adipocytes that are as pure as possible.

Redeposition

This is performed using microcannulas of 7 and 9 cm in length, with smooth ends to avoid vascular injury. This is the basis of the originality of lipostructure and modern methods of adipocyte grafting. Adipocytes are not injected but deposited while removing the cannula. Grafting is done according to different precise plans, using microdroplets, from several micropoints of entrance, in a radial manner, and with the use of microcannulas. There is no formation of 'lakes' or a fatty mass, but microparticles with no confluence. Immobilization lasting some days ameliorates the resorption of adipocytes, the principle of any grafting (cutaneous, cartilaginous, bony) procedure in plastic surgery.

Post-surgery

Pain is minor. Edema, which can be rather important, appears especially during the first 48 hours, and will take from 5 to 15 days to be resorbed. Ecchymosis can be present. Some social discomfort caused by the edema and ecchymosis is therefore envisaged. Sun exposure must be avoided during the first month.

The final results appear during the third month. Even if the result is good, without need of modification, the aging process or drug-related lipoatrophy will impose the necessity of a repeat session after a variable delay. Moreover, in cases of imperfection (depression, irregularity), small modifications can be performed under local anesthesia from the sixth month; supplementary injections and also lipoaspiration are possible. The survival of grafted adipose tissue has been investigated by various histological, biochemical, radiological, and clinical studies. Resorption is variable according to the zone filled. The lips, a very mobile region, constitute the zone that gives the least stable results, with more than 50% resorption. The malar region gives the best results, with about 90% satisfaction, and the temporal region gives intermediate, discouraging results in the case of subcutaneous injection and better results in the case of submuscular injection.

Topography

1. *Forehead.* The improvement of convexity makes the upper third of the face appear younger. Fat deposits are retromuscular, often associated with botulinum toxin.
2. *Temples.* Results are discouraging if injections are not deep enough: they must be at the intra-or submuscular level. It is necessary to overcorrect because the absence of immobilization of the temporal muscle leads to more unpredictable survival.
3. *Cheeks and malar region.* For correction of midjugular concavity and sagging of the malar fat pad,[42,43] injection is made from several points of entrance, allowing crossing tunnels. The deposit does not have to be confluent, and is accomplished in three dimensions. The results are often very good.
4. *Nasolabial groove.* This is difficult to correct, due to its large mobility and significant resorption.[44]

Overcorrection is often necessary. Results obtained by injecting a filler product such as hyaluronic acid, collagen, or slowly or non-resorbable fillers are often better.

5. *Lips.* Results are often discouraging.[42–44] The zone is very mobile and highly vascularized, and often significant resorption occurs. However, overcorrection must be avoided because it is difficult to correct later, and is very unesthetic. Certain authors recommend an intramuscular injection.[45]
6. *Chin.* Results are good.[42,43]
7. *Eyelids and periorbital region.* The procedure is difficult and requires considerable experience. The risks of overcorrection and palpable nodules are important.[32,46,47] It is necessary to analyze the zones where fat is in excess (fatty pockets) and those where fat is missing. These zones are sometimes very close. It is necessary to analyze and treat the whole orbital region: eyelid, lower orbit, external area and upper bony rim, inner area and tear trough. It is also necessary to use microcannulas with a smooth tip in the most precise way possible, to inject only very small quantities, because fat resorption is minimal or non-existent, and to pay attention not to injure important structures (vessels, orbit). Certain authors recommend 20–30 passages to deposit 1 ml[48] (Figures 44.1 and 44.2).
8. *Superciliary region.* This allows augmentation of the projection of the eyebrow.
9. *Nose.* It is used especially to correct a defect after rhinoplasty and principally on the dorsum.[46]

Indications

Cervicofacial aging

Cervicofacial aging is the first indication. Analysis of the facial skeleton allows differentiation of a 'long face', with regression of the fat mass, from a 'short face', where there is a lower fat excess with prolapse.

Fat involution occurs around the orbit, the temporal region, the submalar region, and the near chin region. Additionally, premalar adipose support presents a progressive reduction, with descent of the malar region into the canine fossa, and repositioning of this is often necessary.

Therefore, volumetric reconstruction of the face using adipocyte grafting is indicated:

- as an isolated procedure, in the first stages of aging (Figures 44.3 and 44.4)
- associated with surgery, to complete a cervicofacial facelift at the level of the periorbital region, the mid-third, or the mental region (Figure 44.5)
- to support the long-term results of surgery.

This reestablishment of the volume of the face allows the fullness of youth to be restored and ameliorates softness and smoothness of the face.

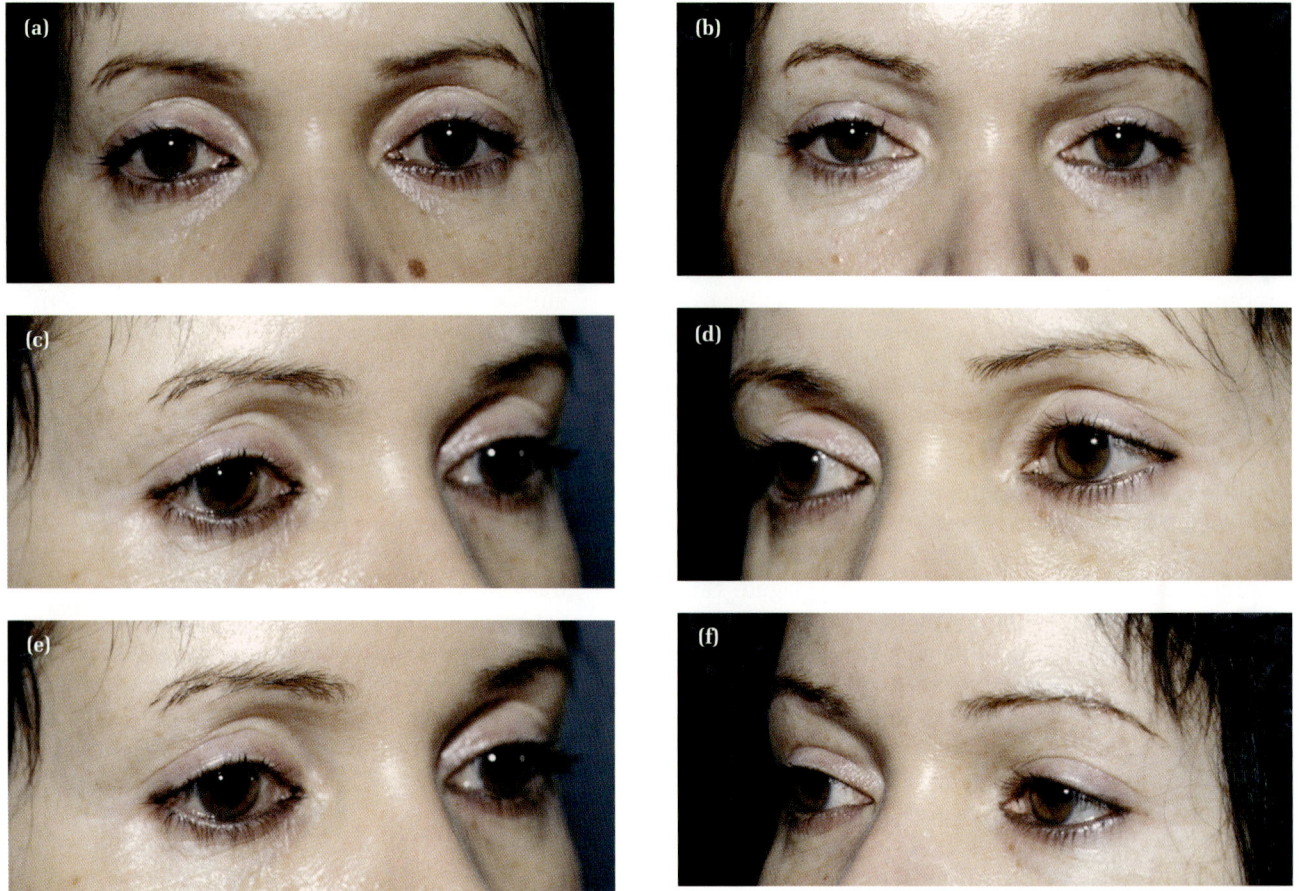

Figure 44.1   (a–f) Contouring after a superior blepharoplasty. Reconstruction using 0.7 ml of fat per side.

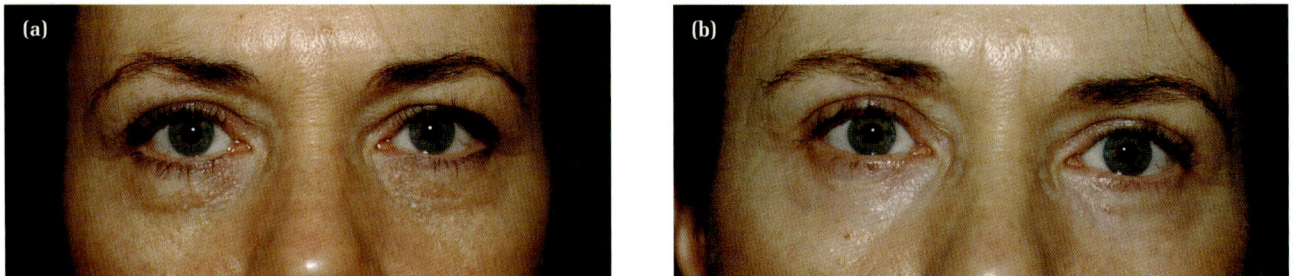

Figure 44.2   (a, b) Periorbicular aging, association of partial excision of a fatty hernia by conjunctival approach and orbicular lipostructure.

In these facial indications, fat injection can be considered as a permanent volumetric filler, with the additional important property of amelioration of skin texture quality.

Reconstructive surgery

Indications are:

- facial atrophy in HIV-positive patients treated by tri-therapy

- genetic facial distortions of the hemiatrophy type (Figure 44.6)
- trauma scar or after surgery (Figures 44.7 and 44.8)
- scarrring due to cutaneous disease or after acne: improvement is attributed to creation of a living fatty 'mattress' (Figure 44.9).

In fact, all loss of substance of the soft tissues can be rebuilt by fat grafting.

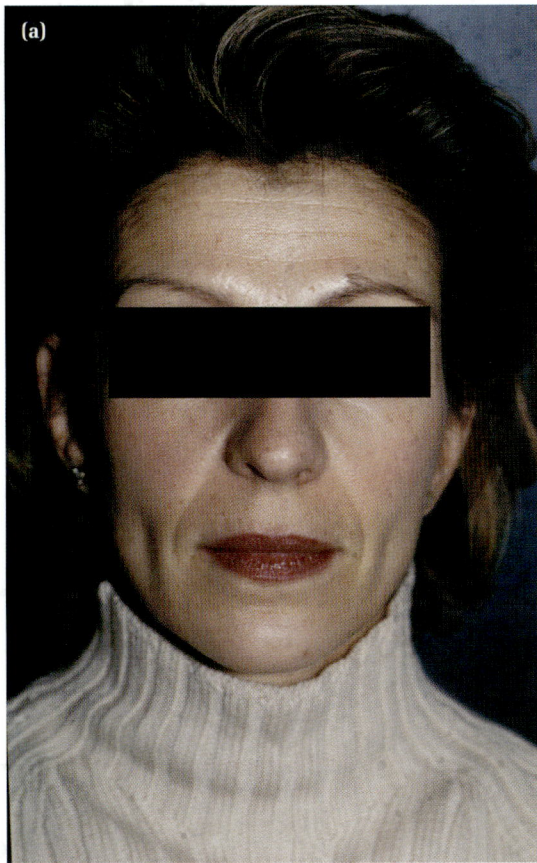

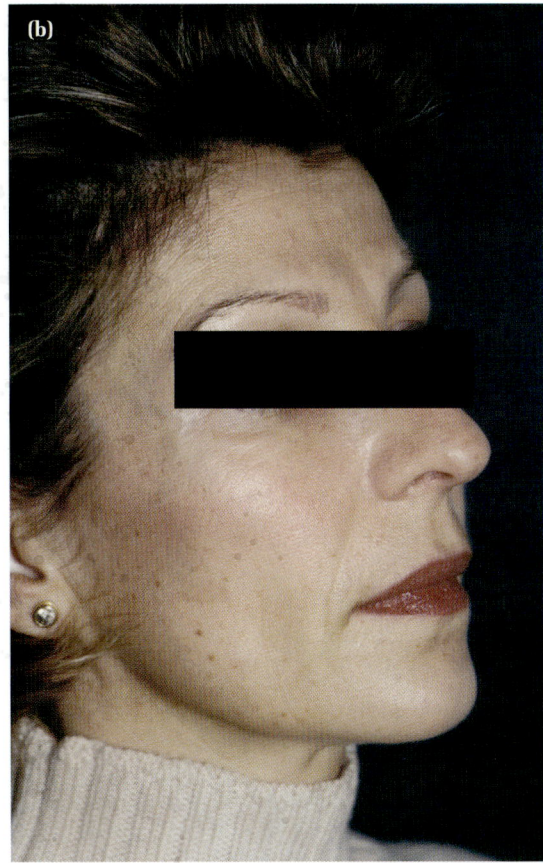

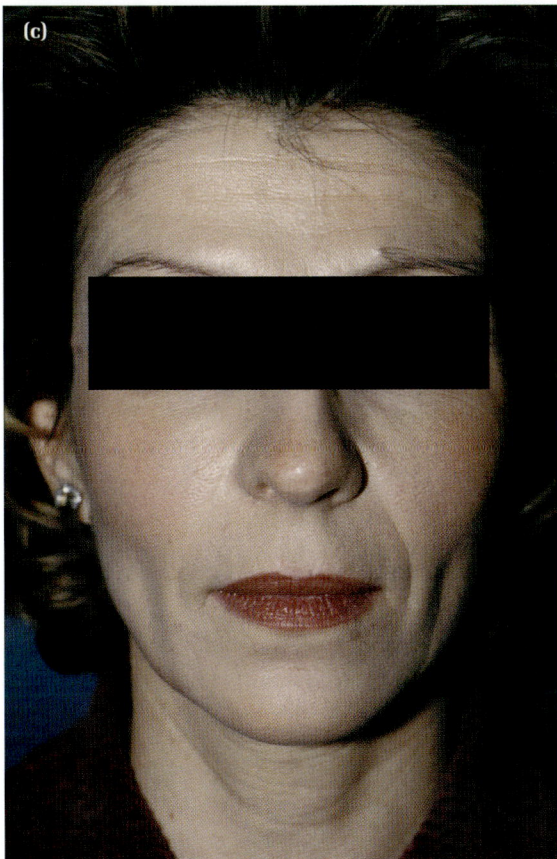

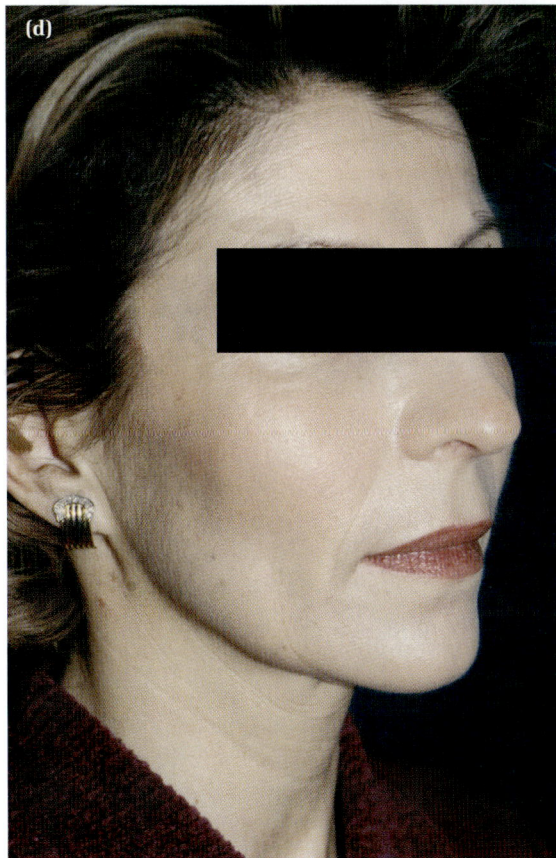

Figure 44.3   (a–d) Rejuvenation by mid-facial lipostructure.

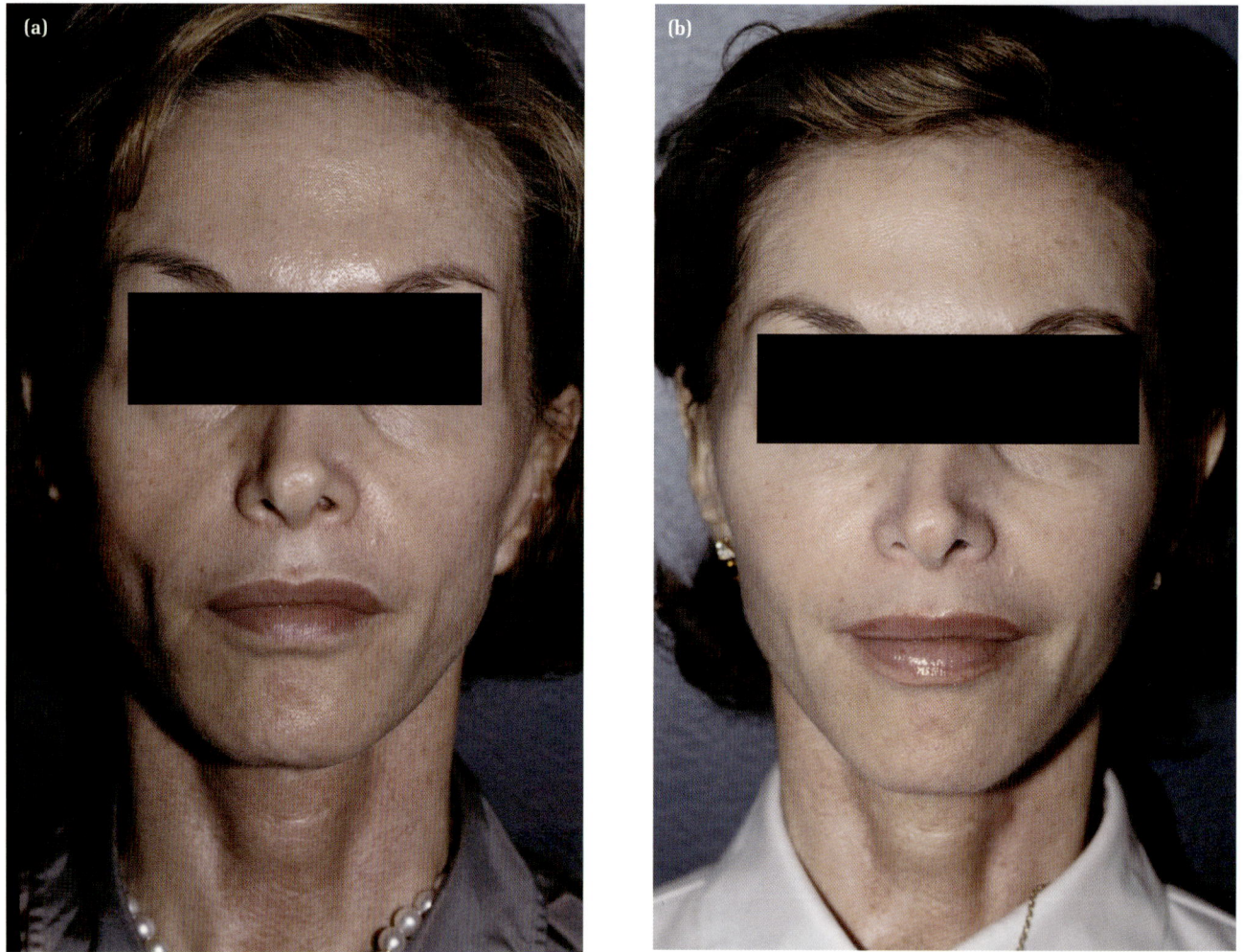

Figure 44.4   (a, b) Diffuse contouring. Orbicular and jaw lipostructure.

Complications

Edema and ecchymosis

These do not really constitute a complication. They are a normal consequence, which is necessary to inform patients about. Numerous passages of the cannula cause an aggression which is often responsible for significant edema.

Nodules, irregularity, or malpositioning

Certain irregularities can occur following lipostructure in cases of poor reinjection technique (not uniform or too superficial) (Figures 44.10 and 44.11).

Necrosis of reinjected tissues (cytosteatonecrosis) is a problem related to revascularization of reinjected tissues. This revascularization starts from the periphery and proceeds toward the center. Grafting is more assured, therefore, when it is done with a small quantity of fat.

Malpositioning is due to poor analysis of the zone of facial atrophy (Figures 44.12 and 44.13).

Complications in subjacent or systemic structures

The progress of the cannula can theoretically be at the origin of subjacent lesions. A strict respect of the technology allows avoiding lesions of the facial nerve of the orbital septum or of Stenon's canal. Several publications show cases of secondary central neurological complications after fat reinjection, either cerebral ischemia or unilateral blindness. Also, a case of occlusion of the central artery of the retina has been reported.[49] The physiopathology of these disturbances is probably a fatty embolism in ophthalmic or cerebral arteries by retrogressive flux via the branches of the external carotid.

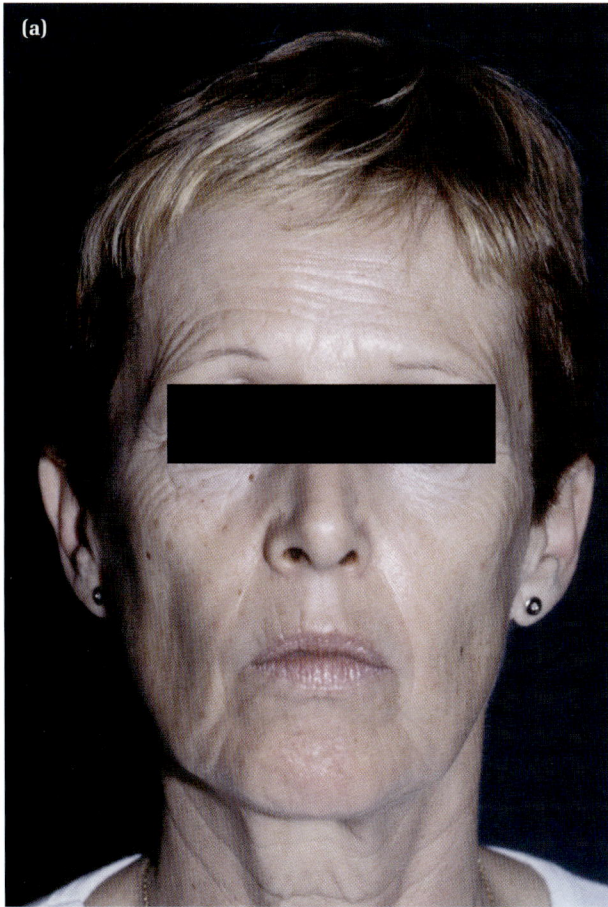

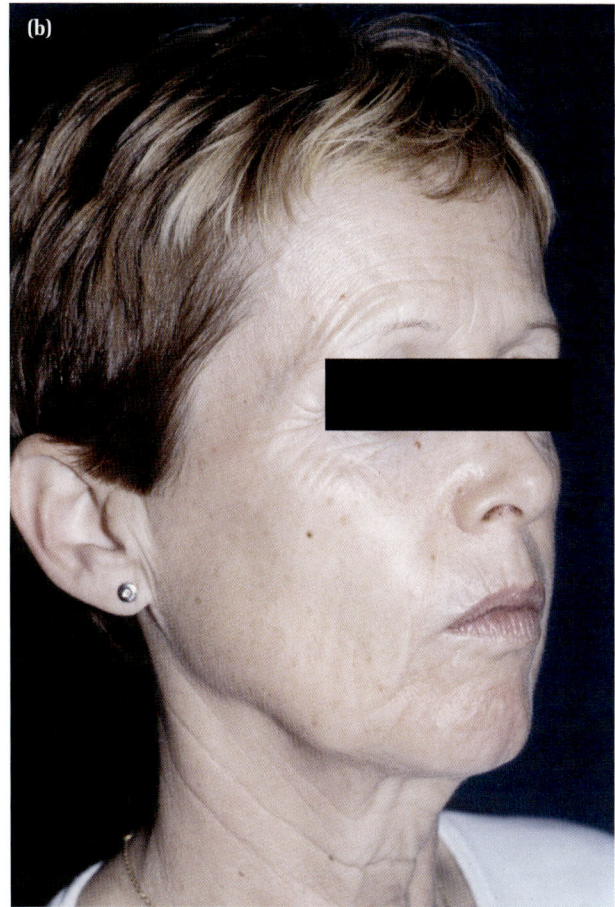

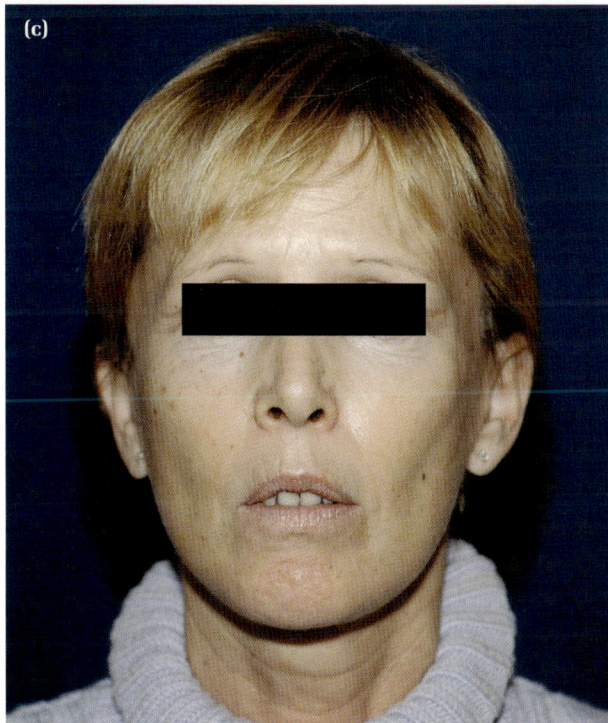

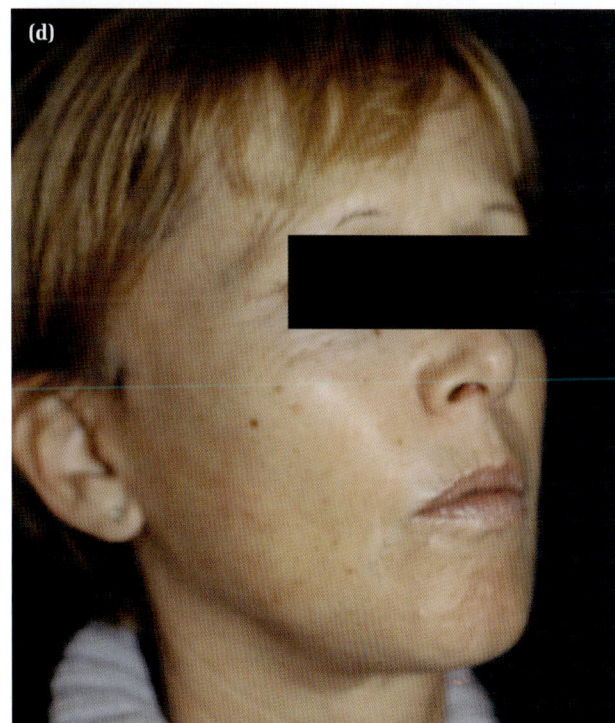

Figure 44.5 (a–d) Lifting plus mid-face and chin region lipostructure.

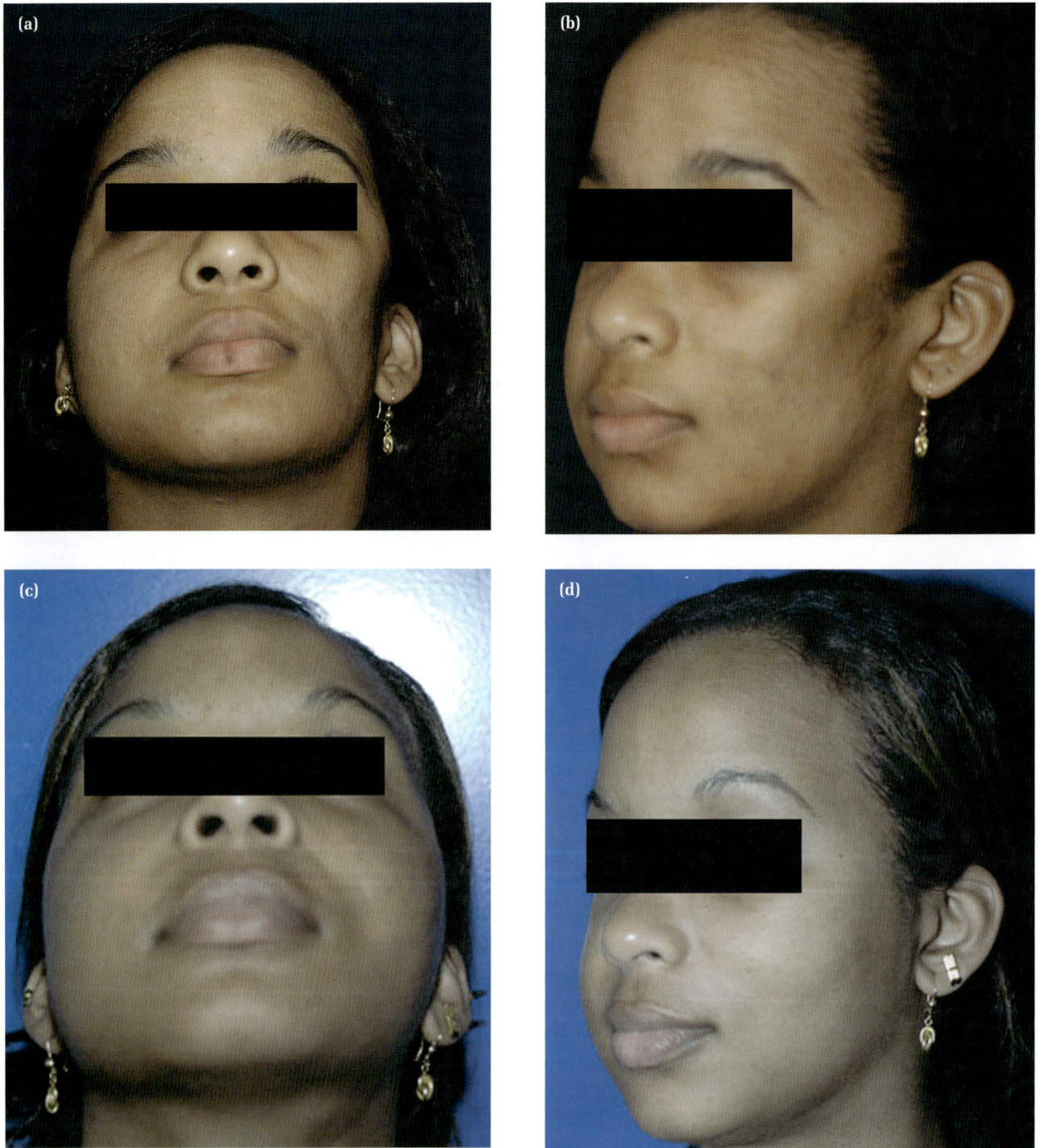

Figure 44.6 (a–d) Left side face atrophy. First step of reconstruction: 40 ml of fat graft.

Infection

This is a theoretical risk. Local consequences are probably the resorption of reinjected fat.

Resorption

The factors of resorption are variable. However, we can identify some of them:

- a too hemorrhagic sample (often in thin patients having little fat under the skin)

- a hematoma or an infection in the receiver site
- undercorrection favored by edema caused by the passage of the cannula
- the migration of reinjected tissue.

The integration of the fat graft depends on the volume grafted in comparison with the receiver site, in practice 100% in the orbital region (small quantities injected between orbicular muscle and periosteum layer) and 20--30% in the lips. Between these two extremes, the

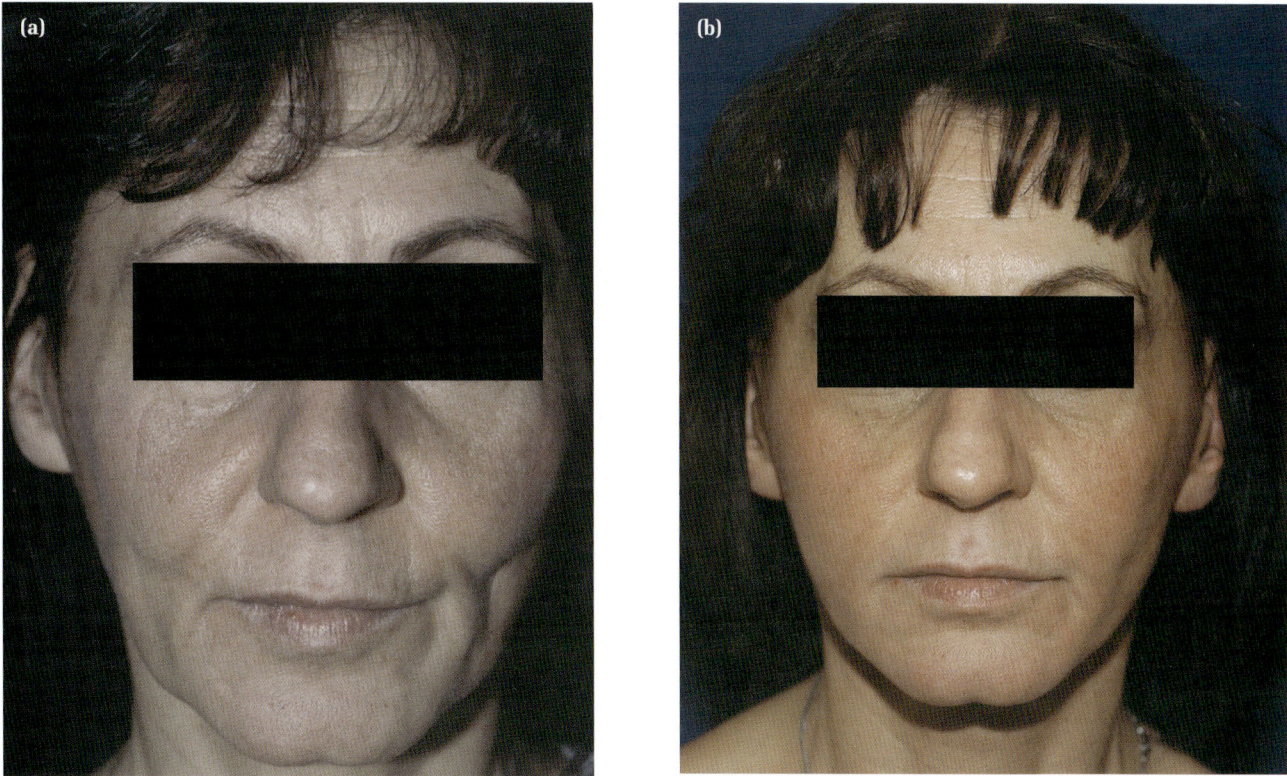

Figure 44.7 (a, b) Facial asymmetry. Association of lifting plus asymmetric lipostructure: 4 ml on the right and 7 ml on the left.

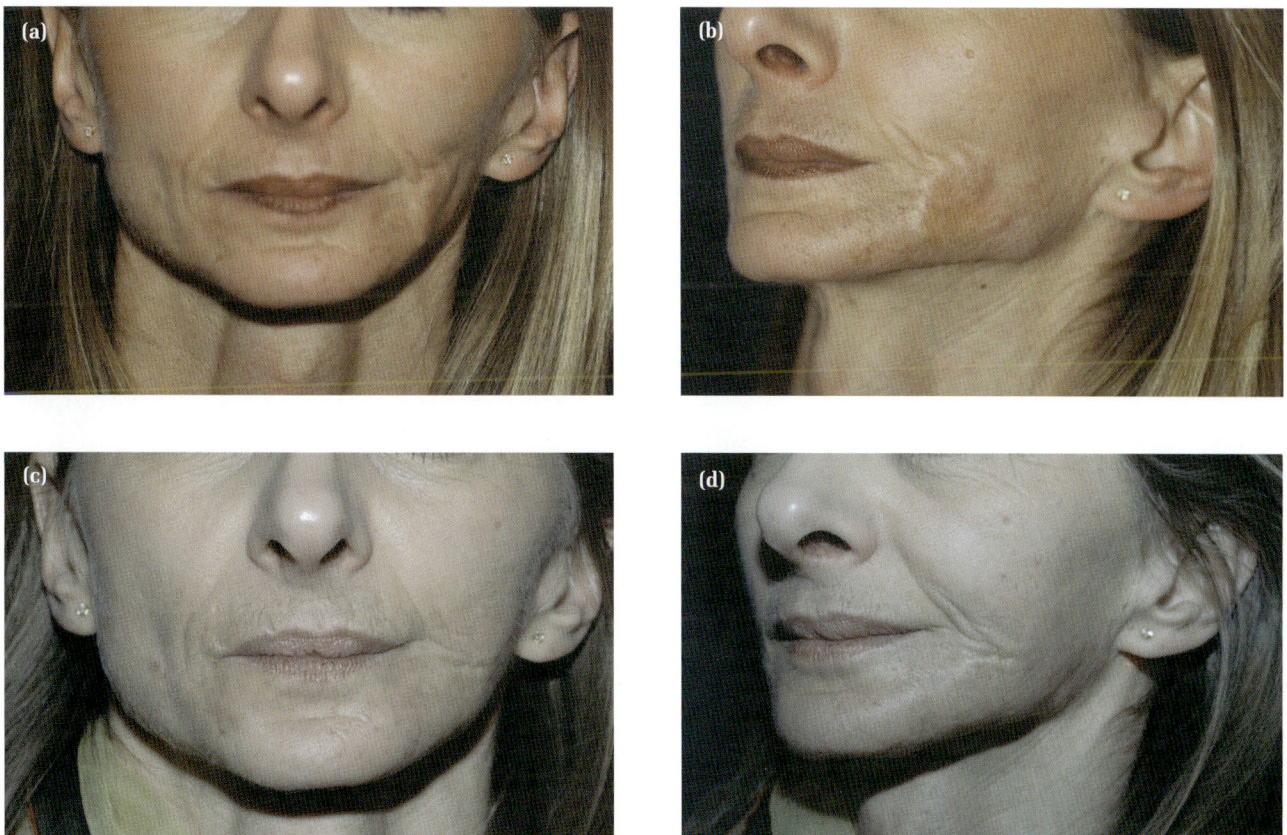

Figure 44.8 (a–d) Scarring after left lateromandibular radiotherapy. Amelioration of skin atrophy using a fat graft.

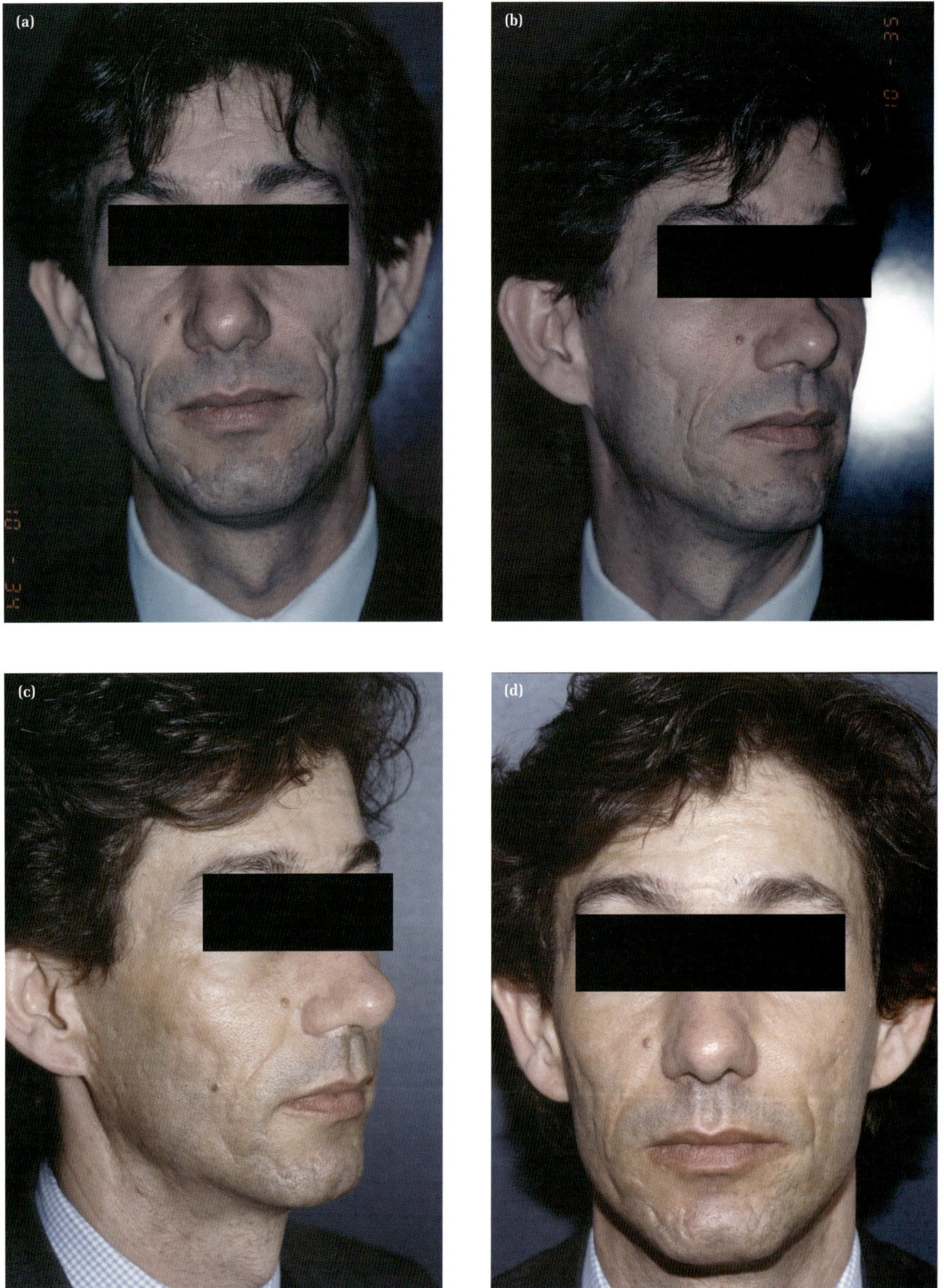

Figure 44.9   (a–d) Significant acne scars. Association of jaw fat graft plus CO_2 ultrapulse laser.

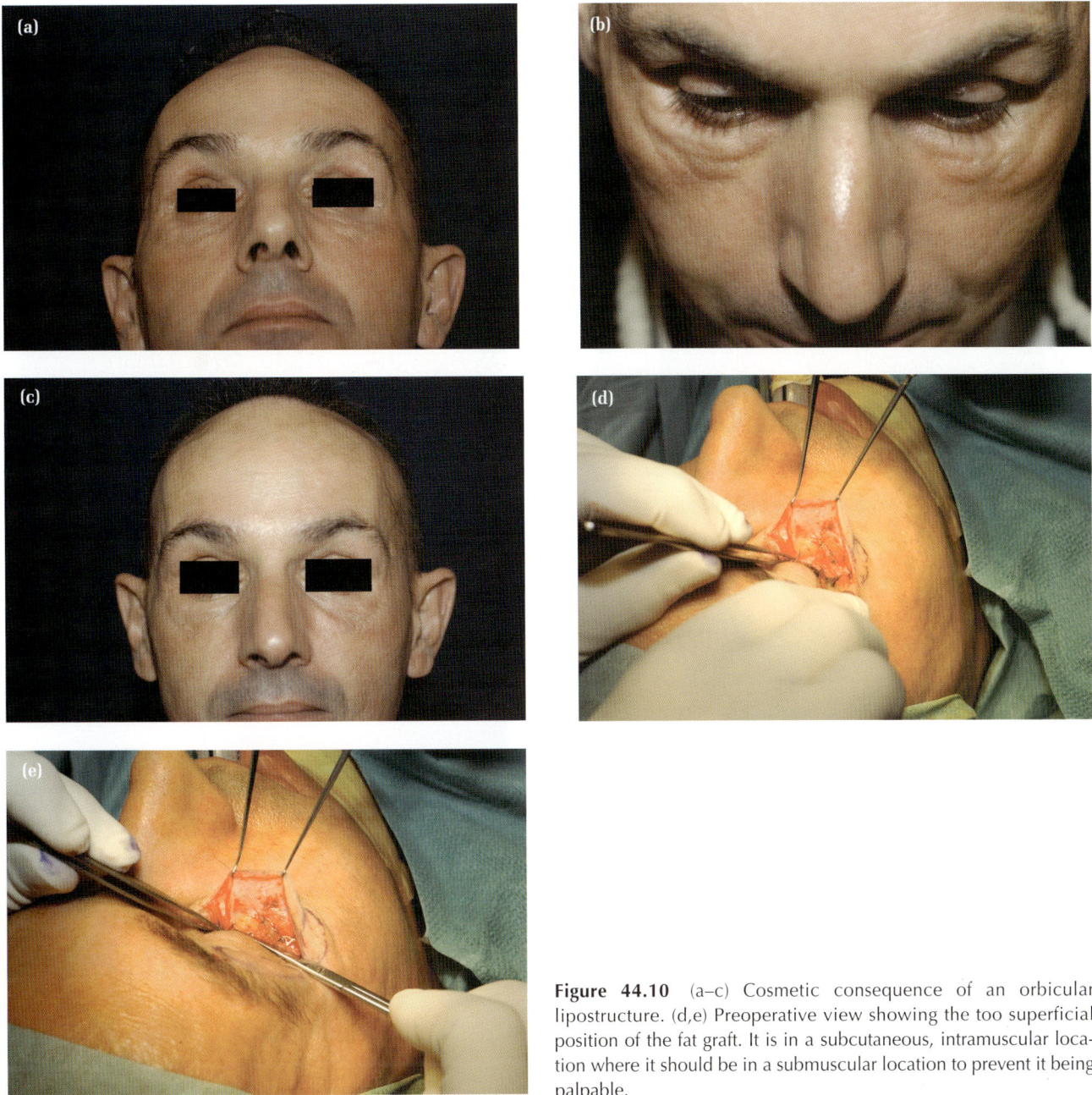

Figure 44.10 (a–c) Cosmetic consequence of an orbicular lipostructure. (d,e) Preoperative view showing the too superficial position of the fat graft. It is in a subcutaneous, intramuscular location where it should be in a submuscular location to prevent it being palpable.

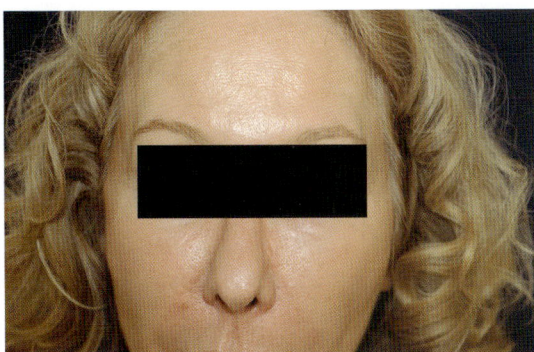

Figure 44.11 Left inferior lid nodule. This patient was operated for excess graft in the submuscular position.

percentage of fat tissue depends on: the purity of the adipocytes and their volume; atraumatic deposition character; the quality of the receiver zone; the possibility of immobilizing the graft. The vascularization of the receiver zone can be changed by local radiotherapy or by tobacco addiction.

Hypertrophy of reinjected fat

In certain cases, it is possible to note an enlargement of the reinjected fat due to weight gain. Fulton et al[42] in 1998 presented four cases in which histological analysis found adipose tissue of normal aspect enclosed by a fibrous capsule.

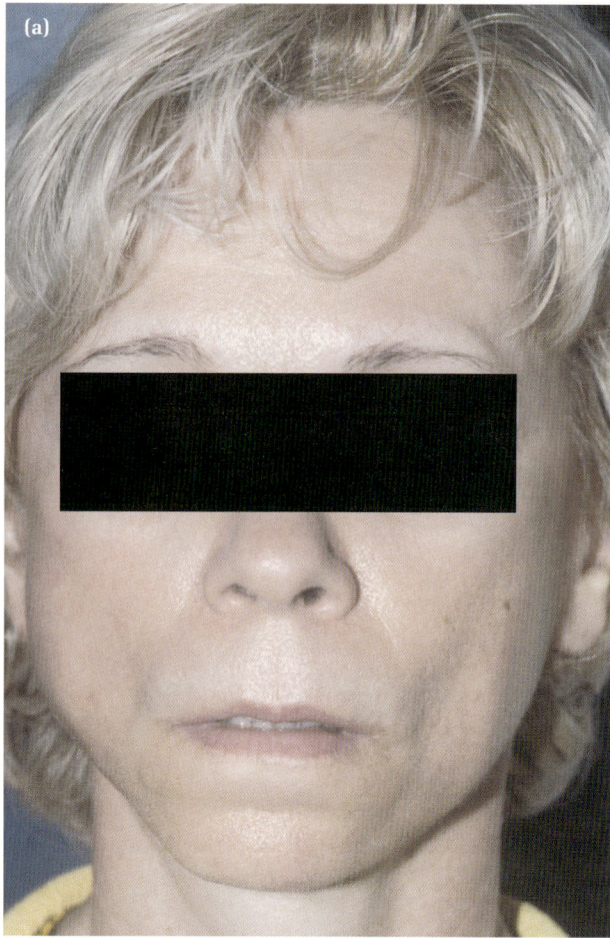

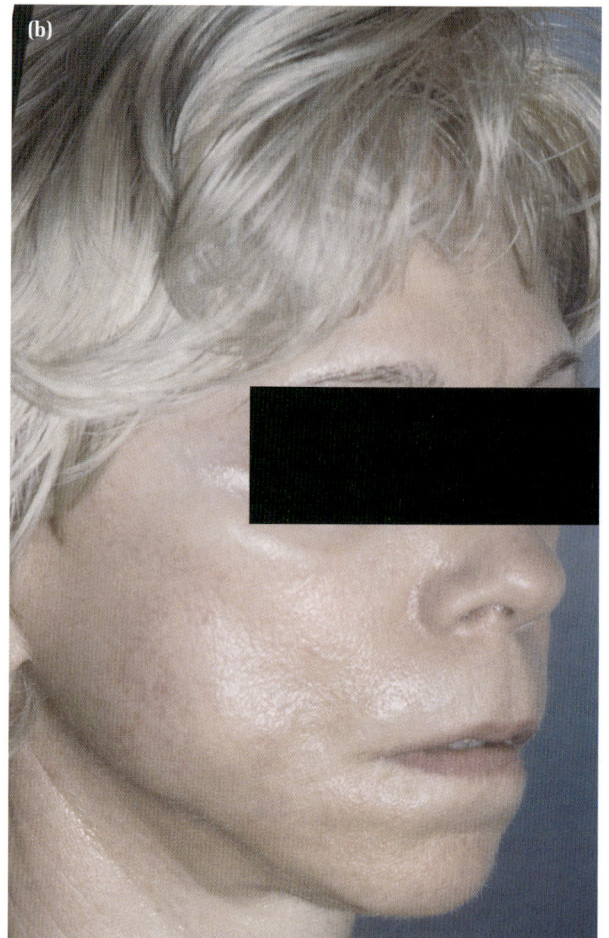

Figure 44.12 Right jaw fat graft, very anterior and very low.

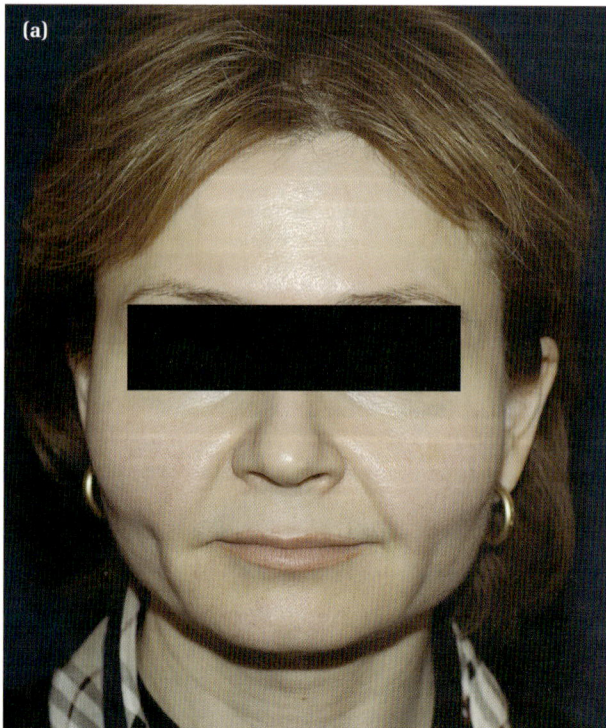

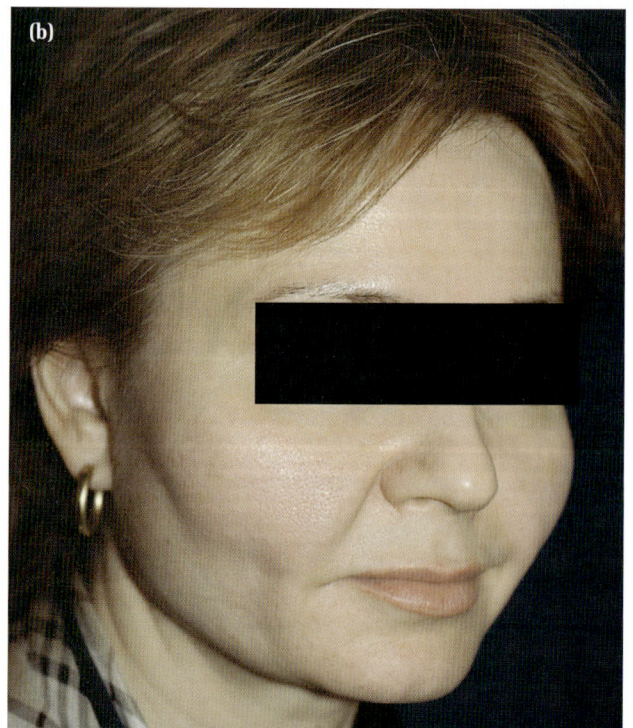

Figure 44.13 *(Continued)*

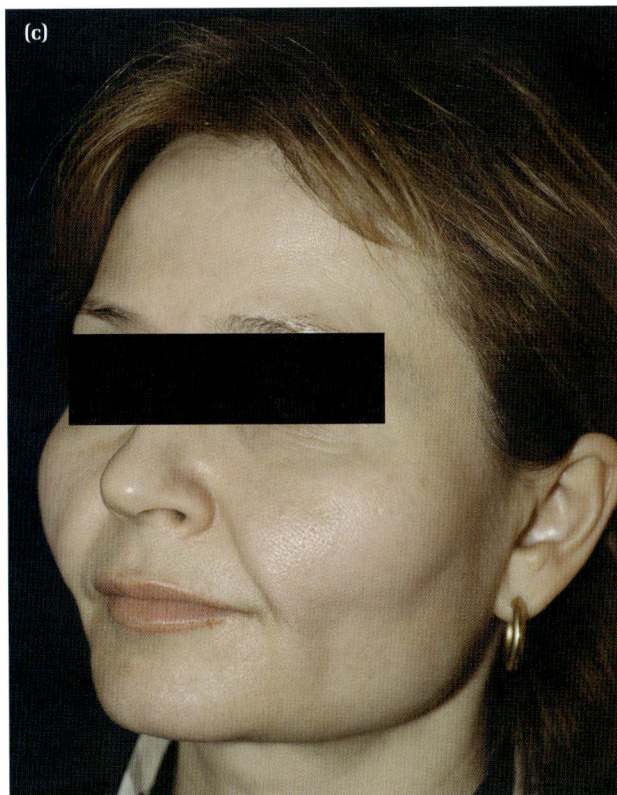

Figure 44.13 (a–c) Poor cosmetic results of a fat graft which is very volumetric and very anterior in a round face.

Future perspectives

Adipocytes and more particularly preadipocytes[50,51] are being increasingly used in tissue engineering. Yuksel et al[52] showed in the rat the creation of de novo adipose tissue after injection of non-adipocytic cell forerunners and adipocytic growth factors (insulin and insulin-like growth factor 1, IGF-1) in the abdominal wall. De Ugarte et al[53] introduced adipose tissue as a source of stem cells. From the mesenchymal stem cells extracted from some adipose tissues, we can develop adipocytes, osteoblasts, chondrocytes, myocytes, and neuron-like cells.[51,54,55] Numerous studies are currently ongoing to investigate the beneficial aspects of preadipocytes and constitute pivotal research and development.

References

1. Little J. Applications of the classic dermal fat graft in primary and secondary facial rejuvenation. Plast Reconstr Surg 2002; 109: 788–804.
2. Pitanguy I, Pamplona D, Weber H et al. Numerical modeling of facial aging. Plast Reconstr Surg 1998; 102: 200–4.
3. Gonzalez-Ulloa M, Flores E. Senility of the face: basic study to understand its causes and effects. Plast Reconstr Surg 1965; 36: 239–46.
4. Pessa J, Zadoo V, Mutimer K et al. Relative maxillary retrusion as a natural consequence of aging: combining skeletal and soft-tissue changes into an integrated model of midfacial aging. Plast Reconstr Surg 1998; 102: 205–12.
5. Pessa J, Chen Y. Curve analysis of the aging orbital aperture. Plast Reconstr Surg 2002; 109: 751–5; discussion 756–60.
6. Coleman S. Facial recontouring with lipostructure. Clin Plast Surg 1997; 24: 347–67.
7. Trepsat F. Volumetric face lifting. Plast Reconstr Surg 2001; 108: 1358–70; discussion 1371–9.
8. Amar R. Adipocyte microinfiltration in the face or tissue restructuration with fat tissue graft. Ann Chir Plast Esthét 1999; 44: 593–608.
9. Neuber GA. Fett transplantation. Verl Dtsch Ges Chir 1893; 22: 66.
10. Lexer E. Freie Fett transplantation. Dtsch Med Wochenschr 1910; 36: 640.
11. Brunning P. Contribution à létude des greffes adipeuses. Bull Mem Acad R Med Belg 1919; 28: 440.
12. Peer LA. Loss of weight and volume in human fat graft, with postulation of a 'cell survival theory'. Plast Reconstr Surg 1950; 5: 217.
13. Eitner E. Fettplastik bei Gesichtsatrophie. Med Klin 1931; 27: 624.
14. Boering G, Huffstadt AJ. The use of derma-fat grafts in the face. Br J Plast Surg 1967; 20: 172–8.
15. Sawhney CP, Banerjee TN, Chakravarti RN. Behaviour of dermal fat transplants. Br J Plast Surg 1969; 22: 169–76.
16. Czerny V. Plasticher Ersatz der Brustdrüse durch ein lipom. Zentralb Chir 1895; 27: 72.
17. Lexer E. Die gesamte Wiederherstellungschirurgie. Leipzig: JB Barth, 1931.
18. Billings E Jr, May JW Jr. Historical review and present status of free fat graft autotransplantation in plastic and reconstructive surgery. Plast Reconstr Surg 1989; 83: 368–81.
19. Bames HO. Augmentation mammaplasty by lipotransplant. Plast Reconstr Surg 1953; 11: 404.
20. Scrocher F. Fettgewebsverpflanzung bei zu kleiner Brust. Munchen Med Wochenschr 1957; 99: 489.
21. Laubier H. Über Enukleation mit Fettimplantation. Ztschr Augenh 1910; 23: 426.
22. Lambert L. Un cas de greffe graisseuse extra-pleurale. Bull Mem Soc Chir Paris 1913; 39: 1196.
23. Koll IS. Transplantation of fat in prostatic and kidney surgery. J Am Med Assoc 1917; 68: 536.
24. Green JR. Repairing bone defects in cranium and tibia. South Med J 1947; 40: 289.
25. Grandin P, Deroubaix P. Traitement d'un volumineux kyste paradentaire du maxillaire inférieur par greffe de graisse. Rev d'Odonto Stom 1954; 1: 1087.
26. Egyedi P. Utilization of the buccal fat pad for closure of oro-antral and/or oro-nasal communications. J Maxillofac Surg 1977; 5: 241–4.
27. Illouz YG. Adipoaspiration and 'filling' in the face. Facial Plast Surg 1992; 8: 59–71.
28. Fournier P. Microlipoextraction et microlipoinjection. Rev Chir Esthet Lang Fr 1985; 10: 40.
29. Fournier P. Facial recontouring with fat grafting. Dermatol Clin 1990; 8: 523–37.
30. Bircoll M, Novack BH. Autologous fat transplantation employing liposuction techniques. Ann Plast Surg 1987; 18: 327–9.
31. Bircoll M. Autologous fat transplantation to the breast. Plast Reconstr Surg 1988; 82: 361–2.
32. Ellenbogen R. Free autogenous pearl fat grafts in the face—a preliminary report of a rediscovered technique. Ann Plast Surg 1986; 16: 179–94.
33. Coleman SR. Structural fat grafts: the ideal filler? Clin Plast Surg 2001; 28: 111–19.
34. Coleman SR. Hand rejuvenation with structural fat grafting. Plast Reconstr Surg 2002; 110: 1731–44; discussion 1745–7.

35. Coleman SR. Long-term survival of fat transplants: controlled demonstrations. Aesthetic Plast Surg 1995; 19: 421–5.

36. Aboudib JH Jr, De Castro C, Gradel J. Hand rejuvenescence by fat filling. Ann Plast Surg 1992; 28: 559–64.

37. Shafik A. Perianal injection of autologous fat for treatment of sphincteric incontinence. Dis Colon Rectum 1995; 38: 583–7.

38. Guerrerosantos J. Autologous fat grafting for body contouring. Clin Plast Surg 1996; 23: 619–31.

39. Pereira LH, Radwanski HN. Fat grafting of the buttocks and lower limbs. Aesthetic Plast Surg 1996; 20: 409–16.

40. Stampos M, Xepoulias P. Fat transplantation for soft tissue augmentation in the lower limbs. Aesthetic Plast Surg 2001; 25: 256–61.

41. Lewis CM. Correction of deep gluteal depression by autologous fat grafting. Aesthetic Plast Surg 1992; 16: 247–50.

42. Fulton J, Suarez M, Silverton K, Barnes T. Small volume fat transfer. Dermatol Surg 1998; 24: 857–65.

43. Fulton J, Parastouk N. Fat grafting. Dermatol Clin 2001; 19: 523–30, ix.

44. Eremia S, Newman N. Long-term follow-up after autologous fat grafting: analysis of results from 116 patients followed at least 12 months after receiving the last of a minimum of two treatments. Dermatol Surg 2000; 26: 1150–8.

45. Colic M. Lip and perioral enhancement by direct intramuscular fat autografting. Aesthetic Plast Surg 1999; 23: 36–40.

46. Ellenbogen R. Fat transfer: current use in practice. Clin Plast Surg 2000; 27: 545–56.

47. Jauffret JL. Utilisation de la graisse autologue en chirurgie plastique et esthétique: la technique de SR Coleman. Thèse de Doctorat d'État en Médecine, Marseille, 1998.

48. Donofrio L. Structural autologous lipoaugmentation: a panfacial technique. Dermatol Surg 2000; 26: 1129–34.

49. Dreizen NG, Framm L. Sudden unilateral visual loss after autologous fat injection into the glabellar area. Am J Ophthalmol 1989; 107: 85–6.

50. Katz AJ, Llull R, Hedrick MH, Futrell JW. Emerging approaches to the tissue engineering of fat. Clin Plast Surg 1999; 26: 587–603, viii.

51. Patrick CW Jr. Tissue engineering strategies for adipose tissue repair. Anat Rec 2001; 263: 361–6.

52. Yuksel E, Weinfeld AB, Cleek R et al. De novo adipose tissue generation through long-term, local delivery of insulin and insulin-like growth factor-1 by PLGA/PEG microspheres in an in vivo rat model: a novel concept and capability. Plast Reconstr Surg 2000; 105: 1721–9.

53. De Ugarte DA, Ashjian PH, Elbarbary A, Hedrick MH. Future of fat as raw material for tissue regeneration. Ann Plast Surg 2003; 50: 215–19.

54. Van RL, Roncari DA. Complete differentiation in vivo of implanted cultured adipocyte precursors from adult rats. Cell Tissue Res 1982; 225: 557–66.

55. Huss FR, Kratz G. Adipose tissue processed for lipoinjection shows increased cellular survival in vitro when tissue engineering principles are applied. Scand J Plast Reconstr Surg Hand Surg 2002; 36: 166–71.

45 Chin lipofilling

Ahmad Halabi

History

Free fat autografts were used as early as 1893 to fill a soft tissue defect. Abdominal fat autografting to correct deficits in the chin was reported in 1909. Chin augmentation using bony osteotomy techniques started only in the mid-1940s.

Introduction

The chin is one of three parts that establish facial symmetry and balance; these three parts, from top to bottom looking at a profile, are the forehead, the nose, and the chin; additionally, the malar area has a role in the balance but not in the symmetry of the face.

The chin has a prominent role in esthetics and facial balance, and in some contexts it can define the character of the face and perhaps sometimes that of the person; for example, power and strength have been associated with a long chin.

Any change in one of these three parts of the face leads to a radical change in the profile; in some cases even a simple chin augmentation can correct the asymmetry of a mildly protruding nose where a rhinoplasty has been planned as the only solution. A successful but mischosen rhinoplasty will never bring profile symmetry and satisfaction to the patient when their physician thinks that the nose alone is the origin of their profile asymmetry as well as facial balance.

Frequently, facial disharmonies may be corrected using relatively simple operative procedures, with no increase of operation time, postoperative morbidity, or financial cost compared to rhinoplasty, and the patient will readily accept this.[1]

With the aging process, the soft and hard tissues of the chin become atrophied, and the soft tissues fall, together with the labiomental fold; hence, mentoplasty using autogenous fat is one operation carried out in esthetic surgery as a rejuvenation intervention. This can be used alone or in combination with other procedures of profiloplasty, especially neck liposuction (Figure 45.1), which gives definition to the mandibular angle and participates in augmentation of the chin.

Implantable material or mandible osteotomies to add fullness to the chin area are reserved for moderate to severe microgenia.

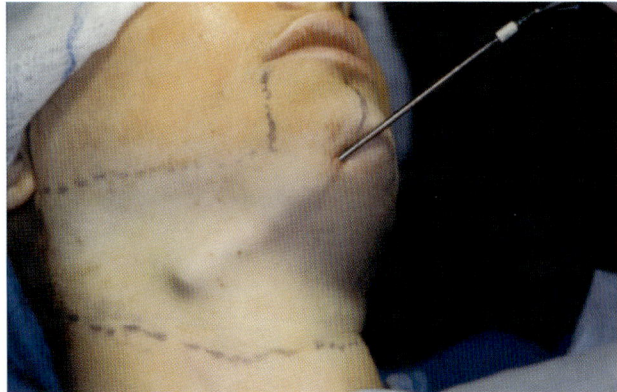

Figure 45.1 Combination of neck liposuction and chin lipofilling.

Esthetic analysis of facial profile

The normal profile comprises not only the symmetry of each of the three profile parts, but also a harmonious relationship between them. Figure 45.2 shows the relationships of the forehead to the nose and the chin, and how the normal frontal bone projects forward.

To evaluate outcomes of esthetic facial plastic surgery objectively, many photogrammetric profile analysis methods can be used (computerized or manual).

Anatomy

The chin is composed of bony skeleton and soft tissue.

The bony skeleton is formed by three structures: the symphysis menti, which is the junction of the two halves of the mandible, the mental protuberance, which is an elevation over this junction, and the mental tubercles, which lie at the inferior margin. The latter two structures form the projection of the chin.

The soft tissue comprises the skin, subcutaneous tissues, and mentalis muscle (the margin of the chin is the region below the labiomental angle). These layers have variable thickness depending on the mentalis muscle, which is usually small, originates from the mandible below the incisors, and continues in the chin pad until its insertion into the skin of the chin. The mentalis muscle can be hypertrophied, but this does not enhance the projection of the chin. The seventh cranial

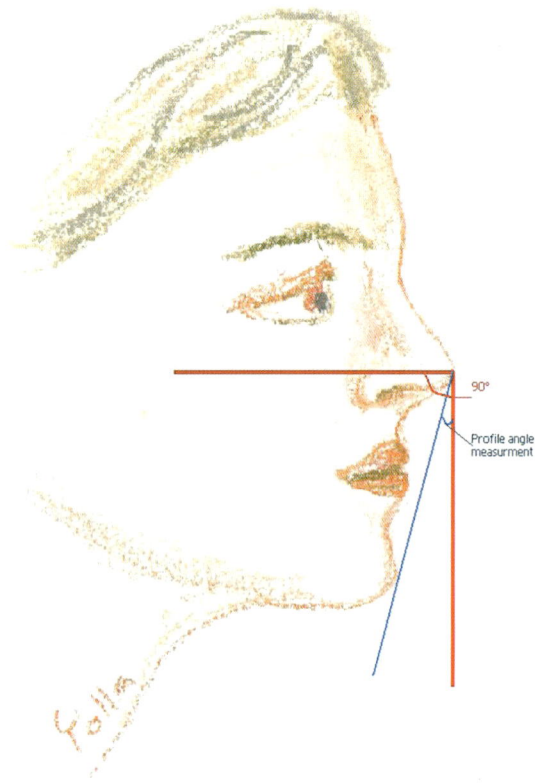

Figure 45.2 Measurement of the profile angle.

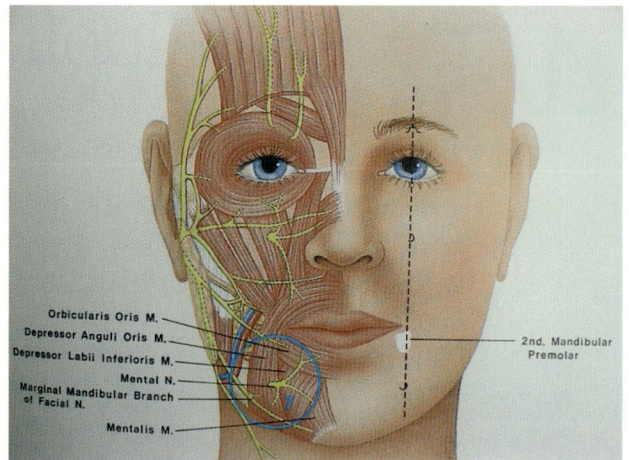

Figure 45.3 Facial danger zone: mentalis nerve region (reproduced with permission from reference 3).

nerve innervates this muscle. Muscle fusion occurs at the midline, where a median fibrous raphe separates it.

Chin relation to the lip

A strong muscular relationship exists between the lip and the chin: the depressor muscles are inserted on the mental tubercles and interdigitate with the orbicularis oris muscle. Any changes in the chin can affect this relationship, and as a consequence can affect the lip.

Physiology

With aging, there is a diminution in skin elasticity, thickness, melanocyte numbers, Langerhans cell numbers, elastic fibers, and collagen, as well as connections between the epidermis and dermis, which causes increased susceptibility to shear forces.[4] At the level of the bony structure of the chin there is a reduction in volume, and the protrusion diminishes.

Danger zones

Two nerves can be injured during chin lipofilling procedures:

- mental nerve: a sensory nerve, the third division of the trigeminal nerve (fifth cranial nerve)
- marginal mandibular branch of the facial nerve.

The mentalis nerve region which must be respected is 1.5 cm around the mental foramen, situated below the second premolar on the mandible, along a vertical line connecting the supraorbital foramen, mid-pupil, and infraorbital foramen (Figure 45.3).[3]

Mental nerve injury can happen during chin lipofilling when the danger zone is not respected. If dissection of the nerve occurs at its foraminal origin by the cannula contacting the bone during the fat injection procedure, this can cause permanent numbness and hypoesthesia of half of the chin and of the outer and inner surfaces of the lip. If the nerve is subjected to only traumatic traction, a transitory hypoesthesia may occur.

Marginal mandibular nerve injury is very rare, but can happen if the lipofilling area being treated extends too laterally and posteriorly to the depressor anguli oris muscle in the mid-mandibular area, to a level 2 cm posterior to the oral commissure.[3] Injury to this nerve leads to paralysis of the depressor anguli oris muscle, and as a result the lip of the affected side rides up over the lower teeth.

Indications for chin lipofilling

Indications include:

- mild to moderate microgenia
- chin drop
- profiloplasty: when rhinoplasty with lump resection changes the harmonious profile of the face
- rejuvenation of the face: chin augmentation is one of the procedures done in combination with other soft tissue augmentation of the face
- in other cases when other augmentation techniques are recommended but contraindicated
- if the patient asks for a 'soft' intervention.

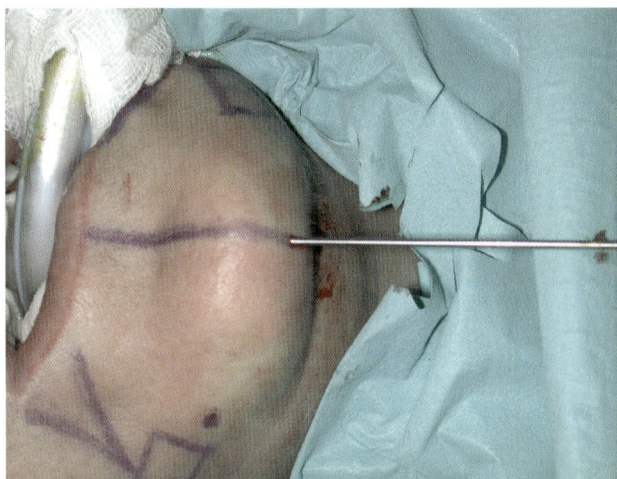

Figure 45.4 Division of the chin into two parts by midline mark and midline injection of fat graft.

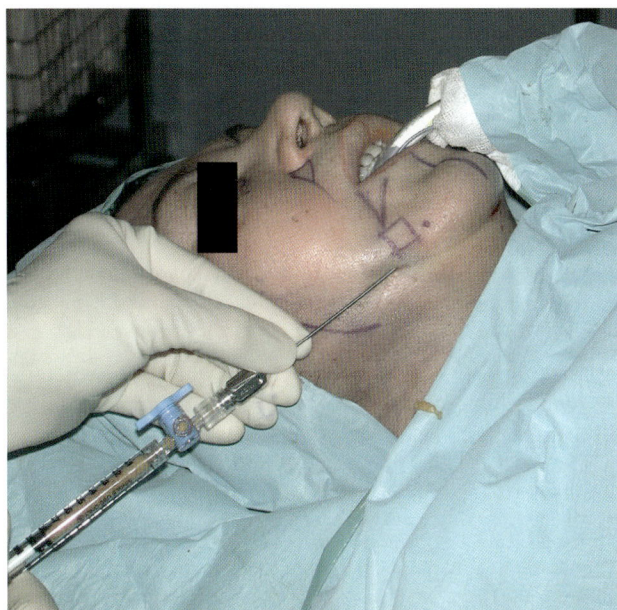

Figure 45.5 Beginning injection in lateral chin sites.

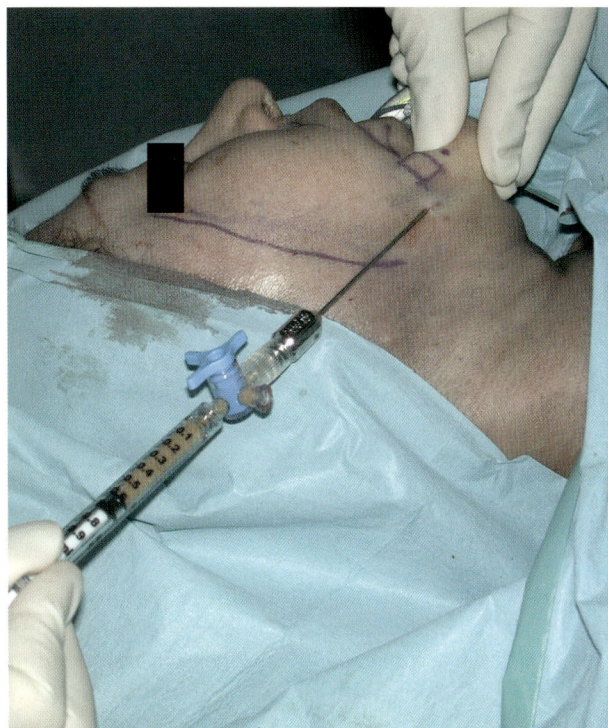

Figure 45.6 Intramuscular injection, holding soft tissues of the chin between index finger and thumb.

- gentle fat manipulation: any trauma to fat cells during their aspiration, transport, or injection can significantly affect the survival of these cells, with the consequence of resorption of such non-viable cells, which gave initially good results, shortly after their transfer
- blood must be removed completely from the graft, otherwise it facilitates rapid resorption of the fat cells.

Technique

The usual region for fat harvesting is the trochanteric area, i.e. inner thigh, for women and the abdominal region for men. Other regions such as the periumbilical area, medial knee, and buttock can be used as well.

Local anesthesia is usually employed, unless the patient prefers general anesthesia or in the case of associated neck liposuction; the donor region is infiltrated with a standard solution of 200 mg of lidocaine, 1 mg of epinephrine, and 5 mEq of sodium bicarbonate dissolved in 1 l of (epinephrine has no negative effect on the fat graft as thought in the past).

We divide the chin into two parts, left and right, using a midline mark (middle of the lower lip and not the teeth, which can deviate in some individuals) (Figure 45.4).

Three microincisions are made, two laterally and one in the medial line. Injection is started first in one of the lateral sites (Figures 45.5–45.7) then in the other,

Contraindications against lipofilling

Contraindications include:

- severe microgenia
- labial incompetence (except for lump correction or very mild lipofilling where there is no effect on the labiomental muscular system)
- chin region skin infection
- severe autoimmune disease.

Principles

In lipofilling of the chin, as well as other areas in general, very important rules must be respected to achieve long-term results:

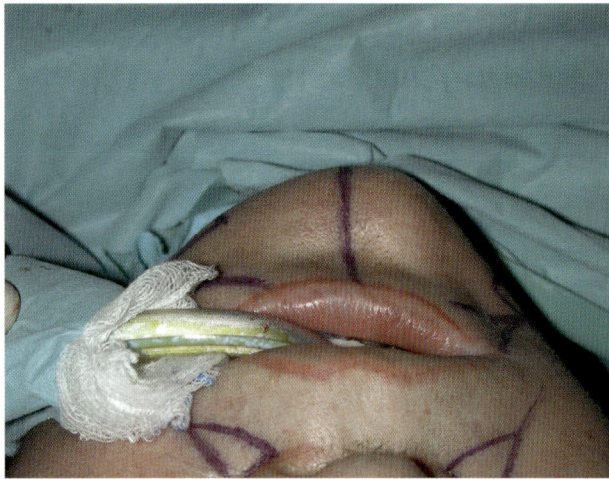

Figure 45.7 Comparison after completing one side of chin filling.

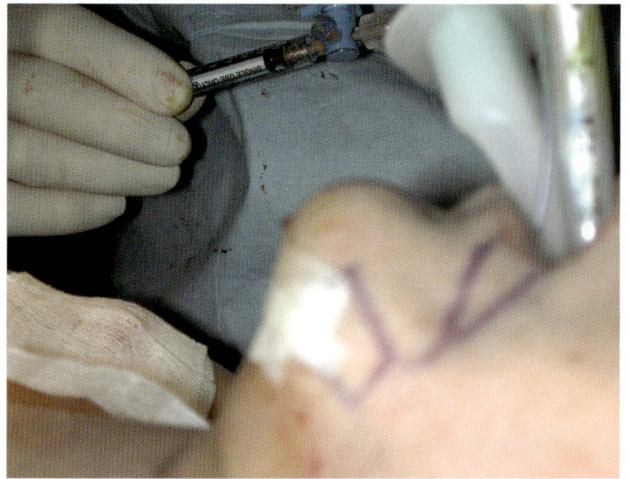

Figure 45.8 Fat graft fixation immediately post-operation.

and we finish by injecting the middle region (Figure 45.4). The injections are done in the form of microdeposits in the deep muscular layer where vascularization is better and the possibility of survival of the fat graft is greater.

Finally, fixation of the chin region with Steri-Strip™ for several days is carried out to limit excessive movement of this region (Figure 45.8).

Conclusion

Chin lipofilling is an easy technique compared with other chin augmentation techniques; results are satisfactory if preoperative indications are well studied. In many cases it may be combined with neck liposuction to ameliorate the submental line and give definition to the chin.

Chin lipofilling can also be used to correct a minor defect or asymmetry due to other surgical techniques of genioplasty.

References

1. Simons RL. Adjunctive measures in rhinoplasty. Otolaryngol Clin North Am 1975; 8: 717–42.
2. Luo JC, Gui L, Zhang ZY et al. [Chin augmentation with bone transplantation from the mandible]. Zhonghua Zheng Xing Wai Ke Za Zhi 2004; 20: 104–5. [in Chinese]
3. Seckel BR. Facial Danger Zones; Avoiding Nerve Injury in Facial Plastic Surgery. St Louis: Quality Medical Publishing, 1994: 47.
4. Gampper TJ. Facial fat grafting. www.emedicine.com, 26 May, 2006.
5. Chang EW. Genioplasty. www.emedicine.com, 15 February, 2008.

46 Fat transfer in facial malformations and after trauma

Jean Louis Foyatier and Ali Mojallal

Introduction

The face is perceptible in three dimensions, i.e. as a volume. This volume is translated into areas of light and dark. These different zones of light and dark constitute esthetic subunits of the face (Figure 46.1). In volumetric reconstruction, it is imperative to respect these esthetic subunits. When the volume defect is linked to bony and/or muscular defect with functional deficit, it is necessary to start treatment with the correction of these structures. The restoration of volume by transfer of adipose tissue is then the final step.

The aim of the transfer of adipose tissue in these pathologies is to correct contour outlines, to fill loss of volumetric substances, to restore the harmony of volumes, and to resurface the skin, due to the dynamic qualities of such tissue.

Etiologies of volumetric disturbances

All *traumas*, which can be of variable intensity originating from a wound, due to scar atrophy, loss of substance, fatty atrophy, distortion of the facial skeleton, and so on, can result in facial outline modification.

All *congenital or acquired malformations* of types Romberg, Apert, and otomandibular dysplasia, labiopalatine cleft, Crouzon, dentofacial dysmorphosis, and so on, can result in modifications of the facial outline and can benefit from volumetric restoration using a morphological procedure.

The *consequences of surgery*, including surgical scars and tumor surgeries, and the consequences of radiotherapy, chemotherapy, steroid therapy, and so on, can lead to changes of facial outline. Lipodystrophy can also be encountered after treatment of human immunodeficiency virus (HIV) by antiprotease therapy.

Method of treatment

Previously, we treated these defects of the facial outlines using heavy surgical techniques ranging from skin

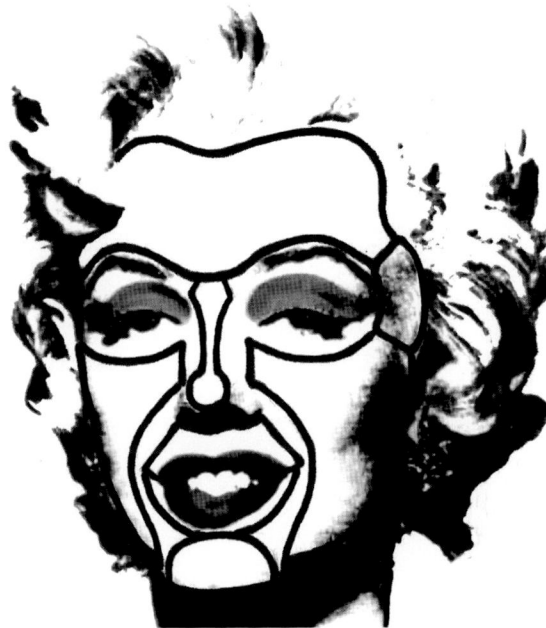

Figure 46.1 Esthetic subunits of the face

or bone grafting to use of pedicle flaps or microsurgical free flaps. Today we consider that treatment of a volume defect, with the exception of any functional deficit, should first proceed by transfer of adipose tissue.

Treatment of combined lesions

It is important to note that in these outcomes of trauma or malformation of the face there is not just a volume defect. According to the pathology and determined lesions, we recommend accomplishing above all the functional treatment and all necessary interventions of plastic surgery to correct functional problems, form, or texture, and only as a last measure should lack of volume be treated by the transfer of fat tissue.

For example, in scarring due to facial burns (Figure 46.2), treatment starts with the repair of scarred zones by changing the skin of every esthetic subunit of the

389

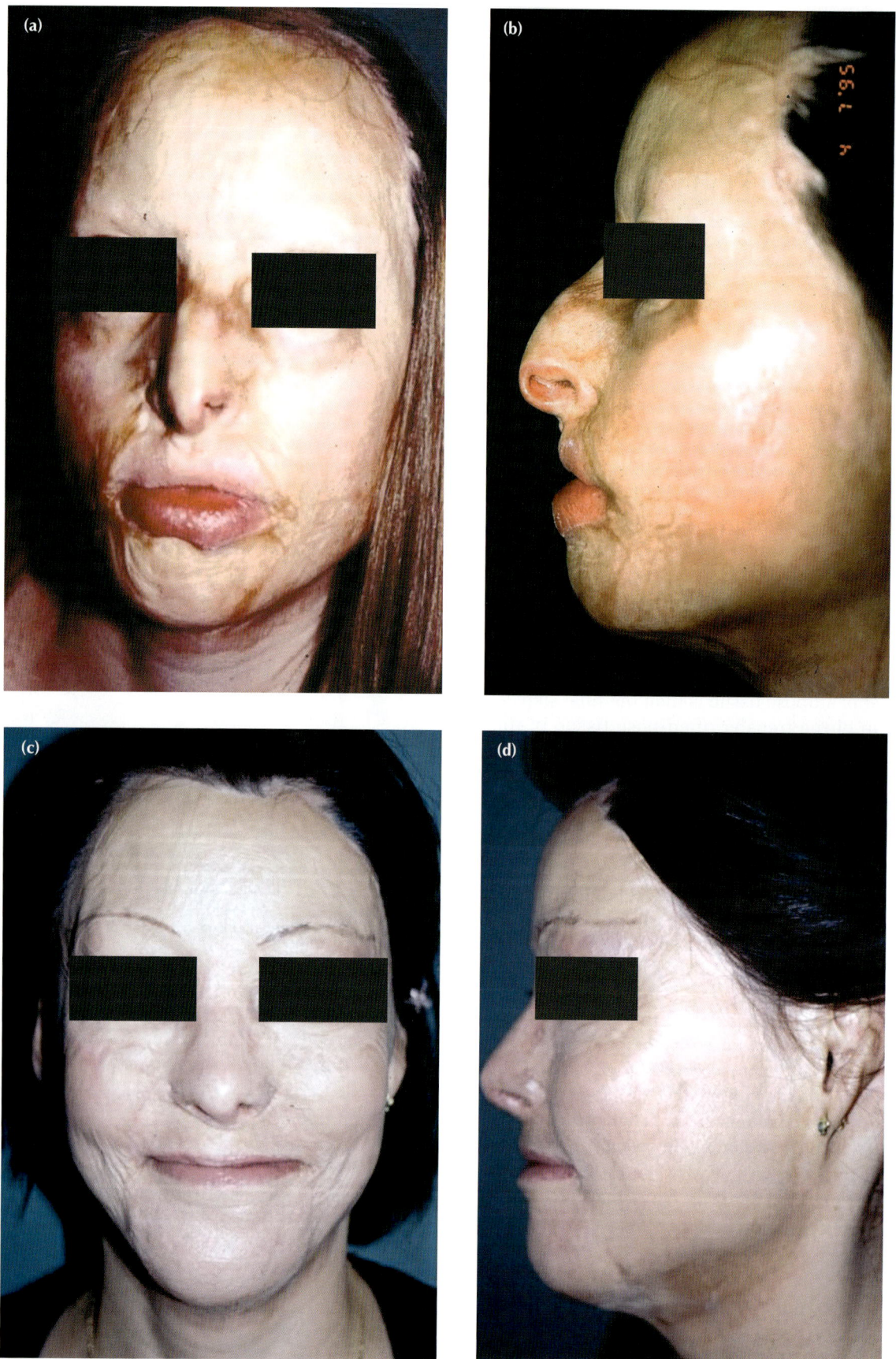

Figure 46.2   (a, b) Late facial burns sequelae. Treatment started by replacing the skin of each aesthetic subunit of the face using a supra-clavicular expanded full thickness skin graft. 18 months after the skin replacement, the volume restoration was performed, notably at the level of the chin, the lateral cheek and the malar area, with a structural fat grafting of 9 ml into the chin pad, 8 ml at the level of each lateral cheek, and 7 ml at the level of the deep malar fat on both sides. (c, d) The results 2 years after the end of treatment.

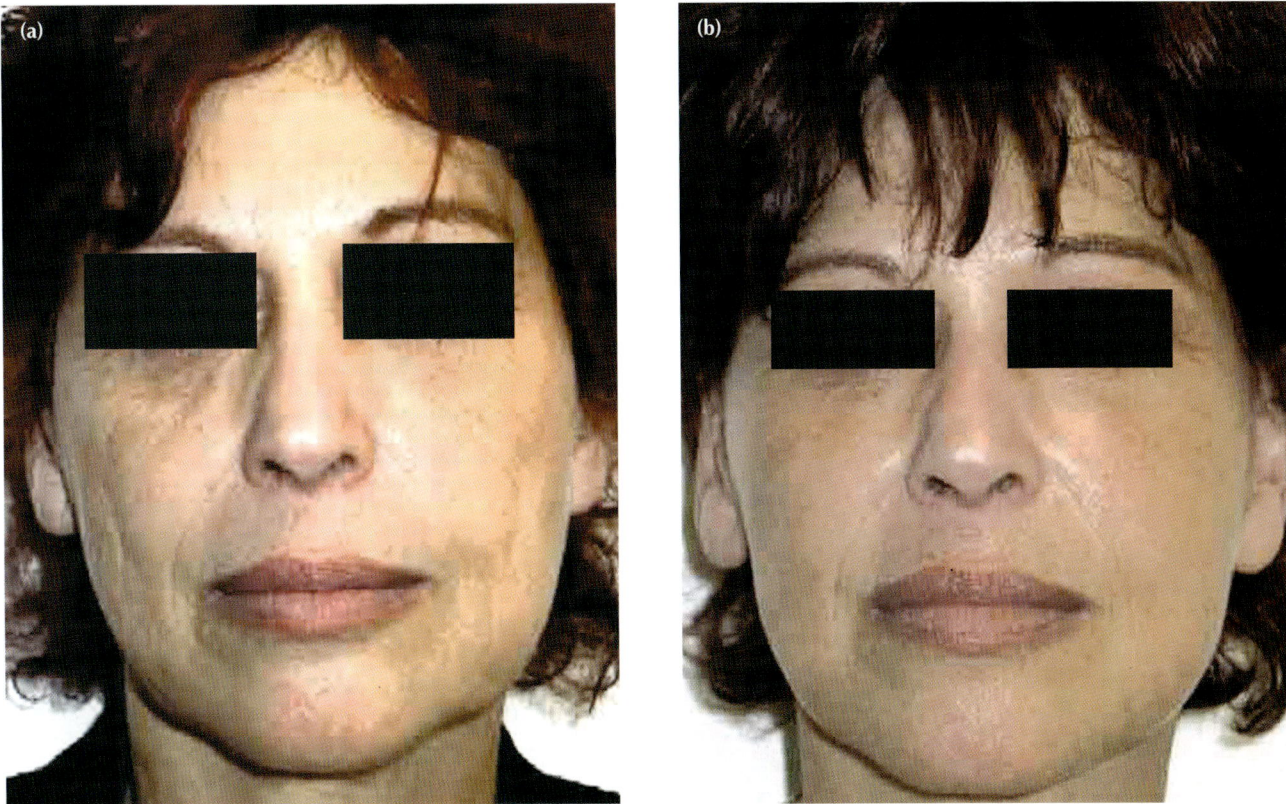

Figure 46.3 Facial trauma sequelae with an inappropriate fixed position of a right zygomatic bone fracture. The patient asked also for a facial rejuvenation procedure. Treatment was done by a cervicofacial facelift combined with a full face fat grafting in the same procedure with injection of 10 ml at the level of the right lateral cheek, 15 ml into the right malar area, 9 ml into the left lateral cheek and 8 ml into the left malar area. (a) Preoperative view; (b): result after 1 year. We can see easily the volume increasing effect of fat and also the skin quality enhancement.

face. Every subunit of burnt skin is replaced with a supraclavicular full thickness skin graft after skin expansion. Having acquired a change of texture of the affected zones, one or several session of transfer of adipose tissue will complete the results and bring volume to the affected zone (Figure 46.3).

Technique

According to the submit to be corrected, one or two incisions are made with a no. 11 scalpel, allowing access to the different zones. The cannula is introduced until it reaches the limit of the incision and injection is made by withdrawing the cannula. For a more superficial fat injection, an 18 gauge needle can be used. It is important to accomplish a multitude of tunnels which criss-cross, to deposit adipose tissue in the form of a three-dimensional network. All grafting procedures start into the deep layer first and after all layers are grafted. For the eyelid region, especially the tear trough and the sulcus marginalis, it is necessary to stay absolutely at a depth in contact with the bone, because any superficial injection at this level is a source of changeability. In the glabellar region, injection must be carefully done, ensuring that it is not intravascular; some cases of blindness by fatty embolism have been reported in the literature.

Tissue fibrosis and multiple sessions

In pathologies of facial dysmorphosis, there are often tissue dystrophies with poor vascularization and some deep adherences, especially after radiotherapy. There is then an augmented resistance to the injection of adipose tissue.

To avoid ischemia of transplanted adipose tissue, it is recomended in these cases not to overcorrect, or even to accomplish the transfer of adipose tissue in several sessions.

The first session often prepares the receiver bed for subsequent sessions. The provision of growth factors and stem cells augments vascularization and ameliorates local atrophy, so subsequent sessions give better results. The injected fat will improve the skin suppleness and texture over time.

Results according to esthetic subunits

In a retrospective study that we carried out in 100 patients for the comparison of results acquired according to esthetic subunits, a significant difference between the lateral cheek and deep malar fat region and the lips was found. Results acquired according to esthetic subunits were:

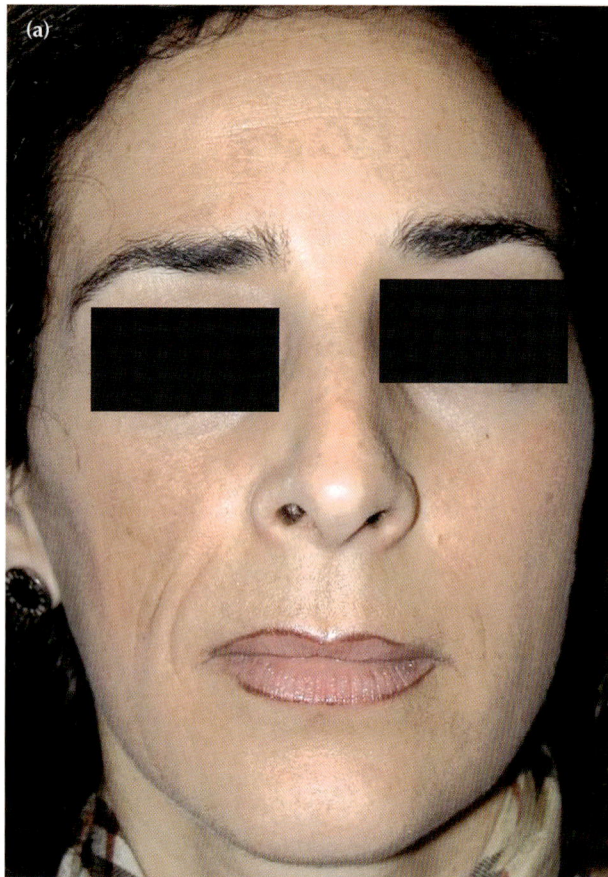

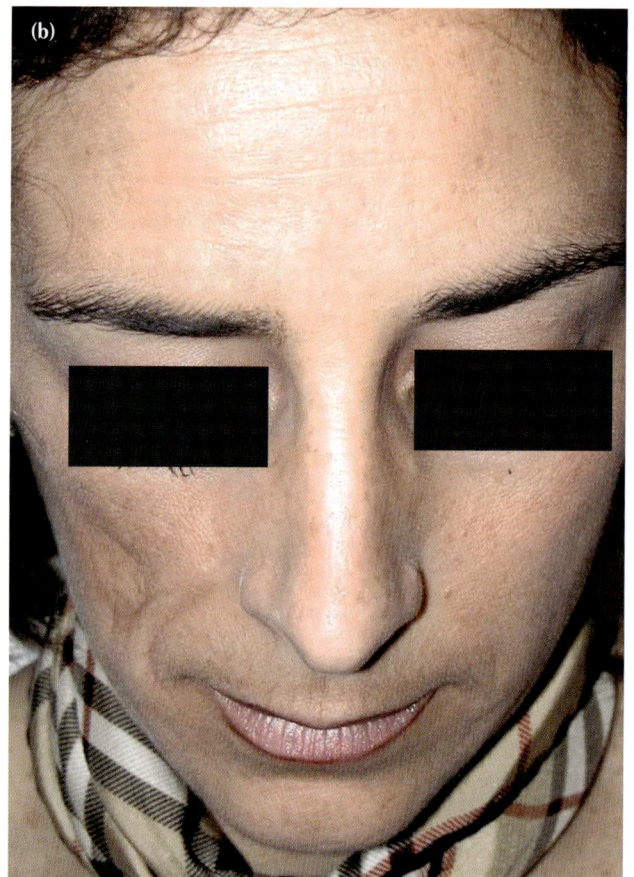

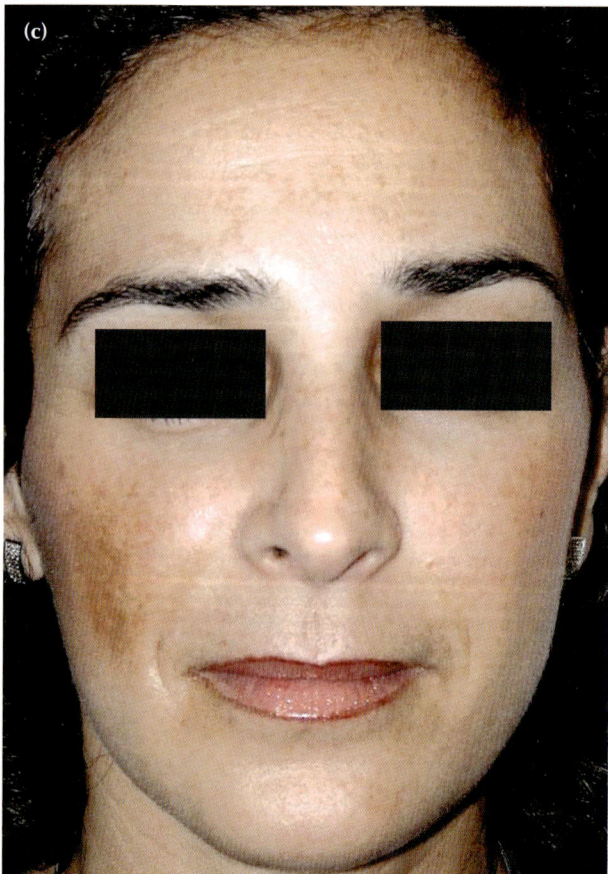

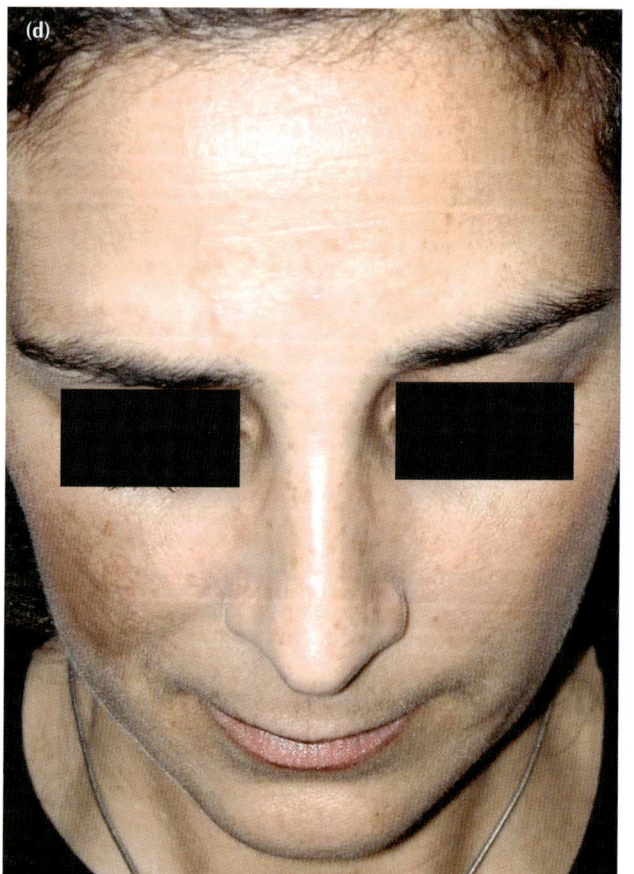

Figure 46.4   Sequelae of an angioma of the right cheek treated by radiotherapy 15 years previously. (a, b) Preoperative aspect; (c, d) 12 months after a fat grafting procedure with injection of 14 ml of fat at the level of the right lateral cheek.

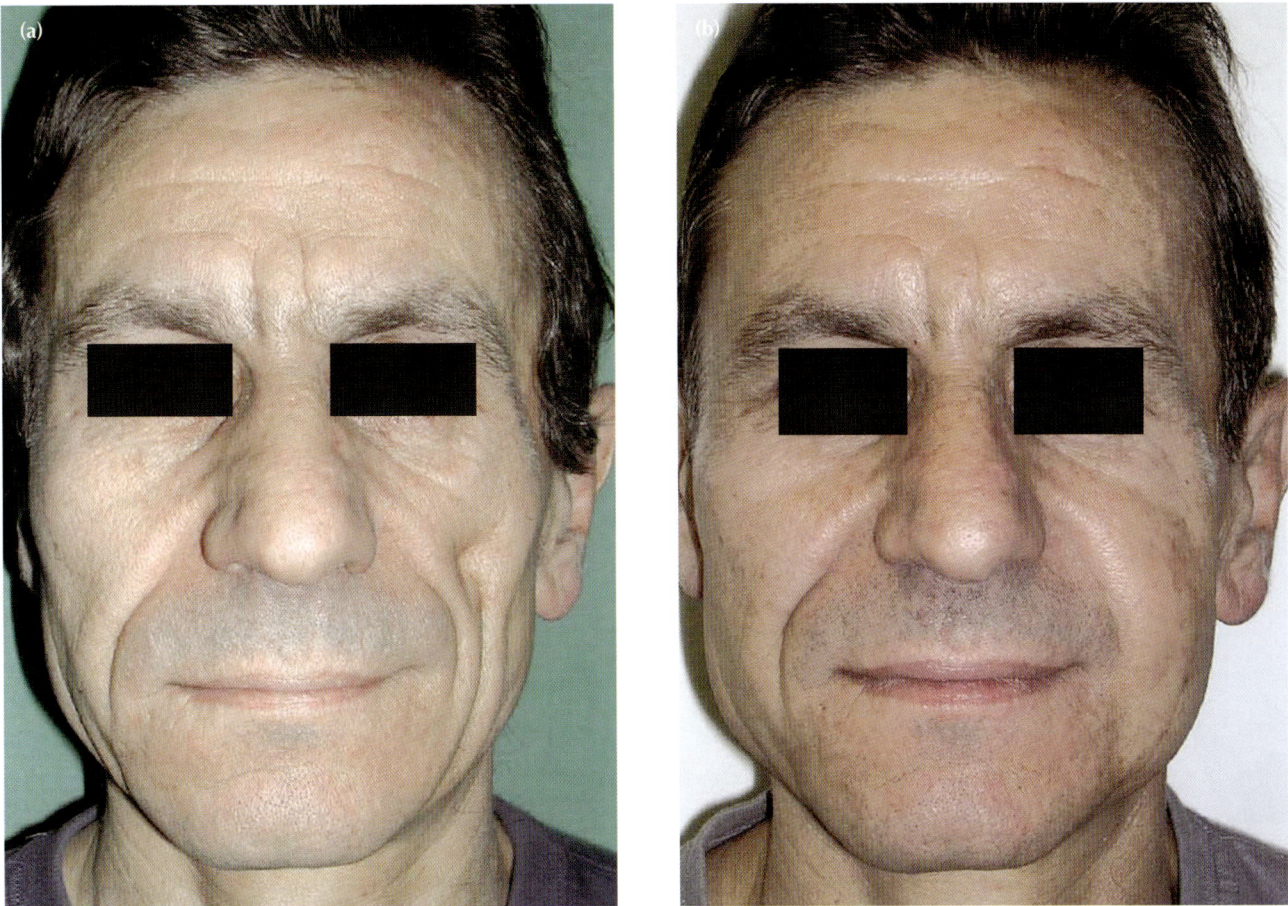

Figure 46.5   Trauma of the left cheek with a local lipoatrophic area. (a) Preoperative photograph; (b) result 2 years after structural fat grafting of 20 ml of fat into this area.

- malar region, 89% good results
- lateral cheek, 84%
- chin, 75%
- labiomandibular fold, 73%
- naso-labial groove, 63%
- forehead, 60%
- eyebrows, 55%
- nose and glabella, 50%
- temple, 36%
- lower lip, 34%
- upper lip, 31%

These variations in result may be explained by the particular anatomy of each zone. Rohrich and Pessa have described the results for fatty compartments in the face. We can agree that the best clinical results in our series have been obtained in the zones where there is a deep fat compartment.

Improvement of skin quality after fat transfer

In the course of time and the increasing numbers of patients treated by this technology, we have noted that the skin over an area injected by adipose tissue shows an improvement of its intrinsic qualities (texture, suppleness). Adipose tissue is considered to be not only a simple product of passive filling, but also an active element which, over a period of time according to the intervention, brings about qualitative improvements in neighboring tissues. These phenomena are linked to the presence of 'stem cells', which can generate other related cells, and also the presence of vasoactive elements, the origin of augmented neovascularization as determined after the treatment of radiotherapy lesions.

Some postoperative clinical cases and photographs are introduced (Figures 46.2–46.8).

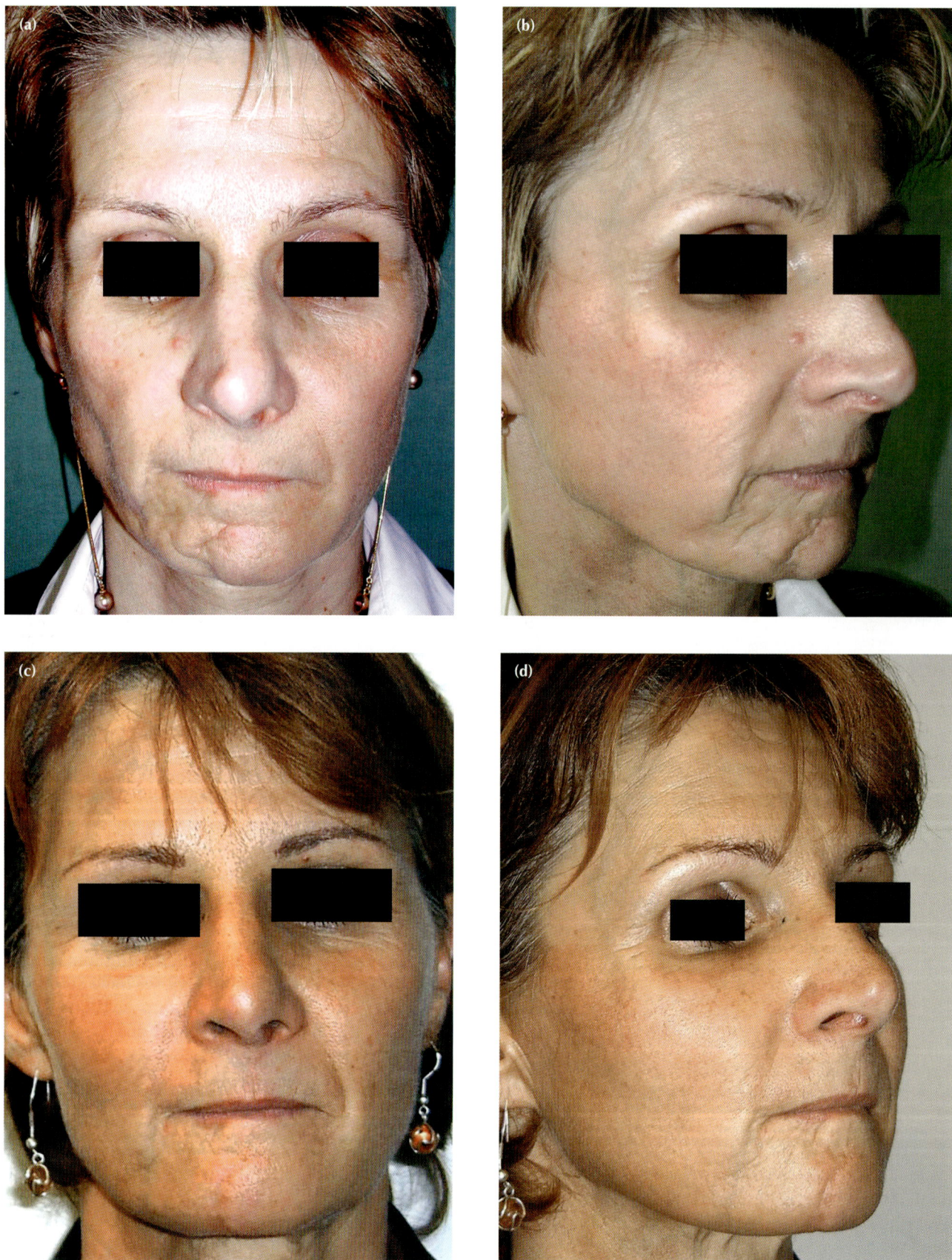

Figure 46.6   Right-sided Romberg's syndrome (a, b). Correction was done with three sessions of structural fat grafting with respectively 5, 6 and 4 ml injected at the level of the right deep malar area; 7, 5 and 5 ml into the right lateral cheek; 4, 3 and 3 ml at the right mandibular border; and 5, 4 and 4 ml into the lateral chin and jowl areas. For the first procedure, the adipose tissue was harvested from the abdominal region. The second and third procedures were carried out 8 and 14 months later, and the adipose tissue was harvested from the trochanteric region. (c) Postoperative frontal view and (d) postoperative oblique view 2 years after the last procedure. Note the improvement of the skin around the chin and in the entire lateral cheek area: the preoperative contour defect and wrinkles around the jowl have disappeared.

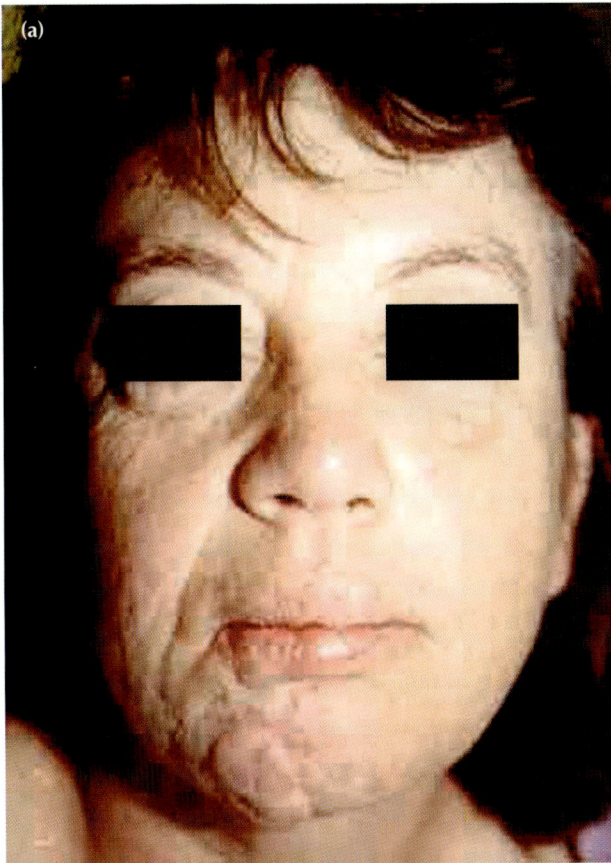

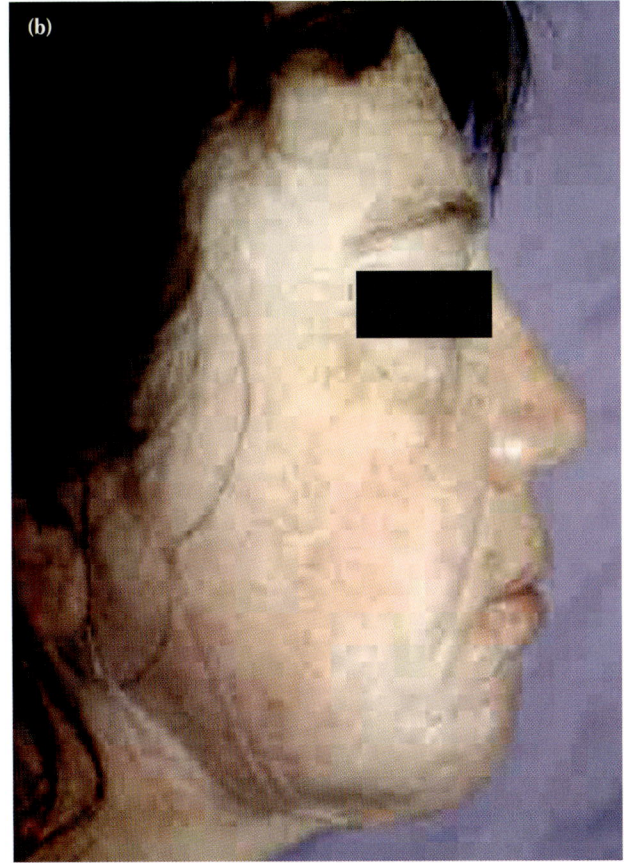

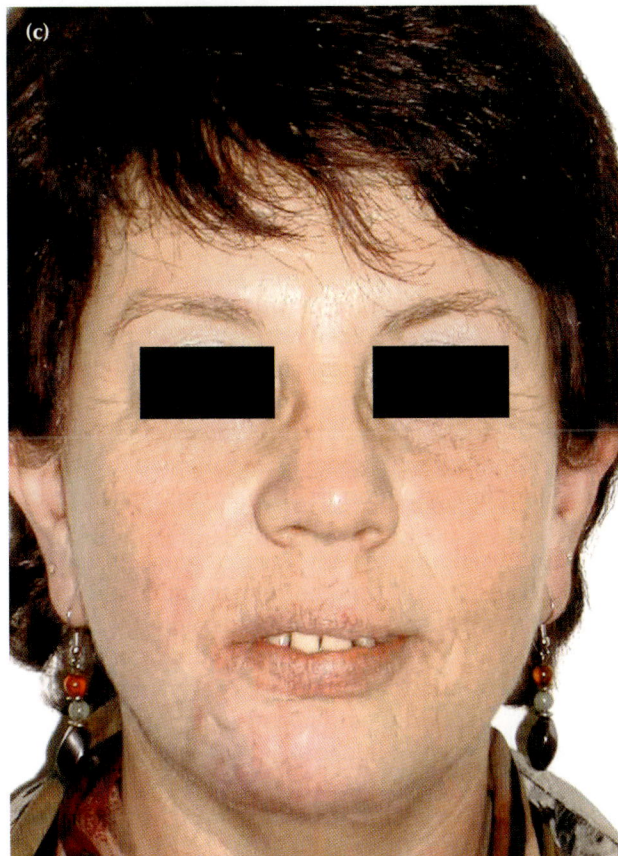

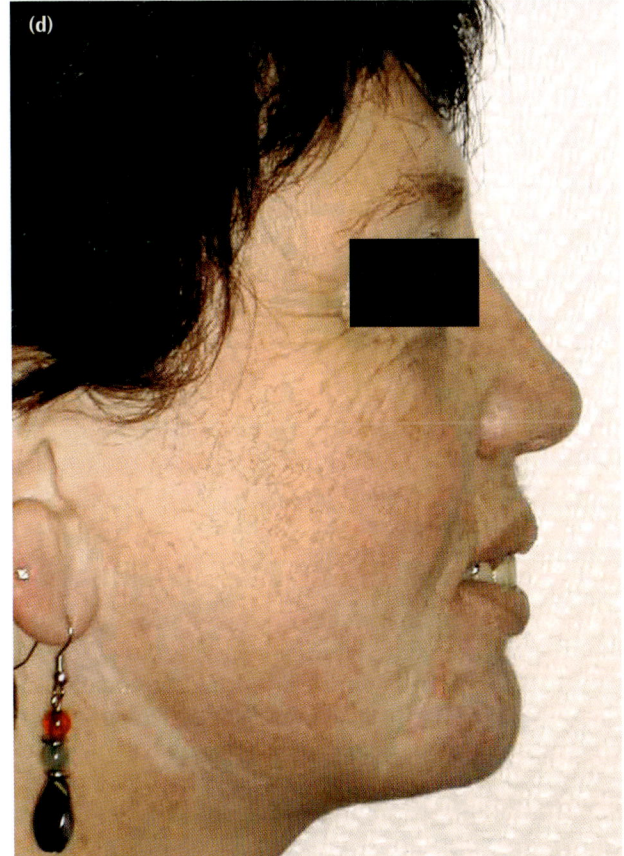

Figure 46.7   (a, b) Facial trauma sequelae, with multiple scars of the chin, neck and the right lateral cheek. (c, d) Results 1 year after a cervicofacial facelift and structural fat grafting into the chin (8 ml, lateral cheek (9 ml on each side), and malar area (8 ml on each side).

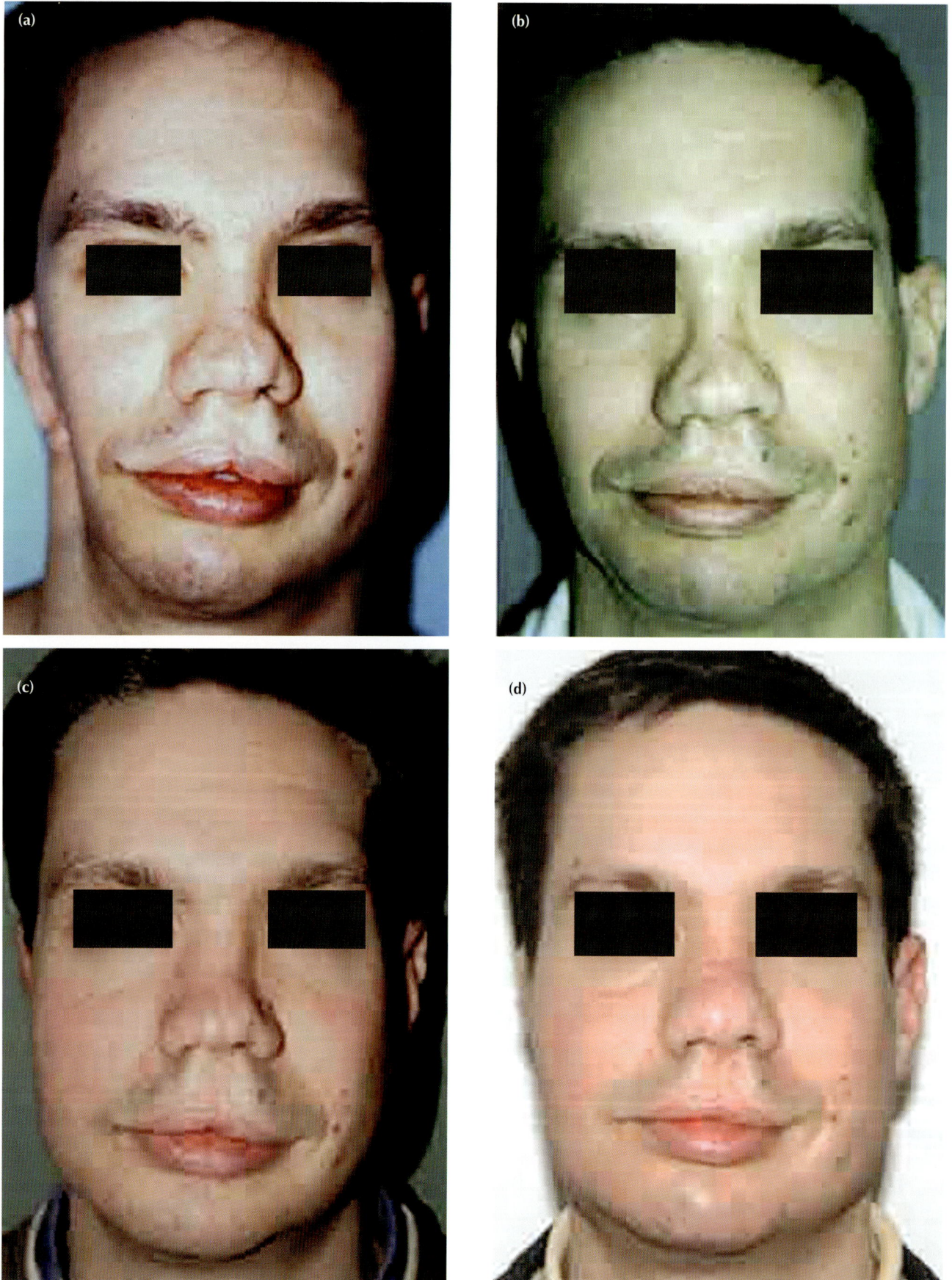

Figure 46.8 (a) A 25-year-old patient has a right hemifacial microsomia: preoperative aspect. (b) Results 1 year after a fat tissue grafting procedure with 43 ml into the entire right hemiface; (c) 10 months later, a second procedure of fat grafting with 36 ml into the right hemiface has been done. 2 years after the second procedure, a third session of fat grafting with 29 ml was performed. (d) The result 2 years after the last procedure.

Filling a volume defect

↓

Bony and functional deficit

Yes ← → *No*

↓   ↓

Functional and bony reparation   Structural fat grafting R 1–3 times

Negative results   Positive results

↓   ↓

Reconstruction with free muscular or adipose-fascial or demo-fascial flap   ± →   Continue with structural fat grafting to improve the result

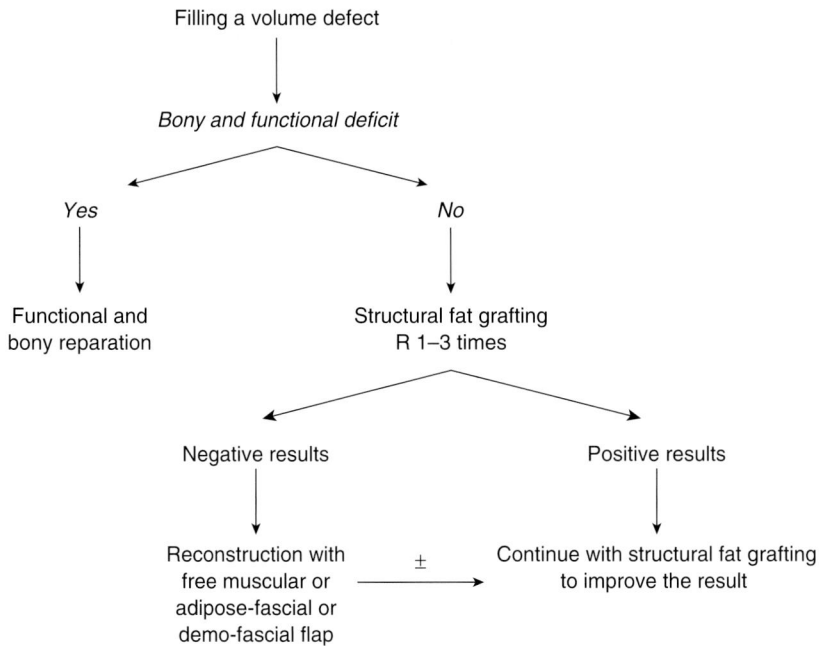

Figure 46.9 Fat grafting for facial repair.

Bibliography

Amar RE. Adipocyte microinfiltration in the face or tissue restructuration with fat tissue graft. Ann Chir Plast Esthet 1999; 44: 593.

Coleman SR. Facial recontouring with lipostructure. Clin Plast Surg 1997; 24: 347–67.

Coleman SR. Structural fat grafts: the ideal filler? Clin Plast Surg 2001; 28: 111–19.

Coleman SR. Structural fat grafting: more than a permanent filler. Plast Reconstr Surg 2006; 118: 108S–120S.

Colic MM. Lip and perioral enhancement by direct intramuscular fat autografting. Aesthetic Plast Surg 1999; 23: 36–40.

Donofrio LM. Structural autologous lipoaugmentation: a panfacial technique. Dermatol Surg 2000; 26: 1129–34.

Ellenbogen R. Free autogenous pearl fat grafts in the face—a preliminary report of a rediscovered technique. Ann Plast Surg 1986; 16: 179–94.

Ellenbogen R. Fat transfer: current use in practice. Clin Plast Surg 2000; 27: 545–56.

Fournier PF. Liposculpture: The Syringe Technique. Paris: Arnette Blackwell, 1991.

Fournier PF. Facial recontouring with fat grafting. Dermatol Clin 1990; 8: 523–37.

Hurwitz PJ, Sarel R. Facial reconstruction in partial lipodystrophy. Ann Plast Surg 1982; 8: 253–7.

Inigo F, Rojo P, Ysunza A. Aesthetic treatment of Romberg's disease: experience with 35 cases. Br J Plast Surg 1993; 46: 194–200.

Mojallal A, Foyatier JL. Autologous fat transfer in post-trauma sequelae. Experimental study demonstrating skin quality improvement. Personal communication at International Symposium on Fat Injection, Fondazione G. Sanvenero Rosselli, Milan 2007.

Rigotti G, Marchi A, Galiè M et al. Clinical treatment of radiotherapy tissue damage by lipoaspirate transplant: a healing process mediated by adipose-derived adult stem cells. Plast Reconstr Surg 2007; 119: 1409–22.

Rohrich RJ, Pessa JE. The fat compartments of the face: anatomy and clinical implications for cosmetic surgery. Plast Reconstr Surg 2007; 119: 2219–27: discussion 2228–31.

Rohrich RJ, Sorokin ES, Brown SA. In search of improved fat transfer viability: a quantitative analysis of the role of centrifugation and harvest site. Plast Reconstr Surg 2004; 113: 391–5; discussion 396–7.

Teimourian B. Repair of soft-tissue contour deficit by means of semiliquid fat graft. Plast Reconstr Surg 1986; 78: 123–4.

47 Fat transfer in breast and thorax reconstructive surgery

Ali Mojallal and Jean Louis Foyatier

The breast

Mammary pathologies requiring volumetric restoration include malformations and distortions acquired after surgery for cancer.

Malformations

Congenital malformations of the breast can have serious psychological consequences for teenagers, justifying the offer of a surgical procedure. We differentiate two major types of malformation: an anomaly of volume, and an anomaly of form and symmetry. Malformation characterized by an anomaly comprises principally the Poland syndrome and the tuberous breast.

The Poland syndrome corresponds to a clinical entity which links mammary hypoplasia and thoracic malformation of variable degree; minimal expression is agenesis of the sternal part of the pectoralis major muscle. In these cases, fat transfer allows treatment of zones difficult to correct using other techniques, notably the relief of the anterior axillary region.

As in breast reconstruction after cancer, by analysis of the distortion compared with the breast defined as ideal, we can imagine and accomplish a corrective intervention by combining different basic techniques. These interventions, which are sometimes intense, although changing considerably the morphology and influencing the psychology of the patient, often gave imperfect results. For these reasons, the provision of adipose tissue transfer as a complementary or as a unique treatment can be of major benefit in such cases. Our experience in this field has shown that it is possible to correct, completely or partly, the lack of volume in Poland syndrome in several sessions using fat transfer, even in the most difficult cases (Figure 47.1).

The consequence of surgery for cancer

The transfer of adipose tissue in reconstruction of the breast is a technique used nowadays for numerous indications. It can be used each time we wish to correct

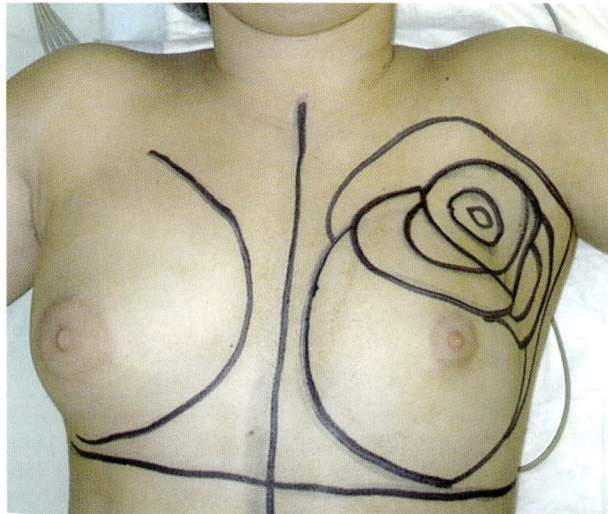

Figure 47.1 Preoperative planning and preestablished marking of the breast and axillary pillar regions to be fat grafted.

a defect that is located on a reconstructed breast. For the breast (in reconstructive surgery), the position of submammary groove, the median axis, the position of the nipple-areolar complex and the volume and projection of the different quadrants of the breast must be compared with the other side. The superomedial quadrant is the most difficult to correct by classical techniques, and also the most visible in the décolleté of the patient. Defects after mammary reconstruction are particularly marked at the level of the internal and superomedial part of the breast, the décolleté region. This region, however, is the most important for the patient, because it is the most visible, and that which 'participates' most in the patient's social life. Until the technique of fat grafting was introduced, there was no method of correcting the décolleté region satisfactorily.

Additional adipose tissue grafting can be used to improve the result of autologous breast reconstruction using latissimus dorsi muscle, transverse rectus abdominis muscle (TRAM), DIEP flap or with breast implant reconstruction methods. However, fat grafting must be accomplished during a separate session, in general 5–6 months after mammary reconstruction.

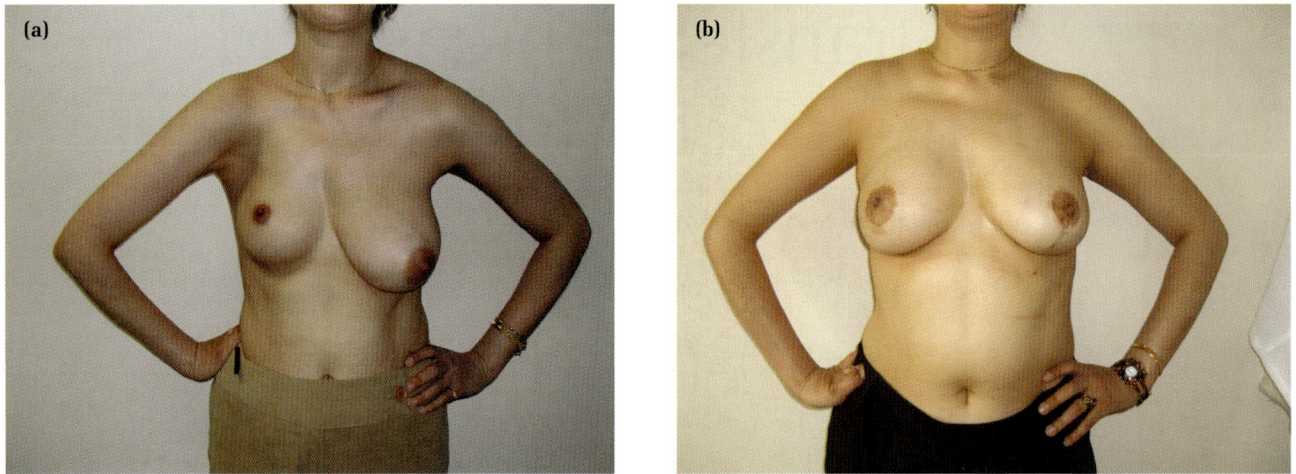

Figure 47.2   A 32-year-old woman presented with right-sided Poland syndrome (a). The first session of fat grafting used 180 ml at the level of the anterior axillary pillar, 6 months after a breast augmentation by silicone breast implant has been carried out. 1 year later, a second session of fat grafting using 240 ml at the level of the anterior axillary pillar combined with nipple-areolar-complex reconstruction has been carried out. (b) The result 1 year after the last procedure.

Techniques

It is often necessary to use large quantities of adipose tissue to fill the region of the anterior axillary pillar or other regions of the breast. For reconstruction of the anterior axillary pillar, the left hand stops the entrance of the cannula into the axillary zone and the right hand manipulates the cannula to inject the fat as a three-dimensional lattice.

In the case of breast reconstruction using a flap, the transfer of adipose tissue can introduce important volume, and can contribute to support the purely autologous nature of reconstruction by ameliorating the volume, form, and projection of the reconstructed breast. Adipose tissue in this case takes the place of the breast silicone implant placed behind the flap. The technique of fat grafting into the breast is nowadays considered suitable for application in a breast which has had a total mastectomy. Since the breast parenchyma has been removed, the minimal changes to the adipose tissue do not warrant any subsequent surveillance. In the case of a conservative breast treatment (after tumorectomy, lumpectomy), this technique is under study by a defined proctocol using evaluative mammography, echography, and magnetic resonance imaging (MRI) before and after surgery. In these cases, and also in the cases of a normal breast augmentation, fat transfer can be indicated. But, as some experimental studies showed that fat tissue promotes the tumorogenesis, fat grafting into a post lumpectomy or in a normal breast must be done only under strict radiological control and in a specialized center. Radiological studies show that the calcification found after this technology differs from neoplastic microcalcification.

It is obvious that, due to the large volumes of adipose tissue needed for injection in to the breast, absolute respect of the principles of micrograft injection using numerous tunnels and multiple sessions is imperative.

Fat grafting combined to a breast reconstruction by implant

Regardless of the initial pathology, the transfer of adipose tissue can be combined with a mammary implant. This complementary treatment must be carried out at a different time. In this case, the injection of fat allows correction of the contour of the prosthesis, reshaping of the décolleté region, recreation of the axillary pillar in Poland syndrome, correction of the double outlines of the third segment in the tuberous breast, and better definition or lowering of the submammary groove in the tuberous breast or in a case of reconstruction. In all these situations, it is necessary to remain vigilant during the intervention so as not to pierce the prosthesis. To achieve this, the prosthesis is dislocated and protected by one hand, and adipose tissue reinjected by the other hand. It is also necessary to accomplish numerous sessions by introducing small quantities per session, because the space around the prosthesis is often minimal.

It seems that, due to its anti-inflammatory nature, adipose tissue will diminish the rate of implant capsular contraction.

Fat grafting combined to an autologous breast reconstruction

The transfer of adipose tissue can also be associated with mammary reconstruction using a flap. After

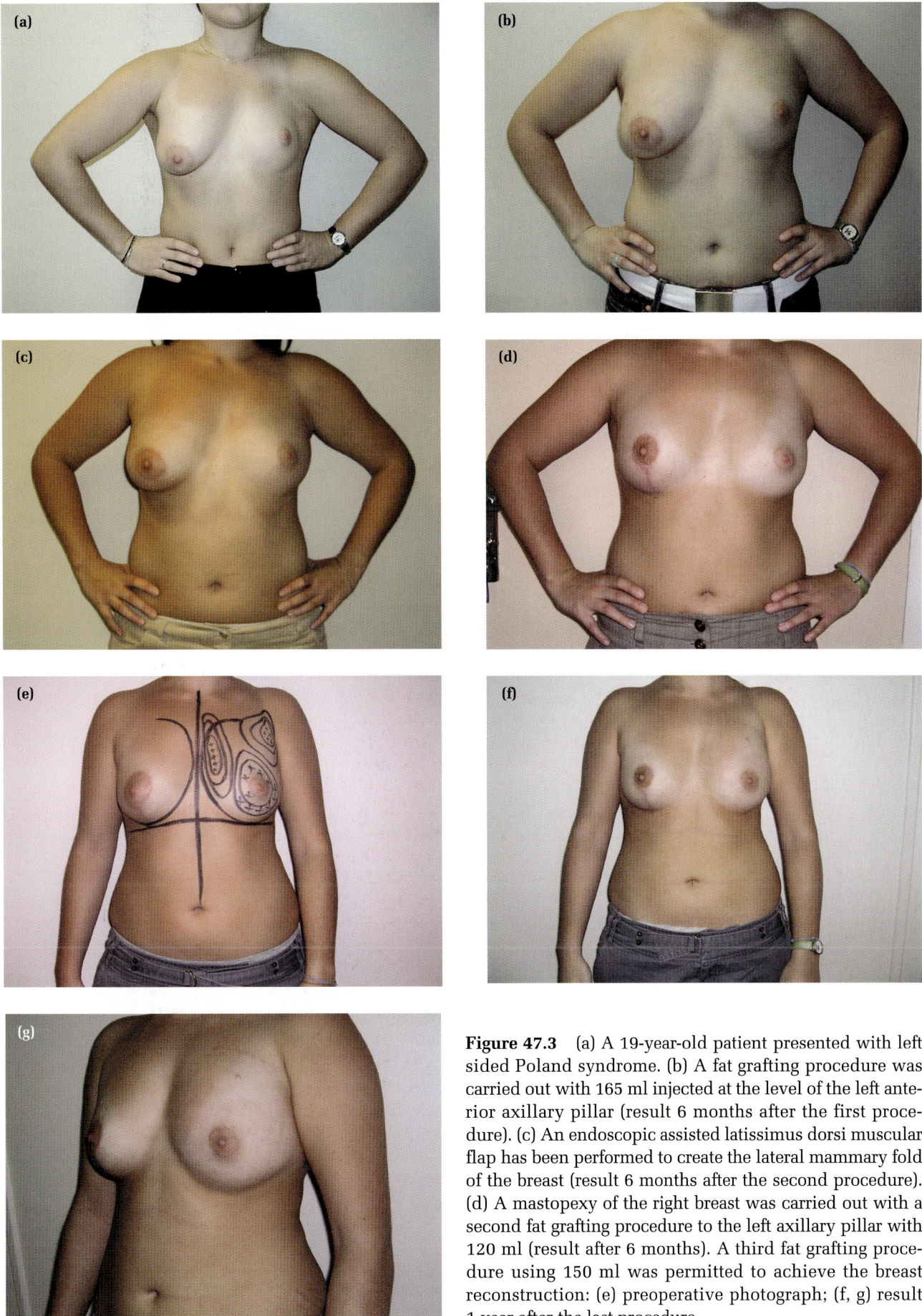

Figure 47.3   (a) A 19-year-old patient presented with left sided Poland syndrome. (b) A fat grafting procedure was carried out with 165 ml injected at the level of the left anterior axillary pillar (result 6 months after the first procedure). (c) An endoscopic assisted latissimus dorsi muscular flap has been performed to create the lateral mammary fold of the breast (result 6 months after the second procedure). (d) A mastopexy of the right breast was carried out with a second fat grafting procedure to the left axillary pillar with 120 ml (result after 6 months). A third fat grafting procedure using 150 ml was permitted to achieve the breast reconstruction: (e) preoperative photograph; (f, g) result 1 year after the last procedure.

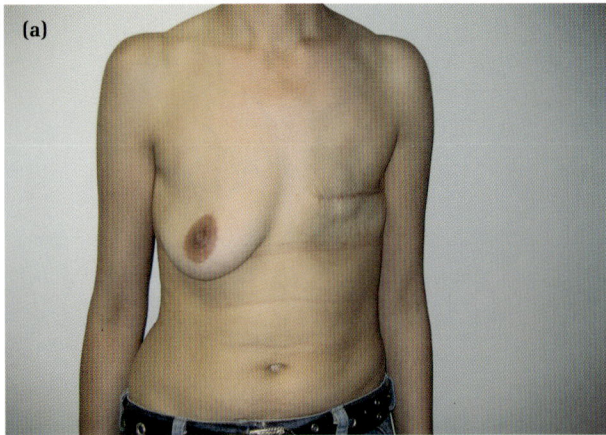

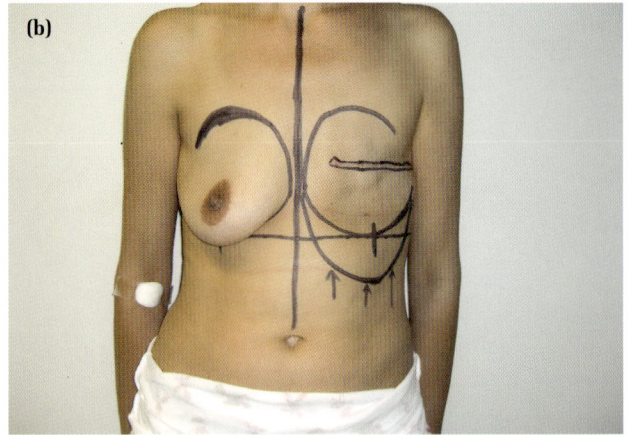

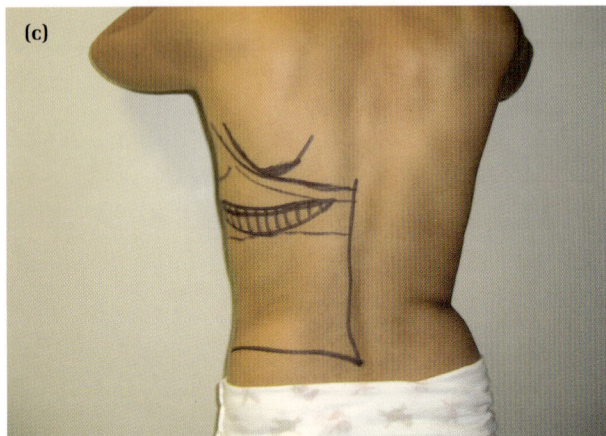

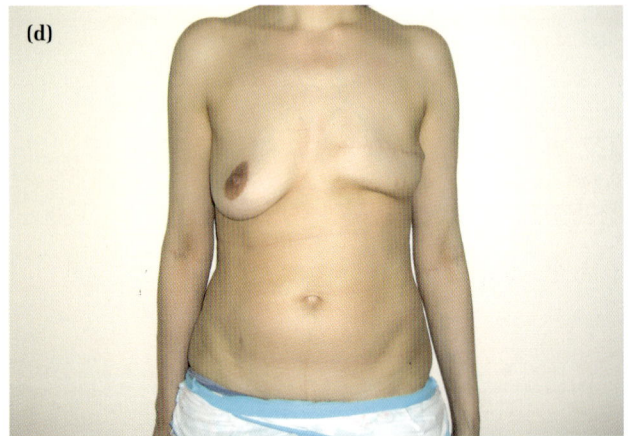

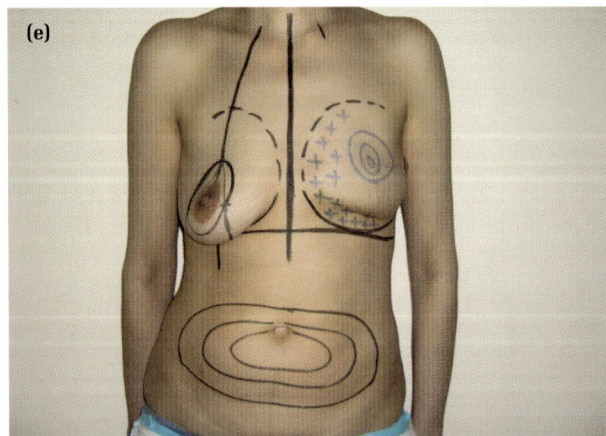

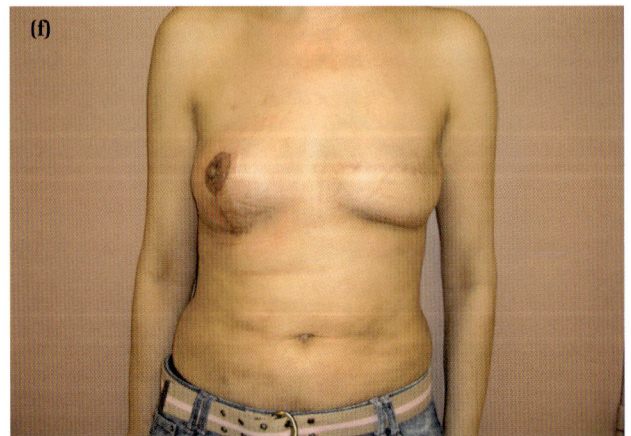

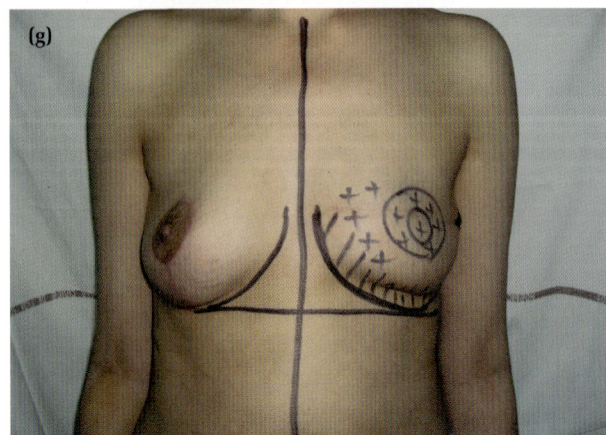

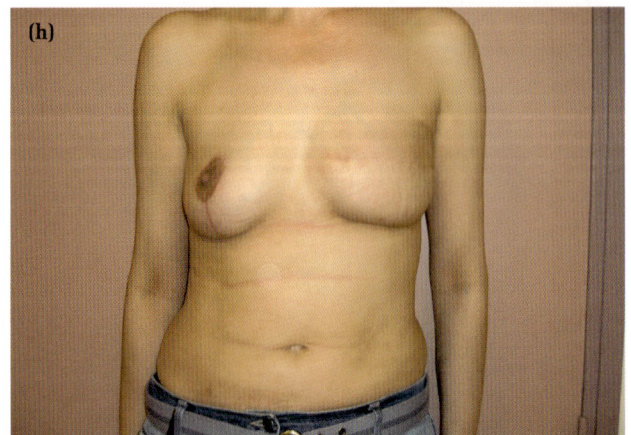

Figure 47.4

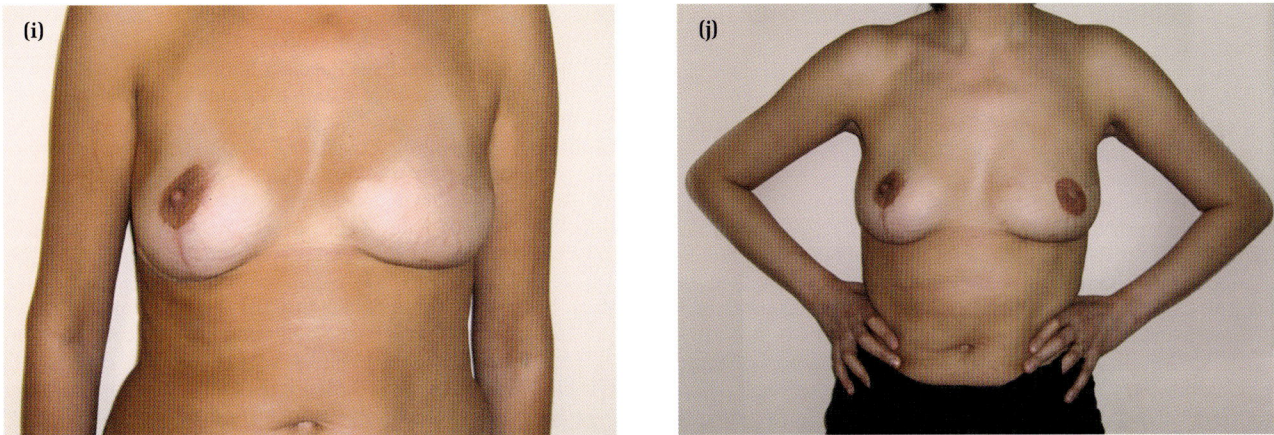

Figure 47.4   (a) A 45-year-old woman underwent mastectomy and left axillary node removal for an invasive breast cancer. Autologous breast reconstruction was performed using a latissimus dorsi muscular flap, associated with a thoracoabdominal advancement flap; (b, c) preoperative photographs; (d) result 1 year after the first procedure (d). Next, a mastopexy of the right breast was performed associated with structural fat grafting into the left reconstructed breast. This first procedure of fat grafting with 250 ml allowed augmentation of the volume of the reconstructed breast and also lowering of the left inframammary fold: (e) preoperative photograph: (f) postoperative result of the second operation after 15 days; and (g) after 6 months, before a second structural fat grafting procedure using 240 ml; (h) result after 4 months and (i) after 7 months. A third structural fat grafting was performed using 215 ml into the reconstructed breast, associated with the nipple-areolar complex reconstruction by tattoo and CV local flaps; (j) result 1 year after the last procedure.

latissimus dorsi muscle, TRAM, or DIEP (deep inferior epigastric perforator) flap surgery, the adipose tissue brings a significant supplementary benefit in cases of localized defects not corrected by the flap, or by increasing the volume of the reconstructed breast. The most difficult part of the breast to reconstruct by a flap is the upper pole and the superomedial part of the breast. Fat grafting is a simple and reliable technique for treating defects at this level; in particular, there is no other simple way to improve the esthetic result in this area. In these cases, the vascularized flap represents an ideal site to receive the fat injected, so the volume of fat grafted per session can be augmented.

Modification of the base of the breast and lowering the inframmatory fold

We have noted that using fat tissue grafting a lowering of the inframammary fold (IMF) is possible. For this, it is necessary to inject the fat from the former IMF to the expected neogroove. During this time, it is difficult to undermine the skin of this zone adherent to the aponeurosis of the lower part of pectoralis muscle and the upper part of the rectus abdominis muscle. During the first procedure, it seems to be difficult to shape the lower part of the breast above the IMF, but a few months after the intervention, there is an involution of the contour of this zone. The volume of this part of the breast can then be adjusted during further procedures (see Figures 47.4 e-h).

Improvement of the skin quality

It is not rare to see radiotherapy-induced lesions as telangiectatic or dystrophic plaque in the upper pole

of the breast. We have been able to prove the amelioration of these lesions after fat transfer in an experimental study. This improvement is linked to the presence of multipotent, vasoactive 'stem cells' in the adipose tissue injected, and also stimulated by adipokins (the adipocyte's secreted hormones).

The thorax

The funnel chest or thorax (pectus excavatum) is the most frequent congenital malformation of the thoracic wall. It is a complex malformation involving the sternocostal plate, and is characterized by a depression of the long vertical axis, in general at the median, variably deep and symmetrical. All modern studies have consensus that functional disability associated with funnel thorax does not exist or is minimal in the great majority of cases. The aim of intervention is therefore purely morphological or cosmetic, and it is logical to correct funnel thorax using fillers, because the radical technique of sternochondroplasty is intense, the morbidity is not negligible, results are unstable, and it frequently recurs. Previously, dermal grafting, dermal-fat grafting or omentum flap, and more often non-vascularized bony and cartilaginous graft fragments, were used, which were inevitably subjected to necrosis due to the large volume needed and the non-favorable and poorly vascularized tissular environment. For these reasons, correction by preformed silicone prosthesis has more recently become the standard treatment for these malformations. However, with the availability of fat grafting techniques, a new alternative was realized which appears to be of benefit for minor forms of central or lateralized deformity.

Bibliography

Bames HO. Augmentation mammaplasty by lipo-transplant. Plast Reconstr Surg 1953; 11: 404.

Bircoll M, Novack BH. Autologous fat transplantation employing liposuction techniques. Ann Plast Surg 1987; 18: 327–9.

Bircoll M. Cosmetic breast augmentation utilizing autologous fat and liposuction techniques. Plast Reconstr Surg 1987; 79: 267–71.

Bircoll M. Autologous fat transplantation to the breast. Plast Reconstr Surg 1988; 82: 361–2.

Castello JR, Barros J, Vazquez R. Giant liponecrotic pseudocyst after breast augmentation by fat injection. Plast Reconstr Surg 1999; 103: 291–3.

Chavoin JP, Grolleau JL, Lavigne B et al. Chirurgie des malformations du thorax. In: Encyclopédie Médico-Chirurgical. Techniques Chirurgicales, Paris: Elsevier, 1998: 45–671.

Delay E, Jorquera F, Pasi P, Gratadour AC. Autologous latissimus breast reconstruction in association with the abdominal advancement flap: a new refinement in breast reconstruction. Ann Plast Surg 1999; 42: 67–75.

Delay E, Gounot N, Bouillot A, Zlatoff P, Rivoire M. Autologous latissimus breast reconstruction: a 3-year clinical experience with 100 patients. Plast Reconstr Surg 1998; 102: 1461–78.

Gradinger GP. Breast augmentation by autologous fat injection. Plast Reconstr Surg 1987; 80: 868–9.

Grolleau JL, Chavoin JP, Costagliola M. Chirurgie des malformations du sein. In: Encyclopédie Médico-Chirurgical. Techniques Chirurgicales. Paris: Elsevier, 1999: 41–940.

Haik J, Talisman R, Tamir J et al. Breast augmentation with fresh-frozen homologous fat grafts. Aesthetic Plast Surg 2001; 25: 292–4.

Hang-Fu L, Marmolya G, Feiglin DH. Liposuction fat-fillant implant for breast augmentation and reconstruction. Aesthetic Plast Surg 1995; 19: 427–37.

Har-Shai Y, Lindenbaum E, Ben-Itzhak O, Hirshowitz B. Large liponecrotic pseudocyst formation following cheek augmentation by fat injection. Aesthetic Plast Surg 1996; 20: 417–19.

Hartrampf CR, Bennett GK. Autologous fat from liposuction for breast augmentation. Plast Reconstr Surg 1987; 80: 646.

Maillard GF. Liponecrotic cysts after augmentation mammaplasty with fat injections. Aesthetic Plast Surg 1994; 18: 405–6.

Rosen PB, Hugo NE. Augmentation mammaplasty by cadaver fat allografts. Plast Reconstr Surg 1988; 82: 525–6.

Fat transfer in lower limb reconstructive surgery

Ali Mojallal, Michael Veber, and Jean Louis Foyatier

Atrophy of the lower limb represents a reduction of volume of the member in single or combined tissues: muscular and/or subcutaneous and/or cutaneous. To be didactic, we have classified atrophy of the lower limb into two categories: general atrophy or localized atrophy. General atrophy can occur for various reasons: it can be of congenital or secondary origin in poliomyelitis, iatrogenic, traumatic, or due to an attack to the tibial nerve (internal sciatic popliteal nerve) and/or the external sciatic popliteal nerve, it can be unilateral or bilateral, and it can affect the entirety or part of the lower limb.

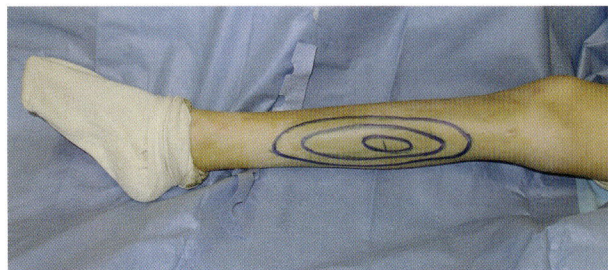

Figure 48.1 Preoperative location of zones to be injected: definitive mapping of the leg.

Surgical technique

In the case of localized atrophy, injection is carried out in the center and depth of the atrophic zone. The injection of adipose tissues can be accompanied by liposuction in the periphery of the affected zone to diminish the visual aspect of the depression, which can be accentuated by the fatty thickness around the atrophic area. In the case of injection into a scar and the adherent area, it is useful to use a dissecting cannula with a V-shaped cutting end to dissect the subcutaneous fibroses. This maneuver must be done with a maximum of precaution to avoid penetration of the thin skin cover in this area. In the case of circular atrophy, the injected zones are located at the level of the relief notable visually when facing the patient, such as external or internal side of the calf or the supramalleolar zone.

The injections respect a defined area marked on the patient before the intervention. Injection starts from the depth and moves towards the outer surface (Figure 48.1) in both intramuscular or subaponeurotic injections.

Liposuction of the contralateral lower limb, in case of excess weight, can complete the procedure, to diminish any visual difference in volume of both lower limbs.

Post-surgical care

The average period of hospitalization is 48 hours, with 5 days of anti biotics therapy using penicillin M. Mobilization of the patient is allowed the day following the intervention, without support for 15 days, and then with the use of progressive supports. Anticoagulant treatment using low molecular weight heparin is continued for 15 days.

The distinction of lower limb atrophy into two categories allows analysis of patients to be simplified. It is important to take into consideration every etiology to refine the method of management.

The restricting factor in the treatment of atrophy of the lower limb is often the cutaneous elasticity. In most cases it is difficult to expand the skin, and sometimes we are in direct contact with some fibrotic tissue. Our method of injection is from the depth towards the outer surface in either pure subcutaneous or subaponeurotic injection. In effect, the muscular lodges of the lower limb are considered to be a little elastic despite the rigidity of the aponeuroses.

For treatment of a circular atrophy of the lower limb, it is necessary to assimilate the lower limb with a cylindrical model, with height h and radius r.

Comparison of the calculated volume of the limb and that of the healthy limb shows a large difference. This large volume difference is difficult to compensate entirely, especially since the survival of transplanted tissues is not 100% and since overcorrection and/or renewal of the grafting can be envisaged. It is therefore necessary to analyze the treatment plan thoroughly in a preoperative consultation with the patient, including desired volume, number of sessions, and alternative choices in case of failure, and to establish accurately the zones to be injected by marking on the patient.

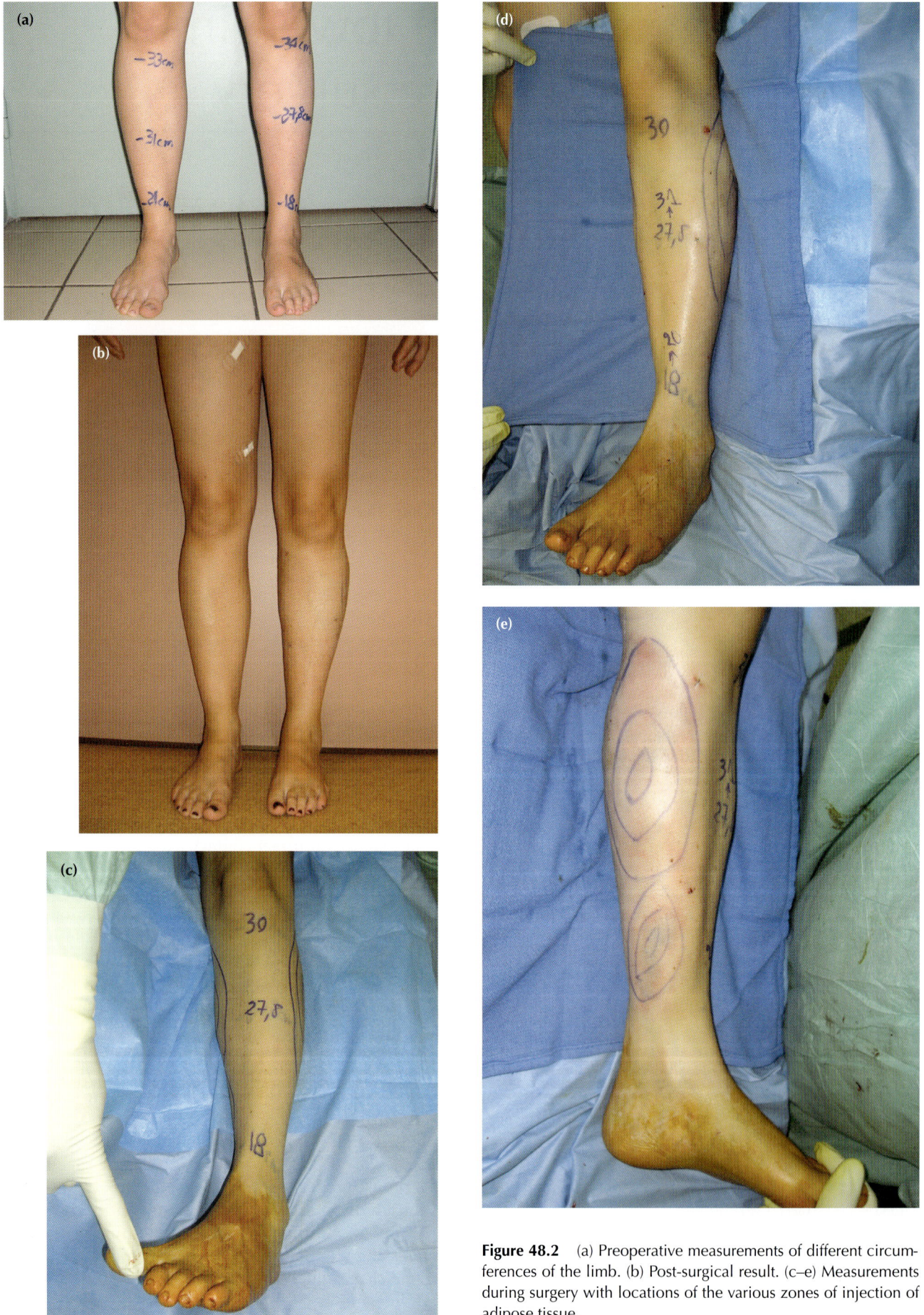

Figure 48.2 (a) Preoperative measurements of different circumferences of the limb. (b) Post-surgical result. (c–e) Measurements during surgery with locations of the various zones of injection of adipose tissue.

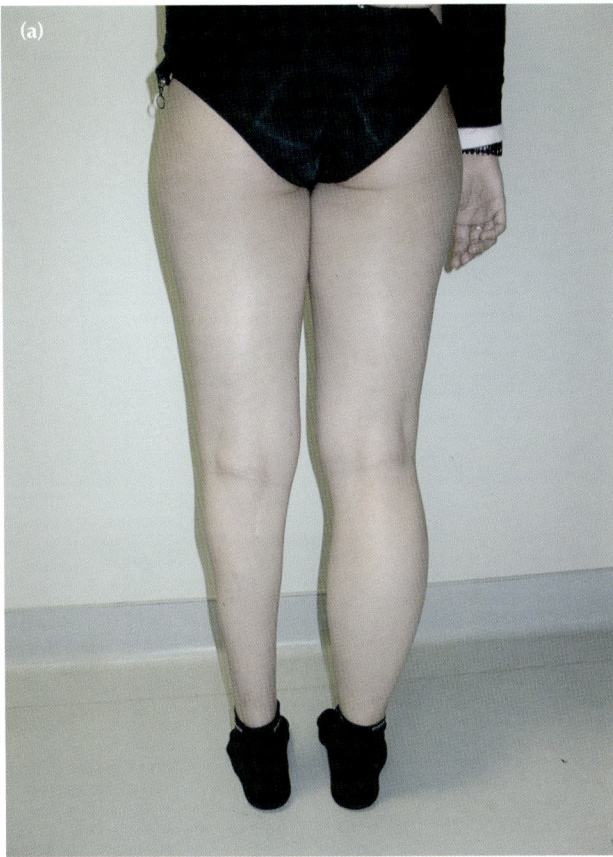

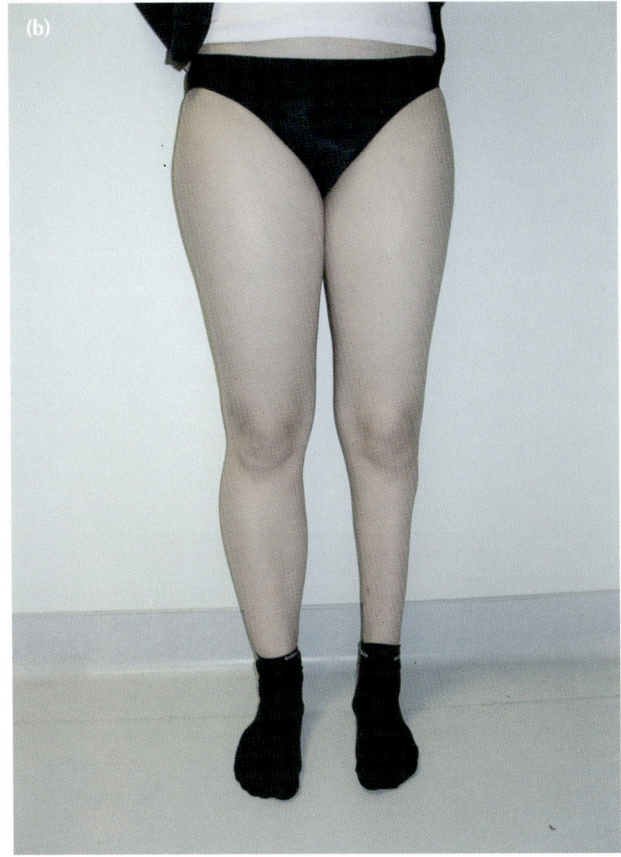

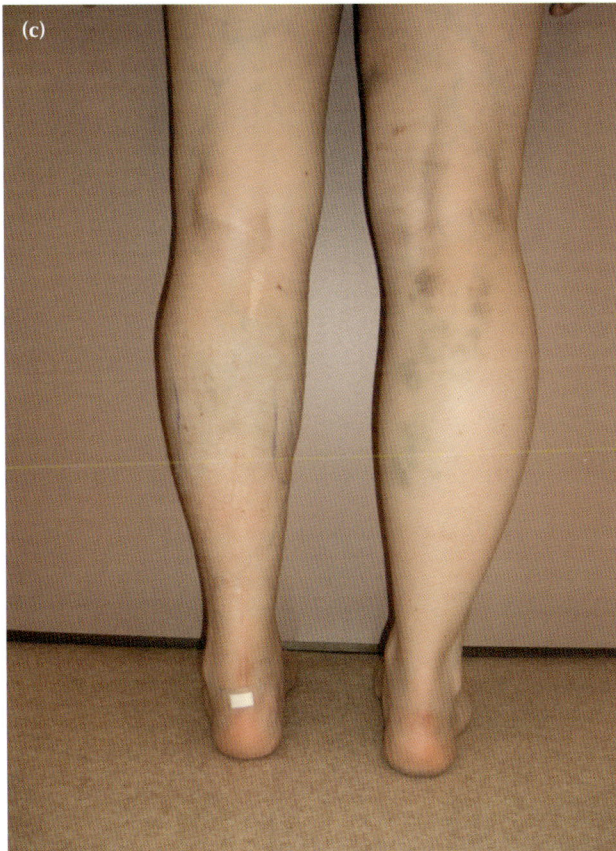

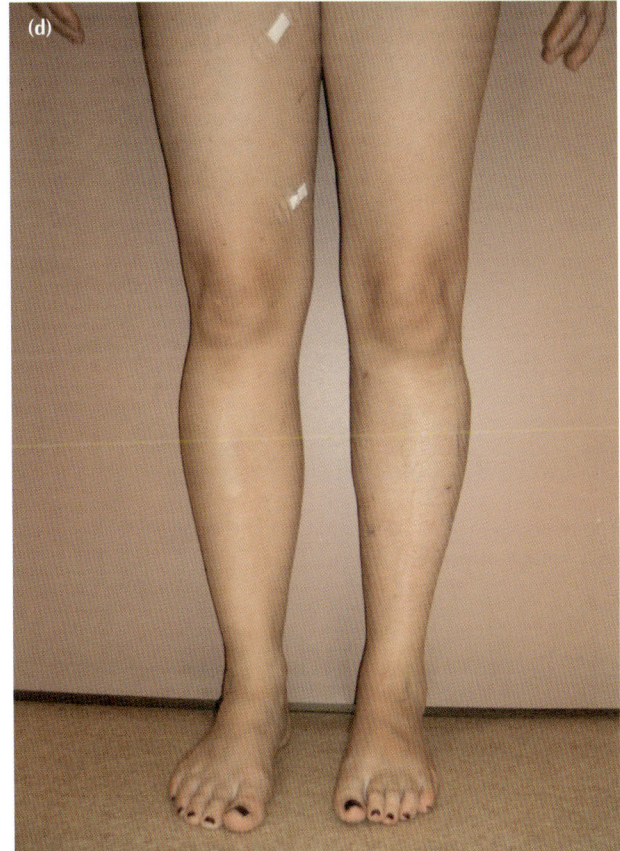

Figure 48.3   A 22-year-old woman with after effects of iatrogenic 'spinnaker' lesion (internal sciatic popliteal nerve). (a, b) Before the intervention, (c, d) result after three injections (140, 170, 185 ml) over 2 years.

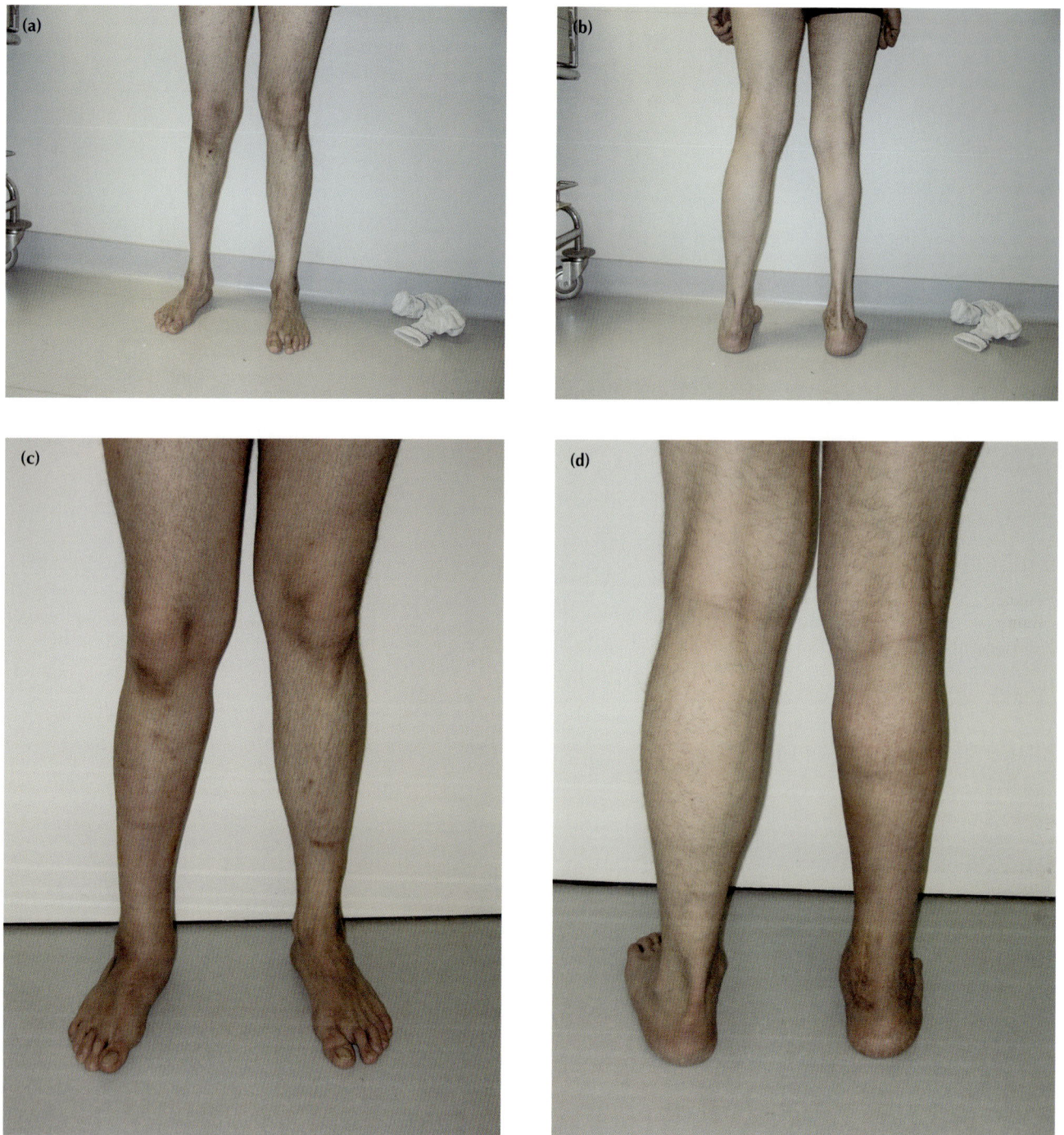

Figure 48.4   (a, b) A 31-year-old man with congenital atrophy of the right calf. (c, d) Results after two sessions of injection (100, 126 ml) of adipose tissue.

As the quantity of adipose tissue injected will be less than that estimated, it is necessary to concentrate the volumetric correction on the lateral and medial axes of the leg, to accentuate the visual effect of correction, or on the zones which give more plasticity, for example the middle third of the calf.

The objective evaluation of results by measurement (in centimeters) is efficient in cases of circular atrophy, and is easily done during the consultation. It allows the permanence of the result to be assessed, and the best donor sites for the transfer of adipose tissues to be established.

In the case of injection under a skin graft, it is necessary to analyze the suppleness of the skin and the plan of cutaneous sliding. It is then necessary to inject small quantities and to repeat sessions to avoid any risk of necrosis of the skin graft.

Another solution is the use of silicone implants. Numerous studies have shown complications related to this technology, such as breakage, protrusion, capsular

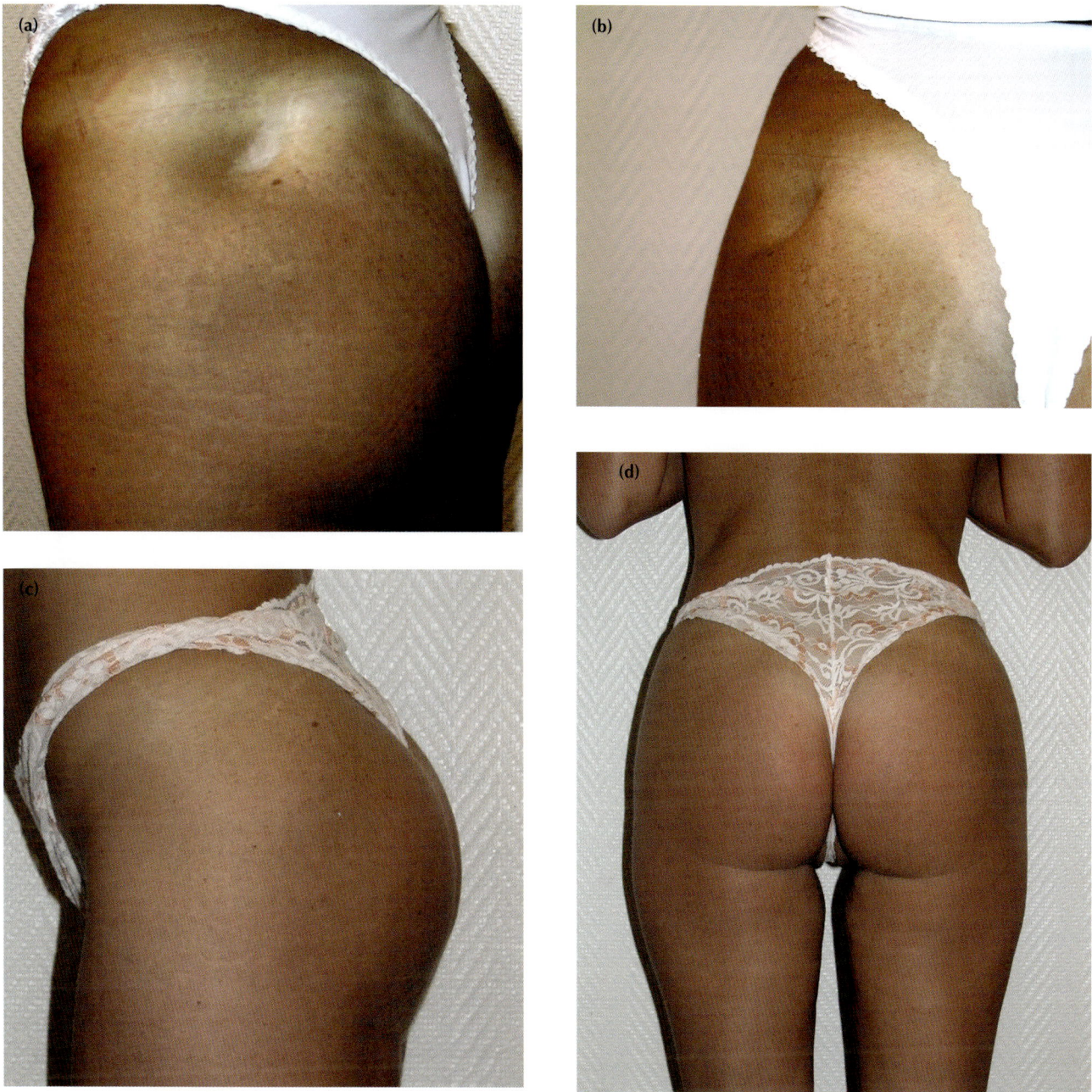

Figure 48.5 (a, b) A 25-year-old woman with localized atrophy following intramuscular injection. (c, d) Result after one session of transfer of adipose tissue (40 ml) showing repair of secondary scar.

contraction, or even cases of deep venous thrombosis due to compression caused by the implant. This last solution is in our opinion the choice to be made in cases of absence of results after three or four sessions of transfer.

Additionally, the transfer of adipose tissue contributes to an increase of elasticity of the cutaneous bed, which is complementary to amelioration of contours in the case of silicone implant installation.

It is now assumed that the provision of stem cells and growth factors within the adipose tissues allows, besides an improvement of the quality of the skin, an increase of the output ratio of sample/final injection. This aspect allows the transfer of adipose tissue to previously irradiated skin.

One of the major interests of current research into the transfer of adipose tissues is preadipocyte culture. Indeed, the perfection of this technology would notably allow palliation of the problem of too-weak fatty reserves in certain patients, or restriction of the rate of resorption of grafted adipose tissues.

In summary, Figure 48.8 demonstrates a schema for indications of use of the transfer of adipose tissues in atrophy of the lower limb.

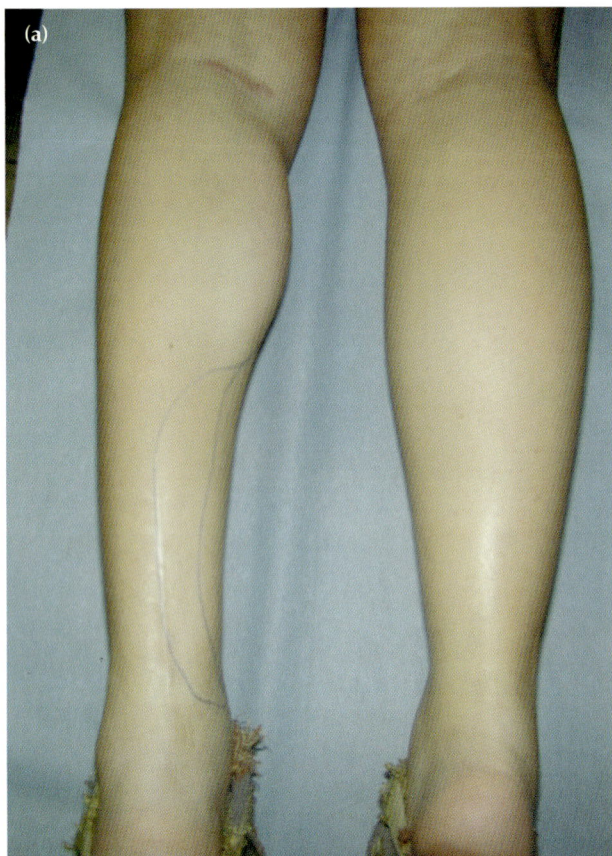

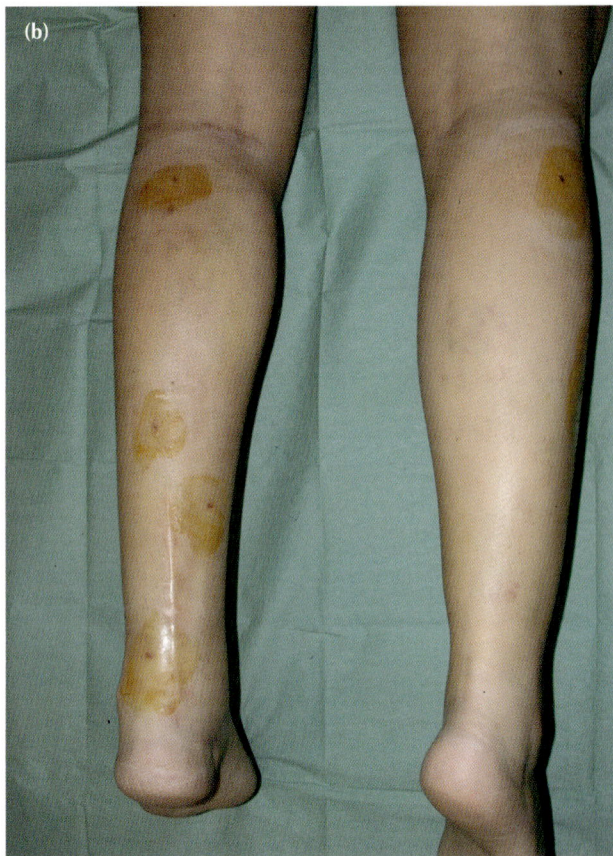

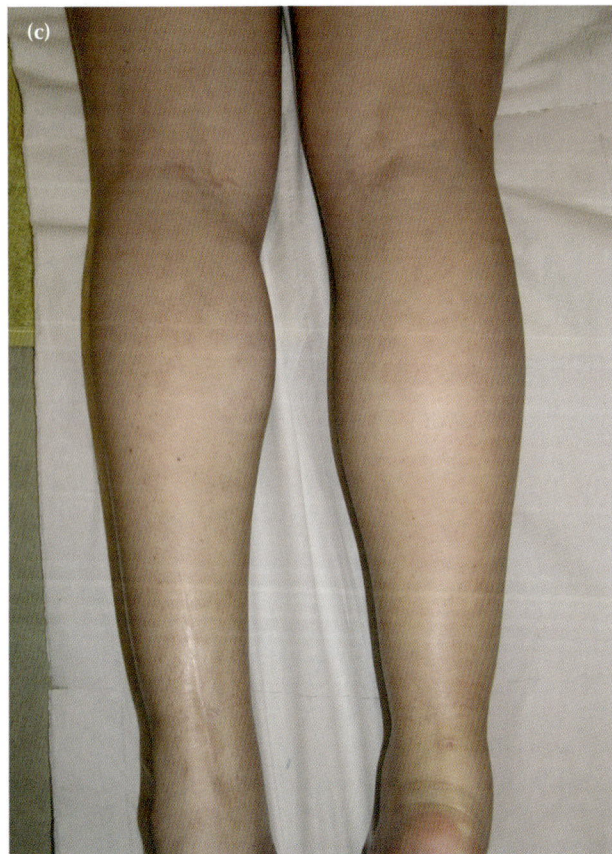

Figure 48.6   (a) A 35-year-old woman showing after effects of poliomyelitis of the left leg and before augmenting leg by implant. (b, c) Result after one session of transfer of adipose tissue (48 ml) located in the distal part of the leg. Photographs taken during procedure (b) and 1 year afterwards (c).

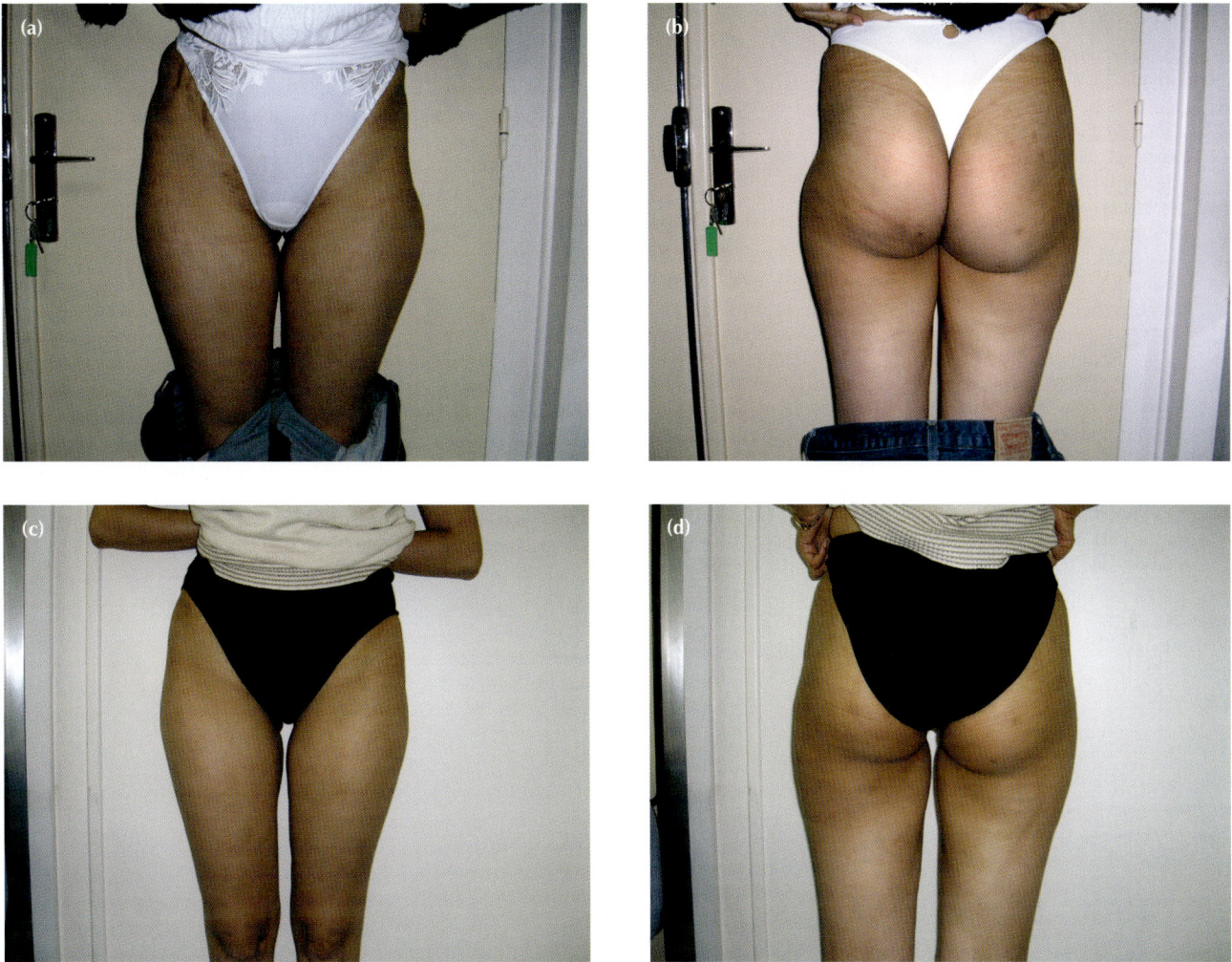

Figure 48.7 (a, b) A 22-year-old woman with lipodystrophy of the left hip after orthopedic surgery of the pelvis. (c, d) Result 1 year after one session of transfer of adipose tissue (90 ml) located in the proximal part and lipoaspiration of the distal part of the hip.

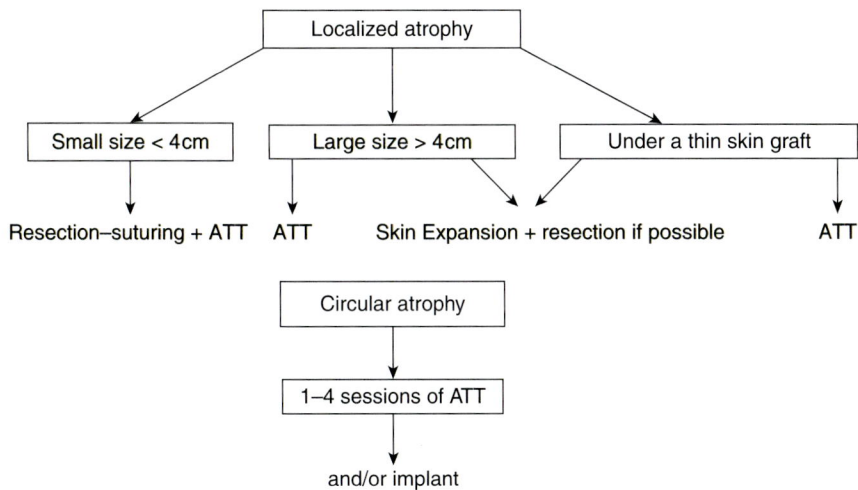

Figure 48.8 Decision-making tree for treatment of atrophy of the lower limb. ATT, adipose tissue transfer.

Bibliography

1. Mojallal A, Foyatier JL. Historical review of the use of adipose tissue transfer in plastic and reconstructive surgery. Ann Chir Plast Esthet 2004; 49: 419–25.

2. Peren PA, Gomez JB, Guerrerosantos J, Salazar CA. Gluteus augmentation with fat grafting. Aesthetic Plast Surg 2000; 24: 412–17.

3. Coleman SR. Structural fat grafts: the ideal filler? Clin Plast Surg 2001; 28: 111–19.

4. Chang KN. Surgical corrections of post liposuction contour irregularities. Plast Reconstr Surg 1994; 94: 126–36.

5. Most D, Kozlow J, Heller J, Shermak MA. Thromboembolism in plastic surgery. Plast Reconstr Surg 2005; 115: 20–30.

6. Lewis CM. The current status of autologous fat grafting. Aesthetic Plast Surg 1993; 17: 109–12.

7. Karacalar A, Orak I, Kaplan S, Yildirim S. No-touch technique for autologous fat harvesting. Aesthetic Plast Surg 2004; 28: 158–64.

8. Valeriani M, Mezzana P, Madonna Terracina FS. Liposculpture and lipofilling of the gluteal-trochanteric region: anatomical analysis and technique. Acta Chir Plast 2001; 43: 95–8.

9. Stampos M, Xepoulias P. Fat transplantation for soft tissue augmentation in the lower limbs. Aesthetic Plast Surg 2001; 25: 256–61.

10. Jackson IT, Simman R, Tholen R, DiNick VD. A successful long-term method of fat grafting: recontouring of a large subcutaneous postradiation thigh defect with autologous fat transplantation. Aesthetic Plast Surg 2001; 25: 165–9.

11. Lewis CM. Correction of deep gluteal depression by autologous fat grafting. Aesthetic Plast Surg 1992; 16: 247–50.

12. Murillo WL. Buttock augmentation: case studies of fat injection monitored by magnetic resonance imaging. Plast Reconstr Surg 2004; 114: 1606–14.

13. Mojallal A, Foyatier JL. The effect of different factors on the survival of transplanted adipocytes. Ann Chir Plast Esthet 2004; 49: 426–36.

14. Mojallal A, Breton P, Delay E, Foyatier J-L. Greffe d'adipocytes: applications en chirurgie plastique et esthétique. EMC Techniques chirurgicales – Chirurgie plastique reconstructrice et esthétique. Paris: Elsevier, 2004: 45–125.

15. Gutstein RA. Augmentation of the lower leg: a new combined calf-tibial implant. Plast Reconstr Surg 2006; 117: 817–26.

49 The different products and their pharmacology

Pierre J Nicolau

Injectable filling agents are most commonly classified according to their duration within the human tissues, as short- or moderate-lasting agents: 3–12 months, or long-lasting or permanent fillers, whose duration is at least 12–18 months.

However, they can also be considered according to the reactions they induce within human tissues. Any implantation of a device into the human body starts a reaction of identification, isolation from the host tissues, and, if recognized as dangerous, its removal. This is the foreign body reaction.

Foreign body reaction

It starts with an inflammatory reaction which occurs in two steps: first, an acute inflammatory reaction with neutrophil polynuclear cells, then, over 2 weeks, chronic inflammation with lymphocytes or monocytes, according to the type and location of the implant.

The host must recognize the foreign body. This recognition is based on monocytes, which will adhere to the firm substrate. This adhesion is the most important aspect of the cellular interaction.[1,2]

Through adhesion, cellular responses are activated. It is a complex process, implying protein adsorption on the surface of the foreign body. These proteins start a specific recognition by cell surface receptors, then a non-specific interaction between cell surface molecules, the adsorbed proteins, and the implanted material.[3] The more proteins that are found on the surface of the implant, the more efficient will be the resulting cellular adhesion, spreading, and proliferation.[4] Macrophages fuse into giant cells to try and phagocytose large size particles.[5,6] It appears that this cellular fusion, and hence the formation of foreign body giant cells (FBGCs), is an adaptation to the difficulties of eliminating foreign bodies, while 'inefficient' cells go into self-destruction (apoptosis) in a first step. Apoptosis is proved by cell prints on the protein layer.[4] To summarize, macrophages adhere, phagocytose, or fuse into FBGCs. If not phagocytosed and eliminated, the implant will be isolated by fibroblasts with a strong fibrous collagenous capsule, and will gradually be replaced by fibrocytes. Each

foreign particle will finally be encapsulated independently from the others.[7,8] Or, if there is no adhesion and no phagocytosis, there is destruction without remnants of the useless protective cells, and the foreign body will be isolated by a thin fibrillar membrane, which is relatively poor in cells.

Nevertheless, many factors will modify thes reactions.[9]

Size and volume of implant

Particles over 40 μm are not phagocytosed.[10] The smaller is the size, the faster is the phagocytosis.[11] Also, the smaller is the size, the more inflammation[6] and the more migrations there will be,[12] particles being carried away by phagocytes. For fluid implants, either liquid or gel, such as silicone or acrylic gels, the reaction at the host/implant interface will diminish within 3–4 weeks, but will be reactivated in an acute manner for each droplet that becomes detached from the main mass.[13] Thus, the inflammatory reactions induced by these fluids can last for years, and follow the eventual migration or displacement of the implant. The same can be seen with solid implants, such as Teflon® paste.[14,15]

Morphology of implant

Irregular shapes induce more macrophage activation.[16,17] Spherical shapes induce less enzymatic activity.[18,19] Smooth surfaces induce less inflammatory reaction,[11,20] but more collagen secretion.[10,21,22] The fibrous capsule is thicker on a flat surface than on the edges.[23] This is why Bioplastique®, Dermalive®, and Dermadeep®, made of irregular shaped fragments, show more secondary inflammation than Artecoll® and Artefill®.

Surface area

There is a critical value for a particle surface area, above which the inflammatory response increases spectacularly for a given mass.[18] This notion of 'threshold' surface area is very important, and explains why the largest particles induce more inflammation. As a spherical particle has the smallest surface for the largest mass, it will induce less inflammation than an irregular shaped one. And for the same given mass, 100-μm beads induce 56% collagen, and 40-μm beads induce 78% collagen, as their total surface area is larger.[24] All spherical particles will therefore be more efficient for collagen encapsulation, with less inflammatory reactions than with irregular particles. This is another reason explaining why Bioplastique, Dermalive, and Dermadeep, made of irregular shaped fragments, show more secondary inflammation, which is much more difficult to treat than the one seen with Artecoll and Artefill.

Chemical composition

A vertebrate cell surface has carboxylate anions that most bacteria do not have: a simple and effective means to recognize alien organisms. Therefore, the more carboxylate anions there are on a surface, the less cell spreading and fusion into FBGCs there is.[2] Hydrophobic implants (ethylmethacrylate, EMA) induce more fibronectin adsorption (protein surface deposition, for foreign body recognition) and more macrophage adhesion.[1,6,25] Carboxylic groups (hydroxyethylmethacrylate, HEMA) activate the C3 fraction of complement, inducing specific macrophage recognition[26] and FBGC reaction. This is precisely the chemical composition of Dermalive and Dermadeep.

Electric charge

Positively charged beads attract and/or activate macrophages.[7,27] Positive charges induce greater FBGC formation, induce faster orientation of collagen bundles, and result in thicker connective tissue. This explains the connective tissue formation around resorbable dextran microspheres of Reviderm® and BeautySphere®.

Implantation site

The complication rate is less in the chin and malar area, and greater in the nose and ears.[28] This is related to the thickness and tension of the skin. The fibrous capsule is thicker on the surface towards the skin, and thinner on the inner surface.[23]

Conclusion

Therefore, only non-resorbable gel implants do not induce a strong fibrous encapsulation reaction. There is little cell adhesion at the surface of the bulky implants, a moderate foreign body response, and the formation of a thin fibrillar isolation membrane with few cells. Only these can be considered as strict volume fillers. But this does not guarantee that there will be no unfavorable evolution.

The different products

The injectable products can also be classified according to their physical characteristics and composition:

- tissue-derived resorbable fluids: collagens, hyaluronic acid
- homogeneous resorbable polymer fluid: cross-linked polyvinylic acid: Bioinblue®
- homogeneous non-resorbable polymer fluids: silicone gel or oil, acrylic hydrogels
- suspension of non-resorbable polymer fragments or microspheres in a resorbable fluid: polymethylmethacrylate microspheres and collagen: Artecoll, Artefill; hydroxyethylmethacrylate/ethylmethacrylate fragments and hyaluronic acid: Dermalive, Dermadeep; silicone fragments and polyvinylpirrolidone: Bioplastique
- suspension of slowly resorbable polymer microspheres in a resorbable fluid: polylactic acid microspheres in a mannitol and carboxymethylcellulose solution: New-Fill®, Sculptra®; calcium hydroxyapatite microspheres in a carboxymethylcellulose gel: Radiance®, Radiesse®; dextran microspheres in hyaluronic acid: Reviderm, Philoderm® BeautySphere
- suspension of slowly resorbable polymer microspheres in non-resorbable fluid: polyvinylhydroxide microspheres + polyacrylamide gel: Evolution®

Acrylic polymers

Solid acrylic polymers

Dermalive and Dermadeep Dermalive (Dermatech, Paris, France) is made of fragments of two acrylic polymers, HEMA and EMA, of 45–65 μm in size, 2%, within 1.4% cross-linked hyaluronic acid in 96.6% saline (CE Mark n° 0120). Dermadeep is made of fragments of the same two acrylic polymers, HEMA and EMA, but of 80–110 μm in size, 2%, within 1.4% cross-linked hyaluronic acid in 96.6% saline (CE Mark n° 0120). As seen above, this association of HEMA and EMA induces a desired neocollagenogenesis effect, but also provides the potential for a strong inflammatory reaction. The irregular shape of the elements reinforces it.

Polymethylmethacrylate (PMMA) Artecoll (RMI, Breda, The Netherlands) (or Artefill (Artes Medical Inc, San Diego, CA, USA)) is made of smooth, round PMMA microspheres, 30–42 μm in diameter, 20%, as a suspension within a solution of partly denatured bovine collagen 3.5%, lidocaine hydrochloride 0.3%, saline 72.2% (CE Mark n° 51490TE01). The microspheres' diameter, between 30 and 42 μm, prevents their phagocytosis. Their smooth surface lessens cell adhesion and therefore foreign body reaction, and the collagen vehicle keeps them apart long enough to prevent a mass effect by agglutination.[11] They end up well isolated from the host tissue by a strong fibrous capsule, in which will persist some FBGCs.

Acrylic polymer gels

Polyacrylamide gels Royamid®, Formacryl®, Interfall® (Contura SA, Montreux, Switzerland, and Kiev, Ukraine), and Aquamid® (Contura International SA, Soeborg, Denmark) are all a cross-linked polyacrylamide gel, 2.5%, in 97.5% pyrogen-free water (CE Mark n° 0543). Dr Kebuladze in Kiev, Ukraine, first used polyacrylamide gel in cosmetic surgery by the end of the 1980s. The gel is hydrophilic, biocompatible, and non-toxic in its cross-linked form. According to the manufacturer's specification, 1 g of pure polyacrylamide absorbs 50 ml of 1% saline. Thus, 1 ml of 5% gel can theoretically bind up to 2.5 ml of normal saline.[29] The surface of the bolus of the gel does not favor protein adsorption, and therefore cell adhesion. The gels do not chemically induce a strong foreign body reaction. After 3–4 weeks, only a thin fibrillar membrane surrounds them, but if they break up into smaller fragments, these will be phagocytosed and start a strong inflammatory reaction. Outline® (Procytech SARL, Martillac, France) is also a cross-linked polyacrylamide gel, 3% in 97% pyrogen-free water (CE Mark n° 0499). According to the laboratory files, 'porosity of the gel has been chosen in order to create a net so that only macromolecules can colonize it, so that cells, especially macrophages, remain outside the gel. It is slowly absorbed over 2 to 8 years, depending on the chosen viscosity, under the action, notably, of non-specific esterases, which gradually shorten the molecular chains'. Allegedly, there would not be any release of toxic acrylic monomers.

Polyalkylimide gel Bio-Alcamid® (Polymekon, Milan, Italy), is an alkylimide polymer gel, 4%, in 96% pyrogen-free water (CE Mark n° 0123). According to the manufacturer, this polymer is different from polyacrylamide as it contains imide–amide groups. Like the other acrylic gels, it shows only limited foreign body reaction. According to a study on its use in human immunodeficiency virus (HIV) related facial atrophy,[30] this implant would be a true injectable endoprosthesis, that could be removable by percutaneous puncture and manual pressure.

Polyvinylhydroxide microspheres + polyacrylamide gel
Evolution (Procytech SARL, Martillac, France) consists of porous polyvinylhydroxide microspheres of 40 μm in diameter, 6%, in a cross-linked polyacrylamide gel 2.5% in 91.5% pyrogen-free water. With the inflammatory potential of porous resorbable microspheres, it is probable that the gel will break up into small droplets or diffuse strands, small enough to be phagocytosed. These characteristics should make it theorically a strong inflammation inducer. No published clinical study is available to date.

Other polymers

Cross-linked polyvinylic acid Bioinblue (Polymekon, Milan, Italy) is a polyvinylic alcohol 8% gel in 92% pyrogen-free water (CE Mark n° 0123). This polymer should not induce inflammatory reactions since it is metabolized into acetoacetic acid within the Krebs cycle. The implant shows slow degradation, and would be replaced in an isovolumetric fashion by neocollagen.

Polylactic acid (PLA) New-Fill/Sculptra (Dermik Laboratories, Berwyn, USA) is made of PLA microspheres, 2–50 μm in diameter, 4.45% in sodium carmellose 2.67%, mannitol 3.87%, to be diluted in 3 ml pyrogen-free water 89% (CE Mark n° 0459). Particles over 40 μm should not be phagocytosed, but their enzymatic degradation makes them porous. So, after a first phase of moderate inflammation when they become porous and slowly degrade into irregular shapes, there follows a secondary stronger inflammatory phase, with many FBGCs, to phagocytose and accelerate the degradation of the implant.[31] Then it will gradually settle down, with disappearance of the particles, leaving a thick fibrous tissue.

Silicone particles Bioplastique (Bioplasty, St Paul, MN, USA, and Geleen, The Netherlands) is made of polymerized irregular shaped silicone particles (polymethylsiloxane), 100–600 μm in size, suspended in polyvinylpirrolidone as a carrier. The size of the particles makes them non-phagocytosable, but their irregular shape will induce a strong foreign body reaction, as it increases the total surface area of the implanted particles. The fluid carrier does not allow the particles to be kept apart, which favors cluster formation and increases the potential for foreign body reaction. Very active granulomas can be seen, with numerous FBGCs, and many phagocytes with asteroid bodies infiltrating all the spaces, even within the recesses of the particles themselves, and surrounded by very thick collagen bundles mixed with fibroblasts and a moderate lymphocytic infiltrate.[32]

Dextran microspheres in hyaluronic acid These include Reviderm and Philoderm BeautySphere (RMI, Breda, The Netherlands), with dextran microspheres 40–60 μm in diameter, 2.5%, mixed with cross-linked hyaluronic acid 2% in pyrogen-free water 95.5% (CE Mark n° 0125). The positive electric charge of the dextran microspheres has a stimulating effect on macrophages, fibroblasts, and connective tissue formation.[7,27] Dextran is also very hydrophilic. Clinically it will induce edema, before starting a strong stimulation of the fibroblasts.[33]

Calcium hydroxyapatite microspheres Radiance/ Radiesse (Bioform Inc, San Mateo, CA, USA) contains calcium hydroxyapatite microspheres 25–40 μm in diameter, 30% in a carboxymethylcellulose gel 70%

(CE Mark n° 0086C). The round microspheres induce less inflammatory reaction and disappear faster than irregular shaped particles.[17] There is a strong potential for bone formation.[1,8,23]

β-TCP microspheres Atlean™ (ABR Developement, Baillargues, France), tri-calcium phosphate microspheres 25–40 μm in diameter, 7% in non-cross-linked hyaluronic acid 1.8% and carmellose 2.7% (CE mark n° 0459). The round resorbable microspheres induce less inflammatory reaction and disappear faster than irregular shaped ones.[17] According to the manufacturer, half of them disappear within a year, leaving a strong collagen network.

Conclusion

Apart from these constant physiologic reactions, some fillers induce specific local modifications: they have a biostimulation effect.

Collagen or hyaluronic acid based fillers are used for their filling effect by the volume injected. They also play an important role in cutaneous metabolism, by stimulating neocollagen formation, by enhancing dermal cohesion, fibrocyte and keratinocyte metabolism,[34] or water retention. They cannot be considered only as volume enhancers, but also as true biostimulators, even if their duration within the tissues is short.

This biostimulation effect is sought and is part of the desired characteristics of some of the implants. Artecoll and Artefill have smooth microspheres whose characteristics will stimulate a strong fibrous encapsulation, isolating completely the beads from the host tissues and assuring long-lasting tolerability in most cases. It is partially the same with New-Fill, Sculptra, Radiesse and Atlean which induce a resorption/replacement of their microspheres by fibrous/osseous tissue, albeit after a strong secondary inflammatory phase.[31] This is also the case with the dextran microbeads of Reviderm and BeautySphere, attracting water then strongly stimulating collagen formation.

The only strictly volumetric implants are the fluid ones: silicone or acrylic gels, which do not first induce a foreign body reaction. Nevertheless, like the others, they have some side-effects, and complications.

References

1. Rizzi SC, Heath DJ, Coombes AGA et al. Biodegradable polymer/hydroxyapatite composites: surface analysis and initial attachment on human osteoblasts. J Biomed Mater Res 2001; 55: 475–86.
2. Smetana KJ, Lukas J, Paleckova V et al. Effect of chemical structure of hydrogels on the adhesion and phenotypic characteristics of human monocytes such as expression of galectins and other carbohydrate-binding sites. Biomaterials 1997; 18: 1009–14.
3. Jirouskova M, Bartunkova J, Smetana KJ et al. Comparative study of human monocyte and platelet adhesion to hydrogels in vitro – effect of polymer structure. J Mater Sci Mater Med 1997; 8: 19–23.
4. Van Wachem PB, Schakenraad JM, Feijen J et al. Adhesion and spreading of cultured endothelial cells on modified poly(ethylene terephthalate): a morphological study. Biomaterials 1989; 10: 532–9.
5. Brodbeck WG, Shive MS, Colton E et al. Influence of biomaterial surface chemistry on the apoptosis of adherent cells. J Biomed Mater Res 2001; 55: 661–8.
6. Tomazic-Jezic VJ, Merritt K, Umbreit TH. Significance of type and the size of biomaterial particles on phagocytosis and tissue distribution. J Biomed Mater Res 2001; 55: 523–9.
7. Mustoe TA, Weber DA, Krukowski M. Enhanced healing of cutaneous wounds in rats using beads with positively charged sufaces. Plast Reconstr Surg 1992; 89: 891–9.
8. Drobeck HP, Rothstein SS, Gumaer KI et al. Histologic observation of soft tissue responses to implanted, multifaceted particles and discs of hydroxylapatite. J Oral Maxillofac Surg 1984; 42: 143–9.
9. Nicolau PJ. Long lasting and permanent injectable fillers: biomaterial influence over host tissue response. Plast Reconstr Surg 2007; 119: 2271–86.
10. Morhenn VB, Lemperle G, Gallo RL. Phagocytosis of different particulate dermal filler substances by human macrophages and skin cells. Dermatol Surg 2002; 28: 484–90.
11. Lemperle G, Morhenn VB, Pestonjamasp V et al. Migration studies and histology of injectable microspheres of different sizes in mice. Plast Reconstr Surg 2004; 113: 1380–90.
12. Pannek J, Brands FH, Senge T. Particle migration following transurethral injection of carbon coated beads for stress urinary incontinence. J Urol 2001; 166: 1350–3.
13. Sanger JR, Kolachalam R, Komorowski RA et al. Short-term effect of silicone gel on peripheral nerves: a histologic study. Plast Reconstr Surg 1992; 89: 931–40.
14. Maas CS, Papel ID, Greene D et al. Complications of injectable synthetic polymers in facial augmentation. Dermatol Surg 1997; 23: 871–7.
15. Flint PW, Corio RL, Cummings CW. Comparison of soft tissue response in rabbits following laryngeal implantation with hydroxylapatite, silicone rubber and Teflon. Ann Otol Rhinol Laryngol 1997; 106: 399–407.
16. Panilaitis B, Altman GH, Chen J et al. Macrophage responses to silk. Biomaterials 2003; 24: 3079–85.
17. Misiek DJ, Kent JN, Carr RF. Soft tissue response to hydroxylapatite particles of different shapes. J Oral Maxillofac Surg 1984; 42: 150–60.
18. Gelb H, Schumacher HR, Cukler J et al. In vivo inflammatory response to polymethylmethacrylate particulate debris: effect of size, morphology and surface area. J Orthop Res 1994; 12: 83–92.
19. Matlaga BF, Yasenchak LP, Salthouse TN. Tissue response to implanted polymers: the significance of sample shape. J Biomed Mater Res 1976; 10: 391–7.
20. Jordan DR, Brownstein S, Gilberg S et al. Investigation of a bioresorbable orbital implant. Ophthal Plast Reconstr Surg 2002; 18: 342–8.
21. Taylor SR, Gibons DF. Effect of surface texture on the soft tissue response to polymer implants. J Biomed Mater Res 1983; 17: 205–27.
22. Allen O. Response to subdermal implantation of textured microimplants in humans. Aesthetic Plast Surg 1992; 16: 227–30.
23. Li DJ, Ohsaki K, Ii K et al. Thickness of fibrous capsule after implantation of hydroxyapatite in subcutaneous tissue in rats. J Biomed Mater Res 1999; 45: 322–6.
24. Lemperle G, Romano JJ, Busso M. Soft tissue augmentation with Artecoll: 10 year history, indications, techniques and complications. Dermatol Surg 2003; 29: 573–87.

25. Okada Y, Kobayashi M, Fujita H et al. Transmission electron microscopic study of interface between bioactive bone cement and bone: comparison of apatite and wollastonite containing glass-ceramic filler with hydroxyapatite and beta-tricalcium phosphate fillers. J Biomed Mater Res 1999; 45: 277–84.

26. Smetana KJ. Cell biology of hydrogels.Biomaterials 1993; 14: 1046–50.

27. Eppley BL, Summerlin D-J, Prevel CD et al. Effects of positively charged biomaterial for dermal and subcutaneous augmentation. Aesthetic Plast Surg 1994; 18: 413–16.

28. Rubin JP, Yaremchuck MJ. Complications and toxicities of implantable biomaterials used in facial reconstructive and aesthetic surgery: a comprehensive review of the literature. Plast Reconstr Surg 1997; 100: 1336–53.

29. Niechajev I. Lip enhancement: surgical alternatives and histologic aspects. Plast Reconstr Surg 2000; 105: 1173–83; discussion 1184–7.

30. Protopapa C, Sito G, Caporale D et al. Bio-Alcamid in drug-induced lipodystrophy. J Cosmet Laser Ther 2003; 5: 1–5.

31. Spenlehauer G, Vert M, Benoit JP et al. In vitro and in vivo degradation of poly(D,L-lactide/glycolide) type microspheres made by solvent evaporation method. Biomaterials 1989; 10: 557–63.

32. Rudolph CM, Soyer HP, Schuller-Petrovic S et al. Foreign body granulomas due to injectable aesthetic microimplants. Am J Surg Pathol 1999; 23: 113–17.

33. Lemperle G, Morhenn V, Charrier U. Human histology and persistence of various injectable filler substances for soft tissue augmentation. Aesthetic Plast Surg 2003; 27: 354–66; discussion 367.

34. Prestwich GD, Marecak DM, Marecek JF et al. Controlled chemical modifications of hyaluronic acid: synthesis, applications and biodegradation of hydrazide derivatives. J Control Release 1997; 53: 99.

50 Side-effects, contraindications, and legislation

Pierre J Nicolau

Side-effects and contraindications

We have seen that there are constant physiologic reactions with fillers, but some of them induce specific local modifications: they have a biostimulation effect.

Collagen or hyaluronic acid based fillers are used for their filling effect by the volume injected, but they also play an important role in cutaneous metabolism, by stimulating neocollagen formation, by enhancing dermal cohesion, fibrocyte and keratinocyte metabolism,[1] or water retention. They cannot be considered only as volume enhancers, but also as true biostimulators, even if their duration within the tissues is short.

This biostimulation effect is sought and is part of the desired characteristics of some of the implants: Artecoll® and Artefill® have smooth microspheres whose characteristics will stimulate a strong fibrous encapsulation, isolating completely the beads from the host tissues and assuring long-lasting tolerability in most cases. It is partially the same with New-Fill®, Sculptra®, Radiesse® and Atlean® which induce a resorption/replacement of their microspheres by fibrous/osseous tissue, albeit after a strong secondary inflammatory phase.[2] It is also the case with the dextran microbeads of Reviderm® and BeautySphere®, attracting water then strongly stimulating collagen formation.

Some implants are described as inducing at first little or no inflammatory reaction, but clinical experience has shown that they are responsible for delayed major reactions. In that respect, their biostimulation effect can be considered an unfavorable reaction leading to complications. This is the case with Dermalive® and Bioplastique®.

The only strictly volumetric implants are the fluid ones: silicone or acrylic gels, which do not first induce a foreign body reaction. Nevertheless, like the others, they have some side-effects, and complications.

Acrylic gels

Acrylic polymer gels marketed to date include:

- polyacrylamide gels (PAAG): Royamid®, Formacryl®, Interfall® (Contura SA, Montreux, Switzerland, and Kiev, Ukraine), Aquamid® (Contura International SA, Soeborg, Denmark)
- polyalkylimide gel: Bio-Alcamid® (Polymekon, Milan, Italy).

They induce light tissue reaction and formation of a thin fibrillar membrane. This is why it was not thought that they would be responsible for so many complications. This thin membrane is not a proof of the perfect tolerability of the product, but means only that, as a bulk implant, it does not induce a strong foreign body reaction. It does not mean that no foreign body reaction could ever occur: this depends on many factors.

Displacement and breaking up of the gel

For Evstatiev,[3] it is not true that the hydrogel is resistant to diffusion and migration. On the contrary, he has shown that the hydrogel diffuses into areas with minimal resistance and moves downward with time. De Cassia Novaes and Berg say that one should avoid injection in the corner of the mouth because of the weight of the gel.[4] This was also reported by Huo et al[5] in 2002, who found that the shape and location of the implant was not stable. The injected hydrogel disseminates in all directions and in all tissues. As there is no strong fibrous capsule around it to immobilize it within the tissues, the gel can easily migrate, under the action of local muscles and gravity. Milanov et al[6] found gel in the axilla, originating from retromammary injection. Migration in the subclavicular area, inside the pectoralis major muscle, disseminated within the glandular tissue of the breast, has also been reported.[7–9] Christensen et al in 2004[10] write that gel has been seen within the pectoral muscle, and confined by a membrane of macrophages or interspersed in minute amounts among the collagenous fibers. However, in their 2005 publication,[11] they state that 'gel migration has not been reported', although in 2000, Milanov et al[6] noted migration of retromammary gel as early as 20 days post-injection, as proved by ultra-sonography. They conclude that the main cause of changes in the tissues 'is PAAG migration to the mammary tissue, subcutaneous fat, and tissues lying farther from the injection site'.

In its displacement, it will break up into smaller amounts. Christensen et al[12] have described, in all histologically examined cases, three features: a cellular membrane with a thickness of up to 1 mm, a thin rim of macrophages, and interdigitating strands of gel within the connective or fat tissue. This fragmentation of the gel mass by fine connective tissue bands is also found by Adamyan et al.[7]

These fragments or droplets will be recognized as foreign bodies, due to their size, and will arouse the inflammatory process. If the fragments are phagocytosed, they will provoke cellular death, and hence sterile abscess formation, which will increase the inflammatory response. Gel has been found in macrophages and in foreign body giant cells (FBGCs).[9,12] Sterile abscesses are found in the axillae of all patients with inflammation of the breasts following PAAG enlargement.[3,7] This fragmentation might be facilitated by the dehydration of the gel,[3,8] whose end result is a granular mass.[9,12] Macrophages have been found within the bulk of the implant.[7,9,11]

Infection

Inflammation at the point of original puncture for gel administration has been observed,[7] even before pus formation. It is therefore possible to believe that it could be an entry point for bacteria. Nevertheless, when the gel is injected subcutaneously, it will be in contact with skin annexes, and local bacteria. Not surprisingly, Christensen et al have found bacteria, non-pathogenic in humans, in all of the 28 biopsies examined from patients with nodules following PAAG injections to the face.[11] It is not possible yet to confirm that these non-pathogen agents are responsible for the inflammatory reaction. These biopsies showed a heavy inflammatory reaction, with macrophages, lymphocytes, and foreign body giant cells, together with fragments or droplets of the gel, either isolated or phagocytosed. To us, this seems to be the most probable reason for strong inflammation, growth of non-pathogenic bacteria possibly being the trigger. More studies are needed.

Toxicity

Polyacrylamides are said to be non-toxic in their macromolecular, cross-linked form. However, a consensus conference in 2002 stated that PAAG fillers can partially degrade, and carcinogenic and mutagenic monomers can be released (the European Committee on Quality Assurance and Medical Devices in Plastic Surgery, Proceedings of EQUAM V Consensus Conference, July 2002[13]).

An experimental study by Huo et al[5] has shown that polyacrylamide gels are toxic for the kidneys. Their conclusion is that hydrophilic polyacrylamide gel has obvious cytotoxicity and is not a suitable material as a soft tissue implant, resulting in poor shape and texture.

Bulk injections for large volumes: the breast complications example

As early as the year 2000, Milanov et al[6] started questioning the use of PAAG for breast augmentation. Pshenisnov et al[8] describe 24 cases of women who underwent breast enlargement with PAAG. All patients complained of deformity of the breast, pain, palpable nodules, and discharge from the nipple. Cheng et al[9] in 2002 state that multiple breast indurations or lumps are the most common complication following PAAG augmentation mammoplasty, presenting as indurations, nodular formations, pearl-like masses, or firm ball-like lumps. Induration masses, degree II–III in Baker's classification, are usually found at different depths and in various sizes, multiple or single, localized or diffused, and have a smooth, round shape in breasts. This is quite in opposition to Christensen et al,[12] who claim in 2003: 'furthermore, capsule shrinkage caused by the development of a thick, firm, disfiguring connective tissue capsule, which may be found around silicone prostheses, has never been reported or observed'.

Hematomas, lactorrhea, unsatisfactory contour, nipple sensation changes, infection, mastodynia, and skin necrosis are part of the multiple related complications.[6–8]

Radiological findings prove that gel migrates into the breast tissue and the infraclavicular region. Ultrasonography shows a honeycomb appearance with ill-defined borders with the breast tissue, confirming the finger-like diffusion.[9,13] Radiologically, it is not possible to differentiate fibrotic reaction from carcinoma, and the ultimate diagnosis relies on histology, as clinically this appearance of nodules with nipple discharge is quite worrying.

All these findings have brought Adamyan et al[7] to refuse further participation in a Russian Ministry of Health's clinical trial. Considering the multiplicity of symptoms, they have classified them in a 'polyacrylamide mammary syndrome'.

Removal of material

Huo et al, in 2002,[5] could not entirely remove the gel, in contrast to the manufacturer's claims that it could be removed by puncture and manual pressure. Attempts to remove it by aspiration, either syringe or vacuum-assisted, were not always sufficient. As described by Cheng et al,[9] when the cannula punctures the PAAG mass, normal saline with antibiotics is injected and the masses are softened by massage, then the implanted gel and blood conglomeration are drawn out using a 10-ml syringe or negative suction. This procedure should be repeated several times, because injected PAAG masses are separated by many thin fibrous capsules. In many cases, removal of the material has required a direct surgical approach.[3,5–9,14]

Other polymers

Cross-linked polyvinylic acid, Bioinblue® (Polymekon, Milan, Italy), is metabolized in acetoacetic acid, and is slowly degraded over 12–18 months. The manufacturer states that it is gradually replaced by collagen. No studies could be found to date.

Conclusion

The use of polyacrylamide hydrogels is now forbidden in Russia and in Bulgaria[3] for bulk injections.

In Switzerland, the Institute for therapeutic products has issued a recommendation that the use of non-resorbable products, including Aquamid®, should be limited to serious conditions, as in reconstructive surgery. The recommendation of non-use for cosmetic purposes is based on the known risk of disfiguring complications (nodules, swelling, discoloration).[15]

It seems that more studies are needed prior to continued use of polyacrylamide gels as large volume enhancers, notably in human immunodeficiency virus (HIV) related facial atrophy.

It seems appropriate to leave the last words to Cheng et al:[9]

> In order to keep up with advancing technology, many young surgeons are enthusiastic to apply new techniques and materials in aesthetic plastic surgery, but plastic surgeons should be aware of the side effects and complications associated with the new developing technique, equipment, and biomaterial, especially when there is deficient scientific data support, inadequate experience on clinical observation, and operative technique, and abuse without correct indication for new things. Furthermore, it should be emphasized that only qualified plastic surgeons and defined medical centers are permitted to use PAAG injection for cosmetic purposes.

Legislation: US and European comparative

The US Food and Drug Administration (FDA), under the authority of the Federal Food, Drug, and Cosmetic Act (FFD&C), was the first to regulate medical devices,

with the 1976 Medical Devices Amendments. The Safe Medical Devices Act (SMDA) of 1990, the Medical Devices Amendments of 1992, and the Modernization Act (FDAMA) of 1997 considerably modified the FFD&C again. These laws rule on medical devices manufactured, imported, or offered to importation in any state or territory of the United States, the District of Columbia, or Puerto Rico.

In the European Union, rules are given in the European Council Directives: Directive 90/385/EEC relating to Active Implantable Medical Devices (AIMD), Directive 93/42/EEC relating to Medial Devices of 1993 (MDD), Directive 98/79/EC of 1998 relating to In Vitro Diagnostic Medical Devices (MDD IVD), and Directive 2000/70/EC relating to plasma and human blood.

These laws offer a classification of medical devices, but also regulate the manufacturers' quality systems, and post-market controls.

Classification of medical devices

The FDA devices classification process is fairly different from those described in the various European directives.

The FDA asks specialist groups for advice and recommendations concerning the classification of medical devices. Based on these recommendations, the appropriate class is determined by the FDA, which classifies or reclassifies the device by means of a regulation. FDA regulations are based on device class. There are three classes: I, II, and III. Class I devices need the lightest controls, while class III devices need the most rigorous. All devices have to go through General Controls, classes II and III have to comply with Special Controls, and class III devices need a Premarket Approval (510k).

The regulation on proposed classification is then published in the federal register to be submitted to public discussion, prior to final agreement. The FDA then publishes a final regulation classifying the device.

A manufacturer who wants to market a device in any class must prove that it is substantially equivalent to a device already marketed, and to which a class has already been attributed. For a device found to be not substantially equivalent to a device already marketed, the manufacturer must submit a Premarket Approval Application (PMA) in order for the FDA to determine its class.

The European Union (EU) classifies medical devices under 18 rules, published in annex IX of the MDD. Their aim is to help manufacturers determine to which of the four classes their device belongs. Therefore, the manufacturers decide for themselves the device's classification.

Rules cover different combinations of the following criteria:

- duration during which the device is in contact with the patient (temporary, short, or long period)
- invasive or non-invasive device (for instance: used for blood filtration or in contact with the skin)
- the degree of invasiveness (penetration through a body orifice or surgical implantation)
- the part of the body affected by the device (central cardiovascular system)
- active or non-active devices (function depending on an energy source)
- special cases (for instance: devices containing a drug, or tissues of animal origin or their derivatives).

Rules 1–4 concern non-invasive medical devices (MDs), 5–8 invasive MDs, 9–12 active MDs, and 13–18 special cases.

Four classes are determined; I, IIa, IIb, and III, according to the established risk:

- class I: low potential risk (surgical instruments, non-invasive MDs, invasive MDs, for temporary use)
- class IIa: moderate potential risk (sterile and/or with measuring function class I MDs, contact lenses, dental prostheses, short-duration invasive MDs, surgical type invasive MDs)
- class IIb: high potential risk (long-term implantable devices: Artecoll®, Radiesse®)
- class III: critical potential risk (long-term implantable devices in contact with the heart or the central nervous system, resorbable implantable devices: hyaluronic acid, mammary implants).

When a device is meant for more than one use, or if more than one rule might apply, it is then considered to belong to the higher risk class.

Table 50.1 shows a comparison between US and EU classification systems.

Conformity evaluation: quality systems

In the EU there are six different methods of evaluating the norms of conformity to obtain CE Marking. They are described in annexes II–VII of the MDD. However, nowhere in the directives is a specific quality system recommended for use. The manufacturer is free to choose which quality system it will use to demonstrate that its product is conforming to the applicable essential demands.

Manufacturers who design devices and sell their products in the USA must choose a conformity evaluation method which uses a full quality system, i.e. a method ensuring control of the concept. FDA demands this for most class II devices, all class III devices, and those using a software component.

Table 50.1 Classification of medical devices

US FDA Device Classification	European Council Directive 93/42/EEC (MDD)
Class III	Class III
Class III	Class IIb
Class II	Class IIa
Class I	Class I

Clinical evaluation

Under FDA rules, it is mandatory to perform experimental studies when it is considered that a medical device for human use presents a high risk, class III, in order to collect all data pertaining to its safety and efficiency. The PMA application must contain sufficient information to reasonably assure the FDA of the safety and effectiveness of the device. This requires valid scientific data to demonstrate that the device is safe and effective for its intended use. In most cases, this includes well-controlled clinical studies; full reports of safety and effectiveness; and data regarding the manufacture of the device. Clinical studies to support the Premarket Approval Application must be done in accordance with the Investigational Device Exemption (IDE) regulation.

In order to carry out experiments in new devices for use in humans, the FDA may exempt manufacturers from some of the requirements. This exemption is called Investigational Device Exemption (IDE). IDE applicants have to give the FDA proof that all tests will be done under the review of an Institutional Review Board (IRB), that appropriate informed consent will be obtained, and that appropriate data will be filed and reports made. Concerning low risk devices, it is not necessary to produce such information to the FDA; nevertheless, IRB approval is required.

As for the EU, rules are defined in annex X of the MDD. As a general rule, confirmation that the requirements concerning the characteristics and performance of a device under normal use conditions is required. Side-effects evaluation must be based on clinical data, particularly with regard to implantable devices and class III devices.

The validity and relevance of the clinical data are based upon:

- either a compilation of relevant scientific literature currently available, concerning the intended use of the device and the techniques it employs, and, if needed, a written report containing a critical evaluation of this compilation
- or the results of all clinical investigations performed.

As it is not mandatory for manufacturers themselves to perform appropriate clinical studies, injectable devices can be marketed in Europe whose dangers might only appear several months or years later.

Post-market surveillance

For both MDD and MDD IVD, the manufacturers must proactively monitor the performance of their product following its production.

In the USA, the FDA may order manufacturers to conduct post-market surveillance studies to gather safety and efficacy data for certain class II and class III devices. Manufacturers must set a method for proactive data retrieval concerning the efficacy of the device, in order to make sure that it satisfies the demands of safety and efficiency, and that improvements can be made, if needed.

MDD IVD creates a European data bank, accessible to the competent authorities, keeping the data pertaining to manufacturers' approval, data on certificates emitted, modified, completed, suspended, or refused, and data obtained through the surveillance procedure, in a standardized format.

Monitoring report

As far as the EU is concerned, the manufacturer should set up and keep up to date a system which permits one to identify events relating to the health or safety of the patients or the user, and to take the appropriate corrective measures. These events principally include those that may have caused or contributed to a death or serious injury.

The same applies to the USA where the FDA requires manufacturers and importers to report to them whenever the firm becomes aware of information that reasonably suggests that one of its marketed devices:

- has or may have caused or contributed to a death or serious injury, or
- has malfunctioned and that the device or a similar device marketed by the manufacturer or importer would be likely to cause or contribute to a death or serious injury if the malfunction were to recur.

Distributors must keep files of complaints and make these files available to the FDA when required. The establishments that use these devices must make a report on 1 January, each year, but it is up to them to choose if they wish to make two annual reports.

References

1. Prestwich GD, Marecak DM, Marecek JF et al. Controlled chemical modifications of hyaluronic acid: synthesis, applications and biodegradation of hydrazide derivatives. J Control Release 1997; 53: 99.
2. Spenlehauer G, Vert M, Benoit JP et al. In vitro and in vivo degradation of poly(D,L-lactide/glycolide) type microspheres made by solvent evaporation method. Biomaterials 1989; 10: 557–63.
3. Evstatiev D. Late complications after injections of hydrogel in the breast. Plast Reconstr Surg 2004; 113: 1878.
4. De Cassia Novaes W, Berg A. Experiences with a new non-biodegradable hydrogel (Aquamid): a pilot study. Aesthetic Plast Surg 2003; 27: 376–80.
5. Huo M, Huang J, Qi K. Experimental study on the toxic effects of hydrophilic polyacrylamide gel. Zhonghua Zheng Xing Shao Shang Wai Ke Za Zhi 2002; 18: 79–80.
6. Milanov NO, Donchenko EV, Fisenko EP. Plastic contour correction with polyacrylamide gels. Myths and reality. Ann Plast Reconstr Aesthet Surg 2000; 4: 63–9.
7. Adamyan AA, Svetukhin AM, Skuba ND et al. Polyacrylamide mammary syndrome: clinical features, diagnosis and treatment. Ann Plast Reconstr Aesthet Surg 2001; 4: 20–32.
8. Pshenisnov KP, Makin IL, Omelchenko TE et al. Problems of breast reconstruction following injections of polyacrylamide gel. Ann Plast Reconstr Aesthet Surg 2001; 2: 41–51.
9. Cheng N-X, Wang Y-L, Wang J-H et al. Complications of breast augmentation with injected hydrophilic polyacrylamide gel. Aesthetic Plast Surg 2002; 26: 375–82.
10. Christensen LH, Breiting VB, Aasted A et al. [Reply to: Late complications after injections of hydrogel in the breast]. Plast Reconstr Surg 2004; 113: 1878–9.
11. Christensen LH, Breiting V, Janssen M et al. Adverse reactions to injectable soft tissue permanent fillers. Aesthetic Plast Surg 2005; 29: 34.
12. Christensen LH, Breiting VB, Aasted A et al. Long-term effects of polyacrylamide hydrogel on human breast tissue. Plast Reconstr Surg 2003; 111: 1883–90.
13. Lam WWM, Chu WCW, Tse G et al. Radiological appearance of breast augmentation with injected hydrophilic polyacrylamide gel. Clin Radiol Extra 2003; 58: 61–3.
14. Bui P, Pons-Guiraud A, Kuffer R et al. Les produits injectables lentement et non résorbables. Ann Chir Plast Esthét 2004; 49: 486–502.
15. Institut suisse des produits thérapeutiques, Division Dispositifs Medicaux. Recommandations concernant les produits injectables non-résorbables pour le comblement des rides. Berne, Switzerland: Swissmedic, 22 April, 2002.

Index

Figures in **bold**, *Tables* in *italics*